KK Women's and Children's Hospital

SingHealth

About KK Women's and Children's Hospital

KK Women's and Children's Hospital (KKH) is Singapore's largest tertiary referral centre for obstetrics, gynaecology, paediatrics and neonatology. The academic medical centre specialises in the management of high-risk conditions in women and children.

Driven by a commitment to deliver compassionate, multidisciplinary care to patients, KKH leverages innovation to advance care. The hospital has launched the SingHealth Duke-NUS Maternal and Child Health Research Institute (MCHRI) to support the growth of every woman and child to their fullest potential through research and innovation, to transform national heath in Singapore and the region.

The Academic Medical Centre is also a major teaching hospital for Duke-NUS Medical School, Yong Loo Lin School of Medicine and Lee Kong Chian School of Medicine. In addition, KKH runs the largest specialist training programme for Obstetrics and Gynaecology, and Paediatrics in Singapore. The programmes are highly rated for the quality of clinical teaching and translational research.

KKH was founded in 1858. For more information, visit www.kkh.com.sg

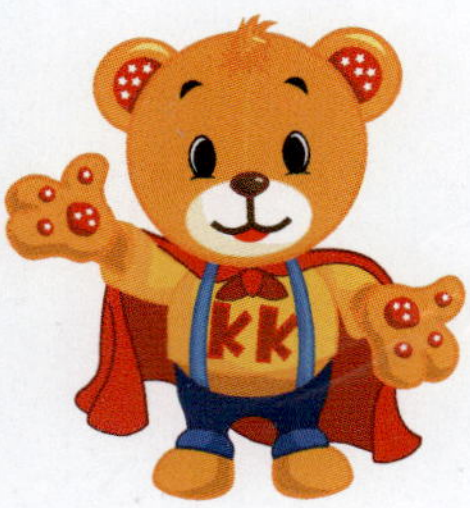

About KK Super Bear

KK Super Bear is KK Women's and Children's Hospital's mascot. He is a brave and playful bear with super powers to help children, the young and young-at-heart stay happy and smile.

THE BABY BEAR BOOK

A Practical Guide on Paediatrics

Fourth Edition

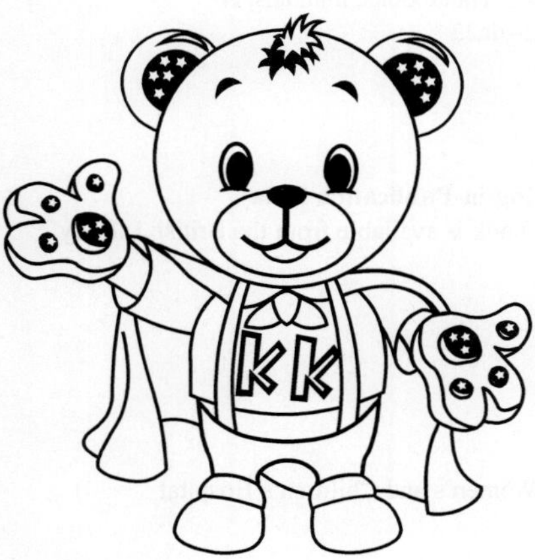

Editors

Chong Kok Wee

Tan Yi Hua

KK Women's and Children's Hospital, Singapore

KK Women's and Children's Hospital
SingHealth

World Scientific

Published by

World Scientific Publishing Co. Pte. Ltd.
5 Toh Tuck Link, Singapore 596224
USA office: 27 Warren Street, Suite 401-402, Hackensack, NJ 07601
UK office: 57 Shelton Street, Covent Garden, London WC2H 9HE

National Library Board, Singapore Cataloguing in Publication Data
Name(s): Chong, Kok Wee, editor. | Tan, Yi Hua, editor.
Title: The baby bear book : a practical guide on paediatrics / editors, Chong Kok Wee, Tan Yi Hua.
Other Title(s): Practical guide on paediatrics
Description: Fourth edition. | Singapore : World Scientific Publishing Co. Pte. Ltd., [2023] |
"KK Women's and Children's Hospital, Singapore."
Identifier(s): ISBN 978-981-12-6628-7 (hardback) | 978-981-12-6715-4 (paperback) |
978-981-12-6629-4 (ebook for institutions) | 978-981-12-6630-0 (ebook for individuals)
Subject(s): LCSH: Pediatrics--Handbooks, manuals, etc.
Classification: DDC 618.92--dc23

British Library Cataloguing-in-Publication Data
A catalogue record for this book is available from the British Library.

For any available supplementary material, please visit
https://www.worldscientific.com/worldscibooks/10.1142/13141#t=suppl

Printed in Singapore

Contents

Foreword

'Paediatrics' comes from two Greek words — παῖς/pais (meaning child) and ἰατρός/iatros (meaning doctor/healer). Paediatrics is a relatively young discipline in medicine's long history — having only been in practice for about 200 years.

As Dr Constance Elaine Field wrote in 1962, the '*emergence of paediatrics as a special branch of medicine in Singapore can probably date back to the year 1921*'. This was when the Singapore General Hospital (SGH/previously known as 'General Hospital' or 'Outram Road General Hospital/ORGH') started providing inpatient medical care for children in Singapore.

It has been 25 years since the paediatric departments from the SGH, Tan Tock Seng Hospital and Alexandra Hospital as well as the neonatal departments from KK Hospital came together in 1997 to form KK Women's and Children's Hospital — our first and only children's hospital in Singapore and in this region.

The *Baby Bear Book: A Practical Guide on Paediatrics*, since its first edition in 2008, has helped to train and equip our healthcare team of doctors, nurses, allied healthcare providers with the know-how and ability to manage and care for our paediatric patients through the years. *The Baby Bear Book* has served as an essential tool to strengthen many of the key components of the 6 medical competencies of 'medical knowledge'; 'patient care'; 'practice-based learning & improvement' and 'systems-based practice', thereby improving 'interpersonal & communications' and 'professionalism'.

Constantly updated and practical clinical guidelines are essential in our 21st century medicine to ensure that up-to-date clinical care is rendered to our paediatric patients in an appropriate and value-driven manner. The 'Appraisal of Guidelines, REsearch and Evaluation (AGREE) Collaboration' developed a checklist in 2003 and key elements that were assessed included 'scope and purpose'; 'clarity and presentation' and 'applicability'. Our Baby Bear Book has consistently met these important key attributes and standards through the years and has provided the necessary guidance for our inter-professional clinical teams here in Singapore.

The practice of paediatrics is a living discipline. As we continue to learn and improve, as well as transform paediatrics, we must continue to not only be evidence-based but be value-driven in our approach to paediatric health and healthcare delivery in Singapore.

Children are our key human resource and capital. They represent our future, and as health and healthcare providers for children and their families, we should and must continue to ensure and secure healthy outcomes and optimise the human potential of all our children, thereby safeguarding our nation's future.

Clinical Associate Professor Ng Kee Chong
Chairman, Medical Board
KK Women's and Children's Hospital

Preface

For the past two decades, *The Baby Bear Book* has been the go-to text for healthcare professionals caring for sick children in Singapore. With an emphasis on the clinical aspects of paediatric care, the fourth edition includes important revisions and new chapters by experienced clinicians to enhance its usefulness in today's practice.

The Baby Bear Book is a practical guide which provides the latest evidence-based information that is relevant to the care of children from newborn through adolescence. Medical and nursing students, as well as paediatric and family medicine trainees, will appreciate the accessibility of information that is concise and useful. Practising paediatricians, family physicians, as well as nursing and allied health practitioners will find the book a pertinent and handy reference in both ambulatory care and hospital settings.

As we continue to update and reorganise *The Baby Bear Book* to keep it relevant, we wish to express our gratitude to the authors who contributed to this edition, and also the editors and authors who worked on previous editions. We are especially thankful for the support rendered by the SingHealth Duke-NUS Paediatrics Academic Clinical Programme. We also want to show our appreciation to our readers around the world who have provided us with helpful suggestions. Most importantly, we are forever indebted to the sick children and their families whom we have served.

We hope the book will benefit you as you continue your invaluable work in healing more patients under your care!

Dr Chong Kok Wee & Dr Tan Yi Hua
Editors of *The Baby Bear Book*, Fourth Edition

Department of Paediatrics
KK Women's and Children's Hospital

Endorsements

Critical information that needs to be readily available when caring for an ill child is encapsulated in this handy book. It is written in a clear and concise way that makes for easy referencing and understanding. The fourth edition of *The Baby Bear Book* should be an indispensable tool in the consultation room of every doctor providing care for children. I would like to warmly congratulate all the contributors and editors for the tireless efforts to bring us this practical guide.

Professor Ivy Ng
Group Chief Executive Officer
SingHealth

The publication of the fourth edition of *The Baby Bear Book* reflects the rapid pace of advancement in the art and science of paediatrics and child health. Not only is there a pressing need to update our approach to many prevailing medical problems in child care, but also the evidence-based guidance for emerging issues. This book will be an important reference in providing the best care to the children and the families, from medical students to the senior doctors.

Professor Ho Lai Yun
Emeritus Consultant, Singapore General Hospital
Master Academic Clinician, Duke-NUS Medical School
Advisor, SingHealth Duke-NUS Paediatrics Academic Clinical Programme

The Baby Bear Book is the go-to for many family physicians in general practice. Designed to effectively diagnose and manage paediatric patients, this comprehensive guide features useful diagrams and concise descriptions of paediatric conditions, presenting family physicians in practice or in training with an essential point-of-care resource or general review. In this present iteration, it is a fabulous resource for all family doctors, and should take pride of place in our consultation rooms.

Adjunct Associate Professor Tan Tze Lee
President
College of Family Physicians Singapore

The Baby Bear Book has been the survival handbook of every paediatric house officer and medical officer since its first inception! I am sure the fourth edition, with new sections on dermatology, mental health and adolescent health, will be an invaluable resource to every primary care provider!

Dr David Ng Chee Chin
Chief Executive Officer
SingHealth Polyclinics

The Baby Bear Book has been the go-to paediatric guide for many doctors over the years. In this latest fourth edition, the authors have updated the comprehensive range of topics and added new chapters, with the book written in its trademark easy to read manner. Both doctors and medical students looking for practical clinical approaches and management, will find this book invaluable. It will help shape the way doctors care for children, both in the hospital and primary care setting, making a difference in clinical care. This updated edition of *The Baby Bear Book* is by far the most practical, handy reference guide and a must-have for doctors who provide care for children.

Dr Karen Ng
Family Physician, Senior Consultant
Deputy Chief Executive Officer
National Healthcare Group Polyclinics

SECTION 1

MEDICAL EMERGENCIES

CHAPTER 1

Recognising the Critically Ill Child

Loi V-Ter, Mervin; Lim Kian Boon, Joel

Introduction

Children are often unable or unwilling to verbalise complaints. In addition, symptoms and signs of sepsis or cardiopulmonary compromise are often vague and subtle in children.

The ability to assess and recognise an ill child early allows for timely interventions and therapy, such as respiratory support, fluid resuscitation or early antibiotics to reverse potentially life-threatening cardiopulmonary instability.

Anatomic and Physiological Considerations

Respiratory arrest is the most common cause of cardiopulmonary collapse in children. This is largely because the paediatric respiratory system is ill-designed to cope with an increased work of breathing. The reasons are multi-factorial and include a relatively large tongue and floppy epiglottis, small airways with increased airway resistance, and increased chest wall compliance due to a cartilaginous chest wall. Respiratory failure is characterised by inadequate ventilation, insufficient oxygenation or both.

Cardiac output is a product of stroke volume and heart rate, and blood pressure is a function of cardiac output and systemic vascular resistance.

Circulatory shock is defined as the failure of the circulatory system to provide oxygen and nutrients to meet tissue metabolic demands. Shock can be classified into compensated, uncompensated or irreversible.

Compensatory mechanisms include tachycardia and increased systemic vascular resistance in an effort to maintain cardiac output and perfusion pressure (blood pressure), respectively. Decompensation occurs when these mechanisms fail and result in end-organ hypoperfusion and hypotension. Untreated, shock states can rapidly deteriorate into failure of multiple organ systems and lead to irreversible shock and death.

The pathophysiology of shock can be divided into distributive, hypovolaemic/haemorrhagic, cardiogenic or obstructive. It is not unusual for one patient to have a number of different pathophysiological patterns of shock, which can evolve depending on the time-course of their disease.

Recognition of pre-shock states is important so that early goal-directed therapy can be instituted. The regimen of resuscitation includes fluid boluses, airway intervention and inotropic support. The key is early shock recognition and prompt action.

History

Functional status of the child is a simple but effective measure of how ill the child is. Questions to ask include:

- Level of activity/play
- Conscious level/irritability
- Feeding/fluid intake
- Urine output

Red flags in the history include:

- High-pitched cry/inconsolable crying
- Grunting
- Cyanosis
- Apnoeic episodes
- Pallor, cool and clammy peripheries
- Shortness of breath or dyspnoea
- Acute change in mentation
- Focal seizures
- Bloody stool in a neonate

There should be a high index of suspicion in the very young or if there is a significant medical history, such as:

- Maternal history of Group B Streptococcus (GBS) infection (for neonates)
- Congenital cardiac defects
- Primary immunodeficiency syndromes
- Chronic steroid usage
- Haematological-oncological disorders on active chemotherapy
- History of adreno-cortical deficiency, e.g. hypopituitarism, congenital adrenal hyperplasia, hypothalamic or pituitary lesions

Vital Parameters

Hypotension is defined as systolic BP:

- <60 mmHg in a neonate
- <70 mmHg in infants (1–12 months)
- <70 mmHg + [2 x (Age in Years)] in children 1–10 years
- <90 mmHg in children older than 10 years

Mean arterial pressure can be calculated as {50 + [2 x (Age in Years)} mmHg.

There is significant inter-individual variability of pulse pressure (systolic minus diastolic BP), increasing with age and generally ranging between 20 and 40 mmHg. A widened pulse pressure is present in distributive shock. A narrow pulse pressure may suggest hypovolaemic or cardiogenic shock.

Unexplained tachycardia may be one of the first signs of compensated shock.

Table 1.1 Table of Normal Heart Rate, Respiratory Rate and Systolic Blood Pressure (BP) by Age

Age	Heart Rate (beats/min)	Respiratory Rate (breaths/min)	Systolic Blood Pressure (mmHg)
Neonate	120–180	40–60	60–80
Infant (1 mth to 1 yr)	110–160	30–40	70–90
Toddler (1–2 yr)	100–150	25–35	80–95
Young child (2–7 yr)	95–140	25–30	90–110
Older child (7–12 yr)	80–120	20–25	100–120

Physical Examination

Clinical states which can rapidly progress and are life-threatening include:

- Severe respiratory distress
- Cardiovascular instability/cardiogenic shock
- Sepsis/septic shock
- Severe dehydration
- Seizures/altered mental state
- Trauma
- Any organ failure, such as renal/hepatic failure

Learn to integrate the signs of an unwell child as no single sign is definitive. If there are concerning features in the history and/or physical examination, consider the following:

- Admit for observation or transport patient to an appropriate care facility after initial stabilisation.
- Call for senior help if there is evidence of severe respiratory distress, poor perfusion and/or hypotension, obtundation/change in mentation, prolonged seizure or cardiac arrhythmias.
- Activate the paediatric Emergency Code Team if there is imminent cardiopulmonary arrest, severe respiratory compromise needing intubation, or if there is difficulty stabilising the patient, e.g. difficult venous access, no response to therapeutic interventions, potential difficult airway.

Investigations

- Blood glucose: Exclude hypoglycaemia or diabetic ketoacidosis (DKA) as a cause for obtundation
- Blood gas analysis: Evaluate for metabolic or respiratory acidosis, sodium/potassium/calcium derangements
- Full blood count, renal panel and group and crossmatch
- Imaging: Chest X-ray (CXR) to exclude pulmonary pathology, cardiomegaly. Computed tomography (CT) of the head if there are concerns regarding intracranial pathology.

Table 1.2 Care of the Critically Ill Child (adapted from RCH, 2021)

Assessment	Clinical Features	Management
Airway		
Patency	If compromised: • Abnormal breath sounds (stridor, stertor, snoring, gurgling, voice hoarseness) • Drooling • Tracheal tug • Dyspnoea • Respiratory distress • Paradoxical breathing • Inability to lie flat	Ensure airway patency Avoid agitating child Optimise head position: • Continue child's adopted posture if possible • Infant: neutral position • Child: head tilt, chin lift • Jaw thrust for suspected cervical injury Consider: • Suction • Oropharyngeal or nasopharyngeal airway • Oxygen (humidified if in respiratory distress) • PEEP if upper airway obstruction ***(If severe, escalate to a senior/ anaesthetist for consideration for endotracheal intubation)***
Breathing		
• Adequacy of oxygenation and ventilation • Respiratory muscle endurance	Vital signs • Tachypnoea or bradypnoea • Oxygen desaturation or cyanosis Effort of breathing • Limited ability to talk/fatigue • Symmetry and quality of chest rise/fall • Increased work of breathing (nasal flaring, grunting, head bobbing, accessory muscle use, retractions) • Auscultation findings (reduced air entry, wheezing or crepitations) • Abnormal breathing pattern (shallow breathing, Kussmaul breathing, Cheyne-Stokes) Secondary signs of inadequate oxygenation or ventilation: • Agitation • Altered mental state • Tachycardia/bradycardia • Pallor • Cool peripheries	Consider: • Elevating head of bed • Oxygen supplementation • Institute specific therapy for the underlying cause of respiratory failure • Medications, e.g. bronchodilators for asthma, diuretics in heart failure, antibiotics for pneumonia, etc. • Arterial/Capillary blood gas • Non-invasive ventilation, e.g. High flow nasal cannulae, CPAP, BiPAP • Invasive mechanical ventilation ***If the child is not breathing, commence bag-mask ventilation and prepare for endotracheal intubation*** Indications for intubation: • Reduced respiratory drive • Loss of protective airway reflexes • Intracranial hypertension • Severe airway obstruction • Respiratory failure/fatigue/apnoea • Shock • To reduce metabolic demand

(*Continued*)

Table 1.2 (*Continued*)

Assessment	Clinical Features	Management
Circulation		
Efficacy of circulation	Heart Rate/Rhythm: • Tachycardia/bradycardia • Arrhythmia Blood Pressure: • Narrow/wide pulse pressure • Hypotension (late sign) Assessment of Perfusion • Pallor/cyanosis • Weak/thready pulses • Flash or delayed capillary refill time (>2 s) • Cool/mottled peripheries Secondary signs: • Reduced conscious level • Reduced urine output • Tachypnoea or bradypnoea Praecordium: • New murmur • Gallop rhythm • Hyperdynamic praecordium	• Determine cardiac rhythm and treat accordingly • Obtain large bore intravenous access x 2 (consider intraosseous access early) • Arterial/capillary blood gas (including lactate if possible) • Fluid resuscitation (10–20 ml/kg bolus of 0.9% sodium chloride for acute resuscitation or over 15–60 min if less acute (up to 40 ml/kg, with caution if suspicious of cardiogenic shock — consider early inotropic support) • Consider blood products for haemorrhagic shock, severe anaemia or coagulopathic states • Consider early antibiotics (within 1 h) • Consider peripheral inotropes/ vasopressors • Correct electrolyte imbalances ***Consider early endotracheal intubation and assisted ventilation in shock (reduces work of breathing and cardiac metabolic demands, especially in cardiogenic and septic shock)*** ***If there are no signs of circulation (no pulse, bradycardia <60/min), commence cardiac compressions***
Disability		
Altered mental state	• Irritable • Lethargic • Asymmetrical pupillary reflexes • Tense fontanelles • Focal neurological deficits • Rapidly decreasing conscious level • Seizures	• Avoid hypoxia or hypercarbia • Avoid hyperthermia • Avoid hypo/hypertension • Correct metabolic derangements (hypoglycaemia, symptomatic hypo/ hypernatraemia or hypo/hypercalcaemia) • Manage seizures Consider intracranial pathologies: • Stroke/haemorrhage • Meningitis/encephalitis/abscess • Ventriculo-peritoneal shunt complications
Exposure		
Assess child, equipment and environment systematically	• Hypo/hyperthermia • Rash, petechiae, purpura • Signs of injury (spinal injury, penetrating injury, flail chest, deformities, open wounds, burns, ongoing bleeding)	• Correct hypothermia • Analgesia/sedation • Secure tubes/lines • Secure haemostasis • Clean open wounds • Stabilise injuries • Consider cervical collar/spinal nursing

- Septic screen including blood and urine cultures if sepsis is suspected. Consider cerebrospinal fluid cultures if an intracranial infection is suspected.
- Liver function test/coagulation profile if suspected liver dysfunction/bleeding diathesis.
- Serum lactate if available. This reflects tissue hypoperfusion and can be used as a marker of response to therapy.
- Metabolic screen if there is unexplained severe metabolic acidosis/hypoglycaemia.
- Drug toxicology screen if suspected.

Monitoring

- Continuous pulse oximetry, heart rate and respiratory rate monitoring.
- Close BP monitoring: Consider invasive BP/central venous pressure (CVP) monitoring if there are concerns about haemodynamic status.
- Continuous cardiac monitoring if there are concerns about rhythm disturbances or myocardial dysfunction.
- Conscious level monitoring.
- Urine output as a marker of perfusion and end-organ function.

Bibliography

1. American Heart Association. (2006) 2005 American Heart Association (AHA) guidelines for cardiopulmonary resuscitation CPR) and emergency cardiovascular care (ECC) of pediatric and neonatal patients: Pediatric advanced life support. *Pediatrics* **117**(5):1005–1028.
2. Advanced Life Support Group. (2016) *Advanced Paediatric Life Support: A Practical Approach to Emergencies, 6th ed.* West Sussex: John Wiley & Sons, Ltd.
3. Mejia R, Serrao K. (2008) Assessment of critically ill children. In: Mejia R (ed,), *Pediatric Fundamental Critical Care Support.* Mount Prospect, Ilinois: Society of Critical Care Medicine.
4. Shann F. (2005) *Drug Doses, 13th ed.* Melbourne: Collective Pty Ltd.
5. Kleinman ME, Chaemeides L, Schexnayder SM, *et al.* (2010) Part 14: Pediatric advanced life support: 2010 American Heart Association guidelines for cardiopulmonary resuscitation and emergency cardiovascular care. *Circulation* **122**(3): S876–908
6. Carcillo JA, Fields AI, American College of Critical Care Medicine Task Force Committee Members. (2002) Clinical practice parameters for hemodynamic support of paediatric and neonatal patients in septic shock. *Crit Care Med* **30**(6):1365–1378.
7. The Royal Children's Hospital. (nd) Clinical practice guidelines on resuscitation: Care of the seriously unwell child. Melbourne, Australia. https://www.rch.org.au/clinicalguide/

CHAPTER 2

Cardiopulmonary Resuscitation

Loi V-Ter, Mervin; Lim Kian Boon, Joel

Introduction

In children, cardiopulmonary arrests are usually a result of progressive respiratory failure or shock. While the survival of children with in-hospital cardiac arrests has improved over the years, with recent local data showing 45.6% survival-to-discharge, survival of children from out-of-hospital cardiac arrests remains poor (3.4%). Despite the improved outcome of in-hospital cardiopulmonary resuscitation (CPR), a substantial proportion of survivors have significant neurological deficits.

The provision of advanced paediatric life support usually takes place in a hospital environment where multiple responders can be rapidly mobilised and are capable of simultaneous actions. Important aspects of a successful resuscitation from cardiac arrest include early high-quality chest compressions, early assisted ventilation and early defibrillation (if indicated).

Assessment

- Recognition of cardiac arrest should take no more than 10 seconds.
- The absence or presence of a pulse is not a reliable determinant of cardiac arrest; other determinants include unresponsiveness, gasping breaths and no spontaneous respirations.
- If cardiac arrest has occurred, activate the Emergency Code Team.

Management (Infant <1 year, excluding newborns; child 1–12 years; adolescents >12 years)

Airway/Breathing

- Open airway by appropriate positioning of head.
- Infant: Neutral head position
- Child: Head tilt-chin lift
- Jaw thrust for suspected cervical injury.
- Clear the airway by brief suctioning of mouth and pharynx, if secretions are present.
- Apply bag-mask ventilation with 100% oxygen (at least 15 L/min oxygen flow).

- Use an appropriately sized oropharyngeal airway only in the unconscious child. (Measure the oropharyngeal airway length from incisors to angle of mandible.)
- Ensure correct mask size, tight seal between mask and face, and assess for effectiveness of ventilation (saturations, chest rise, air entry) but avoid excessive ventilation.
- Deliver each breath with an inspiratory time of about 1 s.
- Ventilation should be synchronised with chest compressions at 30 compressions followed by 2 ventilations [i.e. 30:2 ratio] in un-intubated patients in cardiac arrest [if >12 years old and/or only 1 rescuer]; 15:2 ratio if ≤12 years old and at least two rescuers present. In intubated patients, ventilate asynchronously without interrupting chest compressions (30/min for infants, 20/min for children and 10–12/min for adolescents).
- In a patient with a perfusing rhythm but absent or inadequate respiratory effort, give rescue breathing (30/min for infants, 20/min for children and 12/min for adolescents).

Circulation

- Place on cardiac monitor/defibrillator monitoring.
- Place the patient on a firm board and commence chest compressions if pulseless, or heart rate <60/min in child with evidence of shock (see algorithm on "pulseless arrest").
- High-quality CPR requires chest compressions to be of appropriate depth and rate, with complete chest recoil after each compression, minimal interruptions to the chest compressions and avoidance of excessive ventilation. (If manpower permits, it is a good practice to appoint a CPR coach to supervise and provide feedback for CPR.)
- Use "two fingers" (lone rescuer) or "thumb encircling" technique for an infant, placed 1 finger breadth below the intermammary line (lower half of sternum).
- Use the heel of 1–2 hands for an older child placed at the lower half of the sternum in the midline.
- Push Hard: Depress at least a third of the Anterior-Posterior (AP) diameter of the chest (target 3–4 cm for infants, 4–5 cm for children and 4–6 cm for adolescents).
- Push Fast: Chest compressions of at least 100–120/min.

Endotracheal Intubation

- Endotracheal intubation should be performed by an experienced doctor. (See Appendix III "Useful Formulae" for endotracheal tube (ETT) size formula and lengths.)
- Use of Rapid Sequence Induction (RSI) drugs (See Appendix III "Useful Formulae") facilitates emergency intubation and reduces the risk of complications associated with intubation. RSI should be used only by trained, experienced providers. Patients in cardiopulmonary arrest and/or deep coma do not need RSI; otherwise, intubation should be preceded by oxygenation and RSI agents.
- RSI agents typically consist of an anaesthetic induction agent and a muscle relaxant. Maintenance of oxygenation and ventilation by bag-valve-mask

ventilation should be effective before paralysis is instituted. Use paralytic and sedative agents with caution in a patient with a difficult airway as sedating and paralysing such patients may render bag-mask ventilation more challenging. Plan ahead and consider early escalation to a more experienced provider.

- Both cuffed and uncuffed ETT may be used in infants and children. If cuffed tubes are used, cuff inflating pressures should be monitored and limited according to manufacturer's guidelines. Uncuffed ETTs are recommended for neonates.
- Indications for cuffed ETTs include large ETT leak, poor lung compliance and high airway resistance.
- Use both clinical assessment and confirmatory devices (where available) to verify correct ETT placement.

Indications for Intubation

- Severe airway obstruction
- Airway protection in the presence of poor/absent airway reflexes, e.g. decreased conscious level, prolonged seizures, abnormal brainstem function, bulbar/pseudobulbar palsy
- Apnoea or ineffective respiratory drive
- Respiratory failure not responding to or not suitable for non-invasive ventilation
- To assist with airway toileting

Vascular Access

- To obtain two large bore intravenous access for resuscitation. This attempt should take no longer than 60–90 sec.
- Intraosseous (IO) access into the anterior tibial bone marrow (about 1–3 cm below and medial to the tibial tuberosity) can be used if venous access is difficult. All intravenous medications/blood products can be given intraosseously.
- The endotracheal (ET) route can be used to give lipid-soluble emergency drugs (LEAN-lignocaine, epinephrine/adrenaline, atropine, naloxone) followed by a flush of 5 ml normal saline and five manual ventilations. Optimal ET drug doses are unknown, the general consensus is double or triple the dose of lignocaine, atropine or naloxone. For adrenaline, an ET dose ten times the intravenous dose (0.1 ml/kg of 1:1000 concentration) is recommended.
- Central venous cannulation or a venous cutdown may be performed if expertise is available.
- Drugs and fluids (See Appendix II — Drugs [Cardiovascular]). Use isotonic crystalloids as initial fluid for shock/fluid resuscitation. Give aliquots of 20 ml/kg boluses and assess for response.
- There is no added benefit to using colloids during early resuscitative efforts, and there is an associated risk of mortality with the use of colloids for resuscitation in children with trauma, burns or traumatic brain injury.
- Routine use of sodium bicarbonate is not recommended in cardiac arrest. It may be administered for treatment of tricyclic antidepressant overdose or hyperkalaemia.

- Routine use of calcium is not recommended for paediatric cardiopulmonary arrest in the absence of documented hypocalcaemia, calcium channel blocker overdose, hypermagnesaemia or hyperkalaemia.

Gastric Insufflation

- Insert a nasogastric tube if abdominal distension is marked and/or oxygenation and ventilation are compromised.
- Pass the tube after intubation as it may interfere with gastroesophageal sphincter function, increasing risk of aspiration during intubation

Termination of Resuscitative Efforts

- Details of events and treatment must be recorded. Where there is no response after 20 minutes of adequate resuscitation, the senior doctor should decide how much longer resuscitative efforts should continue.

Special Resuscitative Conditions

Ventilation with a Tracheostomy

- Use the tracheostomy tube for assisted ventilation and watch for adequate chest rise.
- If the tracheostomy tube does not allow effective ventilation even after suctioning, change it.
- If still unable to maintain effective ventilation, attempt alternative ventilation methods such as bag-mask ventilation through the nose and mouth while occluding the tracheal stoma.

Bibliography

1. Fuhrman BP, Zimmerman JJ (eds.). (1998) *Pediatric Critical Care. 2nd ed.* St Louis: Mosby, pp. 115–116.
2. Van de Voorde P, Turner NM, Djakow J, *et al.* (20210 European Resuscitation Council guidelines 2021: Paediatric life support. *Resuscitation* **161**:327–387
3. Topjian AA, Raymond TT, Atkins D, *et al.* (2020) Part 4: Pediatric basic and advanced life support: 2020 American Heart Association Guidelines for Cardiopulmonary Resuscitation and Emergency Cardiovascular Care. *Circulation* **142**(16):S469–523.
4. Choi PT, Yip G, Quinonez LG, Cook DJ. (1999) Crystalloids vs. colloids in fluid resuscitation: A systematic review. *Crit Care Med* **27**:200–210.
5. Ong GY, Ngiam N, Tham LP, *et al.* (2021) Singapore Paediatric Resuscitation guidelines 2021. *Sing Med J* **62**:372–389.

RESUSCITATION ALGORITHMS

ALGORITHM FOR PULSELESS ARREST

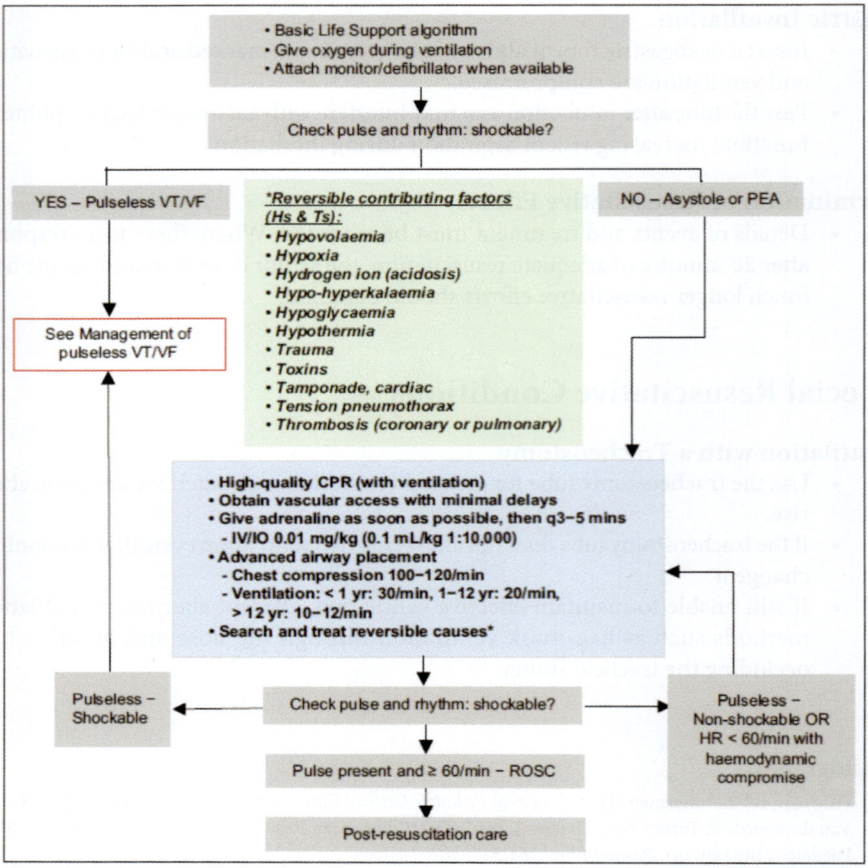

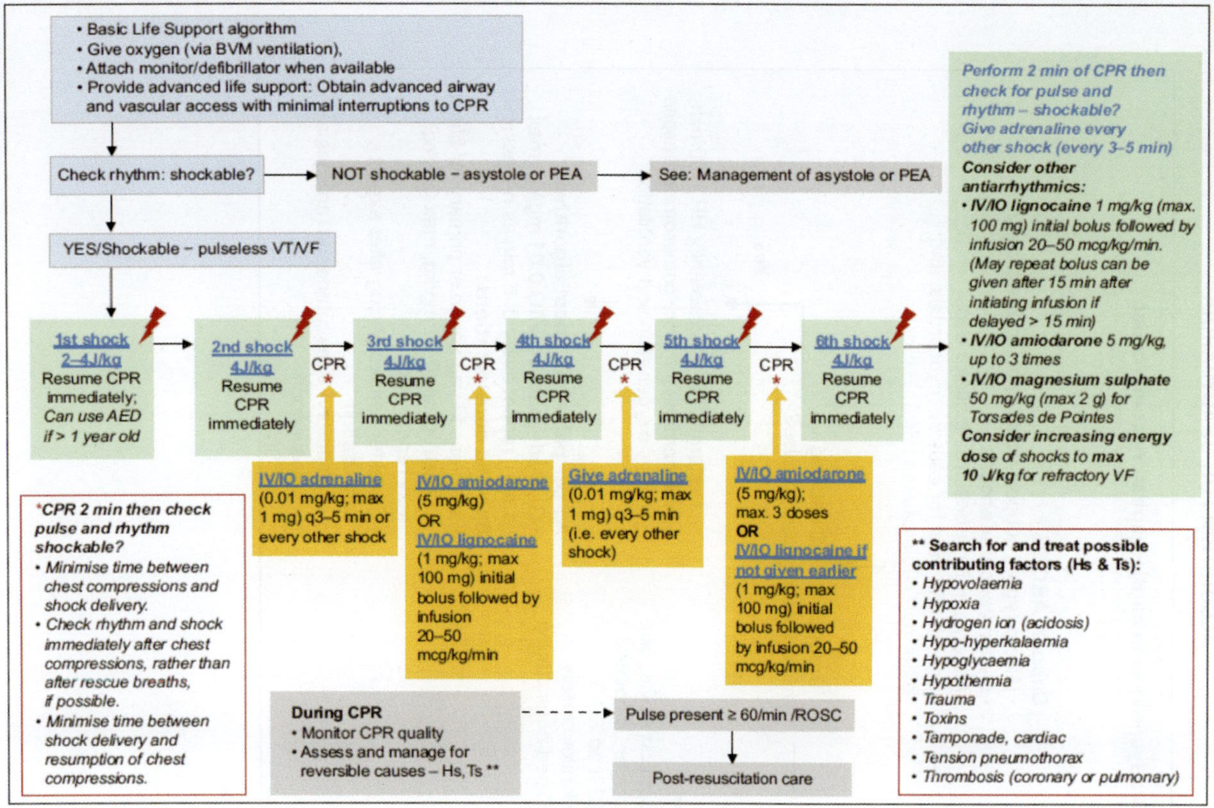

ALGORITHM FOR PULSELESS ARREST (SHOCKABLE)

ALGORITHM FOR BRADYCARDIA

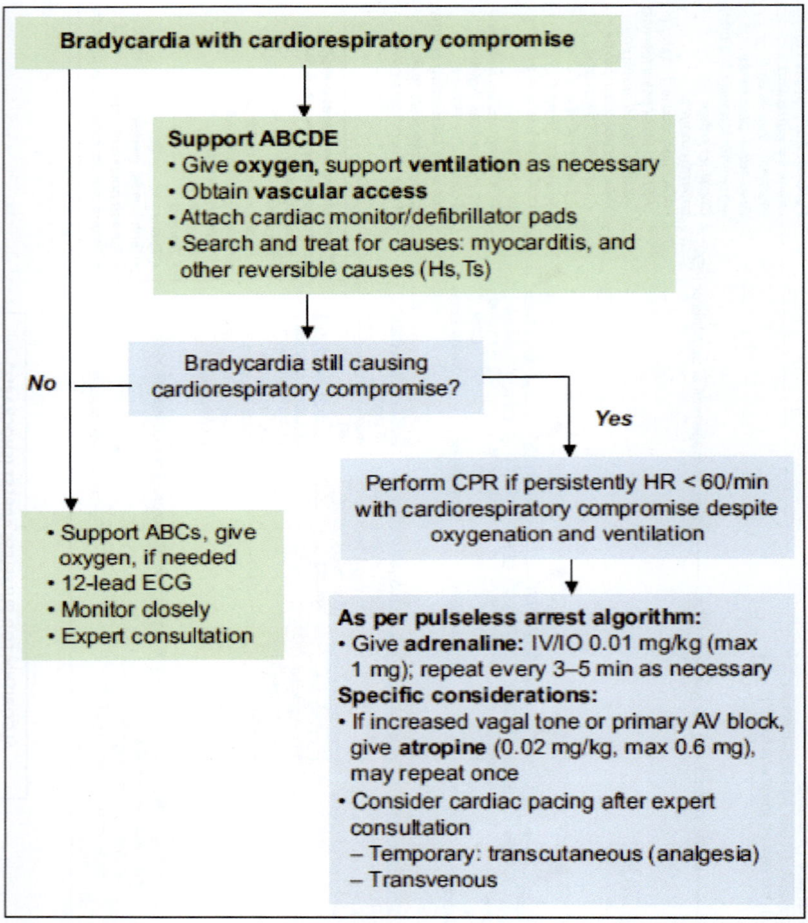

ALGORITHM FOR UNSTABLE TACHYCARDIA WITH POOR PERFUSION

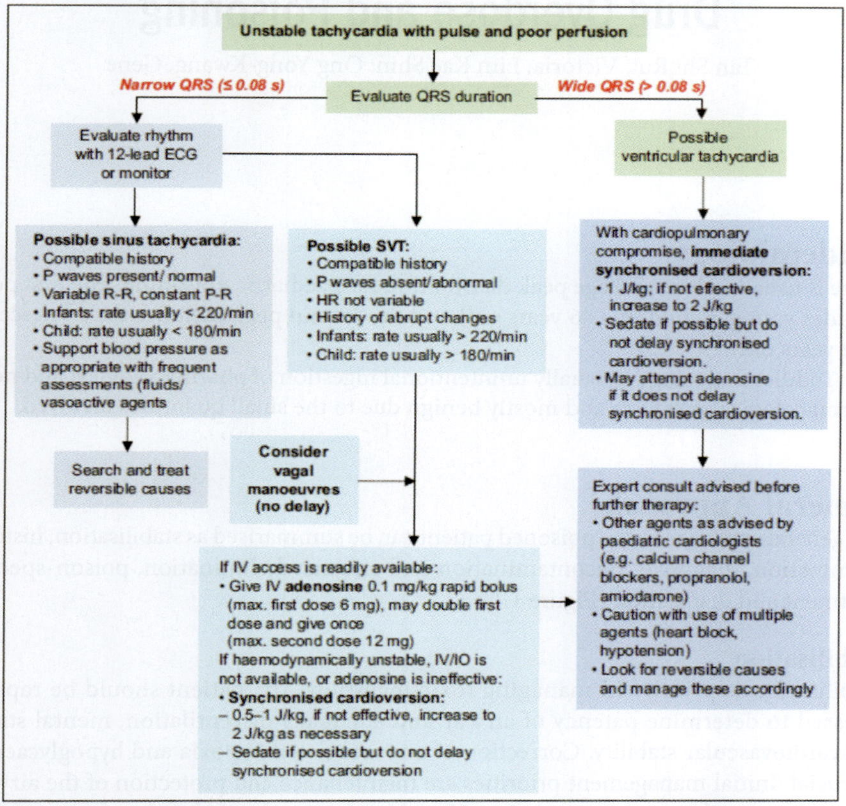

CHAPTER 3

Drug Overdose and Poisoning

Tan Shi Rui, Victoria; Lim Kae Shin; Ong Yong-Kwang, Gene

Epidemiology

There is usually a bimodal age peak distribution for paediatric poisoning. The first peak includes younger children (<6 years old) and the second peak includes the adolescents (>12 years old).

Toddler toxicology is usually unintentional ingestion of pharmacological and non-pharmacological products and mostly benign due to the small quantities involved.

General Approach

The general approach to the poisoned patient can be summarised as stabilisation, history, examination, diagnosis, decontamination and enhanced elimination, poison-specific treatment and disposition (Figure 1.1).

Stabilisation

Stabilisation is priority in managing toxic ingestion. The patient should be rapidly assessed to determine patency of airway and adequacy of ventilation, mental status and cardiovascular stability. Correction of any associated hypoxia and hypoglycaemia is crucial. Initial management priorities are maintenance and protection of the airway, supporting ventilation and circulation. Unstable patients should be placed on a cardiac monitor with measurement of vital signs every 5 to 15 min until the patient is stabilised. The potential for rapid changes in the patient's condition should be considered in making decisions about airway and ventilatory support.

With regard to toxicology, prolonged resuscitation should be attempted in drug-induced cardiac arrest. Extracorporeal membrane oxygenation (ECMO) should be considered if resources and expertise allow.

History

- History and physical examination are performed concurrently with stabilisation.
- History should include

  Who: Patient characteristics, age, weight, relationship to others present and gender

  What: Name and dosage of medication(s) or substance(s) of abuse, co-ingestants and amount ingested

  When: Timing and date of ingestion

Where: Route which toxins was taken
Why: Whether intentional or accidental and associated details

- For paediatric ingestions, thorough history from caregivers is crucial.
- If the toxic ingestion is unwitnessed (time, dose), always manage as for worst-case scenario even if the patient is asymptomatic, especially if the alleged drug is highly toxic.

Advanced Paediatric Life Support: resuscitate and stabilise patient

⇩

GOALS

- Identify the toxin and amount ingested
- Assess the presence and degree of toxicity and potential for toxicity
- Consider if a non-toxicological condition could be the cause of or contributing to clinical presentation

⇩

History	**Physical Examination**	**Bedside point of care testing for unstable patients (if available)**
Important but often: ◆ Unreliable ◆ Unavailable ◆ Incomplete	A focused examination to include: ◆ Vital signs ◆ Arousal levels, Eyes ◆ Muscle tone, Reflexes ◆ Skin, Odours ◆ Look for toxidromes or toxic signs	- Glucose - Blood gas - Electrolytes - Lactate - 12-lead electrocardiogram (ECG) - Urine dipsticks **Laboratory*** ◆ Selective/Progressive ◆ Toxicological testing

⇩

MANAGEMENT

A	Airway
B	Breathing
C	Circulation
D	Disability
	Decontamination
E	Elimination
F	Find an antidote
G	General Management (complications)

Figure 1.1 Assessment and management of a poisoned child.

- Other important historical points from the caregivers include a systemic review, specifically the presence of seizures, agitation, coma, vomiting, headache and shortness of breath.
- Clinicians should be aware that in some cases, the history may be unreliable for teenagers, especially if the toxic ingestion was intentional or if there was ongoing inappropriate substance use. Patients may not know what they ingested, the patient's altered mental status may impede communication, or the patient may intentionally mislead the clinician.

Clinical Examination

- A thorough physical examination should be performed to help with the diagnosis and identify complications.
- Specific attention to vital signs, mental status (depressed or agitated), respiration (depressed, evidence of pulmonary oedema or aspiration), pupils (size, reactivity, presence of nystagmus), skin (diaphoresis or abnormally dry, blisters), bowel sounds (increased or decreased).
- Based on findings from physical examination, the clinician should specifically consider the presence of a toxidrome.
- Note that for young paediatric patients, the classical findings may be different from adolescents and adults. For example, for organophosphate poisoning in young children, nicotinic symptoms may predominate over muscarinic symptoms, and they may present predominantly with muscle weakness with respiratory insufficiency, altered mental status and seizures. The pupils of the organophosphate poisoned young child may not exhibit the classical miosis.

Decontamination

After the patient is stabilised, consideration should be given to removing the toxin. The choice of decontamination should be made based on the clinical status and the suspected toxin. Patients with an inhalation exposure should be removed from the source, with care taken to avoid exposure of the rescuers. When toxic compounds have been splashed into the eyes or onto the skin, copious irrigation should be performed.

Paediatric Gastrointestinal Decontamination

1. Single-dose activated charcoal

The preferred method of GI decontamination. It is indicated as a gastric decontaminant agent if a patient has ingested a potentially toxic amount of a poison up to 1 hour following ingestion.

However, it can be considered for paracetamol toxic ingestion up to 2 hours. Other toxins for which delayed administration can be given include aspirin, digoxin, phenobarbitone, anticholinergics, tricyclics and sustained release tablets.

Dose: 1 g/kg (maximum of 50 g if less than 12 years old).

Drugs which are not absorbable by charcoal — **PHAILS**: Pesticides, Hydrocarbons, Acids/Alkalis, Iron, Lithium and Solvents.

Activated charcoal is contraindicated in patients who are unable to protect their airway. The use of orogastric and nasogastric tubes for administration of activated charcoal in a drowsy or vomiting patient has been associated with pulmonary complications, unless the airway has been secured.

2. Whole bowel irrigation

Whole bowel irrigation (WBI) is not routinely performed in the management of the poisoned patient. WBI is best used in patients who are not vomiting and have normal intestinal function. They are useful in patients with ingestions of highly toxic substances that are poorly bound to activated charcoal, such as iron, lithium or lead, as well as for sustained-release medications (e.g. certain formulations of lithium, theophylline or calcium channel blockers).

WBI is contraindicated in patients with bowel obstruction, gastric haemorrhage, perforation and ileus. It is also contraindicated in unstable patients or inpatients with compromised unprotected airways, haemodynamic instability and intractable vomiting.

The procedure is administered by giving polyethylene glycol bowel preparation at a rate of 1 to 2 L/h in adolescents and 500 ml/h in children through a nasogastric tube, to induce osmotic diarrhoea till rectal effluent is clear (usually about 6 hours). The electrolytes of small children must be closely monitored. For radio-opaque compounds (**CHIPES**: chloral hydrate, heavy metals, iron, phenothiazines, enteric-coated tablets, salicylates/substances in containers, e.g. body packers), continue until repeat radiographs are clear.

3. Gastric lavage

Gastric lavage is not routinely performed in the management of poisoned patients. In certain cases where the procedure is of attractive theoretical benefit (e.g. recent ingestion of a very toxic substance within 1 hour), the substantial risks should be weighed carefully against the sparse evidence that the procedure is of any benefit.

Enhanced Elimination

Enhanced elimination techniques aim to increase the rate of removal of an agent from the body with the aim of reducing the severity and duration of clinical intoxication.

Enhanced elimination techniques are only indicated for poisonings when the following requirements are met: severe toxicity, poor outcome despite good supportive care/antidote administration, slow endogenous rates of elimination, suitable pharmacokinetic properties, benefit exceeds risks, and will not distract from other priorities (e.g. resuscitation, supportive care, decontamination and antidote therapy).

Techniques for enhanced elimination include:

1. Multiple-dose activated charcoal (MDAC)
    - This causes interruption of entero-hepatic circulation and gastrointestinal dialysis for small, lipid soluble molecule drugs with a small volume of distribution and low protein binding.
    - Drugs (ABCD): Antimalarials (quinine), Aminophylline (theophylline), Barbiturates, Carbamazepine, Dapsone.
    - Contraindications: decreased consciousness/anticipated decreased level of consciousness without prior airway protection, bowel obstruction.
    - Give an initial dose of activated charcoal 1 g/kg (children) or 50 g (adolescents) and repeat doses of 0.25 g/kg/h (paediatrics) or 12.5 g/h in divided doses over 2–4 hours.

- Check bowel sounds prior to administration of each dose and reconsider the indications and clinical endpoints for therapy every 6 hours. Multiple-dose activated charcoal should rarely be required beyond 6 hours.
- Complications include emesis (30%), charcoal aspiration, constipation, charcoal bezoar formation, bowel obstruction, bowel perforation (rare) and corneal abrasions. MDAC also risks distracting manpower from resuscitation and supportive care priorities.

2. Urinary alkalinisation
    - Urinary alkalinisation enhances renal elimination of weak acids such as salicylates, phenobarbital and chlorpropamide.
    - Loading dose of IV sodium bicarbonate 1–2 mmol/kg followed by infusing bicarbonate-containing fluids: 3 ampules (150 mmol) of sodium bicarbonate to 1 L of dextrose 5% and run at 250 ml/h (run the IV at 1.5 times maintenance in children).
    - Achieving urinary alkalinisation is impossible if there is total body potassium depletion, even in the presence of normal potassium levels on the renal panel. Potassium supplementation is required.
    - Follow urinary pH hourly. Blood pH, salicylate levels and electrolytes should be monitored regularly. The frequency of monitoring is dependent upon the severity of the clinical situation
    - The goal is to achieve urine pH of 7.5–8.5.

3. Extracorporeal elimination (e.g. haemodialysis, haemofiltration, haemoperfusion, plasmapheresis and exchange transfusion)
    - Effectively enhances elimination of any drug that is a small molecule, has a small volume of distribution, rapid redistribution from tissues and plasma and slow endogenous elimination. Continuous renal replacement therapy (CRRT) has lower drug clearance per unit of time but slow continuous removal may be preferred when the patient is haemodynamically unstable (unable to tolerate rapid solute and fluid loss), the drugs are highly protein/tissue bound toxicant with large volume of distribution with very long plasma half-lives and exhibit 'rebound' phenomenon (e.g. lithium)
    - Indications for haemodialysis/haemofiltration are: carbamazepine (if MDAC is inadequate or infeasible), valproate, lithium, concomitant severe hyperkalaemia, metformin lactic acidosis, methotrexate (if in acute renal failure or leucovorin is not available), paraquat (within 2 hours of ingestion), salicylates, toxic alcohols and theophylline.
    - Exchange transfusion can be considered for severe drug-induced methaemoglobinaemia, or if refractory to IV methylene blue and IV ascorbic acid, if antidote is contraindicated (e.g. methylene blue in G6PD deficiency) or antidotes are unavailable.

Antidotes

- Antidotes are typically given after stabilisation and when the diagnosis was made.

- In certain cases, prompt administration of antidote is imperative. E.g. prompt administration of naloxone may avoid the need for endotracheal intubation in opiate overdose.

Investigations

In general, toxicological testing can serve a number of purposes including:

- Confirming a toxic aetiology and avoiding the need for further diagnostic studies
- Identifying a specific agent
- Assessing the severity of the intoxication
- Assessing efficacy of treatment
- Guiding management decisions
- Prognostication
- Guiding transfer decisions

Disposition

Consider transfer to higher centre in the following circumstances:

- Inability to stabilise patient or deteriorating patient
- Inability to provide patient with ongoing maintenance treatment
- Lack of availability of toxin-specific therapy
- Management and disposition of patients following decontamination is toxin and patient-specific, e.g. interventions such as dialysis, haemodialysis and haemoperfusion.
- All patients who have taken a suicidal ingestion require assessment of suicidal risk prior to discharge, possibly transferring to Institute of Mental Health if still actively suicidal.

Table 1.3 List of Antidotes for Initial Management of Common and Dangerous Poisons (Referral to clinical toxicologists for more detailed management is advised)

Toxin	Antidote/Paediatric dose
Analgesia Poisoning	
Paracetamol	Paediatric dosing for IV N-acetylcysteine Most effective within 8 hr but has significant effects post 8 hr for documented toxicity See section on paracetamol.
Salicylates	IV Sodium bicarbonate1–2 mmol/kg bolus Followed by infusion: 150 mmol Sodium bicarbonate + 40 mmol KCl in total volume of 1 L of dextrose 5% infused to maintain urine output at 1.5–2 ml/kg/hr and urine pH at 7.5–8.5 Repeat IV sodium bicarbonate bolus as necessary, keep serum potassium normal.
Opioid	Correct hypoxia and assist ventilate as main priority IV Naloxone hydrochloride 0.1 mg/kg/dose (max 2 mg/dose). Can repeat up to 0.5 mg/kg or max 10 mg total. Consider infusion in view of short half-life.

(*Continued*)

Table 1.3 (*Continued*)

Toxin	Antidote/Paediatric dose
Cardiovascular drug toxicity	
Calcium channel blocker Beta-blockers	• IV Calcium - IV 10% Calcium gluconate 0.5 ml/kg (max 20 ml/dose) - IV 10% Calcium chloride 0.2 ml/kg (max 10 ml/dose) • IV Glucagon (more effective for beta-blockers than calcium channel blockers) - Paediatric: Initial bolus of 150 mcg/kg and repeat as necessary (max 2 mg/dose up to a max of 10 mg). If effective, may be followed by an infusion of 50–100 mcg/kg/hr (max 5 mg/hr) • High-dose Insulin Euglycaemic Therapy (HIET)–IV Insulin 1 unit/kg with 0.5 g/kg dextrose bolus - Followed by insulin infusion 0.5–2 unit/kg/hr together with a dextrose 10%-saline infusion • 20% MCT emulsion: Intralipid/lipofundin - Bolus: 1.5 ml/kg and may repeat as needed. - Followed by infusion: 0.25 ml/kg/min over 30 to 60 min - Max total dose: 12 ml/kg
Digoxin	Digoxin immune antibody fragment: Empiric dosing: 10–20 vials IV bolus for life-threatening toxicity (See package insert for other dosing regimens)
Tricyclic antidepressants and other sodium channel blockers	IV sodium bicarbonate: 1–2 mmol/kg Repeat boluses titrate to QRS duration (do not exceed arterial pH 7.55)
Cholinergic Poisoning	
Carbamates	IV Atropine 0.05–0.1 mg/kg
Organophosphate	IV Atropine 0.05–0.1 mg/kg Consider IV Pralidoxime 20–50 mg/kg (max 2 g/dose) for Diethyl organophosphate poisoning and specific nerve agent poisoning
Heavy Metals	
Iron	IV Deferoxamine 5–15 mg/kg/hr infusion
Arsenic	PO Succimer (DMSA) 10 mg/kg/dose TDS IM British Anti-Lewisite (BAL) (dimercaprol) 3–5 mg/kg/dose Q4-6H (only if unable to tolerate succimer). BAL is contraindicated in peanut allergic patients.
Lead	<u>Lead encephalopathy:</u> IM BAL (dimercaprol) 4 mg/kg or 50–75 mg/m^2 Q4H; (BAL is contraindicated in peanut allergic patients.) Followed by IV Calcium disodium EDTA 50–75 mg/kg, to be administered 4 hr after BAL (1 g of Calcium disodium EDTA can be diluted with 250 ml dextrose 5% or normal saline. Administer over 8–12 hr or continuously over 24 hr). Succimer (DMSA) (if patient is able to tolerate oral medication) 10 mg/kg/dose TDS, repeat doses are often needed Further management needed for chelation and referral is advised.

Table 1.3 (*Continued*)

Toxin	Antidote/Paediatric dose
Toxic Alcohols	
Methanol Ethylene Glycol	Ethanol (10%): Loading dose 10 ml/kg IV or orally followed by maintenance dose 1–2 ml/kg/hr orally OR IV Fomepizole: 15 mg/kg over 30 min, followed by maintenance dose.
Others:	
Bupivacaine (L.A. toxicity)	20% MCT emulsion: Lipofundin/Intralipid - Bolus: 1.5 ml/kg and may repeat as needed. - Followed by infusion: 0.25 ml/kg/min over 30 to 60 min - Max total dose: 12 ml/kg
Cyanide	- Hydroxocobalamin: IV 70 mg/kg (max 5 g/dose) over 15–30 min. Repeat once 70 mg/kg as needed depending on response (total dose 140 mg/kg or max 10 g). - Sodium thiosulphate: Used in conjunction with hydroxocobalamin or sodium nitrite (synergistic). IV of 25% sodium thiosulphate 1–2 ml/kg; max 50 ml/dose. - Sodium nitrite (not for cyanide toxicity in smoke inhalation): IV 3% sodium nitrite 0.2 ml/kg; max 10 ml. Repeat 2 hr later or as necessary, 0.1 ml/kg; max 5 ml. Watch for methaemoglobinaemia.
Isoniazid	Pyridoxine: IV 70 mg/kg (max 5 g/dose) over 5 min
Methemoglobinemia	Methylene blue: IV 1–2 mg/kg slow infusion, repeat as needed every 30 to 60 min
Sulphonylureas	Octreotide: IV 1–1.5 mcg/kg bolus (max 150 mcg/dose) Q6H or continuous infusion
Drug toxicities with antidotes to be used with caution	
Anticholinergics	Physostigmine salicylate 0.02 mg/kg (max 0.5 mg/dose) slowly over 5 min (may cause bradycardia, respiratory distress and seizures). Its use as an antidote for anti-cholinergic toxicity is controversial due to reports of associated seizures and life-threatening arrhythmias.
Benzodiazepines	Flumazenil IV 0.01 mg/kg (max 0.2 mg). It should not be routinely administered in the patient presenting with coma or altered mental status. Reversal of benzodiazepine effect in mixed drug ingestion involving cyclic antidepressants and chloral hydrate may result in seizures or arrhythmias with fatal outcomes.

Pre-Hospital Paediatric Toxicology — Advice to Caregivers

Primary Prevention

Most poisonings occur when parents or caregivers are home but children may not be supervised.

Advise caregivers to store medicine, cleaning and laundry products, paints/varnishes and pesticides in their original packaging in locked cabinets or containers, out of sight and reach of children.

Caregivers should never refer to medicine as "candy" or other appealing names.One should be reminded not to give or take medication in the dark. They should also check the label each time a child is given medicine to ensure proper dosage as the same drug may come in different concentrations.

Home Management if Toxic Exposure has Occurred

If a child is unconscious, not breathing, or having convulsions or seizures due to poison contact or ingestion, they should be advised to call for emergency services immediately. Caregivers or any one nearby should initiate basic life support if they are able to.

Immediate Management for Home Poisonings

- Toxic ingestion — Advise the caregivers to immediately remove the item away from the child and have the child spit out any remaining substance. Do not induce vomiting or use syrup of ipecac.
- Skin exposures — Remove the child's clothes and rinse the skin with lukewarm water for at least 15 minutes.
- Ocular exposures — Flush the child's eye by holding the eyelid open and pouring a steady stream of room temperature water into the inner corner for 15 minutes.
- Inhalation exposures — The child should be evacuated outside or into fresh air immediately. If respiratory effort is compromised, start cardiopulmonary resuscitation (CPR) and do not stop until the child breathes on his or her own or until someone takes over.

Clinical Presentations

Drug-Induced Bradycardia and Hypotension

- Paediatric advanced life support
  - » Perform CPR if despite adequate oxygenation and ventilation heart rate <60/min with poor perfusion
- Treat reversible causes like hypoxia, electrolyte disturbances
- IV fluids
- Inotropic support
- Atropine
- External or internal cardiac pacing
- Resuscitative Extra-Corporeal Life Support (ECMO)

Drug-Induced Seizures

- The priority still is the management of reversible causes of seizures like hypoxia, hypoglycaemia, electrolyte disturbances and if the history and physical findings are not consistent with toxic seizures, intracranial infections, bleeds, space occupying lesions should be appropriately excluded.

Table 1.4 Causes of Drug-Induced Bradycardia and Hypotension

Calcium channel blockers
Beta-blockers
Digoxin
Opiates
Clonidine
Severe tricyclic antidepressant poisoning
Severe organophosphate poisoning

Table 1.5 Causes of Toxic Seizures

Isoniazid (INH)
Gyromitra mushroom or false morel
Hydrazine
Sulphonylureas — refractory hypoglycaemic seizures
Salicylates
Tricyclic Antidepressants

- Toxic seizures are often transient and no specific treatment is required. However close monitoring may be required depending on the half-life of the ingested toxin and other potential life-threatening conditions, e.g. arrhythmias.
- Benzodiazepines (e.g. diazepam or lorazepam) are usually effective for toxic seizures.
- If benzodiazepines are ineffective, barbiturates such as phenobarbital usually will suffice.
- Phenytoin has no role in toxin-induced seizures and is theoretically harmful in poisoning with substances with sodium channel blockade such as tricyclics. It is also contraindicated in theophylline-induced seizures as it worsens toxicity.
- Pyridoxine may be required only in unusual poisonings such as isoniazid toxicity.
- It is essential that the patients who have or had toxic seizures to be on cardiac monitoring and have a 12-lead ECG performed.

Drug-Induced Altered Mental Status

- Treatment of the most common causes of altered mental status that can be recognised and treated immediately.
- Exclude reversible causes like hypoxia, hypoglycaemia, electrolyte disturbances, sepsis, intracranial pathologies.

Table 1.6 Drugs Causing Altered Mental Status

Clinical Situation/Symptoms
Depressed sensorium with small pupils and hypotension
Opioids Clonidine Phenothiazines Benzodiazepines Barbiturates Nerve agents Organophosphates Carbamates *Classically small pupils are expected in cholinergic poisoning in adults but literature suggests this is variable, with miosis and mydriasis both reported in paediatrics*
Causes of toxidromes with hyperthermia and altered mental status
<u>Sympathomimetic syndrome</u> *(This is usually differentiated from the anticholinergic toxidrome by the presence of marked diaphoresis)* Amphetamines Salbutamol Cocaine <u>Anticholinergic toxidrome</u> Antihistamines Anticholinergic plants (e.g. Dhatura) Antiparkinsonian agents Antiemetics Antispasmodics Antipruritic Cyclic antidepressants <u>Serotonin syndrome</u> Fluoxetine Citalopram Sertraline Bupropion <u>Malignant neuroleptic syndrome</u> *Every class of neuroleptic drug has been implicated, including the low potency (e.g. chlorpromazine) and the newer "atypical" antipsychotic drugs (e.g. clozapine, risperidone, olanzapine)* Antipsychotics, e.g. haloperidol, fluphenazine. Metoclopromide <u>Malignant hyperthermia</u> Succinylcholine General anaesthesia

Table 1.7 Other Drug-Induced Clinical Presentations

Agitated delirium
Anticholinergics Phencyclidine Sympathomimetics (e.g. cocaine) Hallucinogens Alcohol toxicity
Drug-induced acute movement disorders
Dyskinesia Amphetamines Anticholinergics Antihistamines Cocaine Gamma-hydroxybutyrate Dystonia Metoclopramide

Paracetamol Poisoning

I) Toxic ingestion if

a) Single, acute ingestion of ≥200 mg/kg or 10 g (whichever is lesser)

b) Repeated Supratherapeutic Ingestion (RSTI): defined as more than 1 dose of paracetamol ingested in the last >24–72H. (if repeated dosing ≤24 hours, to follow Acute Ingestion pathway)

In symptomatic patients — irrespective of dose, if ≥daily therapeutic dose per day for more than 48 hours.

In asymptomatic patients — cumulative dose of ≥10 g or ≥200 mg/kg (whichever is lesser) within a 24 hour period; or ingestion of ≥4 g/24 hours or ≥100 mg/kg/24 hours beyond 24 hours.

II) Presumed toxic ingestion in

c) Symptomatic patients (even with known time of ingestion)

Clinical Presentation

Early:	Non-specific with nausea and vomiting
24–48 hours:	Tender hepatomegaly with jaundice
Day 4–5:	Acute liver and renal failure
Other features:	Erythema, urticaria, haemolytic anaemia, pancreatitis, haemorrhage (prolonged prothrombin time)

Investigations

Serum paracetamol level: taken at least 4 hours post-ingestion

For acute ingestions, refer to the Rumack–Matthew nomogram

Liver function test (LFT):

- Transaminases (ALT, AST) begin to rise by 12 hours and peak at 72 to 96 hours
- Serum bilirubin (SB) rises more slowly
- Prothrombin time (PT)/International Normalised Ratio (INR) abnormal by 24 to 36 hours

Other investigations: Renal panel/electrolytes, blood gas

Treatment

Activated charcoal 1 g/kg (most useful within 2 hours of ingestion).

Specific antidote: IV N-acetyl-cysteine (NAC)

NAC is indicated if:

- Serum paracetamol level lies above the Treatment Nomogram Line on the Rumack–Matthew nomogram ("Probable Toxicity") for acute ingestion
- Asymptomatic with delayed presentation: ≥200 mg/kg or 10 g of paracetamol has been ingested and serum paracetamol level is not likely available within the 8-hour window. Effectiveness depends on initiation of NAC with maximal benefit within 8–10 hours of acute ingestion, diminishing value after 12–16 hours. If paracetamol levels can be made known within 8 hours, need not start till levels are available.
- Symptomatic — unusual for symptoms to occur if ingestion is less than 8 hours (inaccurate timing or dose reporting).
- Sustained-release (SR) preparation or co-ingestion of agents which affect gastric motility. In such cases, start IV NAC and follow RSTI workflow

Dosage of N-Acetyl-Cysteine (NAC)

For paracetamol poisoning, a total dose of NAC 300 mg/kg body weight was administered over 3 phases traditionally. The current recommended regimen is a 2-bag IV NAC over 20 hours. Reported benefits of this 2-bag regime include significantly reduced non-immune mediated allergic reactions, and it has been shown to be as effective as the 3-bag regimen.

This involves combining the first 2 bags of the traditional 3-course NAC infusion into the loading dose. i.e.

- 1st bag is 200 mg/kg in TOTAL 500 ml (maximum concentration of 22 g over 4 hours, then followed by
- 2nd bag 100 mg/kg over 16 hours.

Please refer to your institution's guidelines for IV NAC infusion and dilution charts for details.

Similar to the 3-bag regimen, the last dose may be repeated if there is ongoing hepatotoxicity. If the initial paracetamol concentration is more than double the nomogram line following acute ingestion, increase NAC dose to 200 mg/kg over 16 hours.

The administration of N-acetyl-cysteine will be dependent on the child's weight for dosing and dilution.

- Phase 1: 200 mg/kg over ≈4 hours
  - » ≤25 kg: Add IV NAC 200 mg/kg in total volume of 100 ml
  - » >25–80 kg: Add IV NAC 200 mg/kg to 500 ml

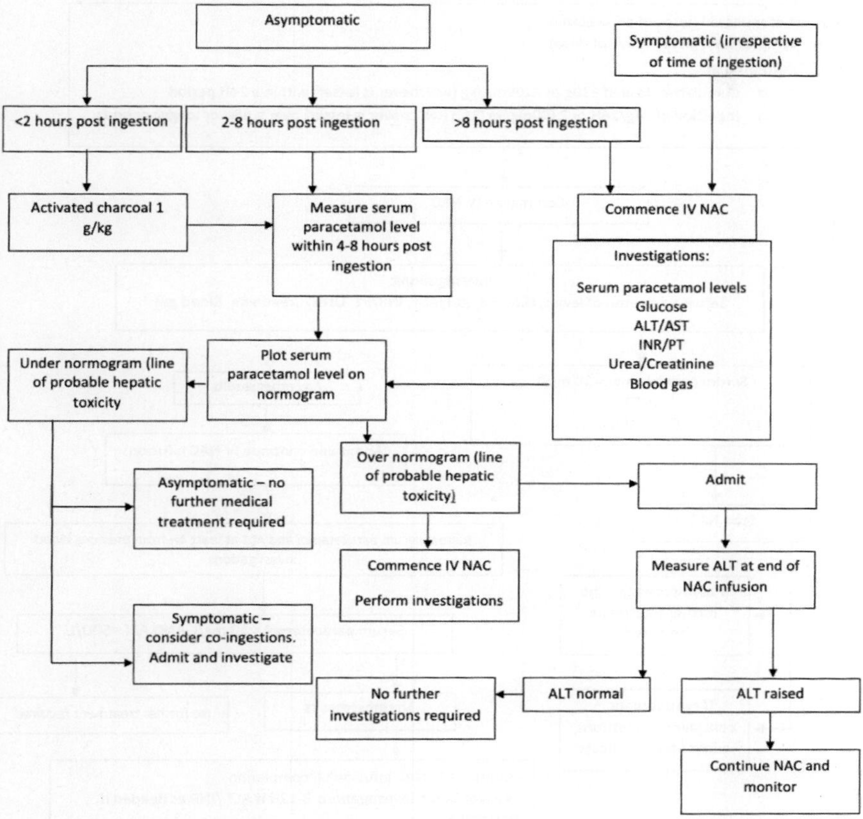

Figure 1.2 Single, acute toxic ingestion of paracetamol.

- » >80 kg: Add IV NAC 200 mg/kg to 1000 ml (in 2 bottles × 500 ml)
- Phase 2: 100 mg/kg over ≈16 hours
  - » ≤ 10 kg: Add IV NAC 100 mg/kg in total volume of 100 ml
  - » >10–50 kg: Add IV NAC 100 mg/kg to 500 ml
  - » >50 kg: Add IV NAC 100 mg/kg to 1000 ml (in 2 bottles × 500 ml)

Total dose: 300 mg/kg
Total duration: ≈20 hours

In all cases, additional maintenance fluids can be given if required, or NAC may be administered in larger volume bags if more convenient. At 18 hours into the NAC infusion (2 hours before completion), send bloods for:

- Paracetamol level
- ALT
- Urea, electrolytes, creatinine (5% of patients with paracetamol toxicity will develop acute renal injury)

The NAC infusion should be discontinued only once the:

- ALT < 50U/L, reached their peak levels and are declining

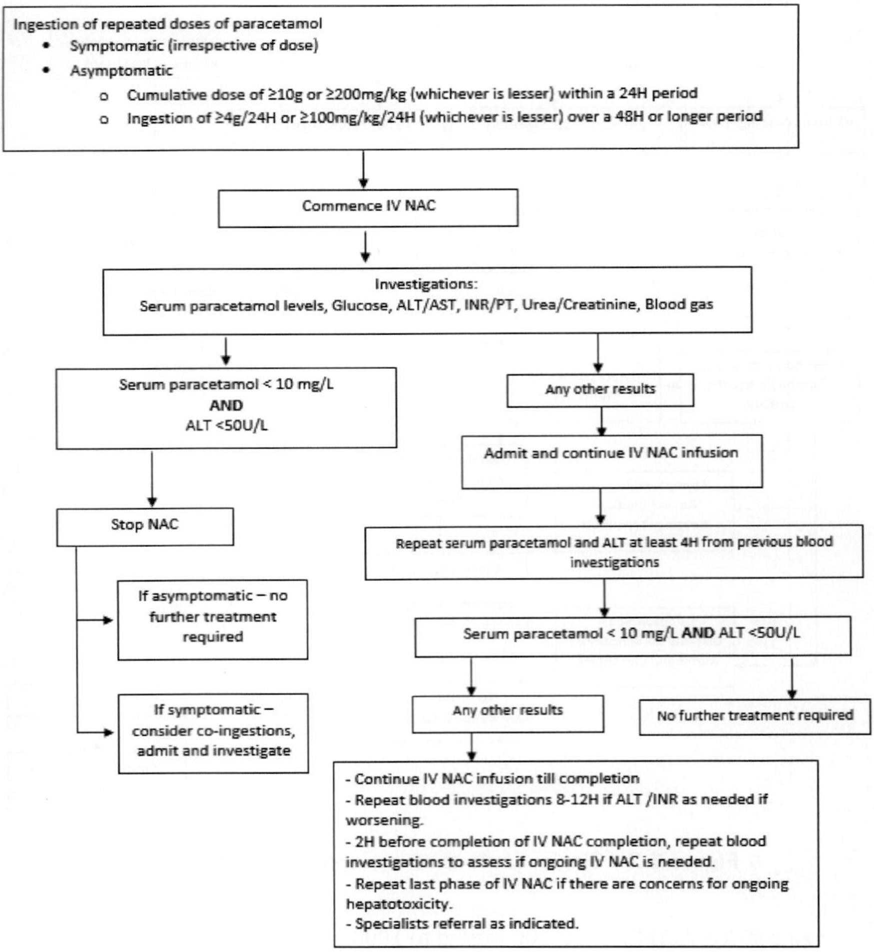

Figure 1.3 Repeated Supratherapeutic Ingestion of paracetamol.

- Urea, electrolytes and creatinine are normal or have normalised (if previously abnormal)
- Paracetamol level has returned to normal (i.e. below <10 mg/dL)

Other Considerations

1) Massive Paracetamol ingestion and its management

Massive paracetamol ingestion is defined by ingestion of ≥30 g or ≥500 mg/kg (whichever is less). Patients should receive IV NAC till completion and increased doses may be needed. Consult clinical toxicologists and intensive care specialists early for further management. Patients may be symptomatic early and present with severe lactic acidosis with or without liver injury (direct effects on mitochondria).

In addition to the standard paracetamol management, if the patient is haemodynamically unstable and with concerns of end-organ dysfunction or refractory

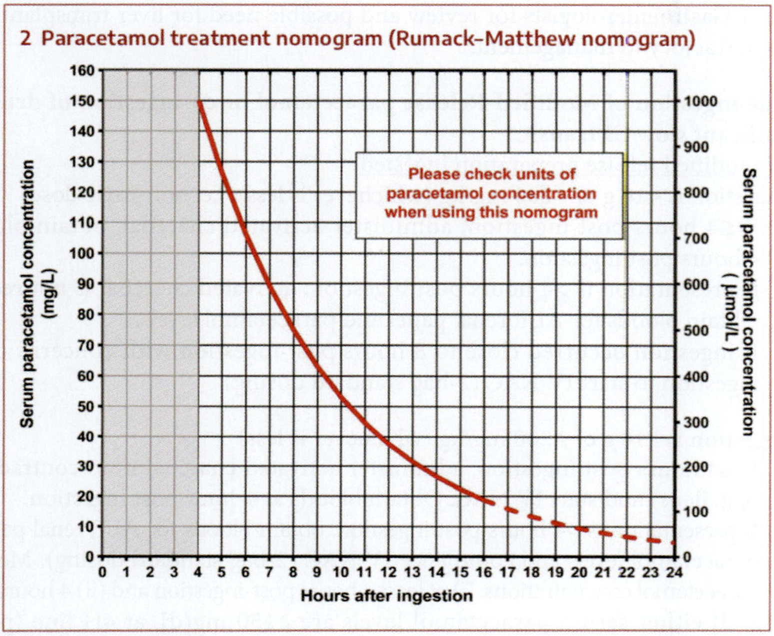

Figure 1.4 Nomogram-relating plasma or serum paracetamol concentration and probability of hepatotoxicity at varying intervals following ingestion of a single toxic dose of paracetamol.

acidosis not responsive to standard resuscitation, consider haemodialysis early. If haemodialysis is needed, IV NAC dosing may need to be adjusted (consult pharmacists/ toxicologists).

Complete IV NAC 2-bag regimen but increased doses needed for the 2nd bag.

If serum paracetamol at 4-hour post ingestion is:

- 2X probable toxicity, i.e. levels are ~300 mg/dL at 4H post ingestion, double the 2nd bag to 200 mg/kg over 16 hours.
- 3X probable toxicity, i.e. levels are ~450 mg/dL at 4H post ingestion, triple the 2nd bag to 300 mg/kg over 16 hours (consult pharmacists/toxicologists)

Repeat paracetamol levels 4H apart to guide need for further decontamination (stat dose of activated charcoal) and IV NAC dose.

At 18 hours into the NAC infusion (2 hours before completion), send bloods for: Paracetamol level, ALT, and Urea, electrolytes, creatinine.

The NAC infusion should be discontinued only when the:

- ALT < 50U/L, reached their peak levels and are declining
- Urea, electrolytes and creatinine are normal or have normalised (if previously abnormal)
- Paracetamol level has returned to normal (i.e. below <10 mg/dL)

The 2nd bag over 16H may be repeated if there is ongoing hepatotoxicity at completion of IV NAC at 20 hours and dosing adjusted to serum paracetamol (should be <10 mg/dL at 20H).

Refer Gastroenterologists for review and possible need for liver transplant if liver injury is refractory to management.

2) Acute ingestion of Modified-Release paracetamol or co-ingestion of drugs that significant slow GI transit.

Dose of modified release preparation ingested

i) If ingestion is <10 g or <200 mg/kg (whichever is less), i.e. non-toxic dose.
- If ≤4 hours post ingestion, administer activated charcoal, obtain bloods at 4 hours post ingestion.
- If presentation is >4 hours post ingestion, activated charcoal is not required. Obtain bloods for ALT, renal panel and paracetamol levels.
- If ingestion occurred close to 8 hours post ingestion with concerns of toxic ingestion to start IV NAC (2-bag standard dosing).

ii) If ingestion is ≥10 g or ≥200 mg/kg (whichever is less)
- If ≤4 hours post ingestion, administer activated charcoal if no contradictions (e.g. ileus) and start IV NAC. Obtain bloods at 4-hour post ingestion.
- If presentation is >4 hours post ingestion, obtain bloods for ALT, renal panel and paracetamol levels and commence IV NAC (2-bag standard dosing). Measure 2 paracetamol concentrations: (i) at least 4 hours post-ingestion and (ii) 4 hours apart.
  - » If either serum paracetamol levels are ≥150 mg/dL at 4H line (possible hepatotoxicity), to complete IV NAC (2-bag standard dosing). If serum paracetamol levels are increasing, consider stat dose activated charcoal and serum levels and ALT re-assessed as needed.
  - » If either serum paracetamol levels are ≥2X probable toxicity, i.e. levels are 300 mg/dL at 4H post-ingestion, double the 2nd bag to 200 mg/kg over 16 hours.

Stopping IV NAC

At 18 hours into the NAC infusion (2 hours before completion), send bloods for: Paracetamol level, ALT, Urea, electrolytes, creatinine.

The NAC infusion should be discontinued only when the:
- ALT < 50U/L, reached their peak levels and are declining
- Urea, electrolytes and creatinine are normal or have normalised (if previously abnormal)
- Paracetamol level has returned to normal (i.e. below <10 mg/dL)

The 2nd bag over 16H may be repeated if there is ongoing hepatotoxicity at completion of IV NAC at 20 hours and dosing adjusted to serum paracetamol (should be <10 mg/dL at 20H).

Bibliography

1. Ministry of Health, Singapore. (nd) Management of acute poisoning, clinical practice guidelines.
2. Cumberland Pharmaceuticals Inc. (nd) 2011 Acetadote® (N-acetyl-cysteine) product monograph, Nashville, TN, USA. www.acetadote.com

3. Sung L, Simon JA, Dayneka NL. (1997) Dilution of intravenous N-acetylcysteine as a cause of hyponatremia. *Pediatrics* **100**:389–391.
4. Marzullo L. (2005) An update of N-acetylcysteine treatment for acute acetaminophen toxicity in children. *Curr Opin Pediatr* **17**:239–245.
5. Kander MZ. (2006) Comparison of oral and IV acetylcysteine in the treatment of acetaminophen poisoning. *Am J Health-Syst Pharm* **63**:1821–1827.
6. Chiew AL, Reith D, Pomerleau A, *et al.* (2020) Updated guidelines for the management of paracetamol poisoning in Australia and New Zealand. *Med J Aust* **212**(4):175–213.

SECTION 2

SURGICAL EMERGENCIES

CHAPTER 4

Neurosurgical Emergencies

Low Yin Yee, Sharon

Common Paediatric Neurosurgical Problems

Head Injury

Head injury is the most common neurosurgical problem encountered in children. Most will have minor head injury, defined by a Glasgow Coma Scale (GCS) of 14 to 15, and will recover fully. However, a small proportion of them will deteriorate and develop severe neurological sequelae, usually from secondary brain injury or the presence of an intracranial haematoma. In the acute setting, the primary aim is to identify this group of children.

The history and clinical findings may provide an indication of the severity of the injury.

- A history of a fall from a height of >1 m or involvement in a road traffic accident is significant.
- The conscious state of the child is an important indicator of the presence of an intracranial lesion. The Paediatric Glasgow Coma Scale (PGCS) is used for assessment (see Table 2.1).

Computed tomography (CT) brain is the procedure of choice for assessment of acute head injury in children. Although there are recent concerns about the relatively high dose of radiation associated with a CT scan in a small child compared to an adult, a CT brain is indicated whenever the presence of an intracranial lesion is suspected, based on history or clinical examination.

Of note, skull X-rays are not useful predictors of the presence of an intracranial haematoma, although they are useful for detecting a skull fracture.

Initial Management

- Assess the ABC — Airway, Breathing, Circulation.
- Prompt ventilatory support and treatment of shock are mandatory to prevent secondary brain injury.

The severity of traumatic brain injury (TBI) is classified using the PGCS as shown in Table 2.2.

The following are guidelines recommended by the Neurosurgical Service, KKH, for the management of head injury. Please consult the on-call neurosurgical team if there is any uncertainty.

Table 2.1 Paediatric Glasgow Coma Scale (PGCS)

Paediatric Glasgow Coma Scale (PGCS)				
	>1 yr old		**<1 yr old**	**SCORE**
Eye Opening	Spontaneously		Spontaneously	4
	To verbal commands		To shout	3
	To pain		To pain	2
	No response		No response	1
Motor Response	Obeys		Spontaneous	6
	Localises pain		Localises pain	5
	Flexion-withdrawal		Flexion-withdrawal	4
	Flexion-abnormal (decorticate rigidity)		Flexion-abnormal (decorticate rigidity)	3
	Extension (decerebrate rigidity)		Extension (decerebrate rigidity)	2
	No response		No response	1
Verbal Response	**>5 yr old**	**2 to 5 yr old**	**0 to 23 mth old**	
	Oriented	Appropriate words/ phrases	Smiles/coos appropriately	5
	Disoriented/ confused	Inappropriate words	Cries and is consolable	4
	Inappropriate words	Persistent cries and screams	Persistent inappropriate screaming	3
	Incomprehensible sounds	Grunts	Grunts, agitated and restless	2
	No response	No response	No response	1
Total Paediatric Glasgow Coma Scale (3 to 15):				

Table 2.2 Severity of TBI

Paediatric Glasgow Coma Scale	Severity of TBI
14 to 15	Mild
9 to 13	Moderate
≤ 8	Severe

Management of Mild Head Injury (GCS 14–15)

- Admission to general ward.
- 2 hourly neurological observations for 6 hours, later reduce frequency to 4 hourly if stable.
- Intravenous drip if child is dehydrated as a result of vomiting.
- Analgesic (paracetamol), anti-emetics (ondansetron) if indicated.
- CT brain if child deteriorates clinically (drop in GCS >2 points is significant).

Management of Moderate Head Injury (GCS 9–13)

- Resuscitate if necessary.
- Early referral to on-call neurosurgical team.
- Urgent CT head, urgent pre-operative blood tests including group and crossmatch (GXM) and coagulation profile.
- Admit to Children's Intensive Care Unit (CICU) or High Dependency Unit (HD), depending on clinical status.
- 1 hourly neurological observations and parameters.
- Keep nil by mouth with IV drip.
- IV anti-emetics (e.g. ondansetron) for vomiting and retching.
- Neurosurgical intervention where indicated.

Management of Severe Head Injury (GCS 8 and below)

- Resuscitate — Intubation and ventilation mandatory. It is important to avoid excessive hyperventilation. Aim for partial pressure of carbon dioxide (pCO_2) 30 to 33 mmHg.
- Early referral to on-call neurosurgical team.
- Ensure patient is fully sedated and paralysed if necessary (patient should not be gagging or moving while intubated).
- Urgent CT brain (with cervical spine if indicated), pre-operative blood tests including GXM and coagulation profile.
- Transfer to operating theatre directly for neurosurgical operation, if indicated, or to CICU. Intracranial pressure (ICP) monitoring is indicated.
- Aggressive neuro-protective measures are indicated; specifics of management are beyond the scope of this chapter.
- Non-accidental injury should be suspected when the history given and/or the clinical findings are suspicious. The presence of a subdural haemorrhage in an infant is highly suspicious.

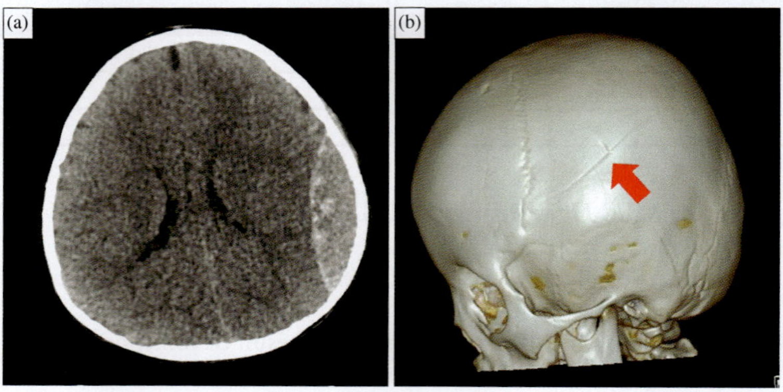

Figure 2.1 A: Representative CT brain image depicting a left extradural haematoma with mass effect in a 6-year-old patient. B: Representative CT image of the 3-dimensional reconstruction of the same patient's calvarium. Red arrow points to the skull fracture overlying the extradural haematoma (Courtesy of Dr S Low).

Post-traumatic Seizures

- Immediate seizure: Seizure occurring at moment of impact usually does not have any long-term sequelae; no need for CT brain or anti-convulsants if the child is well.
- Early or late seizures: Need further investigations and assessment by paediatric neurologist.

Neurosurgical Emergencies

Neurosurgical emergencies are the result ≥1 of the following:

- Rapid disruptive or compressive forces distorting or disrupting part of the nervous system, e.g. intracranial haemorrhage, direct trauma.
- The blood supply to a portion of the brain is interrupted by a thrombus or an occlusion of a vessel, e.g. ischaemic stroke, traumatic carotid artery dissection.
- Loss of perfusion pressure of the entire cerebral hemisphere from decrease in systemic blood pressure (BP) or increased ICP.

Brain Herniation Syndromes

An expanding, intracranial mass lesion exhausts the capability of the brain and cerebrospinal fluid (CSF) to tolerate the added volume within the closed calvaria. The ICP rises, and this causes movement or herniation of brain tissue across the natural boundaries of dura and bone, leading to clinically and anatomically characteristic brain herniation syndromes. These have a profound effect on neurological function, resulting in high morbidity and mortality.

Herniation usually results from:

- Intracranial haemorrhage — Spontaneous or traumatic
- Progressive regional or diffuse brain oedema (usually secondary to cerebral ischaemia, infarction, hypoxia or encephalopathy)
- Disturbance of CSF equilibrium in the setting of raised ICP, e.g. after lumbar puncture in a patient with supratentorial mass lesion

Common Types of Brain Herniation

- **Uncal herniation:**
  - » Classical triad of loss of consciousness, unilateral pupillary inequality (anisocoria) and contra-lateral hemiparesis.
  - » For example, in extradural haematoma involving temporal region.
- **Cerebello tonsillar herniation:**
  - » Seen in rapidly expanding cerebellar mass lesion, e.g. spontaneous cerebellar haemorrhage, or haemorrhage into a posterior fossa tumour.
  - » Increasing drowsiness and sudden respiratory arrest are common presenting symptoms.
- Of note, there are other types of brain herniations that include subfalcine herniation, transtentorial herniation (upward), trancalvarial herniation and central herniation.

Management of Brain Herniation Syndromes

- Transfer to CICU
- Resuscitate as necessary — Intubation and ventilation if GCS ≤8
- Hyperventilation (aim for pCO_2 <30 mmHg)
- Intravenous hyperosmotic therapy (e.g. 20% mannitol, 3% hypertonic saline)
- Urgent CT brain to determine cause once clinically stable
- Surgical management of cause

Acute Hydrocephalus

Hydrocephalus is the result of an imbalance in CSF production and resorption. The time course of ventricular enlargement is usually hours although this can occur over days. There must be clinical signs or evidence of raised ICP. In most instances, the cause of acute hydrocephalus is obstructive in nature and can lead to sudden neurological deterioration. The diagnosis must be suspected early and confirmed by clinical and radiological exams, either CT or magnetic resonance imaging (MRI).

Aetiology of Acute Hydrocephalus in Children

- Shunt obstruction in a child with a known shunt *in situ* (previously put in for CSF diversion)
- Brain tumour obstructing CSF pathways — Posterior fossa (e.g. medulloblastoma), suprasellar (e.g. craniopharyngioma), pineal tumour (e.g. germ cell tumour)
- Acute exudative meningitis
- Head trauma, e.g. epidural haematoma in posterior cranial fossa
- Intraventricular haemorrhage, e.g. ruptured arteriovenous malformation (AVM)

Medical Treatment

- Head position raised to 30°
- Respiratory management — Intubate and ventilate, if GCS <9
- Restrict fluids, osmotic agents, diuretics and BP control.
  *It is important to note the presence of Cushing's reflex
- Response to a rising ICP and not give anti-hypertensives

Surgical Treatment

- External ventricular drain (EVD)
- Shunt — e.g. ventriculoperitoneal (most common), ventriculoatrial or lumboperitoneal
- Endoscopic third ventriculostomy (ETV — In cases of obstructive hydrocephalus)
- Revise shunt (in child with a blocked shunt)
- Mass lesion causing hydrocephalus — EVD/remove mass lesion

Acute Shunt Malfunction

Symptoms

Symptoms consistent with increased ICP (e.g. headaches, nausea and vomiting), which progress to lethargy, stupor and coma. These are signs of brainstem compression, and if untreated will lead to respiratory failure and death. Symptoms can occur rapidly, within a few hours in those who are shunt-dependent. It is important to speak to parents to determine if the child's behaviour is abnormal.

Clinical Findings

- Irritability, progressing to decerebrate posturing
- Gaze impairment or abnormal pupillary responses
- Focal neurological signs

Investigations

- CT or MRI brain (old films may be required for comparison)
- Shunt X-ray series — Skull X-ray anteroposterio (AP)/Lateral, Chest and Abdomen X-ray AP

Shunt tapping (only if ordered by neurosurgeon and to be done by neurosurgical team)

Treatment

- Head up 30 degrees
- Hyperosmotic therapy (to consult neurosurgeon before administering)
- Shunt tapping to release CSF (possible only if blockage is in distal end of shunt)
- Urgent revision of shunt

Child with Ventriculoperitoneal (VP) Shunt and Acute Abdomen

- Inform neurosurgeon
- The shunt may need to be externalised even if no surgery is indicated for the acute abdomen.
- If laparotomy is required, externalisation of shunt can be done at the same setting.

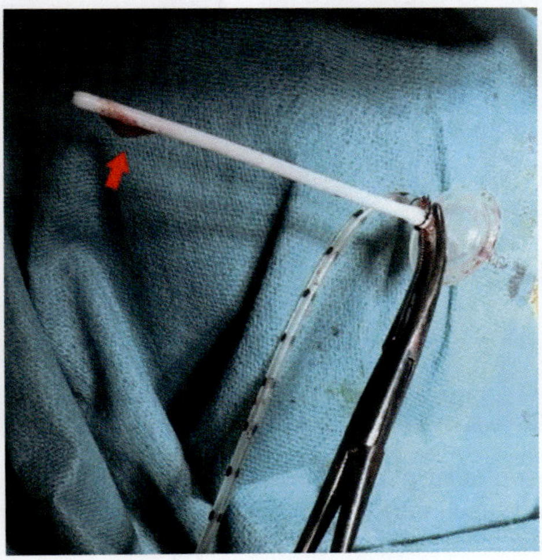

Figure 2.2 Intraoperative photo of a VP shunt that was removed due to shunt blockage. Red arrow points to some tissue blocking the holes in the ventricular catheter, preventing CSF flow from shunt (Courtesy of Dr S Low).

Spontaneous Intracerebral Haematoma in Children

Common Causes

- Intracranial AVM rupture
- Haemorrhage into brain tumour
- Coagulopathy, e.g. haemophilia, leukaemias
- Vasculopathy — Moyamoya disease, vasculitis
- Post-operative haemorrhage into surgical cavity
- Aneurysmal subarachnoid haemorrhage

Management

- Resuscitate as for mass lesion (see 'Brain Herniation Syndromes')
- Urgent CT scan to determine cause
- Check coagulation profile and treat coagulopathy aggressively if present, with transfusion of fresh frozen plasma (FFP)
- Cerebral angiogram and/or MRI/Magnetic Resonance Angiogram (MRA)/CT angiogram if indicated
- Neurosurgical treatment where and when appropriate

Intracranial Infections

- Epidural empyema, e.g. Pott's puffy tumour
- Subdural empyema, e.g. secondary to sinusitis or HIB meningitis
- Intracerebral abscess

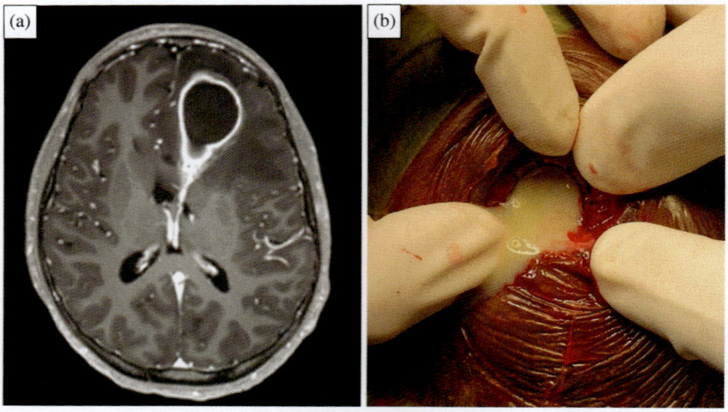

Figure 2.3 A: Representative post-contrast T1-weighted MRI axial image of a patient with an intracerebral abscess in the left frontal lobe. This ring-enhancing lesion is causing perilesional oedema and local mass effect. B: Intraoperative photo taken during drainage of the intracerebral abscess in the same patient via a stereotactic transtubular approach. Note the purulent content of the lesion, consistent with an infective process (Courtesy of Dr S Low).

Management

- Diagnosis confirmed on CT or MRI brain (with contrast)
- Drainage by craniotomy or burrhole aspiration or excision of intracranial abscess
- Appropriate IV antibiotics for 4–6 weeks

Spinal Injuries

- Traumatic spinal injury
- Spinal Cord Injury Without Radiologic Abnormality (SCIWORA)
- Spinal cord compression from epidural (extradural) masses (e.g. haematoma, tumour)
- Intraspinal haemorrhage (e.g. tumour, vascular malformation)
- Spinal infections

Management

- Spinal nursing if instability is suspected
- Intravenous dexamethasone or methylprednisolone where indicated (consult neurosurgeon)
- Urgent MRI spine
- Surgical decompression where indicated
- Surgical stabilisation where indicated

Bibliography

1. Araki T, Yokota H, Morita A. (2017) Pediatric traumatic brain injury: Characteristic features, diagnosis, and management. *Neurol Med Chir* **57**(2):82–93.
2. Kochanek PM, *et al.* (2019) Management of pediatric severe traumatic brain injury: 2019 consensus and guidelines-based algorithm for first and second tier therapies. *Pediatr Crit Care Med* **20**(3):269–279.
3. Kochanek PM, Tasker RC, Carney N, *et al.* (2019) Guidelines for the management of pediatric severe traumatic brain injury, 3rd ed: Update of the Brain Trauma Foundation Guidelines, executive summary. *Neurosurgery* **84**(6):1169–1178.
4. Figaji AA. (2017) Anatomical and physiological differences between children and adults relevant to traumatic brain injury and the implications for clinical assessment and care. *Front Neurol* **8**:685.
5. Chen M, Low DCY, Low SYY, et al. (2018) Management of brain abscesses: Where are we now? *Childs Nerv Syst* **34**(10):871–1880.
6. Osmond MH, Klassen TP, Wells GA, *et al.* (2018) Validation and refinement of a clinical decision rule for the use of computed tomography in children with minor head injury in the emergency department. *CMAJ* **190**(27):E816–E822.
7. Paulsen H, Due-Tonnessen BJ, Lundar T, Lindegaard K-F. (2017) Cerebrospinal fluid (CSF) shunting and ventriculocisternostomy (ETV) in 400 pediatric patients. Shifts in understanding, diagnostics, case-mix, and surgical management during half a century. *Childs Nerv Syst* **33**(2):259–268.

CHAPTER 5

Acute Abdomen

Ong Choo Phaik, Caroline

Introduction

Acute abdominal pain and/or abdominal distension in babies and children is a common undifferentiated problem due to either 'medical' or 'surgical' causes. These range from common, self-limiting illness like viral gastroenteritis to rare life-threatening surgical conditions like intestinal malrotation with volvulus. This chapter provides an approach to diagnosis and management of the paediatric acute abdomen. It describes some common surgical conditions and the rare but important surgical emergencies.

Approach

Clinical assessment with targeted history and physical examination aims to arrive at a working diagnosis (with differentials). For surgical conditions, treatment is often started even before all investigation results are available, to prevent clinical deterioration and major complications. The urgency of investigations, resuscitation and operative management depends on the type of surgical condition.

Clinical Picture

It is helpful to think in age-group categories when considering diagnoses (see Table 2.4). Patients may present with predominantly *pain* or *vomiting* or both. Constant pain

Table 2.3 Surgical and Medical Causes of Acute Abdominal Pain

Symptom Complex	'Surgical' Causes	'Medical' Causes
Constant pain: Possible peritonitis	appendicitis, Meckel's diverticulitis, perforated ulcer	pancreatitis, dengue shock, bowel inflammation from gastroenterocolitis, acute cholecystitis, urinary tract infection
Constant pain: Possible ischaemia	ovarian torsion, ischaemic bowel (incarcerated hernia/closed loop intestinal obstruction)	
Vomiting: Possible intestinal obstruction	pyloric stenosis, malrotation with volvulus	overfeeding, gastroesophageal reflux disease, meningitis
Vomiting with colicky pain: Possible intestinal obstruction	intussusception, adhesive obstruction	gastroenteritis, constipation

Table 2.4 Age-Related Differential Diagnoses* of Patients Presenting with Abdominal Pain and/or Vomiting

Age Group	Baby	Toddler	Child	Adolescent
'Surgical' Cause				
Malrotation with volvulus	Higher	Low	Low	Low
Pyloric stenosis	Higher	Unlikely	Unlikely	Unlikely
Hirschsprung's disease	Higher	Low	Low	Unlikely
Intussusception	Higher	Moderate	Low	Low
Incarcerated hernia	Moderate	Moderate	Moderate	Low
Appendicitis	Low	Low	Higher	Higher
Meckel's diverticulitis/intestinal obstruction	Low	Moderate	Moderate	Moderate
Testicular torsion/ovarian torsion	Low	Low	Moderate	Moderate
Trauma (including child abuse)	Moderate	Moderate	Moderate	Moderate
Choledochal cyst	Moderate	Moderate	Moderate	Low
Solid tumour with bleed	Moderate	Moderate	Moderate	Moderate
Ectopic pregnancy/imperforate hymen	Unlikely	Unlikely	Low	Moderate
'Medical' Cause				
Gastroesophageal reflux disease	Moderate	Low	Low	Low
Acute gastroenteritis	Moderate	Higher	Higher	Moderate
Mesenteric adenitis (with viral illness)	Low	Higher	Higher	Moderate
Urinary tract infection (UTI)	Low	Moderate	Moderate	Moderate
Constipation colic	Low	Higher	Higher	Low
Functional abdominal pain	Low	Low	Moderate	Moderate
Inflammatory bowel disease	Unlikely	Low	Moderate	Moderate
Peptic ulcer disease	Unlikely	Low	Low	Moderate
Hepatitis, pancreatitis	Low	Low	Low	Moderate
Pneumonia	Low	Moderate	Moderate	Moderate
Diabetic ketoacidosis	Low	Low	Low	Moderate
Henoch Schonlein Purpura (HSP)	Unlikely	Moderate	Moderate	Low
Dengue	Low	Low	Low	Moderate
Pelvic inflammatory disease	Unlikely	Unlikely	Low	Moderate

*Only the more common and a few urgent uncommon causes are listed

Legend: Possibility	Higher	Moderate	Low	Unlikely

aggravated by movement suggests peritonitis or ischaemia. Colicky pain may be caused by partial intestinal obstruction. Vomiting is very common in young children when unwell, but persistent vomiting, especially green, suggests intestinal obstruction.

History and Physical Examination

Key points to ask in the history:

- **Abdominal pain** — Intensity, site, characteristic (constant or intermittent), change over time. Associated features, e.g. refusing to move (peritonitis) vs. colicky ('rolling around', drawn-up legs with pallor). Associated abdominal distension.

- **Vomiting** — Colour of vomitus, volume, duration and frequency.
- **Feeding** — Current feeding regimen, appetite, feeding problems, time of last meal and type of feed. If the child potentially needs surgery, instruct nil by mouth (NBM) until review.
- **Urine output** — Indicator of hydration status.
- **Bowel output** — Constipation, diarrhoea, presence of blood or mucus in stools.
- **Relevant prior history** — Solitary or repeated events, any previous surgery, recent travel history, immunosuppression.
- **Medications and allergies** — Antispasmodic medication, antibiotics, analgesia, traditional medicine.

The temporal sequence of symptoms (e.g. timing of pain in relation to changed bowel habits) is important to differentiate between common differential diagnoses like appendicitis and gastroenteritis.

Physical examination is directed towards establishing a working diagnosis and assessment of general status to guide resuscitation. Abdominal examination may be difficult in young children and requires patience. Sedation and opioid analgesia may mask signs of peritonitis. The full abdominal examination includes checking the inguinal hernia orifices, external genitalia and perineum. Gentle per rectal examination is necessary in some situations. If inexperienced, defer this until a senior doctor is available, to reduce the need for repeat examination.

Investigations

Good clinical judgement should be used when ordering investigations to avoid unnecessary patient distress, radiation risk and cost.

Common Screening Tests

- **Full blood count** — Anaemia from hidden gastrointestinal blood loss, white blood cell differential count for bacterial/viral infections, thrombocytopenia in dengue or very ill neonates.
- **C-reactive protein (CRP)** — Useful as an infective marker.
- **Renal panel** — Hydration status, electrolyte derangements, especially with vomiting, or for pre-operative assessment.
- **Urinalysis +/– Urine culture** — Pyuria (UTI), proteinuria (HSP), ketosis (dehydration), crystals/haematuria (urinary stone disease).
- **Abdominal X-ray (AXR)** — Supine AXR is preferred. If intestinal obstruction is suspected, request additional erect (or lateral decubitus view). Look for soft tissue masses, calcifications (appendiceal faecolith, urinary stones), bowel distension, bowel gas distribution and bowel wall thickness.

Other Tests as Indicated for Specific Situations

- **Liver function tests, amylase** — When liver or pancreatic disease is considered.
- **Prothrombin time (PT)/activated partial thromboplastin time (APTT) and group and crossmatch** — Required for pre-operative assessment in major surgery.

- **Chest X-ray (CXR)** —Lower lobe/aspiration pneumonia, pleural effusion. Erect CXR for free air (in older children)
- **Abdominal ultrasound** — Commonly ordered for suspected appendicitis, pyloric stenosis and intussusception. Useful screen for solid organ masses and choledochal cysts. Limited accuracy in obese patients, patients with gaseous bowel distension. Does not exclude solid organ injury for abdominal trauma.
- **Computed tomography (CT) scan** — Associated with radiation risk. Requested when the abdominal ultrasound is unable to provide the necessary information.
- **Contrast study** — Upper gastrointestinal (GI) study is the procedure of choice to rule out malrotation with volvulus.
- **Air enema** — Therapeutic procedure for intussusception performed by the radiologist under fluoroscopy guidance, without sedation. (See section on intussusception).
- **Meckel's scan** — Radioisotope scan that is done electively and patient requires 24 hours pre-scan H2-antagonists. Diagnostic accuracy is about 80–85%.

Management

- **Fluid resuscitation** — Children with surgical acute abdomen are often dehydrated from hidden third space loss, particularly with intestinal obstruction. Resuscitate with intravenous saline 10 ml/kg boluses in addition to maintenance fluids. Monitor heart rate and urine output to assess response to resuscitation. Replace specific losses and correct electrolyte imbalance.
- **Intestinal decompression** — Nil by mouth, insert appropriate size nasogastric tube for hourly aspiration and continuous passive drainage until intestinal function is re-established. Replace nasogastric losses using ml for ml saline mix (normal saline containing potassium).
- **Surgery** — Once confirmed, the surgeon will discuss surgical options with the parents/caregiver. Preparation for emergency surgery involves the following: obtain written informed consent from parent/legal guardian; inform the anaesthetist on-call; trace all pending investigations; ensure blood products are available if required; continue to monitor and resuscitate as necessary until definitive surgery.
- **Pain management** — During initial assessment, limit use of strong sedation and opioid analgesia until diagnosis is established and definitive management decided. It is dangerous to just give painkillers without treating the underlying surgical condition.

Surgical Conditions

Malrotation and Volvulus

- Typically occurs on Day 3 to 5 in an otherwise well baby. Majority present in infancy.

- Bilious (green) or yellow vomiting may be the *only* presenting complaint, so a high index of suspicion is needed. Older children may present with recurrent abdominal pain and vomiting with failure to thrive.
- Although uncommon, it is essential to exclude this condition in a vomiting infant, as failure to recognise volvulus can result in gangrene of the entire small bowel, life-threatening sepsis and short gut syndrome.
- Abdominal signs are often absent. A red and shiny abdomen indicates imminent gangrene requiring urgent laparotomy without waiting for contrast study.
- Abdominal X-ray may be normal or may show an abnormal gas distribution pattern. Upper GI contrast study is diagnostic with abnormal duodenojejunal position indicating malrotation and cork-screw appearance signifying volvulus of small bowel.
- Emergency laparotomy is needed to untwist the bowel and perform Ladd's procedure — widening of the small bowel mesentery, repositioning the bowel (small bowel on right; colon on left side of the abdomen) and appendicectomy.

Intussusception

- Commonly occurs between 6 months and 3 years old.
- Typically idiopathic and preceded by upper respiratory tract infection (URTI) or febrile illness. In recurrent cases and older children, need to consider pathological lead point such as Meckel's diverticulum or intestinal polyp.
- Classic history of intermittent severe abdominal colic with up-drawing of legs, pallor and vomiting of undigested food. Red-currant jelly stools are unusual and indicate intestinal ischaemia from delayed presentation.
- Physical examination — Normal or occasionally may have abdominal distension or a palpable mass in the right hypochondrium (RHC).
- Abdominal X-ray — Usually non-diagnostic; occasionally shows RHC soft tissue mass or dilated bowel loops of intestinal obstruction.
- Ultrasound — Confirmatory if target lesion or pseudo kidney sign is seen. Accuracy is operator-dependent; hence, for centres without ultrasound expertise, diagnostic air enema is recommended instead.
- Management — Air enema reduction performed by the radiologist has a high success rate of >85%. Secure venous access and ensure adequate fluid resuscitation before procedure. Prophylactic antibiotics are recommended during the procedure. Air enema is associated with rare risk of bowel perforation.
- Air enema is contraindicated if there is peritonitis. Surgery is first-line treatment for a child presenting in shock with peritonitis or after failed air enema reduction. Surgery may entail laparoscopic or open reduction and/or resection of gangrenous bowel.
- Recurrent intussusception is reported in up to 15% of children, with highest risk occurring within the first 24 hours.

Appendicitis

- Most common surgical emergency in children.

- Classic presentation of peri-umbilical pain radiating to the right iliac fossa, worse on jumping or walking, with associated anorexia and fever. Physical examination reveals right iliac fossa tenderness with rebound tenderness and guarding.
- Younger children often have atypical presentation, with nonspecific central abdominal pain and vomiting of undigested food.
- Other atypical presentations occur in obese patients, cases of retro-caecal/pelvic appendicitis or patients with prior oral antibiotic ingestion where the symptoms and signs are masked until perforation occurs.
- Patients with complicated appendicitis sometimes present late with signs of peritonitis, sepsis and/or intestinal obstruction (dehydration, delirium, generalised tenderness, abdominal distension and bilious vomiting).
- Appendicitis is often misdiagnosed as other common paediatric conditions. Some clues include the following:
  - » *Complicated appendicitis vs. gastroenteritis* — Perforated appendicitis with pelvic abscess may present with fever and diarrhoea, mimicking gastroenteritis. However, abdominal pain and fever start first, followed by diarrhoea after a couple of days; unlike concurrent pain and diarrhoea for gastroenteritis.
  - » *Appendicitis vs. urinary tract infection* — Urine microscopy in appendicitis may show mild pyuria, representing irritation or urine stasis due to the inflamed appendix situated near the bladder. A pelvic abscess may also cause suprapubic tenderness. This should be differentiated from the burning sensation of dysuria related to cystitis.
  - » *Appendicitis vs. ovarian torsion*– Torsion of ovarian cyst occurs in both prepubertal and pubertal girls and requires more urgent investigation and surgery than appendicitis. Pain and nausea is out of proportion to abdominal signs. Ultrasound is diagnostic.
- Investigations: Raised total white cell count and CRP are suggestive but non-specific. Abdominal ultrasound has sensitivity and specificity between 86 and 95% but is operator-dependent. CT abdomen has higher accuracy rate but should not be routine because of radiation concerns and it does not reduce the negative appendicectomy rate in children. If other urgent surgical conditions are excluded, a period of observation and review is appropriate for equivocal cases.
- In centres with relevant expertise, laparoscopic appendicectomy is the procedure of choice for simple appendicitis with a very low rate of conversion to open surgery.
- There is an ongoing multicentre randomised controlled trial for nonoperative antibiotic treatment of simple appendicitis; prior non-randomised trials have early failure rates of 10–12.5% and recurrence rates of 15–27% at 1 year and 40% at 5 years.
- Complicated appendicitis may be treated by immediate laparoscopic appendicectomy or staged (antibiotic treatment followed by interval appendicectomy).
- Surgical options will be discussed by surgeon with the parent/caregiver as part of informed consent taking. Complications after appendicectomy include intra-abdominal abscess, wound infection and intestinal adhesions.

- Average length of stay in our institution for simple and complicated appendicitis is 2 days and 6 days, respectively.

Medication-Induced Paralytic Ileus

- Common in children between 2 and 5 years of age with abdominal colic from gastroenteritis, whom are being treated with antispasmodics. In young children, these ingested medications can exacerbate paralytic ileus associated with bowel inflammation.
- On clinical examination, the abdomen is generally distended, but soft. There may be generalised tenderness. Abdominal X-ray may show generalised small and large bowel distension with some air/fluid levels.
- Differential diagnoses include intestinal obstruction from other causes, e.g. perforated appendicitis with pelvic abscess.
- Treatment requires a period of gut rest with reduced or no feeds and intravenous hydration. A flatus tube to decompress the colon sometimes brings rapid relief of abdominal distension. Majority of cases are self-limiting, resolving in 24 to 48 hours.

Incarcerated Inguinal Hernia

- The diagnosis is evident on physical examination with painful inguinoscrotal mass.
- Differentials include encysted hydrocoele of the cord and torsion of an undescended testis.
- Try to reduce the hernia by gentle traction and pressure. Sedation and analgesia may be helpful; ensure appropriate monitoring and resuscitation.
- An easily reduced hernia can be reviewed in clinic and scheduled on the next elective list. Difficult reductions or special conditions like premature neonates who are at high risk of re-incarceration should be discussed with the surgeon.
- Admission and immediate surgery is required if irreducible. Prolonged incarceration is associated with complications of intestinal obstruction and/or testicular ischaemia and atrophy.

Bibliography

1. Marin JR, Alpern ER. (2011) Abdominal pain in children. *Emerg Med Clin North Am* **29**(2):401–428, ix–x.
2. Ross A, LeLeiko NS. (2010) Acute abdominal pain. *Pediatr Rev* **31**:35–144.
3. Maita S, Andersson B, Svensson JF, Wester T. (2020) Nonoperative treatment for nonperforated appendicitis in children: A systematic review and meta-analysis. *Pediatr Surg Int* **36**(3):261–269.
4. Salminen P, Tuominen R, Paajanen H, *et al.* (2018) Five-year follow-up of antibiotic therapy for uncomplicated acute appendicitis in the APPAC randomized clinical trial. *JAMA* **320**(12): 1259–1265.

CHAPTER 6

Major Trauma

Junaidah Binte Badron

Introduction

Trauma remains to be one of the leading causes of mortality and morbidity amongst the paediatric population. Nearly 1 in 6 children in the United States attend the emergency department for the treatment of injuries. These injuries could result from motor vehicle accidents, submersion incidents, fires, falls and homicides.This poses significant stress on the healthcare system as well as the community as the management of major trauma is resource-intensive.

Historically, the distribution of deaths was described as a trimodal pattern. The first peak happens almost immediately after the injury; usually attributed to severe brain or spinal cord injury, rupture of the heart, aorta or other large blood vessels. The second peak happens up to several hours after the injury. These deaths are usually caused by subdural and epidural haematomas, haemopneumothorax, ruptured spleen, hepatic lacerations, pelvic fractures and multiple other injuries with significant blood loss. The third peak happens several days to several weeks after the injury. This is usually due to sepsis or multiorgan failure. With advancements in medical care that involves the various phases of trauma care, one hopes to alter/improve this distribution of deaths.

Important Anatomical and Physiological Considerations

Table 2.5 Important Anatomical and Physiological Considerations

Component	Anatomy/Physiology	Implications
Airway	Relatively large head	High risk of head and cervical spine injuries
	Large tongue	Could obstruct the airway
	Epiglottis	The floppy epiglottis could obstruct the airway
	Larynx	More cephalad and anterior which could lead to oesophageal intubation
	Cricoid cartilage	Narrowest portion of the airway
	Trachea	Short trachea which could lead to a right bronchus intubation
Circulation	Limited blood volume	Hypovolaemia easily results in shock

(*Continued*)

Table 2.5 (*Continued*)

Component	Anatomy/Physiology	Implications
Disability	Greater head to body ratio, with less myelinated brain and thinner cranial bones	More serious head injuries
Exposure	Greater relative body surface area	Leads to more heat loss, resulting in hypothermia
Secondary survey	Body size	Allows for greater distribution of traumatic injuries
Abdomen	More anterior and lower placement of the liver and spleen, with less protective musculature and subcutaneous tissue	More susceptible to injuries, prone to rupture
	Kidney is less protected and more mobile	More susceptible to deceleration injuries
Spine	C2/C3 pseudo subluxation and spinal cord injury without radiographic abnormality (SCIWORA) in paediatric trauma	Affects interpretation of radiographs and other investigations
Musculoskeletal	Growth plates are still open	Leads to Salter–Harris type of fractures with possible limb length abnormality with healing
	Pliable/less calcified bones	Absence of fracture does not denote absence of soft tissue/internal injuries

Trauma Code Activation

Managing paediatric trauma is a team effort, which involves various disciplines. Coordination between the various stakeholders is important to optimise the outcome of the resuscitative efforts (see Table 2.6).

Management

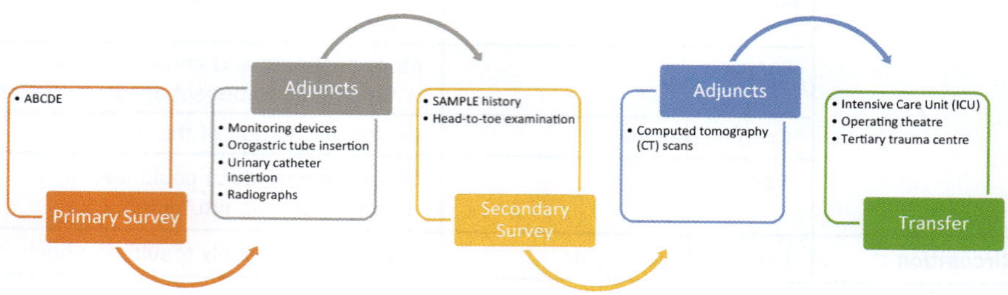

Figure 2.4 Overview of management of major trauma in paediatrics.

Table 2.6 KKH Guidelines for Trauma Code Activation

	Mandatory Criteria to Activate Trauma Code	Trauma Code to be Activated based on Physical Discretion
Cardiorespiratory status	Age-specific hypotension	Tachycardia due to compromised haemodynamics with signs of poor perfusion
	Traumatic cardiac arrest	
	Respiratory distress or failure	
	Transferred patient from another hospital and is receiving blood products, 40 ml/kg bolus or intubated	
Mental alertness		Glasgow Coma Scale (GCS)<14 Motor GCS<6 Observed drop in GCS by ≥2
Mechanism of injury	Fall from height (building/building component)	Road traffic accident
Nature of injury	Gunshot wound to abdomen, neck or chest	Penetrating wounds to the abdomen, neck or chest

Primary Survey

Although it may seem that the primary survey is a series of steps performed one after another, in reality, the various steps are performed concurrently by the various members of the trauma code team.

Airway with Cervical Spine Immobilisation

The airway is assessed for its patency. A quick way is to check for the child's responsiveness. If he is able to speak, there is no total obstruction of the airway. When assessing this component of the primary survey, one has to decide whether a definitive airway is required to be established (see Table 2.7).

When intubating the child, rapid sequence intubation (RSI) should be performed, unless the child is in cardiac arrest.

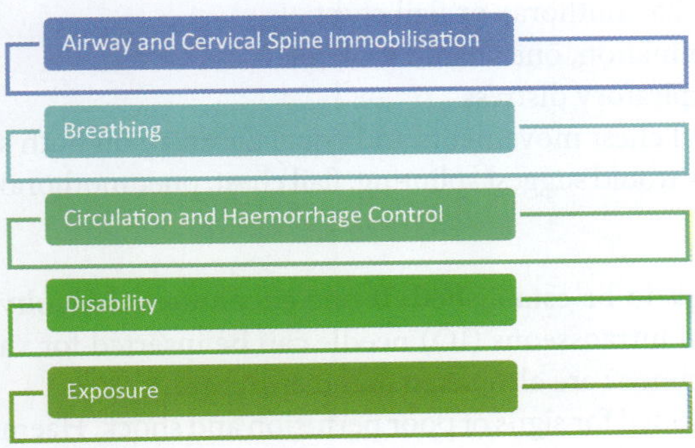

Figure 2.5 Primary survey.

Table 2.7 Criteria for Tracheal Intubation

Respiratory insufficiency
Glasgow Coma Scale (GCS) <8
Suspected raised intracranial pressure (ICP)
Need for prolonged ventilation
Refractory shock

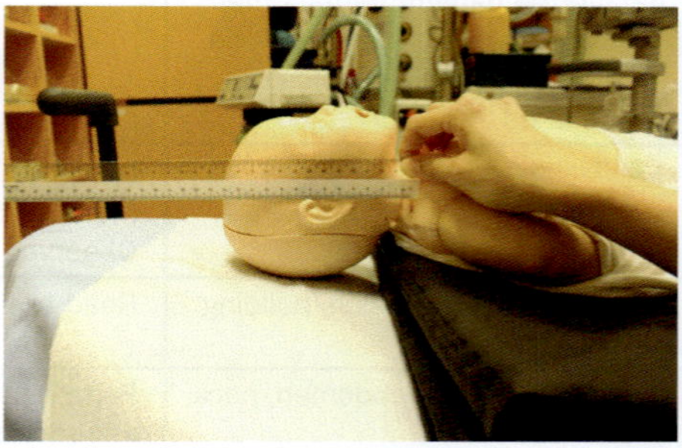

Figure 2.6 Use of a Thoracic Elevation Device (TED).

In addition, the cervical spine has to be appropriately immobilised all the time (unless the spine can be cleared), either with a cervical collar or by manual immobilisation. Younger children have a prominent occiput; hence the neck is prone to hyperflexion. To mitigate this, one can use a Thoracic Elevation Device (TED) or a properly folded blanket. This is usually necessary for children who are younger than 8 years old or weigh less than 25 kg. As demonstrated in Figure 2.6, the spine is well-aligned with the use of the TED.

Breathing

Breathing and ventilation have to be timely assessed as children have greater oxygen consumption, smaller functional residual volume and increased chest wall compliance, predisposing to airway collapse and hypoxia. Furthermore, the diaphragm is easily fatigued and displaced. Urgent intervention is needed to treat tension pneumothorax, open pneumothorax, haemothorax or flail chest.

During the examination, one should look for:

1. Signs of respiratory distress
2. Symmetrical chest movements and equal air entry on both sides of the chest. Asymmetry would suggest splinting, flail chest, pneumothorax or haemothorax

Circulation

Intravenous access has to be established. If one encounters difficulty with peripheral intravenous access, an intraosseous (IO) needle can be inserted for vascular access. At this point, blood specimens are also taken and dispatched.

The patient is assessed for signs of poor perfusion and shock. Haemorrhagic shock is the most common cause of shock in major trauma. In the presence of shock, one should also look for the likely source of bleeding (thorax, abdomen, pelvis and long bones). The

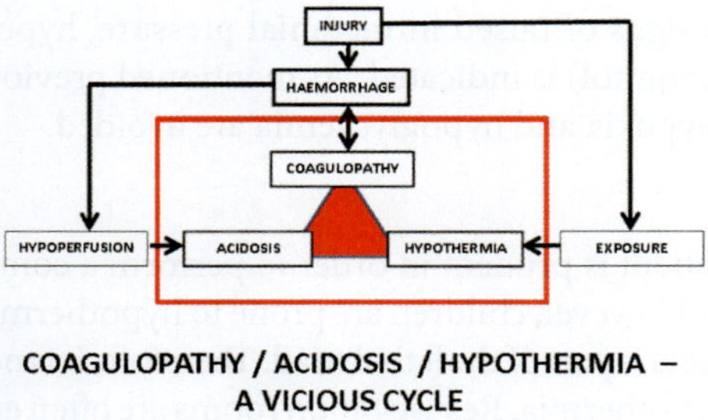

Figure 2.7 Lethal triad of trauma.

management of a child in shock involves fluid resuscitation (commonly crystalloids, usually while awaiting the arrival of blood products) and transfusion with blood products. Patients receive platelets as well as frozen plasma, in addition to packed red cells. This helps to reduce the risk of worsening coagulopathy, which is one of the components of the lethal triad in major trauma.

To ensure blood products are received in a timely manner, one can activate the Massive Transfusion Protocol (MTP) as per your institution's practice.

In addition, intravenous tranexamic acid can be given to the patient to help with haemostasis.

There are also other causes of shock in paediatric trauma patients, which include cardiogenic shock, obstructive shock, neurogenic shock as well septic shock.

Disability

The assessment of disability comprises the following:

1. Glasgow Coma Scale (GCS)
2. Pupillary size and reactivity
3. Full neurological examination, looking for any lateralising sign.

Traumatic brain injury (TBI) is a major contributor of mortality and morbidity in children. The primary goal of management of such patients is the prevention of secondary injury, control of raised intracranial pressure (ICP), maintenance of cerebral perfusion pressure (CPP) and identification of mass lesions needing emergency surgical evacuation.

TBI is classified as mild (GCS 14–15), moderate (GCS 9–13) and severe (GCS ≤8). Indications for computed tomographic (CT) scan includes:

1. GCS ≤13
2. Fluctuating GCS with more than 2 points
3. GCS 14 or 15 plus
   (i) Signs of base of skull fracture: racoon eyes, Battle sign, cerebral spinal fluid (CSF) otorrhea/rhinorrhoea
   (ii) Depressed or compound skull fracture
   (iii) Focal neurological signs or signs of raised intracranial pressure
   (iv) Polytrauma with signs of head injury
   (v) Penetrating skull injury
   (vi) Bleeding diathesis (e.g. haemophilia) or history of intracranial haemorrhage

For patients with signs of raised intracranial pressure, hyperosmolar therapy (3% hypertonic saline or mannitol) is indicated. As mentioned previously, secondary insults such as hypotension, hypoxia and hypoglycaemia are avoided.

Exposure

Full exposure of the patient is prudent in order to perform a complete examination and not miss out any injury. However, children are prone to hypothermia in view of their body surface area. Hypothermia is part of the lethal triad. Therefore, it is necessary to take steps to reduce the risk of the hypothermia. Resuscitation rooms are often equipped with overhead radiant warmers, warming equipment (e.g. the Bair Hugger) as well as fluid warmers.

Adjuncts

1. Monitoring devices, which include electrocardiogram (ECG) leads, blood pressure monitor, pulse oximetry and temperature probe.
2. Orogastric tube to compress the stomach.
3. Urinary catheter to monitor the urine output, which reflects the haemodynamic status of the body.
4. Radiographs (X-rays): Cervical spine (omitted if CT brain/cervical spine planned for), chest, pelvis, others as indicated by the injuries sustained.

Secondary Survey

The secondary survey comprises history taking (SAMPLE) (see Table 2.8) and a full head-to-toe examination. The main aim of the secondary survey is to document the rest of the injuries that are not already noted in the primary survey.

Head and neck

The scalp, skull, facial bones, eyes and neck are examined. Clues to a possible neck injury include cervical spine tenderness, subcutaneous emphysema, tracheal deviation or evidence of laryngeal fractures. The presence of a skull fracture signifies great force and increases the likelihood of intracranial injury.

Chest

Paediatric chest injuries are usually blunt injuries. The compliant chest wall increases the incidence of pulmonary contusion and haemorrhage without overlying rib fractures. However, when rib fractures occur, this signifies a severe injuring force. The list of possible chest injuries is shown in Figure 2.8.

Abdomen

Most paediatric abdominal injuries are blunt injuries. The hypotensive child with penetrating abdominal injuries requires prompt operative exploration. When a child with major trauma presents with signs of hypovolaemic shock, in the absence of other obvious source of bleeding, occult intra-abdominal bleeding has to be considered.

Focused abdominal sonography in trauma (FAST) is a useful modality that can be utilised to detect the presence of haemoperitoneum in such patients. Most solid-organ injuries may be treated conservatively, provided the child remains stable.

Table 2.8 Secondary Survey — History-Taking

S	Symptoms
A	Allergies
M	Medications
P	Past medical history
L	Last meal/menstrual period
E	Events leading to presentation

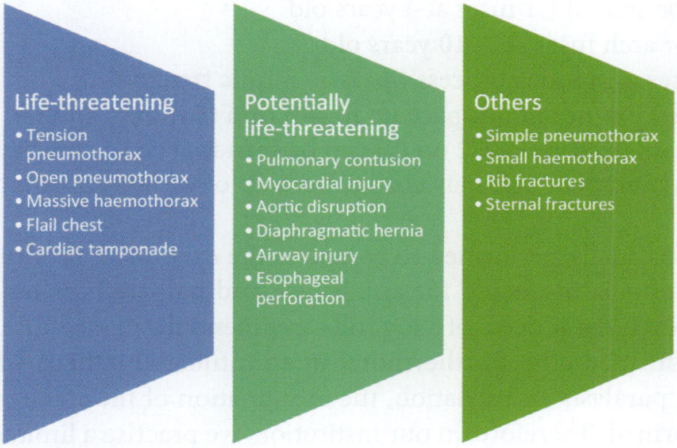

Figure 2.8 Possible chest injuries.

Pelvis/perineum

The pelvic brim should be palpated carefully, looking for the presence of haematomas, tenderness or deformities. The stability of the pelvis is tested by pelvic compression. The flank, scrotum and perineum should be examined for haematomas, lacerations or urethral bleeding. The presence of pelvic fractures indicates significant force, and one should exclude concomitant intra-abdominal or retroperitoneal injury.

Musculoskeletal

Limb swelling, open wounds and limb deformities should be looked for and documented. Peripheral pulses should be carefully assessed, particularly distal to an obvious fracture or dislocation. The possibility of compartment syndrome should be kept in mind. Any limb deformity should be splinted. For an open fracture or a large, deep or heavily contaminated wound, intravenous antibiotics should be administered. The tetanus vaccine status of the patient should also be ascertained. A booster should be given if needed.

Spine

Spinal cord injuries are rare in children. The cartilaginous vertebral bodies are less likely to fracture and the elastic ligaments and horizontal facet joints contribute to increased spinal mobility. This tends to protect the spine by dispersing energy over several segments. There are several unique features of the paediatric spinal column:

- Relatively larger head size, resulting in greater flexion and extension injuries
- Ligamentous injuries are more common than fractures
- Increased flexibility of interspinous ligaments
- Infantile bony column can lengthen significantly without rupture
- Facet joints are flatter with a more horizontal orientation
- Incomplete ossification makes interpretation of bony alignment difficult
- Basilar odontoid synchondrosis fuse at 3–7 years old
- Apical odontoid epiphysis fuse at 5–7 years old
- Posterior arch of C1 fuses at 4 years old
- Anterior arch fuses at 7–10 years old
- Epiphyses of spinous process tips may mimic fractures
- Increased pre-odontoid space up to 4–5 mm (3 mm in adults)
- Pseudo subluxation of C2 on C3 can be seen in 40% of children
- Prevertebral space size may change because of variations with respiration

A log roll is usually performed to complete the examination of the spine. During a log roll, the spine is inspected for any bruise and palpated for tenderness or step deformity. However, the process of a log roll can potentially de-stabilise pelvic fractures and dislodge a formed clot. Furthermore, in an intubated patient who has received medications for paralysis and sedation, the examination of the spine can no longer be accurately performed. Therefore, in our institution, we practise a limited 20° tilt to look for any open wound.

Regular re-assessments of the vital signs should be done. In the event of any deterioration, a repeat of the primary survey should be performed.

Adjuncts

After the secondary survey is completed, appropriate adjuncts such as CT scans can be arranged for and performed.

Transfer

After the relevant investigations have been completed and the haemodynamic status of the patient is stable, the patient is ready for transfer. Prior to transfer, all documentation should be completed and the details should be handed over to the next physician/team managing the patient. A good way to summarise would be using the acronym 'MIST'.

M	Mechanism of injury
I	Injuries sustained
S	Signs (vital signs)
T	Treatment

Bibilography

1. Advanced Paediatric Life Support (APLS) Course Manual 2020, Singapore.
2. The Committee on Trauma & American College of Surgeons. (2018) *Advanced Trauma Life Support (ATLS) Student Course Manual, 10th ed.* Chicago, IL: American College of Surgeons, p. 391.
3. Pek JH, Ong GY-K, Quek ECS, *et al.* (2019) Evaluation of the criteria for trauma activation in the paediatric emergency department. *Emerg Med J*, 36(9):529–534.

SECTION 3

PROCEDURES

CHAPTER 7

Urinary Catheterisation

Chow Wen Hann; Chang Su Ying, Serena; Chan Meng Fai, Joel

Indications

- Investigations (e.g. in-out catheterisation for suspected urinary tract infection)
- Acute urinary retention or bladder/ureter obstruction (e.g. transient myelitis, spinal injury, tumour invasion)
- Monitoring of urine output
- Urinary incontinence (e.g. in neurogenic bladder)
- Prolonged immobilisation (e.g. lumbar fractures) or to aid the healing of open perineal wounds
- Perioperative use for selected surgeries or on regional anaesthesia (e.g. epidural)

Contraindications

- Known urethral trauma
- Acute pelvic fracture
  Note: Consult the paediatric surgical team before placing a catheter in such patients or those with recent genitourinary surgery or known genitourinary abnormality, e.g. hypospadias

Patient Communication and Consent

The following should be discussed with the parent or legal guardian, and where appropriate, the child:

- Procedural steps and analgesia plans
- Verbal consent
- Possible complications, such as pain, haematuria from traumatic insertion, catheter blockage and inability to remove catheter

Equipment Preparation

Prior to the procedure, prepare the following:

- Urinary catheterisation set (alternative: sterile dressing set)
- Antiseptic cleansing solution (e.g. chlorhexidine 0.05% solution)
- 1 vial of sterile water for injection
  The volume of water required to inflate the balloon as stated on the catheter

Table 3.1 Types of Catheters Available

Type of Catheter		Description
One-way catheter		• One drainage channel, no balloon • Available in coated and uncoated types • Short-term use such as collection of urine samples, intermittent catheterisation or instillation of medications • 5 Fr nasogastric tubes can be used for newborns or small infants
Two-way catheter	Silicone elastomer coated latex Foley catheter	• Latex catheters with an external silicone coating and internal elastomer coating • Protection against urethral irritation and encrustation • Suitable for short-term use (most commonly used) • Smallest size 6 Fr (all two-way catheters), not suitable for small infants
	Latex Foley catheter	• Made of natural rubber • High surface friction — more patient discomfort and higher risk of encrustation • Suitable for short term use
	Silicone Foley catheter	• Made purely of silicone • Hypoallergenic and gentle to tissues • Less risk of encrustation and catheter blockage • Suitable for long-term use and patients with latex allergy
Three-way catheter		• Allows for continuous or intermittent bladder irrigation for clearing of blood clots or debris arising from bleeding of the bladder • Not available in paediatric sizes under 16 Fr

- Lignocaine 2% topical syringe gel (10 g)
- 10 ml syringe
- 21 G needle
- 2 pairs of sterile gloves
- 1 Foley catheter (or one-way catheter depending on indication)
- 1 urinary drainage bag and bag holder
- 1 urine collection receptacle
- 1 piece of protective sheet
- Adhesive tape
- 1 polythene bag
- 1 urine specimen container, if required

Pre-Procedural Steps

1. Identify the correct patient (with at least 2 patient identifiers) and confirm the laboratory tests required.
2. Ensure all equipment and relevant urine collection bottles are prepared (refer to checklist above).

Table 3.2 Guidelines for Length of Catheter Insertion and Catheter Size

Age		Weight	Length of Insertion by Gender		Catheter Size
			Female	Male	
0– 5 mth	Newborn/small infant	3–5 kg	5 cm	6 cm	5–6 Fr
6 mth– 1 yr	Infant	6–9 kg	5 cm	6 cm	5–8 Fr
1–2 yr	Toddler	10–11 kg	5 cm	6–8 cm	8 Fr
2–6 yr	Small child	12–14 kg	6 cm	6–9 cm	8–10 Fr
6–12 yr	Child	15–30 kg	6–8 cm	10–15 cm	8–12 Fr
>12 yr	Adolescent	>31 kg	6–8 cm	13–18 cm	10–14 Fr

Choose the most appropriate type and size of urinary catheter for the patient (Table 3.2).
Note: Table 3.2 serves as a reference guide only. It may vary depending upon the patient's body habitus.

Procedural Steps

1. Position the child with the hips flexed and externally rotated.
2. Wash your hands with antiseptic soap and water, put on sterile gloves and clean the perineum with chlorhexidine.
3. Remove gloves and perform hand hygiene. Don a new pair of sterile gloves and set up the sterile drapes.
4. Using lignocaine gel, lubricate the tip of the catheter/feeding tube.

Female Child	Male Child
1) Place a small amount of lignocaine gel onto a sterile cotton ball 2) Place the cotton ball onto the urethral opening 3) Wait 3 to 5 min for an optimal anaesthetic effect 4) Remove the cotton ball and separate the labia majora to expose the urethral opening	1) Lift the penis gently to a 60–90 degree angle 2) Slowly instil lignocaine gel into the urethral opening while holding the penis firmly 3) Remove syringe tip, keep the urethra closed and wait 3 to 5 min for an optimal anaesthetic effect 4) Hold the penis perpendicular to the body and retract the foreskin

5) Pass the lubricated catheter gently into the urethra, 1 cm at a time, until the urine starts to flow freely or until the estimated length needed is reached.
Note: Do not advance the catheter significantly beyond the recommended lengths as this may cause coiling and knotting of the catheter within the bladder, resulting in an inability to remove it.

In-Out Catheterisation Only	Urinary Catheterisation
6) Collect the urine for urine microscopy and culture. 7) Withdraw the catheter after the urine is collected. 8) For an uncircumcised male child, pull the foreskin back to cover the glans penis to reduce the risk of paraphimosis.	6) Advance the catheter a few centimetres further. 7) Inflate the balloon with **sterile water** (required volume is shown on the catheter — do not over inflate). Document the volume of water injected into the balloon. 8) Pull the catheter until resistance (from balloon) is felt. 9) Connect catheter to urine bag. 10) For an uncircumcised male child, pull the foreskin back to cover the glans penis to reduce the risk of paraphimosis. 11) Secure the catheter to the body with adhesive tape.

Troubleshooting Points

1. If there is no drainage of urine upon insertion of the catheter,
   a. Consider the possibility of urethral false passage, especially if it was a traumatic catheterisation. Remove the catheter immediately and inform the senior doctor. A paediatric surgical consult may be required.
   b. The child may be dehydrated or may have just voided prior to catheterisation. You may need to wait a short while for urine to flow.

   IMPORTANT: Do not inflate the balloon when there is no urine flow.
2. If there is pain upon inflation of the balloon, it is likely that the catheter is not in the bladder. Immediately deflate the balloon and insert the catheter further into the bladder.
3. If there is difficulty in removal of the catheter (i.e. concerns of stuck catheter), do not manipulate further but seek help from the paediatric surgical team.

Post Procedure

1. Ensure a closed urinary drainage system at all times to minimise infection.
2. Maintain an unobstructed downhill flow (without kinks) and keep urine drainage bag below urinary bladder to prevent reflux of urine. Ensure regular emptying of urine from urinary bag.
3. Monitor for complications and troubleshoot accordingly (see Table 3.3).

Removal of Urinary Catheter

1. Empty the urinary bag.
2. Prepare equipment (one 10 ml syringe, one pair of non-sterile gloves, one protective sheet).
3. Position patient in dorsal recumbent position, with knees flexed and thighs apart, and place protective sheet under the patient's buttocks.
4. Perform hand hygiene and don the non-sterile gloves.

Table 3.3 Procedural Complications of Urinary Catheterisation

Complication	Monitoring	Intervention
Catheter Associated Urinary Tract Infection (CAUTI)*	Fever Cloudy urine	Remove indwelling catheter. Appropriate antibiotic therapy.
Bladder spasm and pain *Caused by inflammation of bladder and urethral mucosa*	Symptoms of urgency, perineal pain May be associated with irregular bladder emptying and constipation	Anticholinergic medications (oral, transdermal or intravesical). Use catheter with smaller lumen and balloon size. Prevent constipation.
Haematuria *Caused by traumatic insertion*	Significant pain, obstructive features, worsening haematuria	Consult the paediatric surgical team if these symptoms are present. Consider working up for coagulopathy if haematuria persists.
Catheter blockage *Caused by debris, encrustation, catheter kinking, catheter drainage holes blocked by the adjacent bladder wall*	Urinary leakage around catheter	Ensure adequate fluid intake. Perform bladder irrigation under sterile technique to remove encrustation/blood clots. Consider working up for bladder stones if there is recurrent catheter blockage.
Inability to remove catheter *Caused by faulty balloon deflation mechanism or balloon encrustation (especially if saline used to inflate balloon)*		Consult the paediatric surgical team immediately. Possible treatment options: puncture balloon inflation pathway to release water content, ultrasound-guided transabdominal balloon puncture or perforate balloon via cystoscopy.

**Definition of CAUTI:* *Presence of symptoms or signs consistent with UTI, with no other identified source of infection, and urine culture with no more than two species of organisms identified, at least one of which is a bacterium of $\geq 10^5$ CFU/ml. It is considered catheter-associated if this occurs ≥2 days from placement of urinary catheter or within 48 hours of removal.*

5. Attach the syringe to the urinary catheter balloon port and aspirate to deflate the balloon. Ensure that the same volume of water for injection that has been used to inflate the balloon is aspirated fully.
6. Withdraw the urinary catheter gently. If there is any difficulty withdrawing it, try rotating the catheter as you withdraw or inserting the catheter slightly with some lubricant before withdrawing it again.
7. If there is further resistance and inability to withdraw the urinary catheter, do not manipulate it further. Consult the paediatric surgical team.

Video Resources

1. Manzano S, Vunda A, Schneider F, Vandertuin L, Lacroix LE. Videos in clinical medicine. Catheterization of the urethra in girls. (2014) *N Eng J Med* **371**(2):e2.

https://www.nejm.org/doi/10.1056/NEJMvcm1105612?url_ver=Z39.88-2003&rfr_id=ori:rid:crossref.org&rfr_dat=cr_pub%20%200pubmed

2. Lacroix LE, Vunda A, Bajwa NM, Galetto-Lacour A, Gervaix A. (2010) Videos in clinical medicine. Catheterization of the urethra in male children. *N Eng J Med* **363**(14):e19.
https://www.nejm.org/doi/10.1056/NEJMvcm0808873?url_ver=Z39.88-2003&rfr_id=ori:rid:crossref.org&rfr_dat=cr_pub%20%200pubmed

Bibliography

1. KK Women's and Children's Hospital. (2019) KKH clinical practice guideline: Care of patients with urinary drainage systems.
2. Hazinski MF. (2013) *Nursing Care for Critically Ill Child.* St Louis: Mosby.
3. Carlson D, Mowery B. (1997) Standards to prevent complications of urinary catheterization in children: Should and should knots. *J Soc Pediatr Nurs* **2**:37–41.
4. Kopač M. (2013) Formula estimation of appropriate urinary catheter size in children. *J Pediatr Int Care* **2**(4):177–180.
5. Royal Children's Hospital. (nd) Indwelling urinary catheter–insertion and ongoing care nursing clinical guideline. https://www.rch.org.au/rchcpg/hospital_clinical_guideline_index/Indwelling_urinary_catheter_insertion_and_ongoing_care/
6. Rowe J. (2020) Urinary catheter management, Starship Child Health, New Zealand. https://www.starship.org.nz/guidelines/urinary-catheter-management/

CHAPTER 8

Lumbar Puncture

Chow Wen Hann; Chang Su Ying, Serena; Chan Meng Fai, Joel

Indications

- Suspected meningitis or encephalitis
- Intrathecal medication
- Diagnosis or monitoring of conditions including inborn errors of metabolism, neurogenetic conditions and idiopathic intracranial hypertension

Contraindications

- Signs suggestive of raised intracranial pressure (ICP), mass effect, focality (e.g. focal neurological deficits, dropping Glasgow Coma Scale (GCS), hypertension with bradycardia), coma or encephalopathy (GCS <8, rapidly dropping or fluctuating GCS, absent brainstem reflexes)
  - » Neuroimaging after stabilisation
  - » Do not attempt lumbar puncture (LP) regardless of imaging
- Signs of general raised ICP (e.g. papilloedema) but otherwise stable
  - » Neuroimaging
  - » LP may be attempted in consultation with a senior doctor and/or neurologist
- Significant respiratory distress or haemodynamic instability/shock
- Bleeding tendency — platelet count $<50 \times 10^9$/L, coagulopathy and/or anticoagulation/antiplatelet medication
- Congenital spine abnormalities (e.g. tethered cord)
- Local infection at LP site

Patient Communication and Consent

The following should be discussed with the parent or legal guardian, and where appropriate, the child:

- Procedural steps, analgesia and/or sedation plans
- Written consent
- The LP can be complicated, difficult and may require several attempts, especially in young infants. In some instances, LP under ultrasound guidance may be required.
- Possible complications such as headache, backache, bleeding/haematoma, infection, small risk of injury to surrounding structures at puncture site (blood vessels, nerves), and very rarely brain herniation.

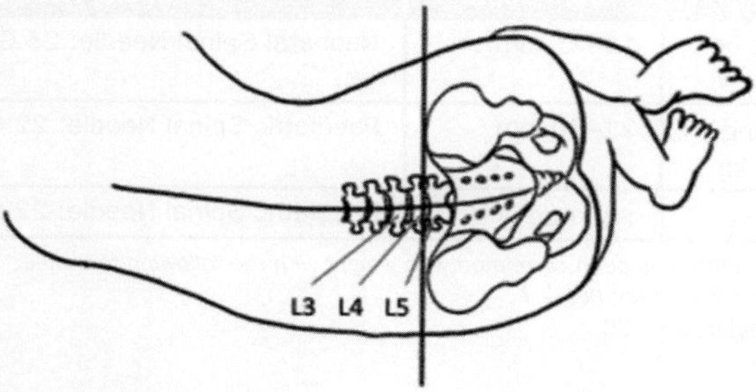

Figure 3.1 Site of insertion when performing lumbar puncture (Illustrated by Dr Sharon Goh/Dr Stella Zhang).

Site Selection

A lumbar puncture can be safely performed at the L3/4 or L4/L5 interspinal space. The 4th lumbar vertebral body is identified by visualising a vertical line between the most superior point of both iliac crests and its transection with the sagittal midline of the spine. (see Figure 3.1)

Equipment Preparation

Prior to the procedure, prepare the following:

- Sterile dressing set and antiseptic swab sticks (e.g. 3M SoluPrep Antiseptic Swab — 2% w/v Chlorhexidine Gluconate and 70% v/v Isopropyl Alcohol)
- Sterile bottles for collection of cerebrospinal fluid (CSF)
- Spinal needles (see Table 3.4)
- Manometer for patient >18 months old, except when administering intrathecal chemotherapy
- Glucometer
- Sterile gloves
- Local anaesthetic cream and sedation, if required

Sedation and Analgesia

Lumbar puncture should be performed under moderate sedation (e.g. IV ketamine or midazolam) for children greater than 6 months old with normal conscious state. Provide adequate analgesia with local anaesthetic cream (e.g. EMLA cream), applied with occlusive dressing over LP site half an hour prior to procedure and/or intradermal lignocaine. In newborns and young infants, oral glucose can be offered as pain relief.

Table 3.4 Choice of Spinal Needles

Age	Median Spinal Cord Depth	Spinal Needle
Neonates to infants up to 7 kg	11–21 mm	Neonatal Spinal Needle: 25 G/Length 25 mm
Infants >7 kg to young children up to 25 kg	21–30 mm	Paediatric Spinal Needle: 22 G/Length 38 mm
Older children >25 kg	>30 mm	Paediatric Spinal Needle: 22 G/Length 90 mm

Note: Median spinal cord depth has been correlated with weight with the following formulae:
Neonates & infants (mm) = 2 x Weight (kg) + 7
Children (mm) = 0.4 x Weight (kg) + 20

Pre-Procedural Steps

1. Neuroimaging (CT/MRI) if indicated (see contraindications).
2. Fundoscopy is necessary for children >18 months old before doing LP to look for any papilloedema (see above).
3. Ensure written consent has been taken.
4. Identify the correct patient (with at least two patient identifiers) and confirm the laboratory tests and/or intrathecal chemotherapy required.
5. Conduct a time out to ensure correct patient and procedure.
6. Ensure all equipment and sterile collection bottles are prepared (refer to checklist above).

Procedural Steps

1. Place the child in a lateral recumbent position with the neck, body, hips and knees flexed. Avoid over-flexing the neck in infants as it may cause airway obstruction and respiratory compromise.
   Alternatively, LP can be performed in an older child slouched in a sitting position.
2. Identify appropriate insertion site at L3/L4 or L4/L5 interspinal space (Figure 3.1).
3. Ensure adequate sedation
4. Wash hands with antiseptic soap and water, put on sterile gloves, clean the area with standard aseptic technique using antiseptic swab sticks and set up sterile drapes.
5. Gently puncture skin with a spinal needle at the identified mark, pointing towards the umbilicus.
6. Gently advance a few millimetres at a time until a 'give' is felt on entering the dura mater. Remove the stylet and CSF should start to drip out.
7. In a child >18 months old (except when LP is done to administer intrathecal chemotherapy), measure the opening pressure by attaching a sterile manometer to the end of the spinal needle (Figure 3.2a). Thereafter, the CSF can be collected by emptying the manometer into the specimen bottle (Figure 3.2b).

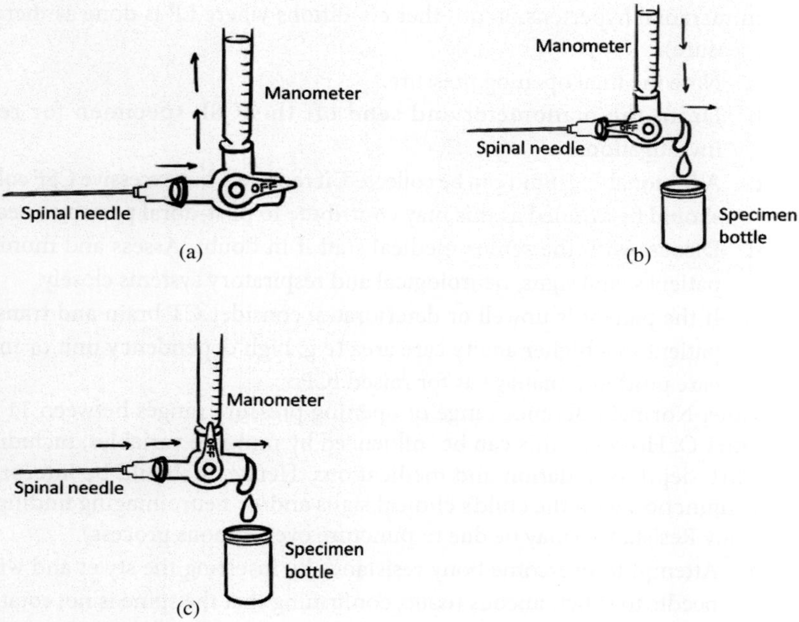

Figure 3.2 Using a manometer during lumbar puncture (Illustrated by Dr Sharon Goh/Dr Stella Zhang). (a) Reading opening pressure, (b) When collecting CSF from manometer tube, (c) Collecting additional CSF specimen

8. Collect the rest of CSF specimen in the specimen bottles by turning the 3-way tap of the manometer (Figure 3.2c).
   a. If the CSF is bloodstained and fails to clear, reinsert the stylet and withdraw the spinal needle. Inform the senior doctor in charge for consideration of more attempts.
   b. If the CSF is turbid, give IV dexamethasone 0.2 mg/kg before or with the first dose of IV antibiotics (this has been proven to reduce severe hearing loss in bacterial meningitis, especially in Haemophilus Influenzae meningitis).
   c. Where indicated, give intrathecal chemotherapy under sterile technique. Ensure aspiration of CSF into syringe before giving intrathecal medication.
9. After collecting all CSF samples, re-insert the stylet and gently withdraw spinal needle. Immediately apply pressure on the puncture site with a sterile gauze and cover it with an adhesive film.
10. Take blood glucose with glucometer.

Troubleshooting Points

1. In the event of raised opening pressure (excluding LP done for idiopathic intracranial hypertension or other conditions where LP is done as therapeutic measure):
   a. Note the final opening pressure.
   b. Drain the manometer and send off this CSF specimen for relevant investigations.
   c. Additional CSF fluid can be collected, if required, but excessive CSF collection should be avoided as this may contribute to post-dural puncture headache.
   d. Discuss with the senior medical staff if in doubt. Assess and monitor the patient's vital signs, neurological and respiratory systems closely.
   e. If the patient is unwell or deteriorates, consider CT brain and transfer the patient to a higher acuity care area (e.g. high dependency unit or intensive care unit) and manage as for raised ICP.

   Note: Normal reference range of opening pressure ranges between 11 and 28 cmH_2O. However, this can be influenced by multiple variables, including age, BMI, depth of sedation and medications. Hence, it should be interpreted in conjunction with the child's clinical signs and/or neuroimaging findings.
2. Bony Resistance (may be due to puncture over spinous process)
   a. Attempt to overcome bony resistance by inserting the stylet and withdraw needle to subcutaneous tissue, confirming that the spine is not rotated, and the puncture site is at midline, reposition child to ensure adequate flexion to open up interlaminar space and gently advance needle more cephalad.
   b. Avoid repeated manipulations as it may predispose to traumatic tap.
3. Poor CSF flow can be improved by:
   a. Rotating spinal needle 90°.
   b. Reinserting stylet and advance needle slightly.
   c. Attempting the procedure at a different site (new needle should be used each time).

Post-Procedure Monitoring and Care

1. Keep the patient supine for 1 hour, after which some movement is allowed, e.g. sitting up in bed to eat a meal or being carried by the parent for feeding. The current evidence shows that a prolonged supine position does not decrease the incidence of post-dural puncture headache.
2. Monitor with hourly parameters for the next 6 hours, especially if sedation was given.
3. In cases of a traumatic tap, nursing monitoring should include looking out for changes in the motor and sensory function of the lower extremities and bladder and bowel dysfunction. The frequency of monitoring should be discussed with a senior doctor.

Table 3.5 Procedural Complications of Lumbar Puncture

Complication	Monitoring	Intervention
Headache (Most common)	Headache occurring hours to a day after LP.	Adequate bed rest and hydration. Analgesia
Mild backache (especially after multiple LP attempts)	Backache within 1 to 2 d after LP.	Analgesia
Bleeding (usually minimal, unless coagulopathy present)	Bleeding at the puncture site. Haematoma: - at skin, resulting in pain (usually resolves in 1 to 2 wk) - at spinal space, resulting in alterations in lower limb neurological function or bladder/bowel dysfunction	Lying flat after procedure reduces bleeding risk. Urgent neurological assessment and neuroimaging where there are concerns of spinal haematoma.
Infection (rare) — puncture site cellulitis, vertebral osteomyelitis, discitis, epidural abscess, bacterial meningitis	Puncture site for erythema and tenderness Neurological deficits Persistent fever	Appropriate antibiotic therapy
Transient dysaesthesia	Abnormal lower limb sensation reported by patient. May occur during the procedure if the needle makes contact with cauda equina nerve roots.	Symptoms should resolve immediately with needle repositioning. Permanent nerve damage is rare.
Cerebral Herniation - occurs in children with raised ICP and an abnormal ICP gradient (e.g. space occupying lesion) - children with uniform increased ICP (e.g. idiopathic intracranial hypertension) may safely undergo LP	Decerebrate posturing, decreasing responsiveness, dilated pupils and vomiting	Urgent neurological assessment and neuroimaging

Video Resources:

1. Srivastava G, Roddy M, Langsam D, Agrawal D. (2012) An educational video improves technique in performance of pediatric lumbar punctures. *Pediatr Emerg Care* **28**(1):12–6.
https://www.nejm.org/doi/full/10.1056/nejmvcm054952
2. Peds cases classic video: An approach to lumbar punctures
https://www.pedscases.com/classic-video-approach-lumbar-punctures

Bibliography

1. Schulga P, Grattan R, Napier C, *et al.* (2015) How to use … lumbar puncture in children. *Arch Dis Child Educat Pract* **100**:264–271.
2. Arthurs OJ, Murray M, Zubier M, *et al.* (2008) Ultrasonographic determination of neonatal spinal canal depth. *Arch Dis Child Fetal Neonatal Ed* **93**:F451–F454.
3. Bailie HC, Arthurs OJ, Murray MJ, *et al.* (2013) Weight-based determination of spinal canal depth for paediatric lumbar punctures. *Arch Dis Child* **98**:877–880.

CHAPTER 9

Central Venous Line Insertion

Cher Yuqin; Ng Si Min, Pamela; Lim Kian Boon, Joel

Indications

- Vascular access to administer inotropes, high osmolality or caustic medications
- Vascular access to perform haemodialysis or plasmapheresis
- Monitoring of central venous pressure

Contra-Indications

- Infection of placement site
- Distortion of anatomy
- Bleeding tendencies — coagulopathy or platelet count < 50×10^9/L → consider performing procedure under fresh frozen plasma or platelet cover
- Thrombosed veins
- Prior injury to the vein
- Uncooperative patient
- For femoral venous catheters, an additional contra-indication includes suspected disruption of the inferior vena cava secondary to abdominal trauma

Patient Communication and Consent

The following should be discussed with the parent or legal guardian, and where appropriate, the child:

- Procedural steps and analgesia plan
- Written consent
- Possible complications, such as pain, bleeding, infection (including blood stream infection), injury to surrounding structures, thrombosis, catheter obstruction/ occlusion requiring line removal or replacement and rarely catheter breakage or wire retention

Site Selection

The *femoral vein* that lies within the femoral triangle in the inguinal-femoral region is a common site used for central venous line placement (Figure 3.3). The relationship of the important structures within the femoral triangle is easily remembered by the acronym VAN:

(Medial) Vein → Artery → Nerve (Lateral)

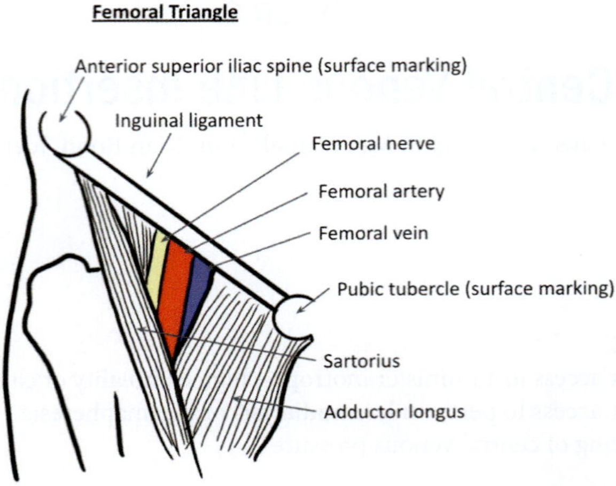

Figure 3.3 Borders and contents of the femoral triangle (Illustrated by Dr Sharon Goh/ Dr Stella Zhang).

The internal jugular vein (IJV) is another possible cannulation site — however, this carries additional risks, such as pneumothorax or injury to the carotid artery or thoracic duct. This should be done only with senior staff supervision *(refer to CICU Handbook on further details on internal jugular vein cannulation).*

Equipment Preparation

- Central venous catheter set — *Refer to CICU Handbook on the type and size of catheter and guide on depth of insertion*
- Sterile procedure set
- Chlorhexidine solution
- Two additional disposable sterile drapes
- Blade (if not provided in the set)
- Silk 3–0 with curved needle
- Gallipot for heparin saline
- Additional 3 ml/5 ml syringes
- Clear adhesive dressing (e.g. Tegaderm)
- Sterile ultrasound sheath with sterile conducting gel
- Heparin saline
- Drawing needle
- Lignocaine 1% solution

Sedation and Analgesia

Central Venous Line (CVL) insertion should be done under moderate sedation (e.g. IV ketamine). Provide adequate analgesia. Local anaesthesia can be given with subdermal administration of 1% lignocaine (0.3 ml/kg, up to 10 ml) to the insertion site.

Pre-Procedural Steps

1. Ensure written consent has been taken.
2. Conduct a time out to ensure the correct patient, procedure and site.
3. *Positioning* of patient: For femoral venous cannulation, lie the patient in supine position, with the hip abducted and slightly externally rotated. Use a hip roll if necessary.
4. Examine the patient: Palpate the femoral pulse or use ultrasound to visualise the vascular anatomy.
5. Ensure that the equipment is prepared (refer to the check list above).
6. Gown up with the shower cap, face mask, sterile gown and sterile gloves.
7. Flush and *prime* all catheter lumens with heparin saline.

Procedural Steps

1. Clean and drape the patient — ensure that the umbilicus can still be visualised.
2. If using ultrasonography, place the ultrasound probe in the sterile sheath.
3. Reassess the insertion site via ultrasonography (preferably) or via surface marking.
4. Ensure adequate sedation and analgesia.
5. Puncture the skin using a needle/cannula, connected to the syringe with heparin saline. The angle of approach should be 30 to 45°, directed towards the umbilicus.
6. Once the vein is punctured, blood should be easily aspirated into the syringe. The blood return should be dark red and non-pulsatile in a venous cannulation. This can be further confirmed by performing a blood gas to assess partial pressure of oxygen, if necessary.
   - If a needle was used, fix the depth and angle of the needle, while gently rotating the syringe to disconnect it from the needle.
     TIP: Do this gently to prevent displacement of the needle.
   - If a cannula was used, fix the needle in place and advance the cannula.
7. *Advance the guidewire* into the needle/cannula.
   TIP: This process should be smooth, with little to no resistance. Avoid forcing the guidewire in if resistance is encountered.
   TIP: Avoid using the 'rear' end of the guidewire, as it may be sharper than the 'front' end and can potentially damage the vessel.
8. Carefully remove the needle/cannula while holding the guidewire in place
   TIP: Hold on to the guidewire at its entry point to the skin to prevent it from slipping out.
9. Using a blade, with the sharp edge *facing away* from the guidewire, make a small incision in the skin approximately 2 to 3 mm at the puncture site, to facilitate passage of the dilator.
10. Pass the dilator over the guidewire and advance it into the vein using a rotating movement, up to a similar depth where backflow was first obtained.
    TIP: Hold the dilator at its midpoint to prevent it from bending and kinking the guidewire.
11. Carefully remove the dilator while securing the guidewire.
    TIP: Anticipate bleeding and use a gauze to apply pressure to the puncture site to minimise bleeding.

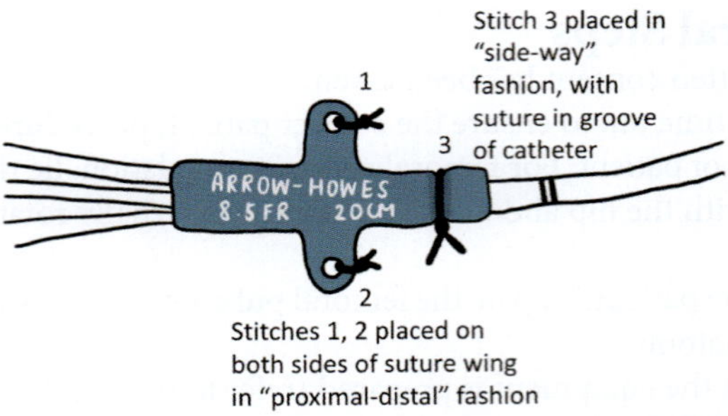

Figure 3.4 Illustration of how to secure a central venous line (Illustrated by Dr Sharon Goh/Dr Stella Zhang).

12. Unlock the distal lumen of the catheter. Pass the catheter over the guidewire.
13. When the catheter tip is about 2 to 3 cm from the skin, carefully withdraw the guidewire until its 'rear' tip has emerged from the distal lumen of the catheter. While holding the guidewire, advance the catheter into the vein and remove the guidewire.
    TIP: Do this slowly; avoid rushing through this step and doing both withdrawal of guidewire and advancing of catheter simultaneously.
    TIP: In general, insert till a depth where the catheter tip should be sited below the liver and diaphragm. *For measurements on depth of insertion, including IJV insertion, refer to CICU Handbook*
14. Check for backflow for each lumen and flush each lumen with heparin saline.
15. Secure the catheter by applying three sutures. (Figure 3.4)
16. Clean and dry the site before applying Tegaderm.
17. Dispose of all sharps safely. Account for all used sharps and guidewires with a witness before disposing.
18. Maintain sterility of the procedure trolley, as the nurses will use the set to connect infusions to the catheter.
19. Order an abdominal X-ray to confirm placement of the central venous catheter.

Post Procedural Monitoring and Care

- Monitor for bleeding/swelling/leaking of infusions/extravasation/signs of infection.
- Maintain sterility when accessing or breaking the line.
- Review the need for the CVL daily — avoid keeping the CVL *in situ* for more than 7–10 days.

Video Resources

1. Video link — Ultrasound-guided placement of femoral venous catheter https://www.nejm.org/doi/full/10.1056/NEJMvcm0801006

Table 3.6 Procedural Complications of Central Venous Line Insertion

Complication	Monitoring	Intervention
Infection (local infection or bacteraemia)	Erythema, swelling, pain, fever, bacteraemia	Remove CVL. Consider line culture and tip culture after line removal. Appropriate antibiotic therapy.
Bleeding/ hematoma	Swelling, oozing from the insertion site	If localised bleeding at the insertion site, apply pressure and reinforce dressing. Reassess the dressing site regularly for further bleeding.
Thrombosis	Inability to draw blood/ flush; swelling of limb	Order ultrasound Doppler to assess. If thrombus is found, remove CVL and consider anticoagulation therapy.
Arterial puncture	Return of pulsatile, bright red blood	Remove CVL and apply pressure on puncture site for at least 15–20 min. In the event of significant puncture with uncontrolled bleeding, consult the vascular surgeons immediately.
Fistula, pseudoaneurysm	Pulsatile swelling with or without bruising	Refer vascular surgeons.
Air embolism	Shortness of breath, chest pain, seizures, loss of consciousness, hemiplegia	Intensive supportive care.
Catheter migration/ embolisation	Visualisation on X-ray, arrhythmias	Remove CVL. In event of embolisation of CVL fragment, consult the interventional radiologist for retrieval.
Cardiac irritation by guidewire *(for IJV cannulation)*	Arrhythmias	Withdraw guidewire and monitor heart rate and rhythm. Continue with procedure if safe to do so.
Retained guidewire	Guidewire fracture on removal or guidewire left *in-situ*	Refer to surgeons or interventional radiology for retrieval and removal.
Pneumothorax/ haemothorax *(for IJV cannulation)*	Respiratory distress, desaturation, difficulty with ventilation, reduced air entry, hemodynamic compromise	Chest drain insertion.
Nerve injury	Paraesthesia, weakness	Serial assessment of motor and sensory function.

Bibliography

1. KK Women's and Children's Hospital. *KKH CICU Handbook*. Singapore.
2. Trieschmann U, Cate UT, Sreeram N. (2007) Central venous catheters in children and neonates — What is important? *Images Paediatr Cardiol* **9**(4):1–8.
3. Scott-Warren V, Morley R. (2015) Paediatric vascular access. *BJA Educ* **15**(4):199–206.
4. Oxford Medical Education. (2016) Central line (central venous catheter) insertion. https://www.oxfordmedicaleducation.com/clinical-skills/procedures/central-line/.

CHAPTER 10

Chest Tube Insertion

Ng Si Min, Pamela; Cher Yuqin; Chan Meng Fai, Joel; Lee York Tien

Indications

- For relief of large or symptomatic pneumothorax.
- Drainage of pleural fluid collections (haemothorax, pleural effusion, chylothorax, empyema), allow collection of samples for investigations.
- Inserted post-operatively to allow drainage of blood/fluid, e.g. post-cardiac operations.
- Part of treatment for empyema thoracis — drainage of pleural effusion and instillation of urokinase.
- Rarely: Instillation of intrapleural antibiotics and pleurodesis agents.

Cautions

- Suspicion of pulmonary tumours/pleural-based malignancy — the lungs may be adherent to chest wall, increasing risk of lung injury during chest tube insertion.
  → Advised to be done under imaging guidance or by surgical team if indicated.
- Bleeding tendencies — coagulopathy or platelet count $<50 \times 10^9$/L
  → Consider doing under fresh frozen plasma or platelet cover

Patient Communication and Consent

The following should be discussed with the parent or legal guardian, and where appropriate, the child:

- Procedural steps, analgesia and/or sedation plans
- Written consent
- Possible complications, such as pain, bleeding, infection and injury to surrounding structures (including lung laceration/perforation)

Site Selection

The *triangle of safety* is defined by the lateral edge of the pectoralis major, base of axilla, anterior border of latissimus dorsi and the 5th intercostal space (Figure 3.5). Enter superior to the rib edge to avoid the neurovascular bundle.

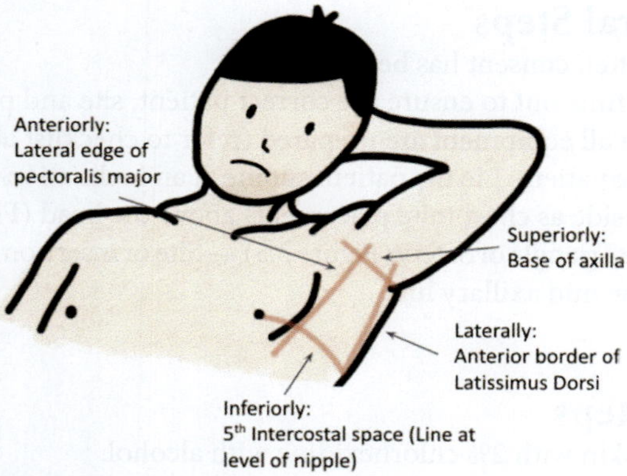

Figure 3.5 The triangle of safety (Illustrated by Dr Sharon Goh/Dr Stella Zhang).

Equipment Preparation

- Chest tube: As a general guide, use smaller sizes for draining air and larger sizes for draining fluid. A sizing guide is as follows:
  - » Newborn: 8–12 Fr
  - » Infant: 12–16 Fr
  - » Child: 16–24 Fr
  - » Adolescent: 20–32 Fr
- Sterile procedure set and drape set
- Chlorhexidine cleansing solution
- 3 ml or 5 ml syringe for drawing up of 1% lignocaine
- 1% lignocaine
- Scalpel
- Artery forceps
- Suture set with silk 3-0, and prolene 3-0 (Optional — as stay suture to facilitate closure of wound during removal of chest drain later)
- Tegaderm with pad
- Hypafix
- Underwater seal

Sedation and Analgesia

Chest tube insertion should be performed under moderate sedation (e.g. IV ketamine) whenever feasible. Local anaesthesia should be given with subdermal administration of 1% lignocaine (0.3 ml/kg, up to 10 ml) to the insertion site.

Pre-Procedural Steps

1. Ensure written consent has been taken.
2. Conduct a time out to ensure the correct patient, site and procedure.
3. Ensure that all equipment are prepared (refer to checklist above).
4. Position the patient: Lie the patient supine at an inclination of 45°, with the arm (ipsilateral side as chest tube placement) above the head (Figure 3.5).
5. Identify the Triangle of Safety (Figure 3.5) — Site of insertion is the 4th intercostal space, in the mid axillary line

Procedural Steps

1. Clean the skin with 2% chlorhexidine with alcohol.
2. Drape the area with sterile dressing towel.
3. Administer procedural sedation with appropriate monitoring.
4. At the site of insertion, infiltrate the skin and the intercostal space with 1% lignocaine.
5. Using a scalpel, make an incision (2–3 cm) in the skin at the superior border of the 5th rib.
   TIP: Avoid making incisions near the inferior border of the rib, as the neurovascular bundle runs here.
6. Using the artery forceps, dissect through the intercostal muscles in the 4th intercostal space, and continue blunt dissection down to the pleura.
   TIP: Direct the dissection towards the chest ('stabbing into the chest') to avoid dissecting along the subcutaneous space and ensure the size of wound is adequate in all layers to accommodate the diameter of the chest tube.
7. On entering the pleural space (you will feel a sensation of a 'give'), ensure the wound is widened with the artery forceps or finger.
   TIP: Be careful not to insert the artery forceps more than 1 cm into the pleural cavity.
8. Prepare the chest tube and remove the trocar. Using the artery forceps, grasp the tip of the chest drain and advance it through the incision into the pleural cavity.
9. Angle the chest tube towards either
   (i) the superior pole of the lung for drainage of air or
   (ii) the xiphisternum for drainage of fluid.
   TIP: Ensure that all exit holes of the chest tube are within the pleural cavity. The correct placement of chest drain in pleural space will be evidenced by fluctuance of moist air and/or fluid in the chest drain.
10. Attach the chest tube to the underwater seal.
11. Place the stay suture with prolene 3-0 into a purse string stitch, and anchor the chest tube to the chest wall using silk 3-0 (Figure 3.6). The stay suture is used to close the wound after the removal of the chest tube.
12. Obtain a chest X-ray (CXR) to ascertain the position of the chest tube.

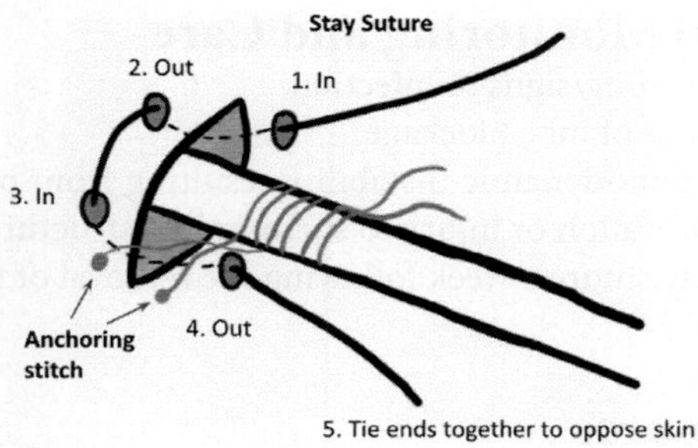

Figure 3.6 Illustration of how to secure a chest tube (Illustrated by Dr Sharon Goh/ Dr Stella Zhang).

Table 3.7 Procedural Complications of Chest Tube Insertion

Complication	Monitoring	Intervention
Bleeding *Excessive bleeding can occur in the event of laceration to major vessels (axillary, intercostal, pulmonary, internal mammary)*	Bleeding from insertion point, e.g. soaking of dressing Increasing/persistently blood-stained drainage from chest tube, especially if exceedingly more than the anticipated effusion/haemothorax volume seen on CXR/CT thorax	Consider checking coagulation profile and platelet levels. Correct as required. Repeat imaging to assess for accumulation of a haemothorax Inform the surgical team.
Infection	Local signs of erythema, pain, swelling, purulent discharge from wound Fever	Appropriate antibiotic therapy. If any purulent discharge, to send for gram stain and culture. Consider removal and reinsertion at alternative site (if the chest tube is still required).
Lung laceration/ perforation/iatrogenic broncho-pleural fistula	Bleeding, respiratory distress Persistent bubbling in chest drain indicates an ongoing air leak from lung/iatrogenic broncho-pleural fistula	Repeat chest imaging. Provide oxygen/respiratory support as clinically indicated. Inform the surgical team to evaluate the need for surgical intervention.
Injury to other organ systems	Signs of hypovolaemia or cardiac tamponade Abdominal distention/ pneumoperitoneum from iatrogenic perforation of diaphragm	Resuscitation as necessary. Inform the surgical team to evaluate the need for surgical intervention.
Tube blockage	Lack of oscillation Acute reduction of drainage Respiratory distress, desaturations, reaccumulation of fluid/air on chest radiograph	Milk along the length of the chest tube. Flush the chest tube with normal saline under aseptic technique. Consider change of tube. Repeat imaging to assess position of tube/residual contents.
Injury to nerve bundle	Horner's syndrome — injury to sympathetic chain (miosis, ptosis, and anhidrosis) Diaphragmatic palsy — injury to phrenic nerve (breathlessness, difficulty weaning from mechanical ventilation; decreased breath sounds and dullness to percussion of the affected side of the chest)	Supportive treatment. Supportive treatment. If symptomatic, may need surgical intervention such as plication of diaphragm and phrenic nerve stimulation.

Post-Procedural Monitoring and Care

- Monitor for bleeding/signs of infection.
- Monitor for signs of tube blockage.
- Monitor for haemodynamic instability resulting from possible complications such as lung laceration or injury to surrounding structures (liver/spleen).
- Remove the stay suture 1 week following the removal of the chest tube.

Additional Resource

1. Video link — OPEN pediatrics by Chris Weldon (Boston Children's Hospital). https://www.youtube.com/watch?v=_6sFa79u6FQ

Bibliography

1. Havelock T, Teoh R, Laws D, Gleeson F, BTS Pleural Disease Guideline Group. (2010) Pleural procedures and thoracic ultrasound: British Thoracic Society Pleural Disease Guideline 2010. *Thorax* **65**(2):ii61–ii76.
2. Cooper J, Browne N. (2019) Chest tube management for pleural disease in pediatrics. *J Pediatric Surg Nurs* **8**(4):118–122.
3. Kwiatt M, Tarbox A, Seamon MJ, *et al.* (2014) Thoracostomy tubes: A comprehensive review of complications and related topics. *Int J Crit Illness Inj Sci* **4**(2):143–155.
4. Oxford Medical Education. (2016) Intercostal drain (chest drain/pleural drain) insertion. https://www.oxfordmedicaleducation.com/clinical-skills/procedures/intercostal-drain/

CHAPTER 11

Bone Marrow Aspiration and Trephine

Cher Yuqin; Ng Si Min, Pamela; Lee Ming Wei

Indications

- Definitive diagnosis of haematologic disorders, such as leukaemia, aplastic anaemia, etc.
- Evaluation of pyrexia of unknown origin
- For staging of lymphomas and solid organ tumours
- To monitor response to cancer treatment

Contraindications

- Infection at site of procedure
- When contraindications to sedation (required for the procedure) are present
- Congenital or acquired coagulopathies, e.g. haemophilia/disseminated intravascular coagulopathy are not absolute contraindications. However, the risk of procedural bleeding needs to be balanced with the need for a diagnostic sample, and the necessary peri-procedural precautions, e.g. administration of factor concentrates, should be taken.
- Thrombocytopenia is NOT a contraindication for Bone Marrow Aspirate (BMA)/ trephine, but post-procedure bleeding should be anticipated and the necessary peri-procedural precautions taken.

Patient Communication and Consent

The following should be discussed with the parent or legal guardian, and where appropriate, the child:

- Procedural steps, analgesia and/or sedation plans
- Written consent
- Possible complications such as pain, bleeding, infection and injury to surrounding structures

Site Selection

Common sites include:

- Posterior superior iliac spine (patient should be placed prone or lateral) (Figure 3.7)
- Anterior tibial surface in infants <12 months old (patient should be placed supine)

Alternative sites may include the anterior superior iliac spine or sternum.

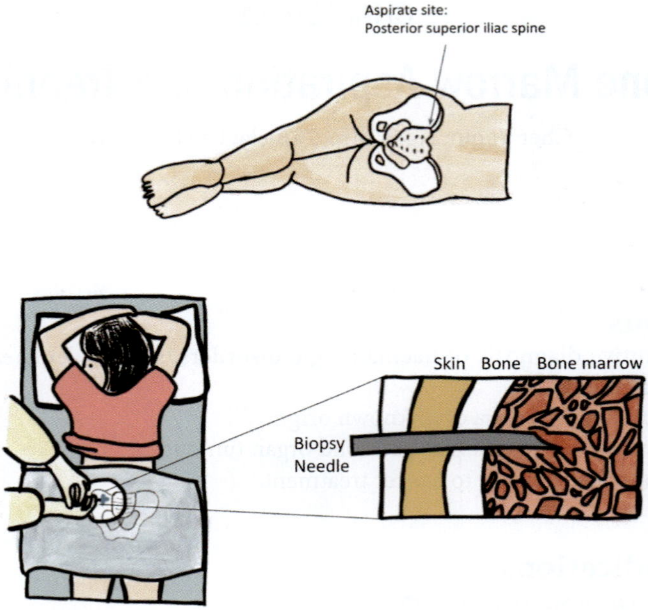

Figure 3.7 Bone marrow aspiration and trephine common site at posterior superior iliac spine (Illustrated by Dr Sharon Goh/Dr Stella Zhang).

Equipment Preparation

- Sterile procedure set
- 3 ml or 5 ml syringe for administration of 1% lignocaine
- 1% lignocaine (50 mg in 5 ml strength)
- 20 ml syringes as needed
- Bone marrow aspirate needle and/or trephine needle
- Specimen tubes/bottles required for sample collection

Sedation and Analgesia

If no contraindications to sedation are present, bone marrow aspiration and trephine should be performed under moderate sedation (e.g. IV ketamine). Provide adequate analgesia, with local anaesthetic cream (e.g. EMLA cream) applied with occlusive dressing over the biopsy site 30 to 60 minutes prior to procedure) and lignocaine infiltrated into the skin and periosteum.

Pre-Procedural Steps

1. Ensure written consent has been taken.
2. Conduct a time out to ensure the correct patient and procedure.

3. Ensure that all equipment is prepared (refer to checklist above) and haematology laboratory technician is available and ready.
4. Position the patient prone, lateral or supine position depending on the site of bone marrow aspiration. Take care to maintain the airway of the patient during the sedation.
5. Locate and identify landmarks carefully as stated in site selection above.

Bone Marrow Aspiration Procedure Steps

1. Administer procedural sedation with appropriate monitoring.
2. Clean the skin with 2% chlorhexidine with alcohol.
3. Drape the area with sterile dressing towels.
4. At the biopsy site, infiltrate the skin and the periosteum with 1% lignocaine.
5. Holding bone marrow aspiration needle with stylet in place, puncture skin and advance through subcutaneous tissue, periosteum and into the marrow cavity using steady, controlled pressure with a twisting motion. When the needle is firmly in place and a slight pressure is felt, the cavity has been entered.
6. Remove the stylet and attach a 20 ml syringe to the needle and aspirate 0.5 ml of marrow.
   - Hand the syringe to the laboratory technologist to obtain bone marrow smears.
   - The laboratory technologist will comment on the quality of smears obtained and if a repeat aspirate should be attempted.
   - Repeat the above step until satisfactory smears are obtained.
7. If the quality of smears obtained is satisfactory, obtain other samples with separate syringes as needed.
8. When sample collection has been completed, withdraw the needle very slowly using a rotatory motion.
9. Using a sterile gauze, apply manual pressure to the bone marrow aspiration site until bleeding stops. An assistant can do this.

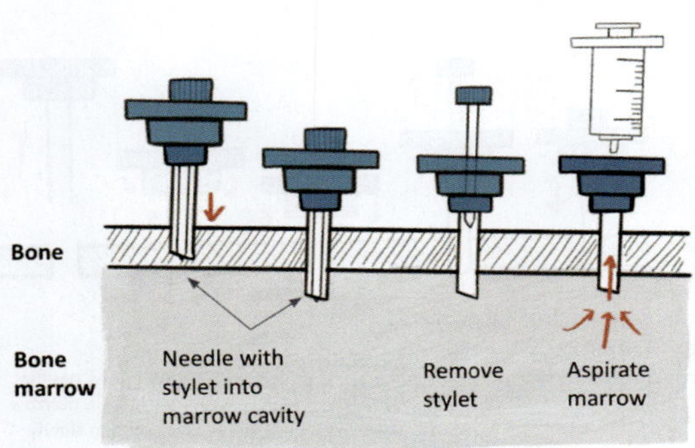

Figure 3.8 Bone marrow aspiration procedure (Illustrated by Dr Sharon Goh/ Dr Stella Zhang).

Bone Marrow Trephine Biopsy Procedure Steps

1. The trephine biopsy can be performed through the same skin incision as the bone marrow aspiration but angled differently such that a different area of the bone marrow is biopsied.
2. Holding the trephine needle with stylet in place, puncture the skin and advance through subcutaneous tissue and periosteum into the cortex of the bone using steady, controlled pressure with a twisting motion.
3. When the needle is in position in the cortex, it should feel firmly anchored and can stand on its own.
4. Remove the stylet and advance the needle further into the marrow cavity another 1–2 cm. There will usually be a slight decrease in resistance when the marrow cavity has been entered.
5. Rotate the trephine needle with three full twists to the right and then to the left without advancing. Rock the needle tip slightly from side to side to loosen the bone specimen from surrounding tissue.
6. Advance the needle slightly another 2 to 3 mm to ensure the bone marrow specimen is captured in place within the needle.
7. Withdraw the needle very slowly using a rotatory motion.
8. Using a sterile gauze, apply manual pressure to the bone marrow aspiration site until bleeding stops. An assistant can do this.
9. To remove the bone marrow specimen from the trephine needle, introduce the stylet through the distal cutting end of the needle to prevent crushing the specimen (Figure 3.10). Drop the bone specimen onto a glass slide provided by the medical technologist.

Post-Procedural Monitoring and Care

- Apply a dry gauze and pressure bandage over the bone marrow aspiration/trephine site.
- Monitor for signs of bleeding and infection.

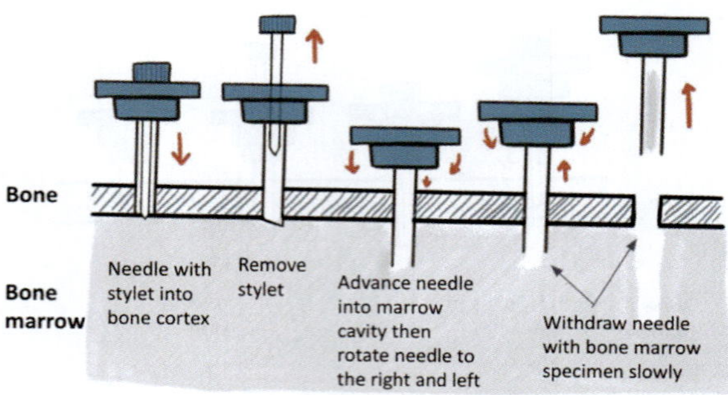

Figure 3.9 Bone marrow trephine biopsy procedure (Illustrated by Dr Sharon Goh/Dr Stella Zhang).

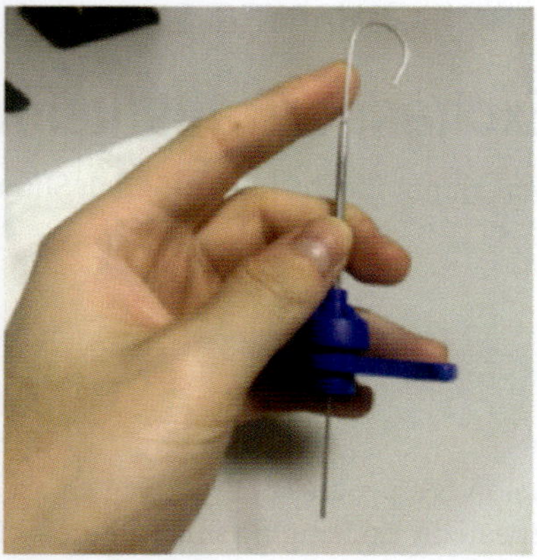

Figure 3.10 Removal of bone marrow specimen from trephine needle.

Table 3.8 Procedural Complications of Bone Marrow Aspiration and Trephine

Complication	Monitoring	Intervention
Bleeding	Bleeding from site, soaked dressing, haematoma	Apply local pressure. Consider checking coagulation profile and platelet levels. Correct as required.
Infection	Erythema, pain, swelling	Appropriate antibiotic therapy
Injury to surrounding structures	Injury to major vessels → retroperitoneal haemorrhage Kidneys/intestinal injury Fracture	Consider imaging to assess Consider referral to the surgical team

Additional Resource

1. Video link — New England Journal of Medicine. https://www.nejm.org/doi/full/10.1056/nejmvcm0804634

Bibliography

1. Abla O, Friedman J, Doyle J. (2008) Performing bone marrow aspiration and biopsy in children: Recommended guidelines. *Paediatr Child Health* **13**(6):499–501.
2. Riley RS, Hogan TF, Pavot DR, *et al.* (2004) A pathologist's perspective on bone marrow aspiration and biopsy: I. Performing a bone marrow examination. *J Clin Lab Anal* **18**(2):70–90.
3. Schaar FE. (1953) Bone marrow aspiration sites in infants and children. *J Pediatr* **43**(3):297–300.

CHAPTER 12

Exchange Transfusion

Chow Wen Hann; Eleah Nolasco Vidal; Shrenik Vora

Definition

- Exchange transfusion is a process of replacing a part of the infant's blood with donor blood by repeatedly exchanging small aliquots of blood over a short period of time.

Indications

- Severe unconjugated hyperbilirubinemia in the newborn due to any cause when intensive phototherapy fails or when there is a high risk of bilirubin encephalopathy.
- Severe anaemia (where there is normal or increased circulating blood volume), especially from haemolysis.

Contraindications

- Haemodynamic instability, as such infants who may not tolerate the fluid shifts.

Patient Communication and Consent

The following should be discussed with the parent or legal guardian:

- Procedural steps
- Written consent
- Possible catheter-related complications, haemodynamic and electrolyte problems

Equipment Preparation

- Infant warmer
- Cardiorespiratory monitor
- Pulse oximeter for oxygen saturation monitoring
- Resuscitation equipment and medication (should be readily available)
- Infant restraints
- Nasogastric (NG)/orogastric tube
- Suctioning equipment
- Equipment for vascular access: Umbilical venous catheter (UVC) or peripheral venous cannula

- Blood warmer
- Sterile exchange transfusion equipment
  - » Two three-way stopcocks with locking connections
  - » 5, 10, 20 ml syringes
  - » Intravenous (IV) connecting tubing
  - » Waste receptacle (empty IV bottle or bag)
- Appropriate blood product (cross-matched blood for exchange transfusion)
- Syringes and tubes for pre- and post-exchange blood investigations

Blood Volume

- Volume of blood for exchange is calculated using an estimate of the neonate's circulating blood volume, i.e. 80 ml/kg.
- Exchange transfusion involves double volume exchange blood transfusion using compatible blood. Hence, total exchange volume is double the circulating blood volume (2×80 ml/kg = 160 ml/kg), maximum 500 ml, as per our institution's practice.

Pre-Procedure Steps

- Ensure written consent has been taken.
- Inform Blood Bank of procedure and retrieve blood product.
- Insert NG tube and aspirate all gastric contents before line insertion.
- Set lines:
  - » If UVC method is used, wet infant's umbilical cord with gauze soaked with normal saline prior to UVC insertion OR
  - » Intra-arterial lines and peripheral venous lines.
- Set up IV drip set (plain dextrose 10% or dextrose 10% with added sodium (no added potassium)).
- Perform blood investigations:
  - » Blood Group Typing — as it will need to be matched with donor blood
  - » Full blood count, reticulocyte count, Direct Coomb's Test — to look for haemolysis
  - » Renal panel, calcium (Ca), magnesium (Mg), phosphate (PO_4) and capillary blood glucose — to check baseline electrolytes and correct them accordingly, as exchange transfusion may aggravate these abnormalities.
  - » Peripheral blood culture if sepsis is suspected, e.g. in a pyrexial infant
- Put infant on cardiac monitoring as there is risk of arrhythmias during the procedure.

Procedural Steps

Exchange transfusion can be performed by either of these techniques:

1) Push–pull technique — using single umbilical venous catheter and 2 three-way stopcocks

2) Iso-volumetric technique (arteriovenous method) — using peripheral arterial catheter for blood draw from infant and a peripheral venous catheter/UVC for infusion of donor blood to the infant.

Push–Pull Technique

1) Insert and secure UVC (see chapter on 'Umbilical artery and vein catheterisation')
2) Connect UVC according to Figure 3.11.
3) Start by withdrawing blood from infant at 10 ml/min.
   a. For infants 2–3 kg, withdraw blood in 10 ml aliquot.
   b. For infants >3 kg, withdraw blood in 20 ml aliquot.
   Note: Amount of blood aliquots may differ based on institutional practice
4) After first withdrawal of blood in appropriate aliquot, proceed to infuse whole blood at the same rate. Continue this process for the whole exchange transfusion.
5) Ensure there are no air bubbles while introducing blood, to avoid air embolism.
6) Put the infant on continuous cardiorespiratory monitoring. Monitor the temperature as well.
7) Midway during the exchange transfusion, do ionic calcium, blood glucose and blood gas. Correct any abnormalities as necessary. Consider calcium gluconate infusion, if required.

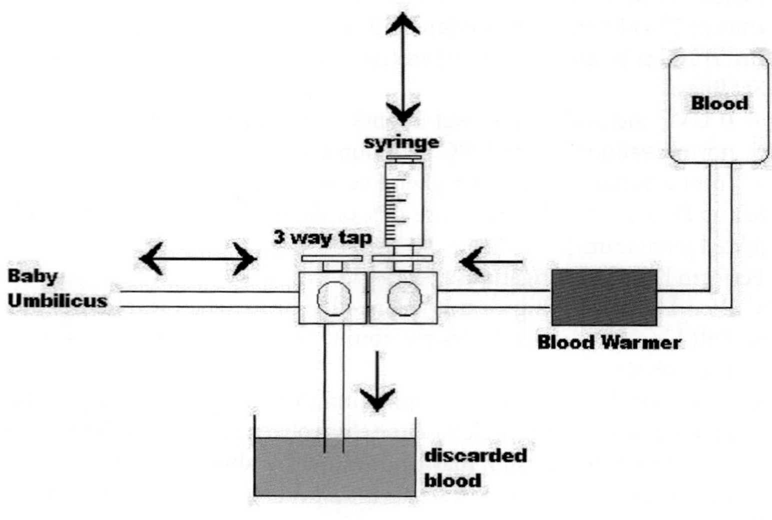

Figure 3.11 Push–pull technique connection.

Iso-volumetric Technique (Arteriovenous method)

UVC + arterial line OR peripheral venous line + arterial line

1) Insert UVC or peripheral IV plug and connect line to the blood according to Figure 3.12.
2) Insert peripheral arterial line and connect a syringe and three-way tap to waste container according to Figure 3.13

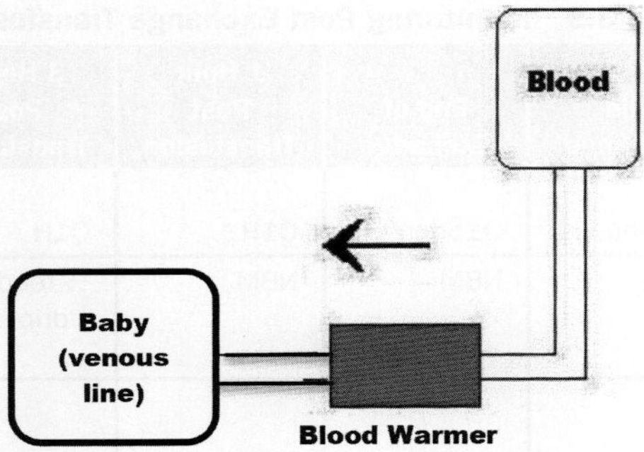

Figure 3.12 Iso-volumetric technique venous connection.

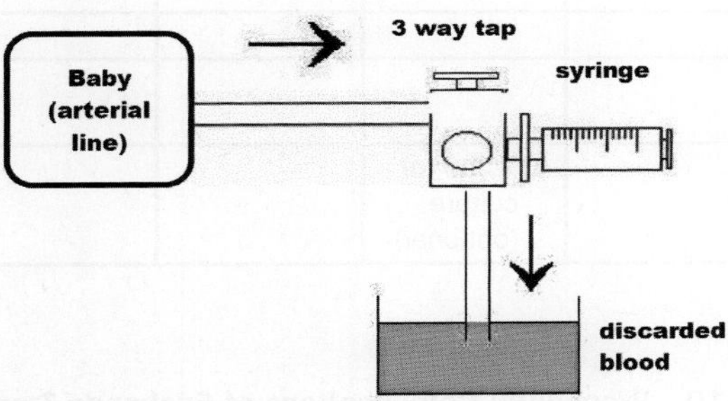

Figure 3.13 Iso-volumetric technique arterial connection.

3) Withdraw and discard blood from arterial side at a rate of 10 ml/min, and infuse blood simultaneously at same rate into venous side. Keep flow as steady as possible and volumetrically equal for infusion and removal.
4) Follow the rest of the steps of push–pull technique until exchange is completed.

Troubleshooting Points

If the infant develops respiratory distress, irritability, cardiac arrhythmias, bradycardia (HR < 110/min) or tachycardia (HR >160/min), pallor or cyanosis during the exchange transfusion, stop the exchange immediately. Assess and resuscitate accordingly and consider transferring to higher acuity care area (high dependency or CICU) for closer monitoring.

Post-Procedural Steps

- Continue intense phototherapy and remove umbilical lines.
- Other investigations and monitoring listed in Table 3.9.

Table 3.9 Monitoring Post Exchange Transfusion

	Mid Exchange	End of Exchange	1 Hour Post Transfusion	3 Hours Post Transfusion	6 Hours Post Transfusion
Vitals Monitoring	Continuous	Q15min	Q1H	Q1H	Q4H
Feeds	NBM	NBM	NBM	½ feeds, ½ drip	Full feeds, off drip if feeding well
Blood gas, ionic calcium	√	√			
Capillary blood glucose	√	√	√		
Serum Bilirubin		√			√
FBC					√
Renal panel/ Ca/Mg/PO4		√			
Others		UVC tip for culture (optional)			

Table 3.10 Procedural Complications of Exchange Transfusion

Complication	Monitoring	Intervention
Catheter-related complications: air emboli, thrombosis, haemorrhage	Haemodynamic monitoring Assess perfusion and pulses regularly	Volume replacement if there is any haemorrhage. Ultrasound Doppler if any concerns of limb ischemia.
Haemodynamic problems: collapse, hypotension or hypertension, bradycardia or tachycardia, arrhythmias	Continuous cardiac monitoring during exchange	Resuscitate accordingly, check and correct any electrolyte abnormalities.
Neurological: intraventricular haemorrhage (preterm babies), seizures	Glasgow coma scale (GCS) monitoring, Fit chart Examine neurology regularly	If there are any seizures, abort them and correct any electrolytes abnormalities. Do cranial ultrasound to look for any haemorrhage. Consider transfer to higher level of monitoring (at least high dependency).

(Continued)

Table 3.10 (*Continued*)

Complication	Monitoring	Intervention
Metabolic/Electrolyte problems: hypoglycaemia, hypocalcaemia, hyperkalaemia, metabolic acidosis	Monitor blood gas and blood glucose as per table above	Ensure IV drip is continued post exchange. Correct hypoglycaemia with dextrose bolus and monitor blood glucose more closely. Correct hypocalcaemia with calcium gluconate. Correct hyperkalaemia as per guidelines, but ensure that baby is not hypoglycaemic before using any insulin/dextrose. Put child on continuous cardiac monitoring and watch for hyperkalaemic changes.
Infection/Sepsis, blood borne infections	Temperature monitoring, trace cultures sent	Should there be suspicion of sepsis, to do full septic workup and cover with meningitic doses of antibiotics before proceeding with exchange transfusion.
Haematological: thrombocytopenia, anaemia, neutropenia, dilutional coagulopathy	Monitor full blood count as above; check coagulation profile if there are bleeding tendencies	If there are any bleeding tendencies, to correct these accordingly.
Gastrointestinal: feeds intolerance, necrotising enterocolitis	Monitor for vomiting or feed intolerance; examine for abdominal distension, abdominal wall changes.	Grade feeds up slowly. If there is suspicion of necrotising enterocolitis, to stop feeds, perform abdominal X-ray and culture and cover with antibiotics. Consider referral to paediatric surgical team.

Video Resources

1) Moeckel D, Julian S, Vachharajani AJ. (2013) Double volume exchange transfusion. *NeoReviews* **14**(10): e536–e538. https://neoreviews.aappublications.org/content/14/10/e536

Bibliography

1. Murki S, Kumar P. (2011) Blood exchange transfusion for infants with severe Neonatal Hyperbilirubinemia. *Semin Perinatol* **35**(3):175–184.
2. Vidal E, Vora S, Alim A. KKH Neonatology. (nd) Clinical practice guidelines: Guideline for exchange transfusion.

CHAPTER 13

Umbilical Artery and Vein Catheterisation

Huang Peiqi; Chow Wen Hann; Kong Juin Yee

Indications for Umbilical Artery Catheterisation (UAC)

- Measurement of arterial blood gases
- Continuous monitoring of arterial blood pressure
- Exchange transfusion

Indications for Umbilical Vein Catheterisation (UVC)

- Emergency vascular access during newborn resuscitation
- Exchange transfusion
- Central venous access for parenteral nutrition
- Infusion of vasopressors or hyperosmolar solutions
- Central venous pressure monitoring
- Difficult venous access
- Balloon Atrial Septostomy (BAS)

Contraindications for Umbilical Vessel Catheterisation

- Omphalocele
- Gastrochisis
- Omphalitis
- Relative contraindications include vascular compromise to lower limbs and buttocks, necrotising enterocolitis (NEC) or peritonitis

Patient Communication and Consent

The following should be discussed with the parent or legal guardian:

- Procedural steps
- Written consent
- Possible complications, such as bleeding, infection, damage to surrounding structures, vascular compromise and catheter malposition requiring line removal

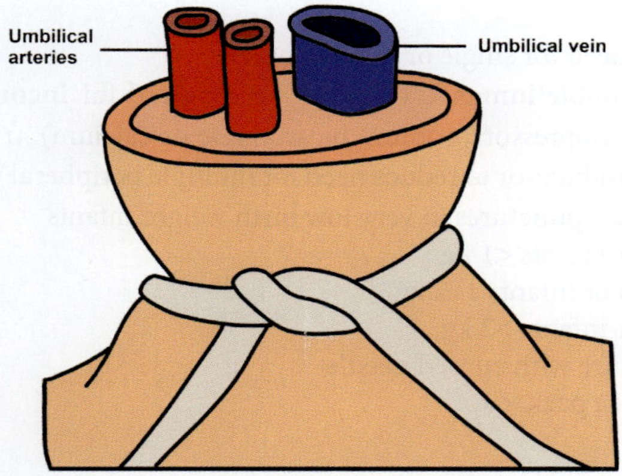

Figure 3.14 Umbilical vessels (Illustrated by Dr Huang Peiqi).

Site Selection

There are usually two umbilical arteries and one umbilical vein (see Figure 3.14).

The umbilical arteries are small, thick-walled and round arteries.

The umbilical vein has a single large thin-walled oval/slit-like lumen.

Equipment Preparation

- Sterile trolley, wiped with alcohol
- Sterile gown set, blue cap, mask and two sets of sterile surgical gloves each for operator and assistant
- Sterile umbilical catheter set, which contains
  - » Thermoplastic tray, McIndoe non-toothed dissecting forceps, Iris forceps, Curved Halstead artery forceps, Straight Halstead artery forceps, needle holder, scissors, Kimguard (sterile wrap), paper hand towel × 4, cord ligature, autoclave tape
- Blade
- 18 G drawing up needle
- 10 ml syringes × 2
- 20 ml Normal Saline ampoule × 1
- 3-way stopcock (red for UAC, blue for UVC)
- Antiseptic swab sticks
  - » For patients <1 kg: 2% chlorhexidine gluconate swab × 3
  - » For patients >1 kg: 2% chlorhexidine gluconate swab with 70% isopropyl alcohol × 3
- Alcohol swab with 70% isopropyl alcohol
- Cord tie
- UAC
  - » 3.5 Fr: For infants <1 kg
  - » 3.5–4 Fr: For infants 1–2 kg
  - » 4 Fr: For infants >2 kg

- UVC
  - » Decide need for single or double lumen.
    - ▪ Double lumen UVCs may be required for incompatible solutions (vasopressors, sodium bicarbonate or calcium), transfusion of blood products or to reduce need for multiple peripheral vascular access and skin punctures in very low birth weight infants
  - » 4 Fr: For infants <1 kg
  - » 4–5 Fr: For infants 1–2 kg
  - » 6 Fr: For infants >2 kg
- Silk 3-0 suture with curved needle
- Sterile Gauze pack × 1

Pre-Procedure Steps

- Ensure written consent has been taken.
- Conduct a time out to ensure correct patient, site and procedure.
- Position and gently restrain limbs as necessary to prevent contamination or interruption of procedure once started.
- Calculate the length of insertion
  - » UAC: (Birth weight in kg) × 3 + 9
  - » UVC: Calculated UAC insertion length/2 + length of stump
- Perform hand hygiene and gown up with a cap, mask, sterile gown and double sterile gloves.
- Prepare tray and equipment.
  - » Cut a hole in the drape approximately the size of the umbilical cord stump.
  - » The nursing assistant will open the items using the No-Touch technique
  - » Connect the catheter to the 3-way stopcock and prime the catheter with normal saline. Ensure there is no leak. Turn stopcock to off position.
  - » Keep the plastic sheath covering the catheter until it is ready to be used.
- Clean the insertion site under aseptic technique.
  - » Clean the umbilical stump as well as clamp thoroughly, furthest from the abdominal wall to the circumferential area of abdominal wall surrounding the stump. Care should be taken for the extremely low birth weight (ELBW) infants and clean ONLY the stump, avoiding excessive scrubbing of the abdominal wall, in order to prevent abrasions or burns on their premature skin.
  - » Place sterile paper at the 6 o'clock region of the stump over the abdominal area to allow the umbilical ties to rest on. This is to keep the string of the ties sterile so that it can be loosened/or tightened whenever needed during the procedure, while maintaining sterility.
  - » Tie the umbilical cord with sterile cord tie using a simple single knot.
  - » The knot should be tight enough to prevent bleeding but loose enough to allow catheterisation of the umbilical catheters.
  - » Hold the cord upright by grasping the cord clamp with a toothed forceps or gloved fingers by the assisting nurse. Cut the cord horizontally 1–2 cm above

the abdominal wall with a scalpel blade to expose a clean smooth surface. Be careful during cutting to avoid abdominal skin injury.

» Place the pre-cut sterile drape over the cut cord, exposing the cord through the hole. The entire length of umbilical tie should be brought up over with the cord to enable access if necessary throughout the procedure.

» Place one drape above the cut cord and another drape below the cut cord, to cover any exposed areas of the abdominal wall. Secure both drapes together with sterile tapes.

» Gently blot any blood with gauze for better visualisation of the lumens.

» Remove the first layer of glove after the cleaning process.

Procedural Steps — Umbilical Artery Catheter

- Identify the three vessels (2 arteries and 1 vein).
- Control any bleeding by adjusting the umbilical tie and blotting the cut surface.
- Use the haemostat to hold the side of cord to stabilise the cord during dilation and insertion. This can be done with an assistant, if available.
- Open the curved iris forceps and gently insert one tip of the iris forceps into the artery lumen, to gently dilate the vessel. Subsequently insert both tips of the closed iris forceps into the artery lumen. Be gentle and do not force it as this may create a false passage in the artery.
- Once in the lumen of the artery, gently allow the spring of the iris forceps to spread apart as the artery then relaxes and dilates. Repeat this until the tip of the forceps is 0.5 to 1 cm deep into the lumen, and the wall is dilated adequately to accommodate the selected catheter.
- Be careful not to disrupt the support of the surrounding jelly.
- Following adequate dilation of the vessel wall, insert the saline-filled catheter into the umbilical artery between the tips of the iris forceps already in the umbilical vessel (Figure 3.15). This can also be done without keeping the iris forceps in the

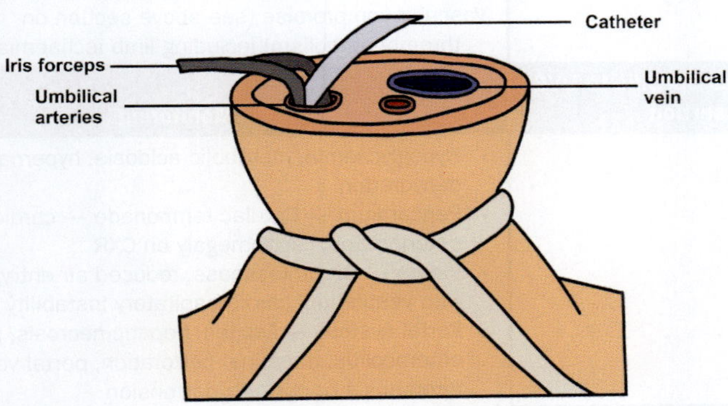

Figure 3.15 Dilation of umbilical artery with iris forceps (Illustrated by Dr Huang Peiqi).

lumen if the vessel is too small to accommodate both. After passing the catheter 1.5 to 2 cm into the umbilical vessel, the indwelling iris forceps can be removed.

- Apply gentle and steady pressure and advance the catheter slowly, while applying gentle traction (counter forces) on the cord to support the body of the cord.
- Insertion should be smooth up till the measured pre-calculated level.
- Once the UAC is in the correct position, arterial blood (in an infant with normal oxygenation) should be easily drawn back with no resistance.
- Flush the line with the primed normal saline to prevent any clotting.
- Proceed with UVC insertion (as below) if required.

Table 3.11 Procedural Complications of UAC and UVC Insertion

Complications Common to both UAC and UVC Insertion	Monitoring
Infection - CLABSI - Omphalitis or superficial skin infection	Signs of infection including fever, shock, acidosis Erythema, swelling, tenderness and discharge around umbilicus
Bleeding	Vessel perforation/false aneurysms → anaemia, pallor shock, collapse
Injury to nearby structures	Perforation of viscera and peritoneum → cardiorespiratory instability, signs of hypovolemia, respiratory distress
Thromboembolism including air embolism and Wharton Jelly embolism	• Haematuria, hypertension, renal failure • Gut ischaemia, necrotising enterocolitis, intestinal perforation • Portal hypertension, hepatic necrosis • Cyanosis or blanching/reduced perfusion of the skin of back, buttock and lower limbs, digital ischaemia or extremity loss • Paraplegia
Line malposition	May lead to any of above complications listed
Complications Specific to UAC Insertion	**Monitoring**
Vasospasm	Vascular compromise (see above section on thromboembolism) including limb ischaemia
Complications Specific to UVC Insertion	**Monitoring**
Extravasation	• Hypoglycaemia, metabolic acidosis, hypernatraemia, dehydration • Pericardium — Cardiac tamponade — cardiorespiratory deterioration, cardiomegaly on CXR • Pleura — Breathlessness, reduced air entry, difficulty with ventilation, cardiorespiratory instability • Portal system — Ascites, hepatic necrosis, necrotising enterocolitis, intestinal perforation, portal vein thrombosis or portal hypertension
Arrhythmias	Arrhythmias noted on ECG monitoring, breathlessness, pallor, cyanosis or collapse

Table 3.12 Troubleshooting Points for UAC and UVC Insertion

Problems Encountered	Troubleshooting	
	UAC	UVC
Inability to advance	• Obstruction may be encountered at different levels: » 2–3 cm: This may be due to the umbilical tie being too tight or the catheter being located at the entry level of the anterior abdomen. May try loosening the umbilical tie and applying 30–60 sec of gentle steady pressure. » 6–8 cm: This corresponds to the level of the bladder or the curvature of the umbilical artery before it enters the iliac artery. May try positioning infant on their side or applying some abdominal pressure.	Resistance may be encountered at 3–5 cm upon insertion. • This may be due to the UVC entering the portal venous system (see below) or impeded blood flow due to angle of the UVC, which may be overcome with simple manoeuvres such as gentle pressure on the abdomen.
Unusual Course	• The UAC may loop caudally back down the contralateral iliac artery or one of the arteries leading to the buttocks. • Consider using a larger stiffer catheter or retracting the catheter, rotating it and readvancing it into the aorta	Insertion to the portal system • There is commonly no back flow of blood once it is in the portal system. Avoid repetitive probing, or trying to advance the catheter tip by force, as this may lead to liver injury. • Pull back the catheter, up to 2 cm level from the tip of the catheter and reinsert it. Try rotating the catheter during insertion. • Try applying pressure on the liver and redirecting the tip of the UVC towards the left shoulder, so as to allow the catheter to slip towards the ductus venosus.
False Passage	• If a pop is felt with a sudden 'release' of the catheter, the catheter may have punctured the vessel wall leading through a false passage in the cord. If so, attempt umbilical artery catheterisation on the remaining artery instead (unless infant has single umbilical artery).	If false passage is suspected, do not attempt further umbilical vein catheterisation. Consider alternative access such as peripheral line or a peripherally inserted central catheter.

Procedural Steps: Umbilical Vein Catheter

- Use the haemostat to hold the side of the cord in order to stabilise it, with care not to accidentally remove the already inserted UAC.
- Remove any clot in the umbilical vein using iris forceps.
- The technique for UVC insertion is similar to that of UAC insertion. Catheter is inserted into the umbilical vein, which is larger and thin-walled compared to the umbilical artery. Efforts to further dilate the umbilical vein are usually not necessary.
  - » If the catheter is being used for emergency access, it should be advanced only as far as required to establish good blood flow, which is usually a depth of 5 cm. Secure the catheter between your fingers or with tape. Avoid inserting the catheter too deeply, as the catheter may enter the portal system instead of the IVC. The inadvertent administration of medication and fluids through the hepatic vessels may result in hepatocellular damage.
- Ascertain the accurate position of the catheters with an X-ray of the chest and abdomen.
  - » Secure the umbilical catheters by suturing them to the umbilical stump while awaiting X-ray confirmation. Leave the fields sterile during this time.
- The ideal position for the UAC tip should be located at T6-9 for a high UAC or L3-5 for a low UAC. The high UAC position is preferred due to association of complications with low UAC placement.
- The ideal position for the UVC tip should be at the diaphragm (T8-9).
- Review the X-ray images immediately to determine if the tip position is satisfactory and adjust if necessary at the same setting. Repeat X-ray is recommended to document the final position of the catheters in the procedure note.
- Following confirmation of the position, secure the umbilical catheters further by putting additional knots along the umbilical lines outside of the body.
- Connect the infusate at the same time.
  - » For UAC, run a patency drip with heparinised saline (typically 0.45% sodium chloride for preterm, 0.9% sodium chloride for term).
  - » For UVC, start desired infusate (heparinised total parental nutrition/dextrose drip).

Post-Procedural Steps

- Dispose of any sharps and perform hand hygiene.
- Document the final position of the catheters, the length inserted and all adjustments made.
- Monitoring: Leave the umbilical catheter site exposed, do not cover with a diaper.
- Readjustment of UVC/UAC after sterile drape is broken is strongly discouraged as this might led to contamination and risk of Central Line Associated Blood Stream Infection (CLABSI). Withdrawal of a line is acceptable if absolutely necessary but pushing in of the catheter is not recommended.

Catheter Removal

- Perform hand hygiene and put on sterile gloves. Prepare sterile dressing set. Swab the area to clean it, then apply drape around catheter site.
- When removing catheter, remove it slowly over 30–60 seconds while the catheter is still occluding the distal end.
- Secure clamping with forceps at the stump of the umbilical vessels concurrently with the removal of the tip of catheter to stop bleeding.

Video Resources

- Video link — Umbilical vascular catheterisation. https://www.nejm.org/doi/10.1056/NEJMvcm0800666?url_ver=Z39.88-2003&rfr_id=ori:rid:crossref.org&rfr_dat=cr_pub%20%200pubmed

Bibliography

1. Cloherty JP, Eichenwald EC, Hansen AR, *et al.* (eds.) (2012) *Manual of Neonatal Care, 7th ed.* Philadelphia, PA: Lippincott Williams & Wilkins, pp. 855–867.
2. Anderson J, Leonard D, Braner DA, *et al.* (2008) Videos in clinical medicine. Umbilical vascular catheterization. *N Eng J Med* **359**(15):e18.

CHAPTER 14

Percutaneous-Inserted Central Catheter Insertion

Huang Peiqi; Chow Wen Hann; Kong Juin Yee

Indications

- Long-term need for intravenous access (e.g. parenteral nutrition or prolonged antibiotics)
- Safe and continuous administration of hyperosmolar solutions (e.g. concentrated dextrose solution) or vasoactive medications (e.g. inotropes)
- Secure vascular access, if peripheral options are limited or exhausted

Contraindications

- Active bloodstream infection
- Thrombus in the targeted vein
- Excessive bleeding tendency
  - » Aim platelets $> 50 \times 10^9/L$
  - » Correct any coagulopathy before proceeding with insertion of percutaneous-inserted central catheter (PICC)

Patient Communication and Consent

The following should be discussed with the parent or legal guardian:

- Procedural steps, analgesia and/or sedation plans
- Written consent
- Possible complications such as bleeding, infection, damage to surrounding structures including pleura and pericardium, catheter occlusion or obstruction requiring line removal

Site Selection

- Select a large bore vessel (Figure 3.16)
  - » Great saphenous veins, antecubital fossa veins are preferable
  - » Other options include small saphenous vein, popliteal vein or scalp vein

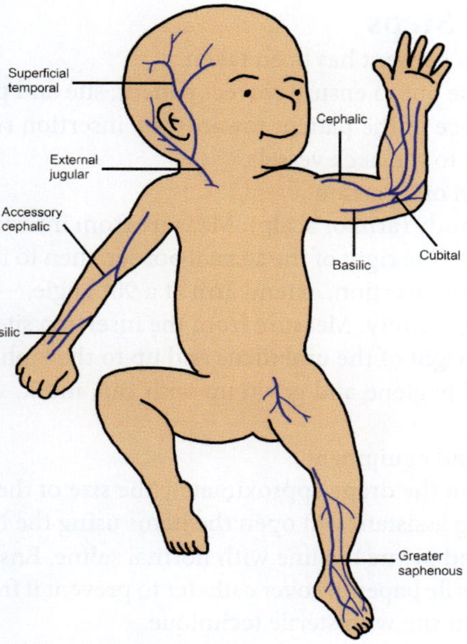

Figure 3.16 Veins used in PICC insertion (Illustrated by Dr Huang Peiqi).

Equipment Preparation

- Sterile trolley, wiped with alcohol
- Sterile gown set, blue cap, mask and two sets of sterile surgical gloves each for operator and assistant
- Long line catheter: Vygon EpicutaNEOcava 24 Fr/2 G catheter (term or later preterm infants) or Vygon Premicath 28 Fr/1 G catheter (<1 kg)
- Jelco cannula set 20 G (optional)
- Sterile neonatal long line catheter set which contains:
  - » Thermoplastic tray, dissecting forceps × 2, Iris forceps (blunt tip), scissors, Kimguard (sterile wrap) × 3, hand paper towel × 4, autoclave tape
- 18 G drawing needle
- 21 G sharp green needle
- 10 ml syringe × 2
- 20 ml Normal saline ampoule × 1
- Sterile measuring tape
- 3-way stopcock (Blue)
- Sterile Gauze pack
- Steristrips × 2
- Tegaderm × 3
- Alcohol swab
- Antiseptic swab sticks
  - » For patients <1 kg: 2% chlorhexidine gluconate swab × 3
  - » For patients >1 kg: 2% chlorhexidine gluconate swab with 70% isopropyl alcohol × 3

Pre-Procedural Steps

- Ensure written consent has been taken.
- Conduct a time out to ensure correct patient, site and procedure.
- Position the face of the patient towards the insertion site, to reduce the risk of line migrating to the neck vessels.
- Estimate depth of insertion.
  - » For upper body (arm or scalp): Measure from insertion site along the course of the vein to the right of the sternal border, then to the 3rd intercostal space. For arm vein insertion, extend arm at a 90° angle.
  - » For lower extremity: Measure from the insertion site along the course of the vein to the right of the umbilicus and up to the xiphoid.
- Perform hand hygiene and gown up with cap, mask, sterile gown and double sterile gloves.
- Prepare tray and equipment
  - » Cut a hole in the drape approximately the size of the limb selected.
  - » The nursing assistant will open the items using the No-Touch technique.
  - » Connect and prime the line with normal saline. Ensure there is no leak.
  - » Fold the sterile paper to cover catheter to prevent it from being contaminated.
- Clean insertion site with sterile technique.
  - » Clean the limb from distal to proximal direction. Clean the upper limb to the axilla and the lower limb to the groin.
  - » Drape the patient. Place the drape with the arm through the hole carefully — ensure it is not too loose to prevent contamination of the insertion site.
  - » Remove external glove after completing the cleaning process.

Procedural Steps

- The 'No-Touch technique' should be practiced throughout the procedure. There should be no direct touching of the insertion site or catheter with the gloved finger. Use the iris forceps to handle the catheter at all times.
- For 24 G catheter (Refer to Figure 3.17 for the following steps)
  - » Access the selected vein with the introducer needle (A). Once blood return is seen, stop advancing the needle.

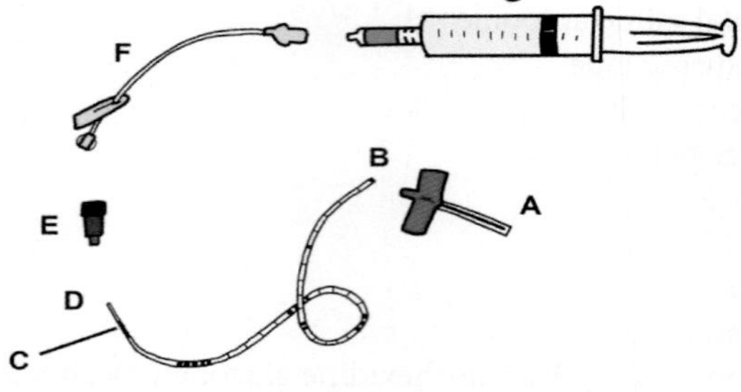

Figure 3.17 Set up for PICC insertion (Illustrated by Dr Huang Peiqi).

   » Insert the catheter (B) through the needle (A) slowly until the pre-measured desired length is achieved. The catheter should advance easily.
      ▪ If there is difficulty advancing the catheter, gently massage the vein or readjust the limb or needle position
   » Partially unscrew the blue connector hub (E) to release the distal end (D) of the catheter. The needle (A) is then removed carefully without injuring the catheter itself.
      ▪ If there is bleeding at the insertion site, use a gauze to apply pressure until the bleeding stops.
   » Carefully reinsert the distal end of catheter (D) back into the blue connector hub (E), ensuring that the black marking (C) is completely hidden inside the blue connector hub.
   » Flush the catheter intermittently with normal saline (F) once it is connected, to prevent back flow or occlusion, with a 10 ml syringe (G). The use of smaller syringes is discouraged as it will generate higher pressure and risk damage to the line.
- For 28 G catheter
   » Access the vein using a 24 G IV cannula.
   » Remove the stylet then feed the catheter through the plastic hub.
   » Flush the inner hub intermittently with saline to clean the clots.
   » Once the estimated length has been achieved, remove the plastic hub without tugging onto the catheter.
- Temporarily secure the catheter with steristrips. Cover the insertion site with gauze while awaiting X-ray confirmation of line position.
- The ideal location for the catheter tip is
   » Upper limb and scalp: Superior vena cava, or the superior vena cava right atrial junction (Figure 3.18)
   » Lower limb: Inferior vena cava
   » Lines that course into the neck or cardiac chambers must be immediately withdrawn and rechecked on a repeat X-ray.
- Once the line position is confirmed to be optimal, secure the line, ensuring all parts of the line and steristrip are covered completely by tegaderm.

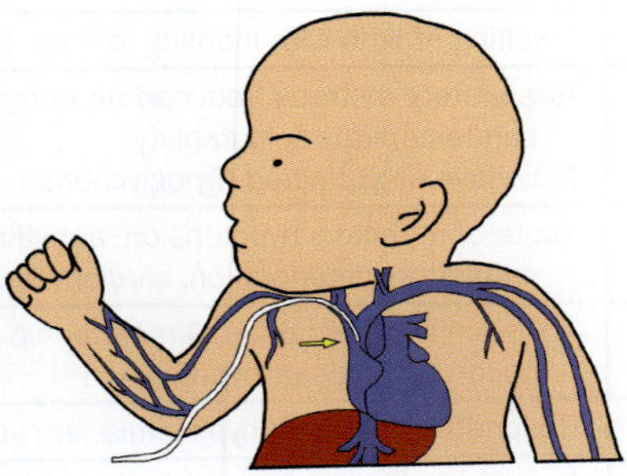

Figure 3.18 Optimal PICC tip placement at the superior vena cava — right atrial junction (Illustrated by Dr Huang Peiqi).

    - » The dressing should not encircle the limb, and the plastic hub should be placed on a small piece of gauze to avoid pressure damage to the skin.
- Prime the infusate and connect to the pump before connecting to the line. This should be done in a sterile manner and the infusate should run immediately to prevent occlusion.

Post-Procedure Steps

- Dispose of any sharps and perform hand hygiene.
- Document the final position of the catheter, the length inserted and all adjustments made.

Additional Points

- If the catheter tip cannot be advanced to the central venous circulation, it may be used functionally as a peripheral line, e.g. line tip terminating in the proximal third of the clavicle. With the catheter tip in this position, it can only be used to administer fluids suitable for peripheral administration.
- The risk of infection is proportionate to the duration of the indwelling catheter. Review for removal of PICC daily.

Removal of PICC

- Perform hand hygiene and put on sterile gloves. Clean and drape the patient, Remove the dressing carefully to avoid injury to the skin.
- Gently pull out the catheter with a slow steady rate to minimise the risk of phlebitis or break of line. Grasp the line and not the hub.

Table 3.13 Procedural Complications of PICC Insertion

Complications	Monitoring
Central Line Associated Blood Stream Infection (CLABSI)	Signs of infection including fever, shock, acidosis and line insertion site erythema, swelling or discharge
Intravascular thrombosis	Swelling of limb with inability to flush line
Pleural and pericardial effusions	Respiratory distress, reduced air entry, difficulty with ventilation, cardiorespiratory instability May have unexplained hypoglycaemia
Cardiac tamponade	Acute or refractory hypotension, arrhythmias, cardiac arrest, respiratory deterioration, cardiomegaly on CXR
Arrhythmias	Arrhythmias noted on ECG monitoring, respiratory distress, pallor, cyanosis or hypotension
Air embolism	Respiratory distress, hypoxemia, arrhythmias, seizures
Arterial cannulation	Pulsation of blood flow, bright red blood
Catheter migration	Delayed migration may lead to any of the complications above

- Document the length of the catheter removed. Compare this with the patient's record to ensure the entire catheter has been removed.
- If the catheter is difficult to remove, do not forcefully remove the catheter as this may cause the catheter to fracture. Consider surgical consultation if it is difficult to remove.

Video Resources

- Video link — PICC placement in the neonate. https://www.nejm.org/doi/10.1056/NEJMvcm1101914?url_ver=Z39.88-2003&rfr_id=ori:rid:crossref.org&rfr_dat=cr_pub%20%200pubmed

Bibliography

1. Menon G. (2003) Neonatal long lines. *Arch Dis Child Fetal Neonatal Ed* **88**(4):F260–F262.
2. Jain A, Shah P. (2013) Peripherally inserted central catheter tip position and risk of associated complications in neonates. *J Perinatol* **33**(4):307–312.
3. McCay AS, Elliott EC, Walden M. (2014) Videos in clinical medicine. PICC placement in the neonate. *N Eng J Med* **370**(11):e17.

SECTION 4

SEDATION AND ANALGESIA

CHAPTER 15

Sedation and Analgesia

Wong Ju Ming, Judith; Lim Kian Boon, Joel; Yeo Siok Hoong, Angela

General Principles of Sedation and Analgesia

1. **Sedation:**
   - To ensure comfort during painful and traumatic procedures through reducing anxiety, pain and/or consciousness with or without inducing amnesia (Figure 4.1).
   - Monitored with the State Behavioural Scale (SBS score).
2. **Analgesia:**
   - Defined as the absence of sensibility to pain (absence of pain on noxious simulation) or the relief of pain without loss of consciousness.
   - Observe the analgesic ladder (Figure 4.2) — optimise lower steps before moving to higher steps.
   - Monitored with the Neonatal Infant Pain Scale (NIPS), Face, Leg, Activity, Cry and Consolability Scale (FLACC), Wong–Baker Faces Pain Rating Scale and Numeric Rating scale as is age-appropriate.
3. Patients weighing >50 kg should be on standard adult doses rather than per kg dosing.
4. Anticipate and treat pain and agitation in patients rather than rescue an already distressed patient — observe the therapeutic window (Figure 4.3).

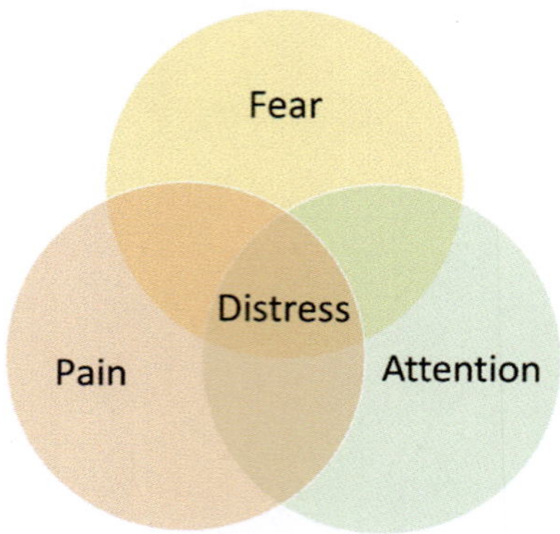

Figure 4.1 Procedural sedation alleviates factors contributing to distress.

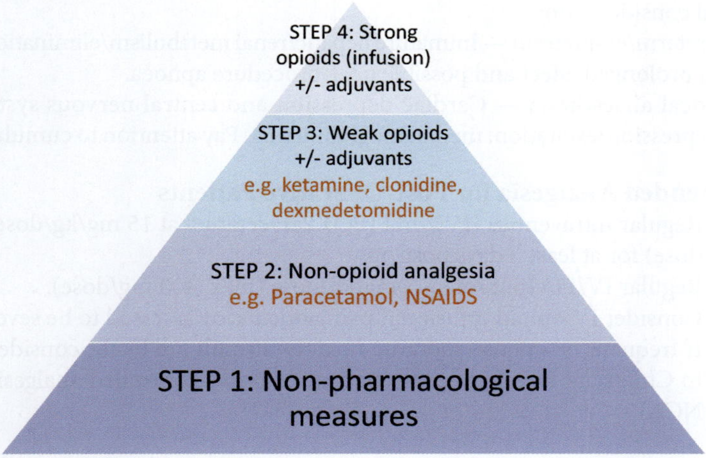

Figure 4.2 Analgesic ladder.

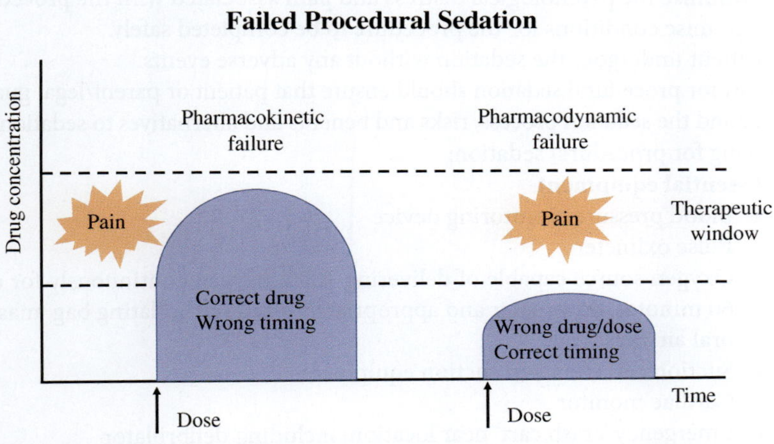

Figure 4.3 Failed procedural sedation due to pharmacokinetic and/or pharmacodynamic failure.

5. Use the minimal amount of sedation/analgesia needed to accomplish the therapeutic goal.
    - Do not use sub-therapeutic doses, which result in inadequate sedation yet exposes the patient to side effects.
    - Use drugs for their primary effect, e.g. primary effect of morphine is analgesia.

6. Special consideration:
   - Preterm/ex-preterm — Immature hepatic/renal metabolism/elimination resulting in prolonged effect and possible post-procedure apnoea.
   - Local anaesthesia — Cardiac depression and central nervous system (CNS) depression/excitation, methaemoglobinemia. Pay attention to cumulative doses.

Recommended Analgesia for Post-Operative Patients

1. Regular intravenous (IV)/oral (PO) Paracetamol at 15 mg/kg/dose (max. 1g/dose) for at least 3 days post-op.
2. Regular IV/PO Ibuprofen 10mg/kg/dose (max. 400 mg/dose).
3. Consider IV opioid infusion if pain anticipated/assessed to be severe.
4. If frequent or intense sporadic noxious stimuli are likely, consider referring to Children's Pain Service for patient or nurse-controlled analgesia (PCA or NCA).

Procedural Sedation

1. **Goals:**
   - Minimise the psychological distress and pain associated with the procedures.
   - Optimise conditions for the procedure to be completed safely.
   - Patient undergoes the sedation without any adverse events.
2. **Consent** for procedural sedation should ensure that patient or parent/legal guardians understand the sedation process, risks and benefits and alternatives to sedation.
3. Preparing for procedural sedation:
   - **Essential equipment**
     - » Blood pressure monitoring device
     - » Pulse oximeter
     - » Oxygen source capable of delivering 100% oxygen continuously for at least 60 minutes, flow meter and appropriately sized self-inflating bag, masks and oral airways
     - » Suction catheters and suction equipment
     - » Cardiac monitor
     - » Emergency 'crash cart' near location, including defibrillator
4. **Roles and responsibilities**
   - All staff involved in sedation should be competent in:
     - » Techniques and modes of sedation
     - » Monitoring physiological parameters
     - » Basic Cardiac Life Support and Bag and Mask skills
     - » Recognising and managing complications
     - » Initiating advanced resuscitation when necessary
   - Doctor's/sedationist's responsibilities:
     - » Sedation pre-assessment
       - i. Current medical history and physical examination record (including airway assessment)
       - ii. Previous sedation encounters

Table 4.1 Continuum of Depth of Sedation

	Minimal Sedation/ Anxiolysis	Moderate Sedation (Conscious Sedation)	Deep Sedation	General Anaesthesia
Responsiveness	Normal response to verbal stimulation	Purposeful response to verbal or tactile stimulation	Purposeful response to repeated or painful stimulation	Unarousable with painful stimulus
Airway	Unaffected	No intervention required	May require intervention	Intervention required
Spontaneous ventilation	Unaffected	Adequate	May be inadequate	Frequently inadequate
Cardiovascular function	Unaffected	Usually maintained	Usually maintained	May be impaired

iii. Current medication (including allergies)
iv. Baseline functional status
v. Last food/liquid intake

» Determine the level of sedation/analgesia required before and throughout the sedation
  i. Consider use of local or topical anaesthesia for painful procedures
» Calculate the amount of drug(s)
» Ensure appropriate equipment and staff available
» Continually monitor for:
  i. Airway patency and respiratory rate
  ii. Level of consciousness (Table 4.1)
  iii. Occurrence of adverse reactions
» Documentation
» Ensure fitness for discharge from sedation monitoring
» Consider referring to Child Life Therapist for procedural support in appropriate cases

- Nurse's responsibilities:
  » Ensure the body weight is current
  » Help to prepare drugs
  » Prepare, perform and document monitoring parameters during and post sedation
  » Assist the doctor in the procedure or resuscitation if necessary
  » Ensuring fitness for discharge from sedation monitoring and providing adequate post-discharge instructions

5. **Discharge Criteria:**
   - Able to independently maintain an airway.
   - Oxygen saturation ≥95% in room air or equivalent to baseline oxygen saturation in room air prior to the procedure.

Sedation In The Children's Intensive Care Unit

Nurse-led sedation protocol indicated for all patients anticipated to remain intubated for >4 hours.

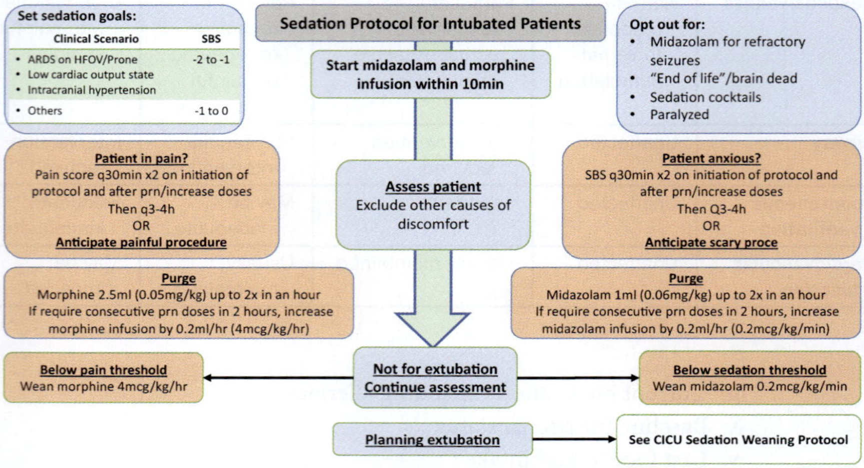

Figure 4.4 Sedation Protocol for Intubated Patients in the Children's Intensive Care Unit (CICU).

- Stable cardiovascular status.
- Easily roused, able to talk (if age appropriate), or is at pre-procedure baseline level of consciousness.
- Able to move/walk with minimal assistance.
- If a reversal agent has been given, monitoring must continue for a minimum of 2 hours before discharge.

Non-pharmacological measures to facilitate minimal medication use:

1. Reducing environmental stimuli such as light and sound (especially at night)
2. Promotion of sleep and maintaining a day-night routine
3. Optimising patient position
4. Swaddling infants or using weighted blankets
5. Comforting touch/massage/rocking
6. Parental involvement in care
7. Regular feeds for infants
8. Ensuring adequate hydration
9. Consider music/play/relaxation/distraction therapy

Weaning Sedation and Analgesia in the CICU

1. A sedation strategy should follow the patient's trajectory, and weaning of sedation and analgesia should begin as soon as it is safe and appropriate to do so.

2. Over-sedation or unnecessarily prolonged sedation should be avoided, as it can lead to tolerance (and iatrogenic withdrawal syndrome), disrupted sleep, delirium, muscle weakness, and prolonged ventilation and immobility.
3. Iatrogenic withdrawal syndrome:
   - The unpleasant signs and symptoms resulting from rapid/abrupt tapering of opioid, benzodiazepines or other drugs with CNS depressant effects.
   - Manifests as symptoms of sympathetic overactivity, sleep–wake disturbance and seizures.
   - Mitigated by use of α-agonist clonidine to block sympathetic activity.
4. Monitored with the Withdrawal Assessment Tool (WAT-1) Scoring.
5. Clonidine withdrawal:
   - Risk of rebound hypertension and increased sympathetic activity with rapid wean/cessation.
   - Also requires gradual weaning, best done after opioid or benzodiazepine wean is complete.
6. Risk Factors for Withdrawal
   - Infants less than 6 months of age
   - Pre-existing cognitive impairment
   - Use of regular opioids/benzodiazepine for 5 days or more
   - Use of >2 agents or high doses (e.g. morphine >40 mcg/kg/h, midazolam >4 mcg/kg/min)

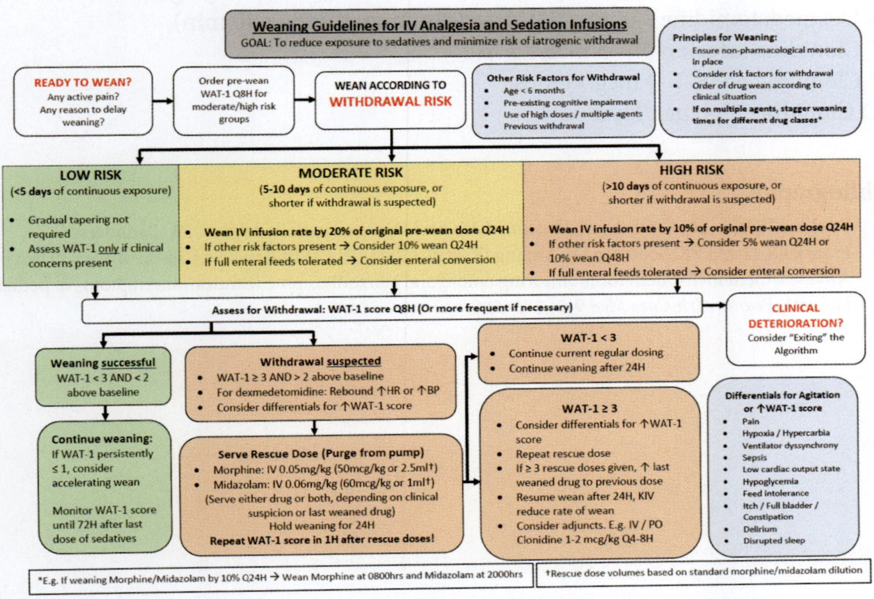

Figure 4.5 Weaning guidelines for IV analgesia and sedation infusions.

- Potent short-acting opiates (fentanyl) may be associated with tolerance within 48–72 hours
- Patients with previous experience of withdrawal

Therapeutic Dosages for Sedation and Analgesia

PO Chloral hydrate 50 mg/kg/dose once for non-painful procedures or 20 mg/kg/dose Q8H for maintenance sedation
IV/PO Paracetamol 10–15 mg/kg/dose Q6H (max. 1 g/dose)
IV/PO Ibuprofen 10 mg/kg/dose Q6H (max. 400 mg/dose)
IV Ketorolac 0.3–0.5 mg/kg/dose Q6H (max. 30 mg)
IV Morphine infusion 10–40 mcg/kg/h (titrate to effect)
IV Morphine bolus 0.05–0.1 mg/kg/dose (max. 10 mg)
IV Fentanyl bolus 0.3–0.5 mcg/kg/dose
Intranasal (IN) Fentanyl 1–2 mcg/kg/dose
IV Midazolam infusion 1–4 mcg/kg/min (titrate to effect)
IV Midazolam bolus 0.05–0.1 mg/kg/dose (max. 4 mg)
PO Mist Morphine (syrup) 0.2 to 0.4 mg/kg/dose (max. 15 mg) Q4–6H with/without 0.1mg/kg/dose (max. 15 mg) Q4H/PRN for breakthrough pain
PO Oxycodone (capsule) 0.1 mg/kg/dose (max. 5 mg) Q4–6H with/without 0.05 mg/kg/dose (max. 5 mg) Q4h/PRN for breakthrough pain
IV Ketamine bolus 1 mg/kg/dose Q15min
IV Ketamine infusion 0.1–0.2 mg/kg/h
IV Dexmedetomidine 0.2–0.7 (up to 1 for procedural sedation) mcg/kg/h
IN Dexmedetomidine 3–4 mcg/kg/dose (duration of action 40 min)
IV Clonidine infusion 0.1–3 mcg/kg/h
IV Clonidine bolus 1–4 mcg/kg/dose
PO Clonidine 2–4 mcg/kg/dose

Bibliography

1. Dorland WAN. (2007) *Dorland's Illustrated Medical Dictionary*. Philadelphia, PA: Saunders.
2. Franck LS, Harris SK, Soetenga DJ, Amling JK, *et al.* (2008). The Withdrawal Assessment Tool-1 (WAT-1): An assessment instrument for monitoring opioid and benzodiazepine withdrawal symptoms in pediatric patients. *Pediatr Crit Care Med* **9**(6):573–580.

SECTION 5

ADOLESCENT HEALTH

CHAPTER 16

The Adolescent Interview: HEADSS Assessment

Kumudhini Rajasegaran; Courtney Davis; Chew Chu Shan, Elaine; Tan Sher Kit, Juliet; Oh Jean Yin

Introduction

Adolescence is generally a healthy period of life in comparison to early childhood and old age. As healthcare professionals in contact with this group of individuals, it is important to understand adolescent development and to have effective communication and consultative skills to better guide treatment and management.

The Home, Education/Employment, Activities, Drugs, Sexuality, Suicide/Depression (HEADSS) assessment is an excellent guide to obtain a bio-psycho-social biopsy and an opportunity to build rapport with the adolescent. It aids in risk assessment as well as helps guide intervention.

Confidentiality

Prior to starting a HEADSS assessment — it is important to address confidentiality and the limits of confidentiality with the adolescent patient and their parent. All information should be considered confidential with several exceptions: (1) Concerns for harm to self/suicidality, (2) Concerns for harm to adolescent (sexual or physical abuse), (3) Concern for harm to others, and (4) Disclosures that require police reporting, including underage sexual abuse/activity and drug use.

Please discuss with your senior colleagues if you are unsure about whether the information disclosed by an adolescent requires disclosure to the parents/guardians or authorities.

HEADSS Comprehensive Adolescent Psycho-Social Screening Interview

Reminder: Discuss confidentiality and limits to confidentiality prior to starting

Home
• Who lives with the patient? Where? Own room? • What are the relationships like at home?

(*Continued*)

Home
• What do parents and relatives do for a living? • Ever institutionalised? Incarcerated? • Recent moves — Running away episodes?
Education (and/or Employment)
• School/grade performance — Any recent changes? Any dramatic past changes? • Favourite/worst subjects • Any years repeated/classes failed? • Suspensions or termination, dropping out history • Future education/employment plans/goals • Any current employment? • Relations with teachers, school attendance • Bullied/bullies • Part-time work
Activities
• With peers (What do you do for fun? Where and when?) • With family • Club/school functions • Sports, regular exercise • Church attendance and club projects • Hobbies — Other home activities • Reading for fun — What? • TV — How much weekly? Favourite shows? • Internet/screen use — video games, social media • Favourite music • Does patient have car, use seatbelts? • History of arrests — Acting out, crime
Drugs
• Used by peers • Used by patient; include alcohol and cigarettes • Used by family members • Amounts, frequency, patterns of use/abuse and car use, while intoxicated • Source — How is it paid for?
Sexuality
• Orientation • Degree and types of sexual experience and acts • Number of partners • History of pregnancy/abortion • Sexually transmitted diseases — Knowledge and prevention • Contraception

(*Continued*)

(*Continued*)

Sleep/Suicide/Self Harm/Depression
• Sleep disorders (usually induction problems, also early/frequent waking or greatly increased sleep and complaints of increasing fatigue) • Appetite/eating behaviour changes • Feeling bored? • Emotional outbursts and highly impulsive behaviour • History of withdrawal/isolation • Hopeless/helpless feelings • History of past suicide attempts, depression, psychological counselling • History of deliberate self-harm (DSH) • History in family or peers • History of drug/alcohol abuse, acting out/crime, recent change in school performance • History of recurrent serious 'accidents' • Psychosomatic symptomatology • Suicidal ideation (including significant current and past losses) • Decreased affect on interview, avoidance of eye contact

CHAPTER 17

Eating Disorders

Oh Jean Yin; Chew Chu Shan, Elaine; Courtney Davis;
Kumudhini Rajasegaran; Tan Sher Kit, Juliet

Introduction

Adolescents are at risk of developing an eating disorder with a lifetime prevalence reported between 6 and 12%. While binge eating disorder is the most common eating disorder, restrictive eating disorders most commonly present for clinical care. Anorexia nervosa is the most commonly known restrictive eating disorder; however, other clinical variants have now been described, including other specified feeding and eating disorders (OSFED) and avoidant/restrictive food intake disorder (ARFID). These conditions will usually present with physical manifestation of malnutrition, growth and pubertal concerns. Bulimia nervosa tends to present in older adolescents with little or minimal physical symptoms.

Anorexia Nervosa

- Restriction of energy intake leading to a significantly low body weight in the context of age, sex, developmental trajectory and physical health.
- Intense fear of gaining weight or persistent behaviour that interferes with weight gain.
- Body image disturbance or persistent lack of recognition of the seriousness of the current low body weight.

Sub Types

- Restricting: Only restriction of intake over the last 3 months
- Binge/purge: Engages in binge eating or purge behaviours (vomiting, laxatives, diuretics) in the last 3 months

Clinical Manifestation

Most adolescents presenting with eating disorders will have the following issues:

- Characteristic cognitive and behavioural signs
  - » Intentional caloric restriction
  - » Preoccupation with weight, food, calories, fat, getting healthy and dieting
  - » Thoughts of 'feeling fat' when weight is normal or low
  - » Fear of gaining weight

  - Feelings of guilt and shame about eating
  - Frequent weighing
  - Weight determines self-esteem
  - Binge-eating
  - Inappropriate compensatory behaviours — including self-induced vomiting, use of laxatives, diet pills, excessive exercise
- Growth and developmental abnormalities
  - Precipitous weight loss or gain or frequent weight fluctuations
  - Failure to gain expected weight or height
  - Delayed or interrupted pubertal development
- Medical consequences of the eating disorder
  - Nutritional deficiencies: acute malnutrition can be a medical emergency
  - Medical instability (see criteria for admission)
- Physical signs that may be seen in anorexia nervosa are listed below.
  - Hypothermia
  - Bradycardia
  - Orthostatic pulse and blood pressure
  - Dull, thinning scalp hair
  - Lanugo hair
  - Emaciated, wears oversized clothes
  - Gastrointestinal side effects: constipation/bloating
  - Flat affect
  - Cold extremities, acrocyanosis
  - Primary or secondary amenorrhea

If an eating disorder is suspected, the first priority is to determine medical stability and to evaluate for complications of an eating disorder. Patients can be medically unstable despite being at a normal body mass index (BMI). Rapid weight loss or poor oral intake prior to admission can lead to medical instability. A close follow-up appointment in 1–2 weeks is recommended, especially if there is rapid weight loss. The most common reason requiring admission is bradycardia.

Medical Instability and Criteria for Acute Admission

- Resting heart rate <50/min
- Electrocardiogram (ECG) abnormalities, e.g. prolonged QTc
- Significant postural and/or haemodynamic changes
- Hypotension
- Systolic BP drop >20 mmHg from lying to standing position
- Diastolic BP drop >10 mmHg from lying to standing position
- Heart rate increase of >30/min from lying to standing position
- Dehydration
- Temperature <35.5°C
- Electrolyte abnormalities

If considering psychological reasons for admission, including acute food refusal or safety concerns, please consider discussing it with the adolescent medicine physician on call.

Suggested Investigations

- ECG
- Full blood count, renal panel, serum calcium, serum magnesium, serum phosphate, random blood glucose, LFT, TFT and in females, serum luteinizing hormone (LH), follicle stimulating hormone (FSH), oestradiol, vitamin D level
- Bone Mineral Density (BMD) — to consult adolescent medicine physician

On admission to the General Paediatric Ward

Place on Eating Disorder (ED) protocol level 1 unless directed by adolescent medicine physician

Refer to the Adolescent Medicine (ADME) team — consisting of adolescent medicine physician, adolescent resource nurse and dietician

- Keep complete rest in bed
- Monitor vital parameters as per ED level 1 depending on medical status
- Continuous cardiac monitoring
- Postural blood pressure and heart rate twice daily
- Blood investigation and/or ECG as above if not already done
- Daily renal panel, serum calcium, serum magnesium, serum phosphate for the first 5 days and then as directed by the ADME team
- Suicide precautions if high risk for suicide or self-harm

Refeeding Syndrome

The clinical manifestations of refeeding syndrome are caused by fatal shifts in fluids and electrolytes into the cells with rapid refeeding of starved patients in a catabolic state. The increased glucose load from refeeding can cause a surge of insulin secretion that stimulates glycogen, fat and protein synthesis. There is activation of the ATPase symporter, which transports glucose into the cells. Magnesium and phosphate are also taken up into the cells, and water follows by osmosis. These processes, coupled with a total body depletion of these electrolytes, result in a decrease in the serum levels of phosphate, potassium and magnesium. Refeeding hypophosphataemia is the most common with a nadir presenting at first few days of refeeding. Monitoring for the clinical signs of fluid shift, such as lower limb oedema, is important in the first few days of refeeding.

Patients who are admitted for medical instability are at risk of the refeeding syndrome. Their nutritional intake and meal plans should be medically supervised and ordered by the dietician to reduce the risk of the refeeding syndrome. Extra food that is not supplied by the hospital is thus strongly discouraged in the first week of admission. Frequent monitoring of serum electrolytes, in particular, serum phosphate, potassium, magnesium is recommended daily, especially for the first 5 days of refeeding.

Goals of Treatment

- Medical stabilisation through nutritional rehabilitation with adequate weight gain and regular eating patterns.
- Monitoring for refeeding syndrome and early recognition of electrolyte abnormalities to prevent progression to refeeding syndrome.
- The average length of hospital stay is 10 to 14 days depending on the degree of medical instability and progress of nutritional rehabilitation.
- Reinforce to the family the seriousness of the condition — mortality rate 1.8–5.9% described.
- Psychoeducation for patient and family.
- Psychological assessment of the eating disorder, family assessment and introduction to outpatient treatment.

Family-based treatment (FBT) or Maudsley approach is now considered first-line treatment for adolescents with anorexia nervosa and is associated with faster and higher rates of recovery as well as lower rates of relapse. In our KKH study, patients with anorexia nervosa treated with FBT had faster and improved rates of weight restoration compared to patients not on FBT.

- Family (parental) involvement and empowering caregivers to renourish their adolescent.
- Non-blaming approach that focuses on rapid weight restoration to reduce physical and psychological effects of malnutrition on the adolescent.
- Best prognosis if there is rapid weight restoration with good engagement with treatment (achieving 2 kg weight gain in first 4 weeks of treatment with weight restoration within 6 months of presentation).
- Optimal care from multidisciplinary team approach
- Emphasises weight and growth restoration and resumption of menses or puberty
- Emphasises cessation of disordered eating pattern and bodyimage distortion with restoration of normal meal patterns that promote health and social norms

Bibliography

1. Lee HY, Hoodbhoy Z. (2013) You are worth more than what you weigh: Preventing eating disorders. *Ann Acad Med* **42**(2):64–65.
2. Lee HY, Lee EL, Pathy P, Chan YH. (2005) Anorexia nervosa in Singapore: An eight-year retrospective study. *Sing Med J* **46**(6):254–256.
3. American Psychiatric Association. (1994) *Diagnostic and Statistical Manual of Mental Disorders, 5th ed.* DSM-IV. Washington, DC: American Psychiatric Association Press.
4. Katzman D. (2005) Medical complications in adolescents with anorexia nervosa: A review of the literature. *Int J Eat Disord* **37**:S52–S59.
5. Academy for Eating Disorders' Medical Care Standards Task Force. (2012) Critical points for early recognition and medical risk management in the care of individuals with eating disorders, 2nd ed.
6. Rosen D. (2010) Identification and management of eating disorders in children and adolescents. *Pediatrics* **126**:1240–1253.
7. Mehanna HM, Moledina J, Travis J. (2008) Refeeding syndrome: What it is, and how to prevent and treat it. *BMJ* **336**:1495–1498.

8. Chew CSE, Kelly S, Baeg A, *et al.* (2021) First presentation of restrictive early onset eating disorders in Asian children. *Int J Eat Disord* **54**(1):81–87.
9. Chew CSE, Kelly S, Tay EE, *et al.* (2021). Implementation of family-based treatment for Asian adolescents with anorexia nervosa: A consecutive cohort examination of outcomes. *Int J Eat Disord* **54**(1):107–116.
10. Davis C, Hong WJN, Zhang SL, *et al.* (2021) Outcomes of a higher calorie inpatient refeeding protocol in Asian adolescents with anorexia nervosa. *Int J Eat Disord* **54**(1):95–101.

CHAPTER 18

Adolescent Sexual Health

Tan Sher Kit, Juliet; Karen Donceras Nadua; Seet Meei Jiun; Lee Hwee Chyen; Courtney Davis; Chew Chu Shan, Elaine; Kumudhini Rajasegaran

Introduction

Adolescent reproductive and sexual health is an important part of adolescent development, which if neglected, may result in unmet sexual and reproductive healthcare needs. Hence, healthcare professionals play an important role in supporting young people's sexual development by providing accurate information and appropriate health services, as well as promoting positive health behaviours.

The domains of sex and sexuality are important components to explore as part of an adolescent's biopsychosocial assessment. Potential topics that may be beneficial to discuss with the youth include his/her sexual history, any history of coercive sexual activity or abuse, prior usage of contraception, menstrual history and history of pregnancy, if applicable, and if he/she has had any prior sexually transmitted infections.

Legal and Ethical Aspects of Sex with a Minor

In Singapore, sexual penetration of a minor below 16 years of age, with or without consent, is considered an offence. The law has also placed a legal responsibility on anyone who is aware of such a case to report it to the police.

Illegal sexual activity with a minor includes

- penile-vaginal penetration
- penile-anal penetration
- digital penetration
- penetration by a foreign body
- performing or receiving oral sex from a minor

As medical professionals, we are legally obliged to make a police report if:

- A minor discloses that he/she has been a participant in these sexual acts, regardless of whether they were consensual or non-consensual, and also regardless of the age of the alleged perpetrator.
- There is an incidental finding of pregnancy in an adolescent or a child, even in the absence of any history of sexual activity or assault.
- There is an incidental finding of a sexually transmitted infection in a child, even in the absence of any history of sexual activity or assault.

The disclosure of sexual activity in adolescents and making a police report can be a difficult process for the adolescents and their families and has to be handled sensitively and contextualised to every adolescent's unique medical and social situation. Junior doctors are advised to get advice from the senior doctor-in-charge and/or adolescent medicine team if unsure on how to manage the disclosure.

When one encounters a teenager who has engaged in sexual activity, screening for sexually transmitted diseases should be carried out after disclosure has been made to both adolescents and parents. Education and counselling on the legal age for sex, safe sex and contraception should be provided. A urine pregnancy test should also be offered to screen for pregnancy.

Sexually Transmitted Infections

Background

A sexually transmitted infection (STI) is an infection passed from one person to another through sexual contact. These infections can be transmitted through vaginal intercourse, oral and anal sex, or skin-to-skin contact. Anyone who is sexually active may be at risk of contracting STIs. All partners should be tested and treated accordingly on epidemiological grounds.

Early detection and treatment of STIs is crucial, as each STI can cause a range of health problems and future complications. These include pelvic inflammatory disease, infertility, ectopic pregnancy and increased risks of certain cancers (e.g. HPV-related pre-cancers or cancers). It is recommended that all sexually active adolescents get screened for STIs, even if asymptomatic at presentation.

Evaluation for STIs

The sexual history of adolescent patients should be routinely obtained from the patients during both acute and routine healthcare encounters. During history taking, adolescents should be screened for risk factors and symptoms of STIs. It is also important to clarify with adolescents when using terms, such as 'sexually active' and 'sexual intercourse', as adolescents may have a differing understanding of these terms and details surrounding their sexual encounters and this may have implications on their STI risk.

Symptoms of STI

Many STIs have only mild symptoms or no symptoms at all. Clinical presentation of STIs in adolescents are similar to those in adults. Symptoms, if present, may include:

- Penile or vaginal discharge
- Dysuria
- Pelvic pain
- Rashes
- Blisters or painless sores on the genital area, anus, tongue or throat
- Painless and/or warty growths on the ano-genital region, groin or thighs
- Jaundice, abdominal pain, nausea, vomiting
- Swollen glands, fevers and body aches

Common STIs

For treatment options, please refer to the Appendix II for Drug Doses.

Chlamydia

Chlamydia trachomatis can be carried in the female cervix, male urethra, and throat and rectum of both sexes. Individuals with chlamydia infections can be asymptomatic or can present with vaginal/penile discharge, abdominal pain, dyspareunia or urinary symptoms. Untreated chlamydial infections can result in cervicitis (women) and epidydimitis (men) and for women, in particular, can lead to pelvic inflammatory disease (PID), infertility, chronic pelvic pain and increased risk of ectopic pregnancy.

Of note, chlamydia, which is often asymptomatic in older adolescent females and women, can present with abnormal vaginal discharge in younger females.

Testing

- Chlamydia PCR (urine, or endocervical/pharyngeal/rectal/urethral swab)

Gonorrhoea

Individuals with gonorrhoea infections may be asymptomatic or may present with urethritis (males) or cervicitis/salpingitis (females). Untreated infections can lead to disseminated gonorrhoeal infections, including that of septic arthritis, pelvic inflammatory disease and potential infertility.

Testing

- Gonorrhoea PCR (urine, or endocervical/pharyngeal/rectal/urethral swab)

Chlamydia and gonorrhoea are always tested together in view of the high prevalence of co-infection.

If chlamydial infection has not been excluded in a patient with confirmed gonorrhoeal infection, or if symptoms are consistent with cervicitis/urethritis/cervicitis in a sexually active adolescent with a high risk of non-adherence to follow up, patients should be treated for concurrent chlamydia and gonorrhoeal infections.

Trichomonas Vaginalis

Primary infections with trichomonas can be asymptomatic or occur with a green–greyish vaginal discharge and itch.

Testing

- Vaginal swab for Trichomonas, Gardnerella, Candida (VP3)

Genital Herpes

Herpes Simplex Virus (HSV) Type II is the most common cause of genital herpes. Primary infections are usually asymptomatic. Secondary infections often present with painful genital ulcers or vesicles, penile or vaginal discharge, fever and lethargy.

Triggers for HSV recurrence can include stress and fatigue. Prodromes can include a tingling, burning sensation at the location of eruption.

Testing

- HSV PCR (vaginal/endocervical/penile swab)

Treatment

Although there is no cure for genital herpes, medications can ease symptoms and reduce the risk of spreading the infection. Please refer to the Appendix II for Drug Doses for more information.

Genital Warts

Genital Human Papilloma Virus (HPV) is the most common sexually transmitted infection. Most HPV infections are asymptomatic, but can also present as warts, typically located on the penile, scrotal, vulva and perianal region. The diagnosis of genital warts is made clinically.

HPV infections and risk of cervical and other HPV-related cancers can be prevented with HPV vaccination, which can be offered to individuals (both male and female) from the ages of 9 to 26 (see Prevention of STIs).

Bacterial Vaginosis

Bacterial vaginosis (BV) is a condition resulting from changes in bacterial flora in the vagina, resulting in an increase in pH and a higher concentration of anaerobic bacterial. It can arise and resolve spontaneously in women, regardless of sexual activity. It is characterised by a whitish vaginal discharge with a 'fishy' odour and is otherwise often asymptomatic.

Syphilis

Syphilis is a systemic infection caused by *Treponema pallidum* and is almost exclusively spread by direct contact with infectious lesions. Syphilitic sores are often found around the penile, vaginal, anal, rectal or oral region. These sores can be painless and firm. <u>If syphilis infection is suspected or confirmed, referral to a specialist is recommended.</u>

Initial Screening

- Treponema Pallidum Antibody (CMIA)

Viral Infections: HIV, Hepatitis B, Hepatitis C

These blood-borne viruses can also be transmitted through mucous membrane exposures and exchange of genital fluids during sexual intercourse. Infections can be asymptomatic for all three viruses. Hepatitis B and C infections may present as acute hepatitis syndrome with symptoms such as fever, abdominal pain, nausea, vomiting and jaundice. HIV infection may present with acute retroviral syndrome with non-specific mononucleosis-like symptoms, such as fever, malaise, lymphadenopathy and skin rash, or diagnosed during a presentation of an opportunistic infection as part of the acquired immunodeficiency syndrome (AIDS).

Testing

- HIV — HIV antibody screen

- Hepatitis B — Hepatitis B immunity profile (HepB surface antigen, HepB surface antibodies) and Hepatitis B Core Total Antibody
- Hepatitis C — Hepatitis C Total Antibody (CMIA)

Treatment is in consultation with paediatric infectious disease physician and gastroenterologist.

Prevention of STIs

- Post-exposure prophylaxis
- Safe sex practices — in particular, barrier methods
- Vaccination

Vaccines are available for prevention of some STIs. These include:

1. Hepatitis B vaccine — this vaccine is initially given as part of the National Childhood Immunisation Program. Immunity during adolescence may wane, and repeat vaccination may be required. Hepatitis B surface antibody levels should be measured in sexually active adolescents and is recommended to be above 10 mlU/ml.
2. Human Papilloma Virus vaccine — both males and females age 9–26 can be given this vaccine. This vaccine is part of the National Childhood Immunisation Program for females and is given in an HPB-school based program for females aged 13–16 years. Males are not included in the National childhood/adult immunisation program and should only be offered HPV9 if high-risk.

Contraception

A minor should be informed of the law in relation to sexual activity. In general, an adolescent is strongly encouraged to involve a parent/guardian in decisions regarding contraception in an open, joint decision-making process.

Adolescents should be informed about all methods of contraception, including emergency contraception (EC) and highlighting the benefits of long-acting reversible contraception (LARC), such as the contraceptive implants and intrauterine devices (IUD). The correct and consistent use of condoms should be advised to reduce the risk of transmission of STIs.

If an adolescent is keen to discuss contraceptive options, consulting with the Adolescent Gynaecology team can be helpful in deciding the most appropriate option.

Adolescent Pregnancy

Worldwide, adolescent pregnancy is a major contributor to maternal and child morbidity and mortality. Pregnant teens are at higher risk of living in poverty, limited employment opportunities, experiencing violence within an intimate relationship, and having daughters whom themselves are at higher risk of teenage pregnancy.

Infant mortality is also significantly higher amongst babies of adolescent mothers than non-adolescent mothers. Infants born to adolescent mothers are at higher risk of numerous medical complications, such as stillbirth, prematurity and low birth weight.

Prevention of unplanned adolescent pregnancies is an increasing global priority for medical and public health professionals. As medical professionals, we can help reduce the risk of adolescent pregnancies through timely identification of adolescents at risk of early sexual activity initiation, and also providing effective sexual health education to this group of youth.

Management

When a diagnosis of pregnancy has been made, the adolescent should be informed in a prompt and confidential manner. A doctor should discuss with the pregnant teen how and when she plans on sharing the news with her parents/trusted adult, as well as the father of the baby.

Appropriate resources and support should be provided and options available to the pregnant teen should be discussed, taking a caring and non judgemental approach. These options include parenthood, future adoption and termination or pregnancy.

In our institution, single pregnant teens who are less than 21 years of age and decide on keeping their pregnancy should be referred to a dedicated clinic for multidisciplinary care and prenatal follow-up.

Termination of Pregnancy

Termination of pregnancy (TOP) or abortion is the removal of pregnancy tissue/products of conception/foetus and placenta from the uterus. Some of the reasons why women request for TOP include unplanned pregnancy, contraception failure, having an abnormal foetus and having a medical condition that will endanger the life of the pregnant woman.

Legal Requirements

There is no defined minimum age for the TOP procedure in Singapore nor is there a legal requirement for parental consent for minors under the age of 16. While parental consent is not required, adolescents should be encouraged to involve their parents or a trusted adult in this decision-making process, unless the adolescent feels that involving a parent in the process would be harmful for their well-being.

Abortion is prohibited after 24 weeks of gestation unless the mother's life is in danger or the pregnant woman is carrying an abnormal foetus that is not compatible with life.

Process

Pre-abortion counselling is mandatory by law for all pregnant women seeking treatment for termination of pregnancy in Singapore. Medical and surgical options can be explored with the adolescent.

An authorised medical practitioner should provide post-abortion counselling to a woman who has had her pregnancy terminated, and it should be done on the day when the abortion procedure is carried out.

Contraception should be discussed and can be started immediately after TOP.

Bibliography

1. Centers for Disease Control and Prevention. (2021) Sexually transmitted diseases. https://www.cdc.gov/std/default.htm.
2. Cunnington A. (2001) What's so bad about teenage pregnancy? *J Fam Plann Reprod Health Care* **27**(1):36–41.
3. Ministry of Health Singapore. (2015) Revised guidelines on termination of pregnancy. MOH Circular No. 17/2015.
4. National Skin Centre Singapore (2013) Guidelines on management of Sexually Transmitted Infections (STI).
5. American Academy of Pediatrics (2018) *Red Book — 2018–2021 Report of the Committee on Infectious Diseases, 31st ed.*
6. Lee RMK, How CH, Rajasegaran K. (2019) Sexual matters among teenagers. *Sing Med J* **60**(9):439–445.

SECTION 6

ALLERGY & IMMUNOLOGY

CHAPTER 19

Anaphylaxis

Goh Si Hui; Lee May Ping, Samantha; Goh Eng Neo, Anne

Definition

Anaphylaxis is a severe systemic hypersensitivity reaction. It is commonly IgE-mediated but can also be induced by other immunological mechanisms or direct mast cell activation.

Diagnosis

Anaphylaxis is a clinical diagnosis. Anaphylaxis is highly likely when *any* **one** of the following two criteria is fulfilled.

1. Sudden onset (minutes to several hours) of an illness with involvement of the skin, mucosal tissue or both (e.g. hives, itching, flushing, swollen lips/tongue/uvula)
   And at least one of the following:
   - Airway/Breathing: Respiratory compromise (e.g. shortness of breath, wheeze, stridor, reduced peak expiratory flow (PEF), hypoxemia).
   - Circulation: Reduced blood pressure (BP) or symptoms of end-organ dysfunction (e.g. hypotonia, collapse, syncope, incontinence).
   - Other: Severe gastrointestinal symptoms (e.g. severe crampy abdominal pain, repetitive vomiting), especially after exposure to non-food allergens.
2. Acute onset (minutes to several hours) of hypotension or bronchospasm or laryngeal involvement after exposure to a *known or highly probable allergen* for that patient, even in the absence of typical skin involvement.

Common Causes of Anaphylaxis

In children, the top cause of anaphylaxis is food, followed by drugs and stinging insects.

- Food: Hen's egg, cow's milk, shellfish, peanut and treenuts, wheat.
  In tropical climates, orally ingested mite-contaminated wheat flour products can trigger anaphylaxis.

- Medications: Non-steroidal anti-inflammatory drugs (NSAIDs), antibiotics (e.g. beta-lactam)
- Stinging insect: Bees, wasps

Approximately 15% of anaphylaxis is idiopathic after thorough history and investigations.

Risk Factors and Co-Factors

- Risk factors for severe anaphylaxis are age (infants, adolescents), concomitant asthma, cardiovascular disease, mast cell disease, consumption of beta-blockers and ACE-inhibitors.
- Co-factors that amplify anaphylaxis are exercise, acute infection, emotional stress, sleep deprivation, pre-menstrual status (in females).

Investigations

Inpatient Investigations

Anaphylaxis is a clinical diagnosis. Serum tryptase level is not required in the diagnosis of anaphylaxis but can be particularly useful in cases of perioperative anaphylaxis, anaphylaxis of atypical clinical presentation or unknown triggers.

Tryptase is best taken at 1 to 2 hours (peak), and not longer than 6 hours, after the onset of reaction. Blood sample is taken in a plain serum tube. Acute tryptase level is compared to baseline level drawn 24 hours after event. Raised tryptase supports the diagnosis of anaphylaxis, although normal levels *do not* exclude the occurrence of anaphylaxis.

In cases of perioperative anaphylaxis, strict serial time-sensitive sampling of serum tryptase levels is essential (Sample 1: immediately after resuscitation. Sample 2: 1 to 2 hours after event, maximum 6 hours. Sample 3, baseline: 24 hours after event).

Outpatient Investigations

Skin prick tests (SPT) and specific IgE levels help to identify IgE-mediated triggers. Tests should only be performed at least 4 weeks after anaphylaxis.

Acute Management

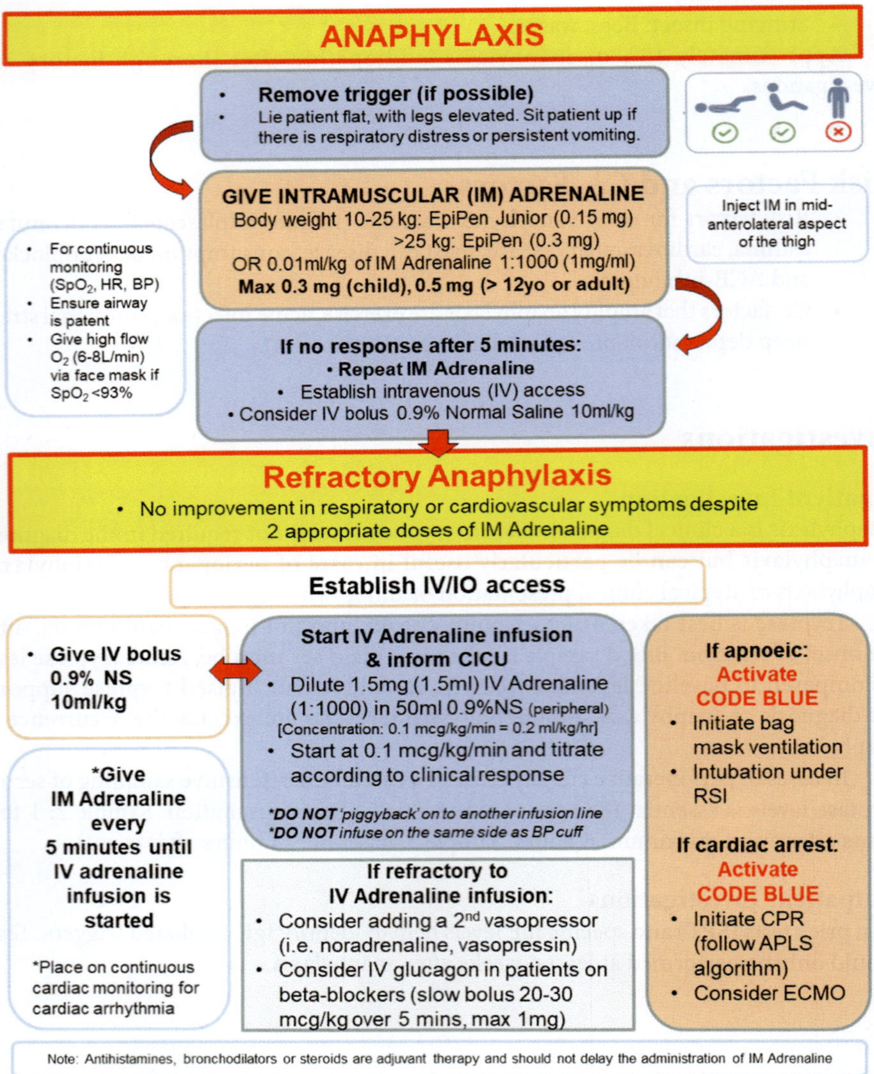

Figure 6.1 Acute management of anaphylaxis.

Further Management

All children with anaphylaxis should be assessed and monitored in the hospital. Biphasic anaphylactic reactions may occur 6 to 12 hours, and up to 72 hours, following event. Prior to discharge, an Allergy Action Plan should be provided to patients and caregivers.

Advice includes how to avoid exposure to likely allergen and how to identify and treat future allergic reactions.

Adrenaline Autoinjector

Patients at risk of anaphylaxis should be provided with at least 1 adrenaline autoinjector.

These include:

- History of anaphylaxis
- Specific foods associated with severe reactions, e.g. nut
- Allergic reaction to trace amounts of allergen
- Allergen is not easily avoided
- Patient with comorbidities, e.g. asthma
- Patients at continuing risk of anaphylaxis, e.g. food-dependent exercise-induced anaphylaxis, idiopathic anaphylaxis
- Limited access to emergency care

Adrenaline autoinjector dose

- EpiPen (adrenaline 0.3 mg) if weight is >25 kg
- EpiPen Junior (adrenaline 0.15 mg) if weight is 10–25 kg
- Or comparable injectable adrenaline product with specific instruction

Bibliography

1. Cardona V, Ansotegui IJ. (2020) World allergy organization anaphylaxis guidance 2020. *World Allergy Organ J* **13**(10):100472.
2. Goh SH, Soh JY, Loh W, *et al.* (2018) Cause and clinical presentation of anaphylaxis in Singapore: From infancy to old age. *Int Arch Allergy Immunol* **175**:91–98.
3. Lieberman P, Nicklas RA. (2015) Anaphylaxis-a practice parameter update 2015. *Ann Allergy Asthma Immunol* **115**:341–384.
4. Sicherer SH, Simons FE, Section on Allergy and Immunology, American Academy of Pediatrics. (2007) Self-injectable epinephrine for first aid management of anaphylaxis. *Pediatrics* **119**:638–646.
5. Muraro A, Roberts G. (2014) Anaphylaxis: Guidelines from the European Academy of Allergy and Clinical Immunology. *Allergy* **69**:1026–1045.

CHAPTER 20

Food Allergy

Chong Kok Wee; Goh Eng Neo, Anne

Introduction

Food allergy is increasingly common in children, with prevalence of up to 10% reported in Westernised countries. Food allergy can be broadly classified into immediate (IgE mediated), delayed (cell mediated) and mixed (IgE and non-IgE mediated). Food allergies involve an immune response and should not be confused with intolerance (e.g. lactose intolerance), toxic (food poisoning) or pharmacologic (e.g. caffeine) adverse reactions.

Immediate (IgE mediated) Food Allergy

The most commonly implicated foods are hen's eggs, cow's milk, peanut, tree nuts, shellfish, wheat, fish, soy and seeds, with the highest incidence locally being hen's eggs. Symptoms of an immediate food allergy occur usually within minutes (up to 2 hours). They range from cutaneous symptoms of hives and angioedema (mild and commonest) to acute vomiting/abdominal pain to anaphylaxis (with cardiorespiratory system involvement).

A clinical diagnosis of immediate food allergy can be made with a history consistent with IgE-mediated food allergy (onset, symptomology) coupled with a positive allergy test. When one or the other is missing or equivocal, the diagnosis should be confirmed by an oral food challenge (OFC) conducted in the hospital by trained personnel. A positive skin prick test or food-specific IgE alone only represents sensitisation and does not equate to clinical allergy. An OFC remains the gold standard for diagnosis of immediate food allergy. The use of component resolved diagnostics (notably IgE to Ara h 2 in peanuts) has increased the reliability of predicting OFC outcomes in recent years.

Egg and milk allergies have a high rate of natural resolution in childhood, whilst peanut, tree nuts, shellfish and seeds usually persist into adulthood.

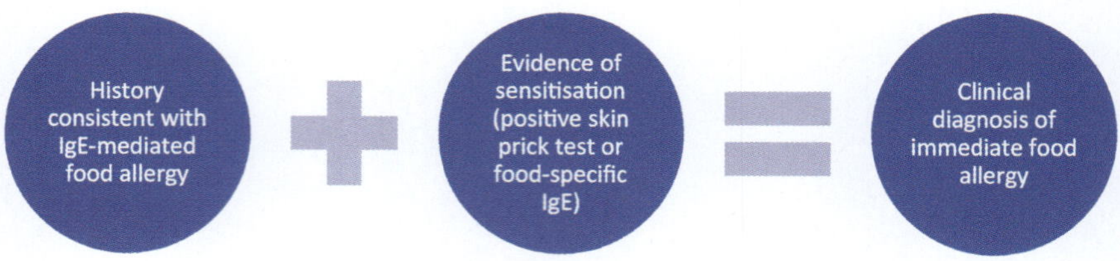

Figure 6.2 Diagnosis of immediate food allergy.

The mainstay of management is strict allergen avoidance and counselling on the recognition and treatment of allergic reactions from accidental exposures. Mild to moderate (cutaneous and gastrointestinal symptoms) symptoms should be treated with a second-generation antihistamine while the first-line treatment of anaphylaxis is intra-muscular adrenaline. A dietitian review is invaluable in the education on allergen avoidance as well as assessing the nutritional status, for early and individualised intervention.

Owing to a growing body of evidence, there is a gradual shift of earlier introduction of 'allergenic food products', especially in high risk, atopic children. These strategies for prevention of food allergies can be discussed with the attending paediatric allergist.

Food immunotherapy (desensitisation) used to be largely performed under research settings in academic centres, but it has been gaining traction and is now offered by allergists experienced in food immunotherapy in an increasing number of countries. Discussing the risks and benefits and setting expectations that it is not a cure to food allergy, are paramount in the decision to embark on food immunotherapy.

Delayed Food Allergy

Delayed food allergy generally presents with gastrointestinal symptoms as it can affect any part of the gastrointestinal tract, ranging from benign allergic proctocolitis to enteropathy and severe enterocolitis.

Table 6.1 Presentations of Delayed Food Allergy.

	FPIAP	FPE	FPIES (Acute)
Age of onset	Days to 6 mth	2 to 24 mth	Days to 1 yr
Clinical Presentation	Intermittent bloody stools in otherwise healthy, thriving infants	Chronic/ intermittent diarrhoea/ vomiting/ constipation, faltering growth	Profuse vomiting, pallor, ± lethargy 1–4 hr post food ingestion. May have diarrhoea 5–10 hr post ingestion. 15–20% present in acute shock
Most common triggers	Cow's milk/ soy through breastmilk or direct ingestion	Cow's milk, soy, egg, wheat	Cow's milk, soy, rice, wheat, fish

FPIAP: food protein-induced allergic proctocolitis; FPE: food protein-induced enteropathy; FPIES: food protein-induced enterocolitis syndrome.

The diagnosis of delayed food allergy is based on:

1. Exclusion of other differentials (e.g. infections, gastrointestinal disorders amongst others).
2. Compatible history suggesting a temporal relationship between new food introduction and a delayed onset of symptoms.
3. Trial of strict dietary elimination of the suspect food allergen (under guidance of physician and dietitian), resulting in resolution of symptoms.
4. Recurrence of symptoms with allergen re-introduction.

Management includes dietary elimination of the offending food, nutritional counselling and support, and regular re-assessments. Treatment of acute FPIES (which may mimic anaphylaxis or septic shock) is aggressive fluid resuscitation. Intra-muscular adrenaline has no role in the treatment of acute FPIES.

The prognosis of FPIAP is good, with most infants achieving tolerance before 1 year of age. The long-term prognosis of the rest of delayed food allergies is also generally good, with most resolving in early childhood.

Bibliography

1. Sicherer SH, Sampson HA. (2018) Food allergy: A review and update on epidemiology, pathogenesis, diagnosis, prevention, and management. *J Allergy Clin Immunol* **141**(1):41–58.
2. Caubet JC, Szajewska H, Shamir R, Nowak-Węgrzyn A. (2017) Non-IgE-mediated gastrointestinal food allergies in children. *Pediatr Allergy Immunol* **28**(1):6–17.

CHAPTER 21

Drug Allergy

Tan Liling, Lynette; Loh Wenyin

Introduction

An adverse drug reaction (ADR) is defined as any noxious, unintended and undesired effect of a drug that occurs at doses used for prevention, diagnosis or treatment.

Drug hypersensitivity reactions (DHRs) are adverse effects of drugs that clinically resemble allergic reactions. Drug allergies are DHRs for which a definite immunological mechanism is demonstrated.

True DHR is uncommon in the paediatric population. Childhood viral exanthems are often misinterpreted as DHR to various medications, such as antipyretics and antibiotics. It is important to confirm the diagnosis of DHR because reported antibiotic allergies are associated with increased use of broad-spectrum antibiotics, longer hospital stays and increased healthcare costs.

Evaluation

The goals of evaluation are either to confirm the diagnosis of a DHR and find a safe alternative or to confirm tolerance to the drug and exclude a DHR. A thorough history is essential in the evaluation of patients with suspected drug allergies.

If a drug-induced allergic reaction is suspected, it is important to distinguish between immediate (<1 hour; sometimes up to 6 hours) and non-immediate (>1 hour) reactions in order to decide on subsequent tests and management.

A useful test for detecting IgE-mediated drug reactions caused by large-molecular-weight biologicals and penicillin is the immediate hypersensitivity skin test. A positive skin prick test (SPT) or intradermal test (IDT) strongly suggests DHR in the presence of clinical reaction. A negative skin test, however, does not exclude DHR, and the patient would benefit from a drug provocation test to confirm diagnosis.

Drug provocation tests (DPTs) remain the gold standard for diagnosis of DHR. DPTs should not be performed if the reaction history is consistent with a severe non-IgE-mediated reaction (e.g. SJS/TEN, DRESS, hepatitis, haemolytic anaemia).

Management

Management would depend on the severity of the reaction. In cases of severe reactions and absence of confirmatory tests, implicated drugs must be avoided.

Table 6.2 Classification of ADRs

Type	Immune Response	Pathophysiology	Clinical Symptoms	Typical chronology
I	IgE	Mast cell and basophil degranulation	Urticaria Angioedema Anaphylaxis	Within 1–6 h after the last intake
II	IgG and complement	IgG and complement-dependent cytotoxicity	Cytopenia	5–15 d after the start
III	IgM or IgG and complement or FcR	Deposition of immune complexes	Serum sickness Urticaria Vasculitis	7–8 d after the start for serum sickness or urticaria 7–21 d after the start for vasculitis
IVa	Th1	Monocytic inflammation	Eczema	1–21 d after the start
IVb	Th2	Eosinophilic inflammation	MPE DRESS	1 to several days after the start for MPE 2–6 wk after the start for DRESS
IVc	Cytotoxic T cells	Keratinocyte death mediated by CD4 or CD8	MPE SJS/TENS Pustular exanthema	4–28 d after the start for SJS/TENS
IVd	T cells	Neutrophilic inflammation	AGEP	1–2 d after the start

MPE: maculopapular exanthema; DRESS: drug rash with eosinophilia and systemic symptoms; SJS: Stevens-Johnson syndrome; TENS: Toxic epidermal necrolysis; AGEP: acute generalised exanthematous pustulosis

Beta-Lactam Hypersensitivity

Beta-lactam antibiotics include penicillin, cephalosporin, carbapenems (e.g. meropenem) and monobactam (e.g. aztreonam). They are the most common cause of drug hypersensitivity reactions in the paediatric population. Clinical history is not reliable as a diagnostic tool, and DPTs remain the gold standard for confirmation or exclusion of beta-lactam hypersensitivity (Figure 6.3). Studies have shown that 90% of children with suspected beta-lactam hypersensitivity do not react at DPT.

Immediate-reading of skin tests (SPT & IDT) may be useful for the evaluation of immediate reactions and delayed-reading of skin tests may be performed for evaluation of non-immediate reactions. However, owing to the low sensitivity of the tests, DPTs may sometimes be performed without prior skin tests, particularly in low risk patients, i.e. mild skin reactions. There is increasing data that this simplified approach is safe in selected patients.

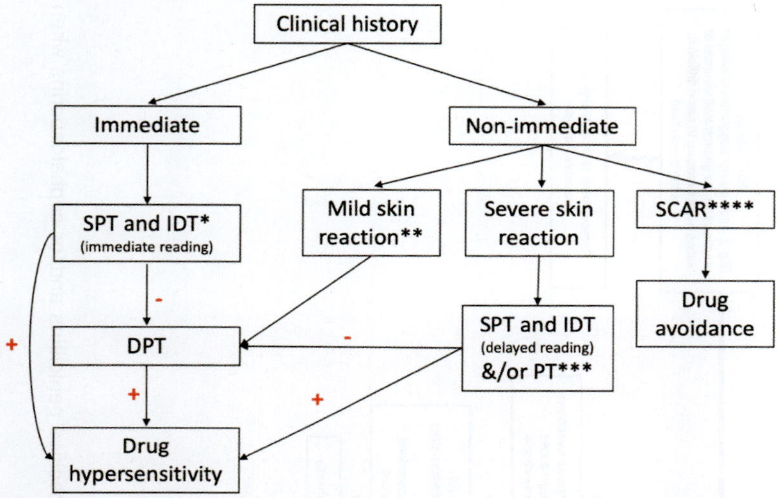

Figure 6.3 Algorithm for the diagnosis of hypersensitivity reactions to beta-lactam antibiotics.

SPT: skin prick test; IDT: intradermal test; DPT: drug provocation test; PT: patch test; SCAR: severe cutaneous adverse reaction such as Stevens–Johnson syndrome, toxic epidermal necrolysis, drug reaction with eosinophilia and systemic symptoms and acute generalised exanthematous pustulosis.

***In vitro* tests (e.g. specific IgE assay) can be considered if skin tests are not possible. However, sensitivity may vary depending on various factors and is generally lower than skin tests.

**Mild maculopapular exanthemas (more or less widespread rash; <1 week duration) or delayed urticaria

***PT is the investigation of choice in contact dermatitis; they may also be useful in maculopapular exanthemas, flexural exanthemas and fixed drug eruptions.

****Skin testing (PT followed by delayed reading IDT) can be considered to evaluate culprit amongst several used drugs.

While various components of beta-lactams are all potentially immunogenic, cross-reactivity related to the common beta-lactam ring is rare in subjects with an IgE-mediated hypersensitivity and rarely described in those with T-cell mediated hypersensitivity. More frequently, cross-reactivity amongst beta-lactams is related to structural similarities amongst their side chain structures. Studies have shown that in patients with IgE-mediated penicillin allergy, cross-reactivity with similar side chain cephalosporin may be as high as 33.3%, whereas cross-reactivity with different side chain cephalosporins was <0.2%. Also, <1% of patients with IgE-mediated penicillin allergy cross-react with carbapenems and monobactam. This suggests that confirmed allergy to a particular drug does not necessarily extend to avoidance of all beta-lactams and further evaluation is strongly recommended.

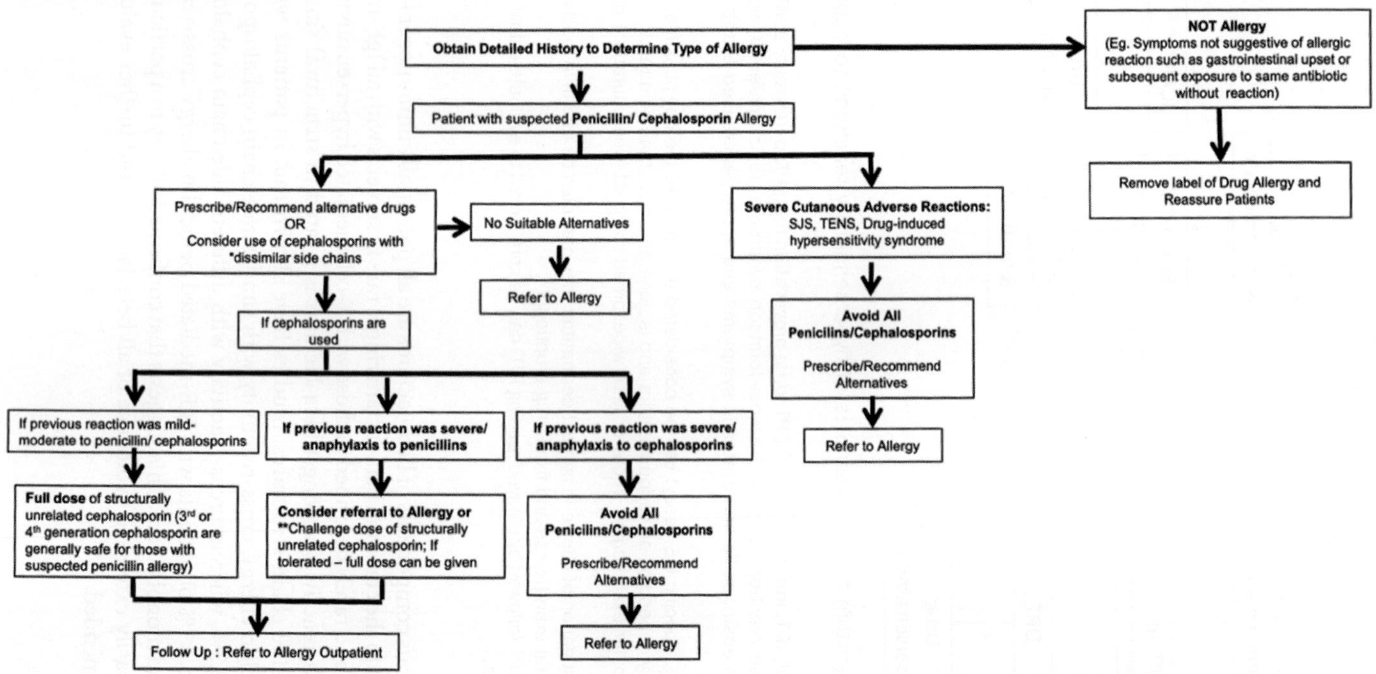

Figure 6.4 Algorithm for patients with histories of hypersensitivity reactions to specified penicillins and/or cephalosporins when immediate referral to an allergist is not feasible.

NSAID Hypersensitivity

Non-steroidal anti-inflammatory drug (NSAID) hypersensitivity can be immune-mediated or as a result of cyclooxygenase (COX) inhibition. A drug provocation test is needed to confirm the diagnosis regardless of the underlying mechanism.

Seven per cent of patients with NSAID hypersensitivity also react to paracetamol.

Patients with cross-reactive NSAID and paracetamol hypersensitivity may benefit from a drug provocation test to a selective COX-2 inhibitor, e.g. celecoxib, etoricoxib.

Perioperative Immediate Hypersensitivity Reactions

Perioperative immediate hypersensitivity reactions (POH) are one of the most complex clinical problems in the evaluation of drug allergy. The combination of the surgical procedure, simultaneous administration of several drugs and numerous differential diagnoses often make determining the trigger(s) very challenging. Perioperative anaphylaxis in the paediatric population range from 1 in 2100 to 1 in 37000. Neuromuscular blocking agents and antibiotics are often reported as the most common causes of POH. Locally, the incidence of perioperative anaphylaxis is 1 in 2500 with the most common identified trigger being antibiotics. The clinical presentation of POH can vary from mild cutaneous symptoms to life-threatening anaphylaxis. Identifying the culprit drug and finding safe alternatives are imperative for safe future anaesthesia and require a systematic approach by both allergists and anaesthetists with investigations performed in a timely manner. Complete evaluation should include measurement of the dynamic tryptase to diagnose perioperative anaphylaxis as well as skin tests (SPT, IDT) to identify the triggering drug and safe alternatives. Drug provocation tests may be performed if skin tests are negative. Skin tests in patients without a history of a drug reaction are not recommended.

Biblography

1. Demoly P, Adkinson NF, Brockow K, *et al.* (2014) International consensus on drug allergy. *Allergy* **69**:420–437.
2. Gomes ER, Brockow K, Kuyucu S, *et al.* (2016) Drug hypersensitivity in children: Report from the pediatric task force of the EAACI Drug Allergy Interest Group. *Allergy* **71**:149–161.
3. Romano A, Atanaskovic-Markovic M, Barbaud A, *et al.* (2020) Towards a more precise diagnosis of hypersensitivity to beta-lactams-an EAACI position paper. *Allergy* **75**:1300–1315.
4. Goh SH, Chong KW, Chiang WC, *et al.* (2021) Outcome of drug provocation testing in children with suspected beta-lactam hypersensitivity. *Asia Pac Allergy* **11**(1):e3.
5. Borges MS. (2010) NSAID hypersensitivity (respiratory, cutaneous and generalised anaphylactic symptoms). *Med Clin N Am* **94:**853–864.
6. Harper NJN, Cook TM, Garcez T, *et al.* (2018) Anaesthesia, surgery, and life-threatening allergic reactions: Epidemiology and clinical features of perioperative anaphylaxis in the 6th National Audit Project (NAP6). *Br J Anaesth* **121**:159–171.
7. Toh T, Foo SY, Loh W, *et al.* (2021) Perioperative anaphylaxis: A five-year review in a tertiary paediatric hospital. *Anaesth Intensive Care* **49**:44–51.

CHAPTER 22

Urticaria

Lee May Ping, Samantha; Ong Lin Xin

Introduction

Urticaria is a condition characterised by the development of wheals (hives), angioedema or both.

Wheal (hive) consists of three typical features:

- A superficial central swelling of variable size and shape, surrounded by reflex erythema
- An itching or sometimes burning sensation
- A fleeting nature, with the skin returning to its normal appearance, usually within 30 minutes to 24 hours

Angioedema is characterised by:

- A sudden, pronounced swelling of the lower dermis and subcutis or mucous membranes
- Tingling, burning, tightness and sometimes painful, rather than itchy
- Slower resolution than that of wheals (can take up to 72 hours)

Acute Urticaria

The most common cause of acute urticaria in children is infection (especially viral), followed by food allergy, drug allergy or idiopathic/spontaneous. Other possible causes include insect stings, latex allergy, plant or animal contacts. Acute urticaria is usually self-limiting. Diagnosis can be made from a detailed clinical history and physical examination and does not usually require any investigations. The only exception is when it is due to IgE-mediated food or drug allergy, where referral to an allergist for further work up is necessary.

Table 6.3 Classification of Urticaria

Types	Definition
ACUTE	Appearance of wheals, angioedema or both, for ≤6 wk duration
CHRONIC	Appearance of wheals, angioedema or both, daily or most days of the week, for > 6 wk duration

Chronic Urticaria

Chronic urticaria typically occurs spontaneously and the cause is usually unknown. It is self-limiting but may persist for many years in some children. Further investigations are usually not necessary and should only be reserved for those with protracted or refractory disease. All patients with chronic urticaria should be followed up by an allergist or dermatologist.

Differential Diagnoses of Chronic Urticaria

- Only wheals (hives):
  - » Urticarial vasculitis
  - » Cutaneous mastocytosis
  - » Autoimmune conditions (i.e. systemic lupus erythematosus, systemic onset juvenile idiopathic arthritis)
  - » Autoinflammatory syndromes (i.e. Schnitzler's syndrome, Cryopyrin-associated periodic syndrome)
- Only angioedema:
  - » Hereditary angioedema (HAE)
  - » ACE-inhibitor induced angioedema

  Note: To rule out other medical causes of oedema (i.e. cardiovascular/renal/hepatic/lymphatic/malnutrition).

Management

The management of urticaria consists of two important approaches. First, the identification and elimination of the underlying causes and avoidance of eliciting triggers (if any). Second, treatment is aimed at providing symptomatic relief. The recommended first-line treatment is with second generation, non-sedating H_1-antihistamines (i.e. cetirizine, levocetirizine, desloratadine, loratadine, fexofenadine, rupatadine, bilastine). Higher

Table 6.4 Chronic Urticaria Subtypes

Chronic Urticaria Subtypes	
Chronic Spontaneous Urticaria (CSU)	**Chronic Inducible Urticaria (CIndU)**
• Spontaneous appearance of wheals, angioedema or both for ≤6 wk due to unknown cause	• Appearance of wheals, angioedema or both for > 6 wk, induced by physical stimuli » Symptomatic dermographism* » Cholinergic urticaria » Delayed pressure urticaria » Heat urticaria » Cold urticaria » Solar urticaria » Vibratory angioedema » Aquagenic urticaria • Can coexist with chronic spontaneous urticaria **commonest cause of CIndU in children*

doses (up to four-fold of standard dosing) and a prolonged course of antihistamines are often required in children with chronic urticaria. Other treatment options such as montelukast, omalizumab and ligelizumab or ciclosporin may be considered in patients with refractory chronic urticaria. At present, there is no role for oral corticosteroids in the management of urticaria and is not recommended except for acute severe exacerbation of chronic urticaria.

Bibliography

1. Zuberbier T, Abdul Latiff AH, Abuzakouk M, *et al.* (2021) The international EAACI/GA²LEN/EuroGuiDerm/APAAACI guideline for the definition, classification, diagnosis, and management of urticaria. *Allergy* **77**(3):734–766.
2. Cornillier H, Giraudeau B, Munck S, *et al.* (2018) Chronic spontaneous urticaria in children — a systematic review on interventions and comorbidities. *Pediatr Allergy Immunol* **29**(3):303–310.
3. Katelaris CH, *et al.* (2019) Position paper — chronic spontaneous urticaria. Australasian Society of Clinical Immunology & Allergy.
4. Khakoo G, *et al.* (2008) Clinical features and natural history of physical urticaria in children. *Pediatr Allergy Immunol* **19**(4):363–366.

CHAPTER 23

Primary Immunodeficiencies (Inborn Errors of Immunity)

Chan Su-Wan, Bianca; Liew Woei Kang

Introduction

Primary Immunodeficiencies (PIDs), now known as Inborn Errors of Immunity (IEI), are a heterogeneous group of more than 400 distinct disorders that impair the normal functioning of the immune system. IEI most commonly manifest as an increased susceptibility to infectious diseases, but they can also present with autoimmunity, autoinflammation, allergies or malignancies. Whilst most IEI are individually rare, they are collectively more common than generally thought, with an estimated prevalence of 1 in every 1200 to 2000 individuals. Most IEI have a well-defined genetic cause, and new genetic disorders causing immune defects are discovered each year.

IEI can be classified into the following 10 groups based on the International Union of Immunological Societies (IUIS) Classification.

Table 6.5 Classification of Inborn Errors of Immunity

International Union of Immunological Societies (IUIS) Classification		
Group		Example
1	Combined immunodeficiencies (CID)	Severe combined immunodeficiency (SCID)
2	Combined immunodeficiencies with syndromic features	Wiskott Aldrich Syndrome (WAS)
3	Predominantly antibody deficiencies	Bruton's Agammaglobulinaemia
4	Diseases of immune dysregulation	Familial haemophagocytic lymphohistiocytosis
5	Congenital defects of phagocytes	Chronic Granulomatous Disease (CGD)
6	Defects in intrinsic and innate immunity	Mendelian Susceptibility to Mycobacterial Disease (MSMD)
7	Autoinflammatory diseases	Familial Mediterranean Fever
8	Complement deficiencies	Properdin deficiency
9	Bone marrow failure	Dyskeratosis Congenita
10	Phenocopies of inborn errors of immunity	Thymoma with hypogammaglobulinemia (Good syndrome)

When to Evaluate for Inborn Errors of Immunity?

Although healthy children may have frequent, monthly self-limiting upper respiratory tract infections each year, children with uncharacteristically recurrent, severe or unusual infections should be evaluated for an underlying IEI.

Common presentations include:

- Recurrent bacterial sinopulmonary infections → antibody deficiency
- Invasive infections, poor wound healing → phagocyte defects
- Severe or disseminated mycobacterial infection → MSMD, CGD, SCID
- Severe fungal or viral infections → SCID, combined immunodeficiency
- Recurrent, severe or unusual herpesvirus infection → NK cell defect
- Severe *Neisseria* infection → complement defect
- Chronic mucocutaneous candidiasis → STAT1 or IL17 pathway defect

Red Flags for Inborn Errors of Immunity

(Adapted from Jeffery Modell Foundation: 10 Warning signs of PID)

Table 6.6 Red Flags for Inborn Errors of Immunity

1	Family history	Positive for early unexplained death, recurrent or severe infections, or specific immunodeficiency diagnoses. Consanguinity, autoimmunity.
2	Frequent infections	Elevated frequency of documented infections including •Four or more new ear infections within 1 yr. •Two or more serious sinus infections within 1 yr. •Two or more pneumonias within 1 yr.
3	Chronic infection	Persistent sinusitis, otitis media, bronchiectasis, recurrent abscess
4	Severe infection	Bacteraemia, osteomyelitis, meningitis, especially if recurrent
5	Complications of infection	Cerebral abscess complicating sinusitis, acute respiratory distress syndrome from common respiratory viruses
6	Site of infection	Unusual sites, e.g. liver or brain abscess
7	Infecting organism	Opportunistic, recurrent or unusual pathogens, e.g. *Aspergillus, Serratia, Nocardia, Burkholderia cepacia*, post-natal severe cytomegalovirus (CMV) infection, disseminated mycobacterium infection
8	Response to therapy	Poor response or recurring infection after antimicrobial discontinuation or needing IV antibiotics to clear infection
9	Other signs	Failure to thrive, severe dermatitis, recurrent diarrhoea with or without colitis, autoimmunity

Children with IEI can also present with non-infectious issues:

- Very early onset inflammatory bowel disease (IBD) (<6 years old)
- Severe eczema (neonatal onset, resistant to therapy, complicated by severe infection)
- Dermatologic manifestations (ectodermal dysplasia, neutrophilic pustular dermatosis, cutaneous granulomas, abnormal skin/hair pigmentation, cold-induced urticaria)
- Early onset autoimmune diseases
- Early onset endocrinopathies
- Haemophagocytic lymphohistiocytosis
- Lymphoproliferative disorders
- Syndromic features (skeletal dysplasia, DiGeorge, ataxia, developmental delay)
- Pulmonary manifestations (pulmonary alveolar proteinosis, pulmonary capillaritis)

How to Evaluate for Inborn Errors of Immunity?

The selection of immunologic tests must be guided by clinical suspicion based on a thorough history and physical examination. A good infection history including sites and microorganisms involved and treatment required, as well as a detailed family history of early childhood deaths, severe infections, autoimmunity and involvement of male relatives, should be obtained. Previous medical records, growth charts and blood counts should be reviewed. A full blood count with differential, immunoglobulin IgG, IgA, IgM and IgE levels, and a human immunodeficiency virus (HIV) screen to rule out secondary causes, would be the first step in the immune evaluation and would help guide subsequent testing.

Table 6.7 Immune Testing

	Quantity	Function	Pattern of Illness
Antibody defects [e.g. X-linked Bruton's Agammaglobulinaemia, Common Variable Immunodeficiency (CVID)] *also check for asplenia	• B lymphocyte number (CD19 or CD20) • Naïve/Memory B cells • Immunoglobulin levels (IgG, IgA, IgM, IgE) • IgG subclass levels	• Class-switching IgM → IgG, IgA • Specific antibodies - to vaccines (e.g. Tetanus, HiB, Pneumococcal, Measles, Varicella) - to previous infections	• Sinopulmonary infection (pyogenic, encapsulated bacteria) • Severe gastrointestinal (Enteroviruses, *Giardia lamblia*) • Autoimmunity (cytopenia, IBD)
Cell-mediated immunity e.g. DiGeorge *also check HIV serology	• Absolute Lymphocyte Counts • T-cell lymphocyte subsets: Total CD3, Helper CD4, Cytotoxic CD8 • Naïve (CD45RA) and Memory (CD45RO) T cells	• Lymphocyte proliferation to mitogens — Phytohaemagglutinin (PHA), Concavalin A (ConA), Anti-CD3 + Anti-CD28	• Pneumonia/ Pneumonitis (pyogenic bacteria, fungi, mycobacteria viruses) • Severe viral infections (CMV) • Gastroenteritis (viruses, *Giardia sp.*) • Dermatitis

Table 6.7 (*Continued*)

	Quantity	Function	Pattern of Illness
Combined Antibody and Cell-mediated immunity, e.g. • Severe Combined Immunodeficiency - Adenosine deaminase deficiency (ADA) SCID • CID with syndromes - Wiskott Aldrich - Hyper-IgM (CD40L deficiency)	• Immunoglobulin levels (IgG, IgA, IgM, IgE) • Full Lymphocyte subsets T: CD3, CD4, CD8 B: CD19 or CD20 NK: CD56 + CD16	• Lymphocyte proliferation to mitogens — Phytohemagglutinin (PHA), Concavalin A (ConA), Anti-CD3 + Anti-CD28 • Specific antibodies to vaccines and previous infections • ADA enzyme • WAS protein (flow) • CD40 Ligand (flow)	• Pneumonia/Pneumonitis (pyogenic bacteria, fungi, mycobacteria, viruses) • Gastroenteritis (viruses, *Giardia sp. Cryptosporidium sp.*) • Disseminated mycobacterium (TB, BCG, NTM) • Severe fungal infections (*Pneumocystis jirovecii*) • Severe viral infections (CMV) • Failure to thrive • Dermatitis
Phagocytes defect, e.g. Chronic granulomatous disease (CGD) Leukocyte Adhesion Defect (LAD) Congenital Neutropenia	• Absolute neutrophil count trends	• Neutrophil oxidation - Nitroblue Tetrazolium (NBT) Test (boys) - Dihydrorhodamine (DHR) (both boys and girls, carriers, AR CGD)	• Atypical/disseminated mycobacteria • *Aspergillus, Nocardia* and catalase-positive organisms • Recurrent skin abscesses • IBD/perianal abscesses (CGD)
Complement, e.g. Final common pathway complement defect, C4 deficiency Hereditary angioedema	• Complements C3, C4 • Individual component assays • C1 inhibitor levels	• Total serum haemolytic complement assay (CH50) • Alternative pathway assays (AH50) • Mannose Binding Lectin level	• Bacterial sepsis (pyogenic infection, esp. encapsulated bacterial infections, e.g. *Neisseria sp.*) • Autoimmune disease (Systemic lupus erythematosus, Glomerulonephritis) • Recurrent angioedema with no urticaria
Innate immunity defect, e.g. IL12–IFNγ pathway defect (MSMD)	• IFN-gamma (IFNγ) Receptor expression (CD119)	• MSMD (IL12–IFNγ) cytokine assay • STAT1 phosphorylation assay	• Disseminated mycobacterium, non-tuberculous mycobacterial infection • Salmonella disease
Asplenia or Hyposplenia, e.g. sickle cell anaemia	• Ultrasound Abdomen • Haemoglobin electrophoresis (HbSS)	• Peripheral blood smear for Howell–Jollybodies	• Sepsis with encapsulated bacteria

Genetic Testing for Disease Confirmation/Search for Cause of Immune Abnormalities

1. Next Generation Sequencing using PID Panels — higher sensitivity for targeted genes
2. Whole Exome/Whole Genome Sequencing — more comprehensive if gene unknown

Important Considerations — Possible Secondary Causes of Immune Deficiency to Exclude

1. Medications (e.g. anti-epileptic, chemotherapeutic, immune-modulatory, steroids)
2. Physiologic losses of immunoglobulins/lymphocytes (e.g. enteropathy, chylothorax)

3. Nutritional deficits and excess, physiologic and psychosocial stress
4. Infection-induced immune suppression (HIV, CMV, sepsis)
5. Anatomical abnormalities (e.g. congenital lung defects, perianal fistulas, ciliary dyskinesia)
6. Atopy, breakdown of skin/mucosal barriers (e.g. poorly controlled eczema, indwelling catheters)
7. Prematurity
8. Other underlying disease conditions

Approach to Recurrent Infections

1. **Recurrent lower respiratory tract infections or bronchiectasis**
    a. Consider impaired respiratory barrier like cystic fibrosis, primary ciliary dyskinesia, congenital cystic adenomatoid malformation (CCAM)
    b. Aspiration pneumonia/gastroesophageal reflux (GER)/swallowing dysfunction
    c. Asthma
    d. Chronic bacteria bronchitis
    e. Inborn Error of Immunity:
        i. Antibody defect, Phagocytic defect, Hyper-IgE syndrome, Combined immunodeficiency, complement deficiency
    f. Immunology Tests:
        i. FBC, Immunoglobulins IgG, IgA, IgM, IgE, Complements C3, C4, CH50
        ii. Vaccine antibodies
        iii. T/B/NK lymphocyte subsets if viral/fungal/tuberculosis (TB)
2. **Recurrent skin abscesses**
    a. Consider impaired skin barrier like atopic dermatitis, ichthyosis, burns, percutaneous catheter
    b. If perianal abscess, consider perianal fistula of Crohn's disease, perianal dermatitis from allergic enteropathy
    c. *Staphylococcus aureus* skin colonisation and auto-inoculation
    d. Inborn Errors of Immunity:
        i. Phagocytes disorders, e.g. Congenital neutropenia, chronic granulomatous disease, leukocyte adhesion defect, Hyper-IgE syndrome, T cell lymphopenia
    e. Immunology Tests:
        i. FBC, Immunoglobulins IgG, IgA, IgM, IgE, Neutrophil oxidation test, e.g. NBT/DHR, nasal/skin swab culture, T Lymphocyte subsets

Important Inborn Errors of Immunity

1. **Bruton's Agammaglobulinaemia (X-linked Agammaglobulinaemia)**
    a. Males, Xq21.3–22, familial
    b. Recurrent sinopulmonary infections, bronchiectasis
    c. Bacteria (*Streptococcus, Pseudomonas*), Severe Enterovirus

d. No palpable lymph nodes or tonsillar tissues
e. Immunology tests
i. All Immunoglobulin classes < 2SDs for age
ii. Lymphocyte subsets < 2% CD19 or CD20 B cells
iii. Absent isohaemagglutinins, poor response to vaccines
iv. Genetics — mutations in BTK tyrosine kinase
f. Treatment with lifelong immunoglobulin replacement

2. Severe Combined Immunodeficiency (SCID)
a. Paediatric Emergency
b. Early presentation — average age at diagnosis <6 months old
c. Family history of early infant death from infections
d. Most frequent manifestations:
i. Interstitial pneumonitis — common respiratory viruses/CMV/ *pneumocystis* pneumonia (PCP)
ii. Disseminated *Mycobacterium bovis* infection
iii. Oral candidiasis
iv. Persistent diarrhoea
v. Failure to thrive
e. Immunology tests
i. Immunoglobulin classes < 2SDs for age
ii. Absent or very low T Lymphocyte subsets CD 3 < 300
iii. Severely reduced T-cell Receptor Excision Circles (TREC) and Naïve T cells
iv. B and NK lymphocyte subsets affected depending on SCID genetics
v. Lymphocyte proliferation to mitogens less than 10% healthy control
vi. Genetics → 15 known SCID gene mutations
f. Definitive treatment by haematopoietic stem cell transplant or gene therapy

3. Chronic Granulomatous disease
a. Hallmark is early onset of severe recurrent bacterial and fungal infections
b. Skin infections; pneumonia/lung abscesses; suppurative lymphadenitis; diarrhoea secondary to colitis; perianal or perirectal abscesses; hepatic or splenic abscesses; osteomyelitis, septicaemia
c. Catalase positive organism: *Staphylococcus aureus, Burkholderia cepacia, Aspergillus sp, Nocardia sp* and *Serratia marcescens*
d. Development of non-infective granulomas in the skin, lung, gastrointestinal or genitourinary tract
e. Immunology tests
i. Neutrophil oxidation tests — NBT or DHR
ii. Genetics — X-linked, Autosomal recessive subtypes
f. Treatment by haematopoietic stem cell transplant, interferon gamma, fungal/TB prophylaxis

Principles of Management of IEI

1. Treat active infection — obtain samples for microbiology, culture-directed antimicrobials
2. Prevent new infections — prophylactic antibiotics, vaccinations, environmental preventive measures, intravenous immunoglobulin (IVIG), if needed
3. Replace deficient components, if possible — IVIG, enzyme replacement for ADA
4. Immunomodulation of inflammation with small molecule inhibitors (e.g. JAK inhibitors), biologics (e.g. Rituximab) or immunosuppressive medications (e.g. steroids)
5. Haemotopoietic Stem Cell Transplant if curative (may not resolve non-haematopoietic involvement of gastrointestinal tract, skin, etc.)

Bibliography

1. Chinn IK, Orange JS. (2019) Immunodeficiency disorders. *Pediatr Rev* **40**(5) 229-242.
2. Tangye SG, Al-Herz W, Bousfiha A, *et al.* (2020) Human inborn errors of immunity: 2019 update on the Classification from the International Union of Immunological Societies Expert Committee. *J Clin Immunol* **40**:24–64.

SECTION 7

CARDIOLOGY

CHAPTER 24

Chest Pain

Tan Teng Hong

Introduction

Chest pain in children is least likely to be cardiac in origin, and often idiopathic (23–45%). It is also rarely associated with life-threatening disease in the paediatric population.

Patients younger than 12 years are more likely to have a cardiorespiratory aetiology of their chest pain compared with older children, who are more likely to have a psychogenic cause. Female patients are more likely to be diagnosed with psychogenic chest pain or costochondritis. Recurrent symptoms occur in 45–69% of patients; up to 19% may have symptoms lasting for >3 years.

History

Table 7.1 Pertinent History in Paediatric Chest Pain

Nature of chest pain	Time of onset and events leading to onset of pain, duration, frequency, nature, intensity, location, radiation, precipitating and relieving factors (including relationship to meals and posture), impact of pain on child's lifestyle and activity level, history of trauma.
Systems assessment	Symptoms of chronic disease, e.g. fever, malaise, fatigue, weight loss, night sweats.
Past medical and surgical history	In particular, any cardiac surgery or disease; previous evaluation, treatment and diagnoses in patients with recurrent chest pain.
Medications	
Family history	In particular of syncope, sudden death or cardiovascular disease.
Social history	Smoking, alcohol or illicit drugs, recent family or peer problems, school performance, including sports and physical fitness, etc.

Physical Examination

A thorough and complete physical examination is fundamental to an accurate diagnosis of chest pain. In particular:

- Vital signs including blood pressure (BP)
- General appearance, i.e. cyanotic, distressed, anxious, sweaty, poor perfusion
- Evidence of trauma (e.g. bruising)
- Rash or joint swelling (collagen vascular disease)

- Abnormal breast enlargement, gynaecomastia in males
- Localised chest swelling or tenderness
- Cardiac findings (abnormal heart sounds, arrhythmias, murmurs, muffled heart sounds, pericardial rub)
- Respiratory findings (depth and rate of breathing, retractions, rhonchi, crepitations, decreased breath sounds, bronchial breathing or pleural rub)
- Abdominal examination (hepatomegaly, tenderness)
- Femoral pulses
- Extremities (temperature, cyanosis, clubbing, oedema)
- Psychological state

Red Flags — Signs and Symptoms

Table 7.2 Red Flags in Chest Pain

Cardiac	• Underlying congenital or acquired heart disease • Arrhythmias • Crushing sternal chest pain with or without radiation to left arm or neck • Exercise-induced chest pain • Persistent tachycardia • Persistent hypertension • Hypotension • Gallop rhythm • Syncope
Respiratory	• Haemoptysis • Dyspnoea • Rales • Cyanosis
Gastrointestinal	• Haematemesis • Haematochezia • Melaena
Others	• Febrile • Life-threatening psychiatric illness, e.g. psychosis or suicidal ideation

Differential Diagnoses

1. Musculoskeletal (very common in paediatric patients; pain is sharp, nagging and localised but may radiate)
    - Costochondritis — mild to severe, localised, reproducible on palpation and coughing; may have a history of recent upper respiratory tract infection (URTI)
    - Muscle strain
    - Trauma
    - Non-accidental injury (child abuse) — especially in younger children
    - Fibromyalgia — pain is continuous and lasts longer than 3 months; tenderness may be elicited over multiple points

- Precordial Catch or Texidor's Twinge — sharp pain occurring at rest, usually over the cardiac apex or left lower sternal edge; short duration; frequency varies; worsens on deep inspiration
- Tietze's Syndrome — observed after minor trauma; localised, moderate and associated with visible swelling; swelling may remit and recur; associated with an elevated Erythrocyte Sedimentation Rate (ESR)
- Slipping Rib Syndrome — occurs when the eighth, ninth or tenth rib overrides the rib above; onset sudden, may radiate to chest or abdomen
- Xiphoid-Cartilage Syndrome — occurs after vigorous running; pain or 'stitch' at insertion of xiphoid into the abdominal musculature; pressure on xiphoid may reproduce the pain
- Others: Tumours, connective tissue disorders, acute chest syndrome in sickle cell anaemia

2. Cardiac
   - Congenital heart disease, in particular:
     » Conditions with left ventricular outflow tract obstruction, e.g. aortic stenosis, hypertrophic cardiomyopathy (HCM)
     » Mitral valve prolapse — chest pain probably results from papillary muscle dysfunction and subendocardial ischaemia
     » Coronary artery anomalies
   - Acquired lesions — cardiomyopathy, endocarditis, myocarditis, acute myocardial infarction (AMI), rheumatic fever, accelerated atherosclerotic coronary artery disease, dissecting aneurysm, pericarditis, Kawasaki Disease
   - Arrhythmias — atrial fibrillation (AF), atrial flutter, supraventricular tachycardia (SVT), ventricular tachycardia (VT)
3. Respiratory
   - Pneumothorax
   - Pneumonia
   - Pleural effusion
   - Pulmonary embolism — especially in adolescent females on oral contraceptives
   - Foreign body inhalation
   - Chronic cough
   - Chronic pulmonary diseases, e.g. cystic fibrosis, chronic asthma (with exercise-induced symptoms)
4. Gastrointestinal
   - Oesophagitis
   - Mallory–Weiss tear
   - Gastroesophageal reflux
   - Hiatus hernia
   - Referred pain from gastritis, peptic ulcer disease, cholecystitis, pancreatitis
   - Foreign body ingestion
5. Psychogenic
   - Hyperventilation syndrome
   - Somatoform disorder
   - Stress

- Depression
- Panic attacks
- Munchausen syndrome

6. Others
   - Breast disease — puberty, menstruation, pregnancy, mastitis may cause pain in females
   - Mediastinal tumours
   - Sickle cell disease with vaso-occlusive crisis
   - Herpes zoster — intercostal neuralgia pain may occur days before appearance of vesicles
   - Cigarette-smoking (with or without chronic cough), cocaine use (palpitations, coronary vasospasm, AMI, caffeine overdose, accidental ingestion or inhaled mercury vapour and trichloroethane aerosol)

Major Threats to Life

- Myocardial ischaemia or infarction
- Pericarditis with tamponade
- Aortic dissection or rupture
- Pneumothorax, pneumomediastinum or pneumopericardium
- Pulmonary embolus
- Perforated or haemorrhaging peptic ulcer

Initial Investigations

- Electrocardiogram (ECG)
  - » Arrhythmias: SVTs, AF, atrial flutter, VTs
  - » Acute ischaemic changes: ST segment depression or elevation, symmetrical T wave inversion or tall, pointed, upright T waves; rarely Q waves
  - » HCM: Left or biventricular hypertrophy
  - » Pericarditis: Decreased QRS voltages, generalised ST segment elevation
- Chest radiograph (CXR)
  - » To exclude pulmonary causes of chest pain, e.g. pneumothorax, pneumonia, pleural effusion
  - » If pulmonary congestion or cardiomegaly present, a thorough cardiac workup is required
  - » Others: Rib abnormalities, fractures, markedly dilated aorta (aortic dissection in patient with Marfan syndrome)

Specific Investigations, If Indicated

- Cardiac: ECG, Holter monitor, exercise stress test, cardiac enzymes (CK, CKMB, Troponin)
- Pulmonary: Computed Tomography (CT) chest, Magnetic Resonance Imaging (MRI) chest, ventilation-perfusion (VQ) scan, lung function test with and without methacholine challenge, bronchoscopy

- Gastrointestinal: Endoscopy, pH probe, abdominal ultrasound, serum amylase, liver function test, upper gastrointestinal series
- Musculoskeletal: Skeletal radiographs, CT spine, MRI spine, nuclear bone scan

Indications for Admission

- Suspected coronary artery disease, pleural effusion, myocarditis, pericarditis or aortic dissection.
- Severe chest pain of unknown etiology.

Indications for Referral to Paediatric Cardiologist

- Severe recurrent chest pain
- Associated with sinister symptoms, e.g. syncope, abnormal heart rhythm (with or without exercise)
- Chest pain during and immediately after exercise, and not clearly musculoskeletal
- Suspicious of congenital or acquired heart disease
- Abnormal cardiovascular examination (e.g. murmur)
- Abnormal initial investigations (ECG, CXR)

Bibliography

1. Kocis KC. (1999) Chest pain in pediatrics. *Pediatr Clin N Am* **16**(2):189–203.
2. Strafford M. (1993) Chest pain. In: Schechter N, Berde CB, Yaster M (eds.) *Pain in Infants, Children and Adolescents*. Baltimore: Williams & Wilkins, pp. 571–586.
3. Pearson GD, Ingall CG, Dorosz JJ, Martin GR. (1998) Chest pain in an urban pediatric cardiology practice. *Am Pediatr Soc Soc Pediatr Res* **43**(4):25.
4. Coleman W. (1984) Recurrent chest pain in children. *Pediatr Clin N Am* **31**(5):1007–1026.
5. Gutgesell HP, Barst RJ, Humes RA, *et al.* (1997) Common cardiovascular problems in the young: Part 1. Murmurs, chest pain, syncope and irregular rhythms. *Am Fam Phys* **56**(7):1825–1830.
6. Selbst SM, Ruddy RM, Clark BJ. (1990) Chest pain in children. *Clin Pediatr* **29**(7):374–377.
7. Swenson JM, Fischer DR, Miller SA, et al. (1997) Are chest radiographs and ECGs still valuable in evaluating new pediatric patients with heart murmurs or chest pain? *Pediatrics* **99**(1):1–3.
8. Bass C. (1991) Unexplained chest pain and breathlessness. *Med Clin N Am* **755**:1157–1173.
9. Crain EF, Gershel JC, Cunningham SJ (nd) *Clinical Manual of Emergency Pediatrics*, Chp 2: Cardiac Emergencies.
10. Leung AKC, Robson WLM, Cho H. (1996) Chest pain in children. *Can Fam Phys* **42:**1156–1164.
11. Selbst SM. (1997) Consultation with the specialist: chest pain in children. *Pediatr Rev* **18**(5):169–173.
12. Brenner JI, Ringel RE, Berman MA. (1984) Cardiologic perspectives of chest pain in childhood: A referral problem? To whom? *Pediatr Clin N Am* **31**(6):1241–1258.

CHAPTER 25

Syncope

Chan Jiahui, Charmaine; Tan Teng Hong

Introduction

Syncope is defined as an abrupt, transient loss of consciousness with the inability to maintain postural tone, followed by a rapid and spontaneous complete recovery. It is presumed to be due to transient global cerebral hypoperfusion. It does not include seizures, shock, coma or other states of altered consciousness, which may be prolonged in duration or due to a mechanism other than cerebral hypoperfusion. Up to 15% of children experience at least one episode of syncope by the end of adolescence.

Thorough evaluation of syncope is warranted to establish the aetiology of syncope with enough confidence to provide a reliable assessment of prognosis, recurrence risk and treatment options. The workup of syncope includes a meticulous history, a detailed physical examination, an electrocardiogram (ECG), risk stratification and appropriately directed investigations.

The age of the patient gives clues to the most likely cause of syncope. Infants should always be aggressively investigated for the cause of syncope, while in adolescents, the most likely causes are vasovagal syncope or orthostatic hypotension.

Causes of Syncope

Life-Threatening Causes

1. Cardiac syncope
   - Most important cause of syncope to exclude.
   - Syncope due to bradycardia, tachycardia or hypotension from low cardiac output, blood flow obstruction, vasodilatation or acute vascular dissection.
   - Arrhythmias
     - Tachyarrhythmias: Wolff–Parkinson–White (WPW), catecholaminergic polymorphic ventricular tachycardia (VT), idiopathic VT/ventricular fibrillation (VF), arrhythmogenic right ventricular cardiomyopathy (ARVC)
     - Bradyarrhythmias: Atrioventricular (AV) conduction disorder, sinus node dysfunction
     - Ion channel abnormalities: Long QT syndrome (LQTS), Brugada syndrome
   - Structural heart disease
     - Coronary artery disease
     - Outflow tract obstruction: E.g. severe aortic stenosis, severe pulmonary stenosis

» Hypertrophic cardiomyopathy
» Dilated cardiomyopathy
» Myocarditis
» Aortic dissection
» Left atrial myxoma
» Prosthetic valve dysfunction
» Severe pulmonary hypertension

2. Heat stroke
3. Anaphylaxis

Reflex Syncope (Neutrally Mediated)

- This is due to increased parasympathetic and reduced sympathetic activity, causing *vasodilation, bradycardia* or both.
- In situations such as standing, venous pooling results in reduced venous return to the heart. The heart may compensate with vigorous cardiac contraction, and it is postulated that this results in increased vagal tone.

1. Vasovagal syncope ('common faint')
   - Most common cause of syncope in children.
   - Triggers can usually be identified, such as stress or pain.
   - Associated with sweating, pallor, nausea or warmth.
2. Situational syncope
   - Reflex syncope associated with a specific action, e.g. micturition, defecation, coughing, sneezing, post-exercise, post-prandial, weight lifting or playing brass instrument.
3. Carotid sinus syncope
   - Uncommon in children; due to carotid sinus hyperactivity, resulting in sinus pause and hypotension.

Orthostatic Hypotension

- Syncope from postural change, related to an abrupt drop in blood pressure (BP).
- Defined as a drop in systolic BP ≥20 mmHg or diastolic BP ≥10 mmHg when standing from a sitting or lying position.
- May be caused by volume depletion, anaemia, pregnancy, drugs (e.g. calcium channel blockers, vasodilators, diuretics).

Other Causes of Syncope

- Metabolic: Hypoglycaemia, hypocalcaemia, hypomagnesaemia, hypoxia, imbalances in the sodium, potassium or chloride levels.
- Drugs

Differential Diagnoses and Mimics for Syncope

- Breath-holding spells

- Neurology: Seizure, migraine
- Psychiatric: Conversion disorder, hyperventilation, malingering

History Taking

It is the most important tool for diagnosis and risk stratification in the evaluation of syncope. The patient, and any eye witnesses, should be asked about the event.

Presyncope: Make note of any prodrome (e.g. nausea, light-headedness, darkening of vision, palpitations, chest pain), triggers (e.g. pain, emotional stress), situations in which the syncope occurred (exercise-induced, postural-related, acute arousal or loud noise).

Syncope: Duration, circumstances of the event, whether there was total loss of consciousness, any seizure-like activity

Post-syncope: Symptoms such as fatigue, dizziness, urine or faecal incontinence, time to recovery

Background Medical History

- History of congenital heart disease or post-cardiac surgery, or primary arrhythmias
- History of syncope/near syncope; history of near drowning
- Metabolic disorder
- Medications/drugs
- Family history of sudden death, arrhythmias, congenital deafness, pacemakers, implantable cardioverter-defibrillators
- Need to consider conditions such as hypertrophic or dilated cardiomyopathies, long QT syndrome, Marfan syndrome, mitral valve prolapse, etc.

Physical Examination

- Vital signs — pulse rate and blood pressure, significant postural hypotension. Syncope and tachycardia on standing up is an indicator of orthostasis and volume depletion.
- Cardiovascular evaluation: Structural cardiac lesions or rhythm abnormalities. Note any clubbing or cyanosis.
- Full neurological evaluation.

Investigations

- Full blood count
- Renal panel and electrolytes, serum glucose
- Urine pregnancy test (female adolescents)

- Arterial blood gases if hypoxia suspected
- ECG — mandatory

Abnormal ECG Findings

Bradyarrhythmia with sinus pauses, high grade atrioventricular (AV) conduction block, ventricular tachyarrhythmia, prolonged QT, delta waves, signs of Brugada syndrome, Epsilon wave (characteristic of ARVC), signs of left ventricular hypertrophy (LVH), signs of right ventricular hypertrophy (RVH), signs of myocardial ischaemia.

Further Tests

If a cardiac cause is suspected, Holter monitoring, echocardiography, transtelephonic ECG, cardiac catheterisation and electrophysiological studies might be indicated. Exercise stress testing is indicated in exercise-induced syncope to exclude provocable ischaemia, chronotropic incompetence or ventricular tachycardia.

If a neurological cause is suspected, may require further investigations with electroencephalogram (EEG), neuroimaging. Psychiatric evaluation may be necessary for conversion disorder or hyperventilation.

Reflex syncope can be diagnosed quite confidently by history alone, with normal physical examination and ECG. Tilt table test may be done in cases of recurrent syncope where reflex syncope is suspected.

Management

Indications for Admission/Further Evaluation

- Red flags for cardiac cause of syncope (see Table 7.3)
- Persistent abnormal neurological findings
- Orthostatic hypotension with continued postural syncope that does not resolve with fluid therapy

Table 7.3 Characteristics with Increased Likelihood of Cardiac and Non-Cardiac Causes of Syncope

More likely cardiac cause	More likely non cardiac cause
Prodrome: Brief or none; complain of palpitations or chest pain	Prodrome: Lightheaded, feeling warm, nausea, darkening of vision
Triggers: Loud noise (LQTS)	Triggers: Pain, dehydration, micturition, defecation, cough, laugh
Syncope on exertion Syncope in supine position	Syncope only in standing position Syncope on positional change
History of cardiac condition	No history of cardiac condition
Abnormal cardiac examination/ECG	Normal cardiac examination/ECG
Positive family history of cardiac condition or sudden death (<50 yr old)	No significant family history

Management of Vasovagal Syncope

- Education about diagnosis, avoidance of triggers (e.g. crowded areas, dehydration), early identification of prodrome, manoeuvres to prevent syncope (e.g. leg crossing, squatting, handgrip and arm tensing)
- Ensure adequate fluid and salt intake
- Medications (seldom required):
  - I) Midodrine: A prodrug that is metabolised to desglymidodrine, a peripherally mediated alpha agonist, to ameliorate the reduction in peripheral sympathetic neural outflow responsible for venous pooling and vasodepression in vasovagal syncope. It is reasonable to be trialled in patients with recurrent vasovagal syncope with no history of hypertension, heart failure or urinary retention. (Class IIa recommendations.)
  - II) Fludrocortisone, beta blockers have not been shown to be effective in paediatric trials on treatment for vasovagal syncope.
  - III) Other drugs, e.g. disopyramide, theophylline, serotonin reuptake inhibitors have been tried.
- Cardiac pacing — has been used in patients with malignant neurocardiogenic syncope (recurrent syncope with significant injury or drug refractory syncope) and documented spontaneous cardio-inhibitory response during monitoring.

Postural Orthostatic Tachycardia Syndrome (POTS)

- This is a clinical syndrome characterised by all of the following:
  1) Frequent symptoms on standing (e.g. light-headedness, palpitations, tremulousness, fatigue, weakness, blurred vision)
  2) Increase in heart rate ≥30/min from supine to standing (or ≥40/min in 12 to 19 years old)
  3) Absence of orthostatic hypotension
- No actual syncope; tends to present from 15 to 25 years old, mostly in females.
- Chronic condition with low quality of life reported.
- Management:
  - » Thorough history and physical examination, and 12-lead ECG
  - » Select patients may benefit from doing a full blood count, thyroid function test, 24 h Holter, echocardiography and exercise stress testing
  - » Multidisciplinary approach
  - » Regular structured and progressive exercise program
  - » Acute decompensation from dehydration: May benefit from short-term IV drip
  - » Medications: Consider fludrocortisone, midodrine, low dose propranolol (Class IIb recommendations)

Bibliography

1. Tadros GM. (2002) Syncope in young patients I: An approach to the patient with syncope. *Hosp Physician* 47–54.
2. Tadros GM. (2002) Syncope in young patients II: Presentation and management of specific causes of syncope. *Hosp Physician* 6–67.
3. Soteriade ES, Evans, JC, Larson MG, *et al.* (2002) Incidence and prognosis of syncope. *N Eng J Med* **347**(72):878–885.
4. Heaven DJ, Sutton R. (2000) Syncope — A scientific review. *Crit Care Med* **28**(10):N116–N120.
5. Morag R. (2001) Syncope: Department of Emergency Medicine, Brooklyn Hospital Centre. *eMed J* **12**(8). http://www.emedicine.com/emerg/topic 876.htm
6. Black KD, Seslar SP, Woodward GA. (2011) Cardiogenic causes of pediatric syncope. *Clin Pediatr Emerg Med* **12**(4):266–277.
7. DiMario FJ, Jr, Wheeler Castillo CS. (2011) Clinical categorisation of childhood syncope. *J Child Neurol* **26**(5):548–551.
8. Fisher J. (2011) Advances in syncope. *J Interv Card Electrophysiol* **32**(3):187–193.
9. Moodley M. (2013) Clinical approach to syncope in children. *Semin Pediatr Neurol* **20**(1):12–17.
10. Moya A, Sutton R, Ammirati F, *et al.* (2009) Guidelines for the diagnosis and management of syncope (version2009). *Eur Heart J* **30**(21):2631–2671.
11. Shen WK, Sheldon RS, Benditt DG, *et al.* (2017) ACC/AHA/HRS Guideline for the evaluation and management of patients with syncope: A report of the American College of cardiology/American Heart Association task force on clinical practice guidelines, and the heart rhythm society. *J Am Coll Cardiol* **70**(5):e39–e110.
12. Sheldon RS, Grubb BP, Olshansky B, *et al.* (2015) Heart Rhythm Society expert consensus statement on the diagnosis and treatment of postural tachycardia syndrome, inappropriate sinus tachycardia, and vasovagal syncope. *Heart Rhythm* **12:**e41–e63.

CHAPTER 26

Cardiac Arrhythmias

Chan Jiahui, Charmaine; Tan Teng Hong

General Principles

- Symptoms may vary depending on the age of the patient. A young child may complain of stomach or chest pain. Older children will be able to give a history of palpitations.
- Urgency of the work-up depends on symptom severity. Children with a history of congenital heart disease or syncope need prompt investigation.
- Obtain a 12-lead electrocardiogram (ECG) with a long rhythm strip for any suspected arrhythmia before making a diagnosis or instituting management.
- In an acute arrhythmia with haemodynamic compromise, a good rule of thumb is to cardiovert for a tachyarrhythmia and resuscitate for bradyarrhythmia.
- In the paediatric population, primary arrhythmias tends to be the result rather than cause of emergencies.
- Children at risk of primary cardiac arrhythmias include those with myocarditis, cardiomyopathy, post-cardiac surgery, congenital heart disease and drug ingestion.
- Urgently treat unstable rhythms — those that compromise cardiac output and those with potential to deteriorate into a lethal rhythm.
- If the arrhythmia is stable, there is time to call the cardiologist to assess patient and advise on treatment.
- Treating a stable patient with an arrhythmia might not only be unnecessary but may also worsen the situation.

Benign Arrhythmias

Sinus Arrhythmia

- This is a normal physiological phenomenon and occurs due to reflex changes in vagal tone during the different stages of respiration — heart rate increases during inspiration and decreases during expiration.
- ECG characteristics:
  - » Variation in PP interval with gradual lengthening and shortening in a cyclical fashion, usually corresponding to the phases of the respiratory cycle.
  - » Normal sinus P wave with no change in P wave morphology.
  - » Constant PR interval.

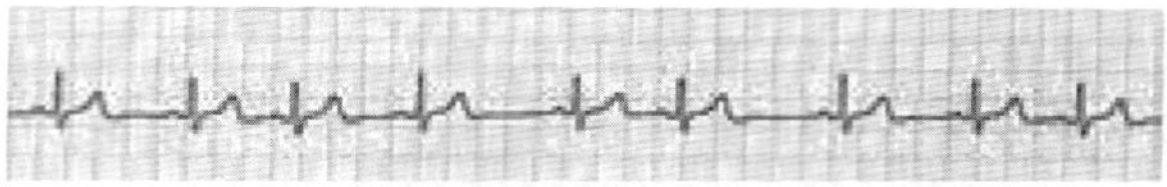

Figure 7.1 Sinus arrhythmia.

- Management: Does not require further evaluation.

Wandering Atrial Rhythm (Wandering Atrial Pacemaker)

- Commonly seen in 25–35% of children, especially during lower heart rate.
- Occurs when there are three or more ectopic foci within the atrial myocardium serving as the dominant pacemaker. Results in an irregularly irregular rhythm.
- ECG characteristics:
  - » ≥ 3 distinctively different P wave morphologies
  - » Ventricular rate not tachycardic for age
- Management: Does not require further evaluation. If heart rate is tachycardic, this is called multifocal atrial tachycardia, which will require further evaluation and treatment.

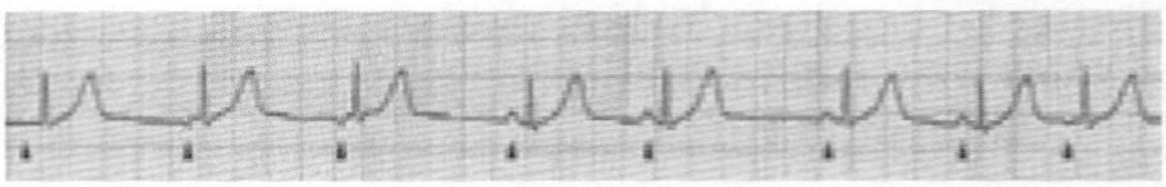

Figure 7.2 Wandering atrial rhythm. Arrowheads indicate position of P waves. Note varying P wave morphology and PP intervals.

Junctional Rhythm

- Can be seen intermittently in sinus arrhythmia, especially during periods of low heart rate. It may be a normal phenomenon in children. Occurs when the electrical activity of the sinoatrial (SA) node is blocked or slower than the automaticity of the atrioventricular (AV) node/His bundle.
- ECG characteristics:
  - » Narrow QRS complex with regular rhythm
  - » Rate 40–100/min (varies with age)
- P waves — frequently not seen. If seen, P wave morphology will be different from that originating from the SA node. It is often seen as inverted in lead II.
- Atrioventricular dissociation may be seen, with QRS rate > P (atrial) rate.

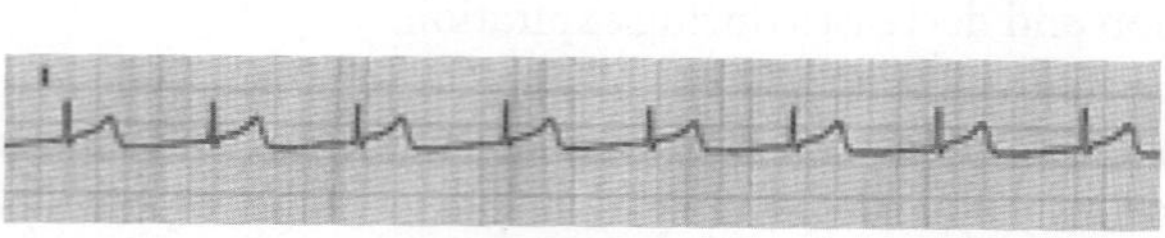

Figure 7.3 Junctional rhythm in an asymptomatic boy. Note the absence of a P wave preceding each QRS complex.The rate here is about 60/min.

- Management: Further evaluation is indicated if the rate is too fast for an escape rhythm, e.g. Junctional Ectopic Tachycardia (JET; rate tachycardic for age), or if it is an escape rhythm due to a diseased SA node, or AV conduction block.

Premature Atrial Contractions (PACs)

- Generally, benign and frequently seen in normal, asymptomatic children. Some patients may complain of palpitations or skipped beats.
- Due to ectopic pacemaker sites in the atria not from the SA node.
- ECG characteristics:
  - » Premature P wave (PP interval is shorter than preceding PP interval). P waves may sometimes be hidden in ST segment, or the preceding T wave, appearing as a 'notch' in the T wave.
  - » P wave morphology different from sinus P wave morphology.
  - » Narrow QRS complexes. In some cases, the PAC can conduct aberrantly, making it difficult to distinguish from PVCs. If the PAC arrives too early, it may not be conducted through to the ventricles, resulting in a 'blocked PAC'.
  - » Sinus pause. This can be compensatory (i.e. 2 × cycle length of 2 sinus PP intervals), less than compensatory or more than 2 sinus beat cycle lengths.
- PACs may be seen in patients who have:
  - » Myocarditis
  - » Tumours
  - » Electrolyte abnormalities
  - » Drugs, e.g. beta agonists, sympathomimetics, tricyclic antidepressants, chemotherapeutic agents, monoamine oxidase inhibitors
  - » Indwelling central venous lines with tip/line in the right atrium
- Management: Further evaluation is not needed unless the PACs are associated with some other condition that warrants investigation or treatment.

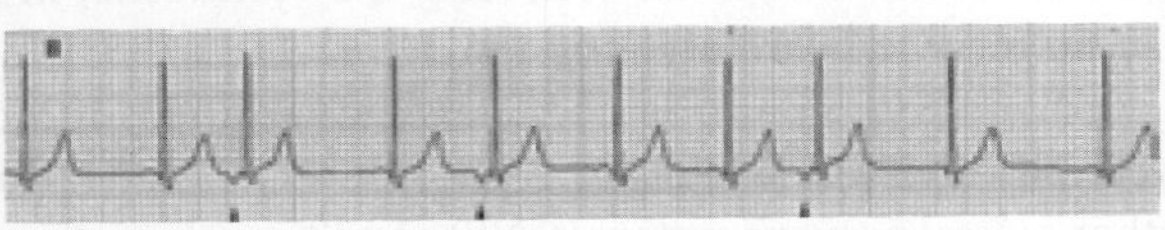

Figure 7.4 Premature atrial contractions. Arrowheads indicate the premature P waves. The AV conduction of the premature beats here is normal.

Premature Ventricular Contractions (PVCs)

- PVCs are very common and frequently asymptomatic and benign. Frequent PVCs may point to an underlying cardiac condition or may result in PVC-induced cardiomyopathies. They may also result in more dangerous cardiac arrhythmias.
- PVCs are due to an ectopic focus in the ventricle that bypasses the His–Purkinje system and directly depolarises the ventricles.
- ECG characteristics:

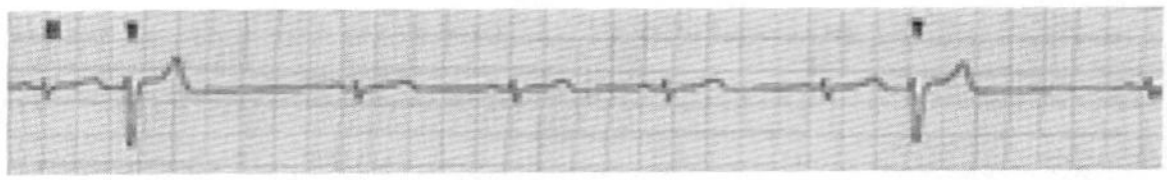

Figure 7.5 Two ventricular premature complexes (arrowheads) are seen in this rhythm.

- » Premature QRS complex (RR interval shorter than preceding RR interval)
- » Wide QRS complexes, with abnormal QRS morphology
- » Discordant ST segment and T wave changes
- » Compensatory pause following the contraction (the next sinus P wave occurs exactly 2 PP intervals after the last sinus beat)
- » Classification: (i) Unifocal or polymorphic; (ii) bigeminy, trigeminy, quadrigeminy, couplet, triplets (≥3 consecutive PVCs at a rate >100/min = VT)

- Management: Refer to cardiology for further evaluation, especially if there is a history or family history of cardiac conditions/sudden deaths, patient is symptomatic with palpitations, syncope or exercise-induced symptoms, abnormal cardiac examination, ECG findings of polymorphic PVCs, frequent PVCs.
- Patients will usually be evaluated with an echocardiography, Holter monitoring, and exercise stress testing.

Bradycardia and Conduction Disorders

Sinus Bradycardia

- Rhythm originates from SA node–P wave upright in leads I, II and aVF
- Rate less than normal for age
- Causes of sinus bradycardia:
  - » Cardiac: Sinus node dysfunction, long QT syndrome, myocarditis, post-cardiac surgery, myocardial infarction
  - » Non cardiac: Hypoxia, obstructive sleep apnoea, infections (relative bradycardia, e.g. malaria, dengue, typhoid fever), raised intracranial pressure and other central nervous system (CNS) conditions, hypothyroidism, anorexia nervosa, hypothermia, drugs (e.g. beta blockers, amiodarone, opioids, dexmedetomidine, corticosteroids)
- Management: Evaluate and treat the cause of sinus bradycardia accordingly.
  - » Unstable sinus bradycardia: Refer to Chapter 2 on Cardiopulmonary Resuscitation

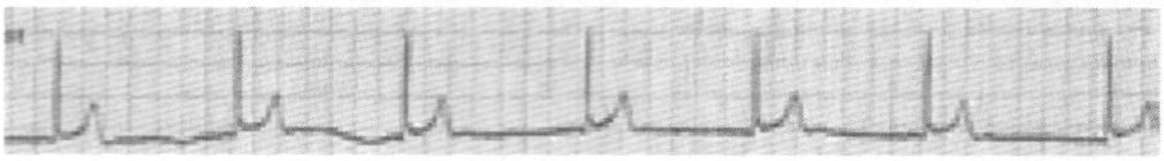

Figure 7.6 Sinus bradycardia.

- » Pharmacological treatment
  - ■ Adrenaline 0.01 mg/kg (0.1 ml/kg of 1:10,000) intravenous (IV) bolus
  - ■ Adrenaline infusion 0.1–1.0 mcg/kg/min
  - ■ Atropine 0.02 mg/kg (min 0.1 mg) IV may be repeated once
  - ■ Isoprenaline infusion 0.01–2.0 mcg/kg/min
- » Pacing, temporary or permanent

Sinus Arrest

- Sudden absence of atrial activity.
- The longest PP interval is not a multiple of the shortest PP interval.
- Escape rhythms of atrial, junctional or ventricular origin are sometimes seen.
- Presents with syncope.
- Indications for therapy are the same as in sinus bradycardia.

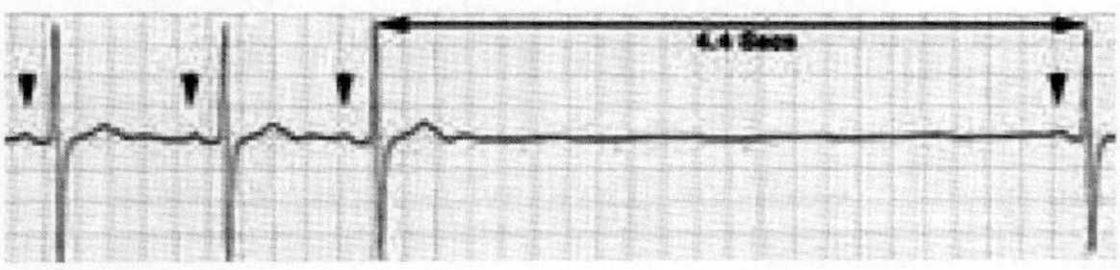

Figure 7.7 Sinus arrest of 4.4-sec duration seen in this Holter recording strip. The vertical arrowheads indicate the position of the sinus P waves.

First Degree Atrioventricular (AV) Block

- Prolonged PR interval (age dependant) due to delay in conduction from atria to ventricles (Table 7.4). All impulses are conducted.

Table 7.4 PR Interval According to Age and Heart Rate and Upper Limits of Normal (ULN)

Rate	0–1 mo	1–6 mo	6 mo–1 yr	1–3 yr	3–8 yr	8–12 yr	12–16 yr	Adults
<60						0.16 (0.18)	0.16 (0.19)	0.17 (0.21)
60–80					0.15 (0.17)	0.15 (0.17)	0.15 (0.18)	0.16 (0.21)
80–100	0.10 (0.12)				0.14 (0.16)	0.15 (0.16)	0.15 (0.17)	0.15 (0.20)
100–120	0.10 (0.12)			(0.15)	0.13 (0.16)	0.14 (0.15)	0.15 (0.16)	0.15 (0.19)
120–140	0.10 (0.11)	0.11 (0.14)	0.11 (0.14)	0.12 (0.14)	0.13 (0.15)	0.14 (0.15)		0.15 (0.18)
140–160	0.09 (0.11)	0.10 (0.13)	0.11 (0.13)	0.11 (0.14)	0.12 (0.14)			(0.17)
160–180	0.10 (0.11)	0.10 (0.12)	0.10 (0.12)	0.10 (0.12)				
>180	0.09	0.09 (0.11)	0.10 (0.11)					

Park MK, Guntheroth WG (2006) *How to Read Pediatric ECGs, 4th ed*. Philadelphia: Mosby.

- Generally asymptomatic and does not progress to a complete heart block. There are exceptions such as in rheumatic fever and endocarditis.
- Causes: High vagal tone (physiological, most common), drugs (e.g. beta blockers, calcium channel blockers), cardiomyopathies, some muscular dystrophies, endocarditis, rheumatic fever.

- Management: Further evaluation not required if history and examination not suggestive of cardiac or systemic disease. Rarely, very prolonged PR interval causing symptomatic bradycardia may benefit from pacing.

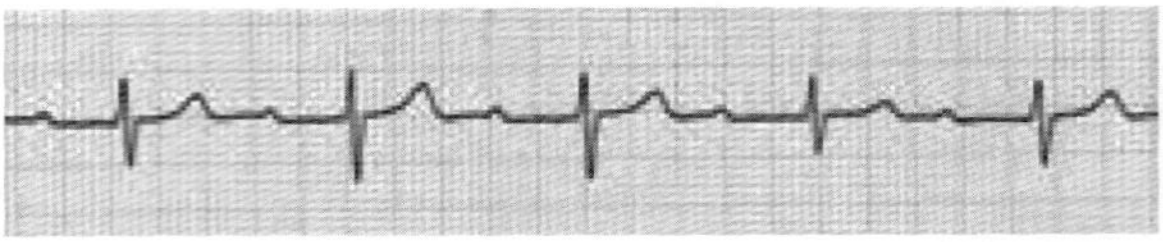

Figure 7.8 First-degree atrioventricular block with a PR interval of 0.4 sec.

Mobitz Type I Second-Degree AV Block (Wenckebach)

- Generally asymptomatic and benign, unlikely to progress to a complete heart block.
- Due to increasing delay in conduction through AV node.
- ECG characteristics:
  - » Progressive PR interval prolongation until a P wave is not conducted.
  - » Irregular rhythm, QRS complexes with 'group beating'.
  - » PP interval is constant.
- Causes: Increased vagal tone (physiological, most common), drugs (beta blockers, calcium channel blockers, digoxin, amiodarone), post-operative cardiac surgery, myocarditis.
- Management: Does not require further evaluation or treatment unless symptomatic.

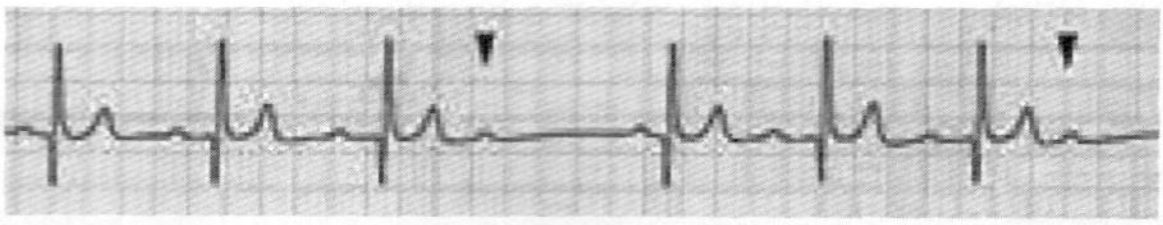

Figure 7.9 Mobitz type I second-degree atrioventricular block. The arrowheads indicate the P dropped beats.

Mobitz Type II Second-Degree AV Block

- Usually caused by a block below the AV node. There is a higher risk of progression to a complete heart block and sudden death. May be symptomatic with light-headedness, presyncope and syncope, although may also be asymptomatic.
- ECG characteristics:
  - » Intermittent non-conducted P waves, *without* progressive lengthening of PR interval.
  - » Constant PP and PR intervals.
- Causes: Drugs (flecainide, procainamide, quinidine), myocarditis, endocarditis, hypothyroidism, hyperkalaemia, infiltrative diseases, e.g. sarcoidosis, neuromuscular disease, post-cardiac surgery.

- Management:
  » Requires close monitoring. Need to evaluate for underlying cardiac disease (echocardiography, consider cardiac MRI)
  » Unstable — refer to management of unstable bradycardia.
  » Stable — if no reversible causes identified, permanent pacemaker is definitive treatment.

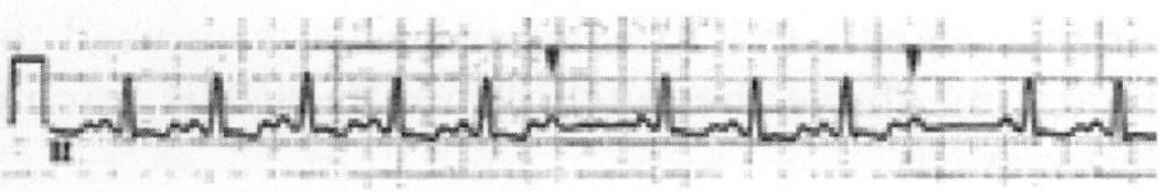

Figure 7.10 Mobitz type II second-degree atrioventricular block. The arrowheads indicate the P waves that were not conducted. Note constant PR interval.

Third-Degree (Complete) AV Block

- Complete absence of atrioventricular conduction, i.e. none of the supraventricular impulses are able to conduct through to the ventricles. Patients may present with fatigue, exercise intolerance, congestive heart failure, presyncope or syncope, or may be asymptomatic. They are at a higher risk of ventricular standstill or sudden cardiac death.
- ECG characteristics:
  » Complete dissociation of P wave and QRS complex.
  » Regular PP intervals, regular RR intervals. Atrial rate higher than ventricular rate.
  » QRS morphology and heart rate vary according to location of the escape pacemaker: the higher the pacemaker, the faster the rate and narrower the QRS complex.
- Causes:
  » Congenital, e.g. babies born to mothers with collagen vascular disease, congenital heart disease, e.g. congenitally corrected transposition of great arteries, genetic.
  » Acquired: Post-operative repair of congenital heart diseasemay require a permanent pacemaker if complete AV block persists more than 2 weeks, myocarditis, rheumatic fever — usually temporary and tend to resolve in < 1 week.
- Management:
  » Refer to Cardiology.
  » Unstable — see management for unstable sinus bradycardia.

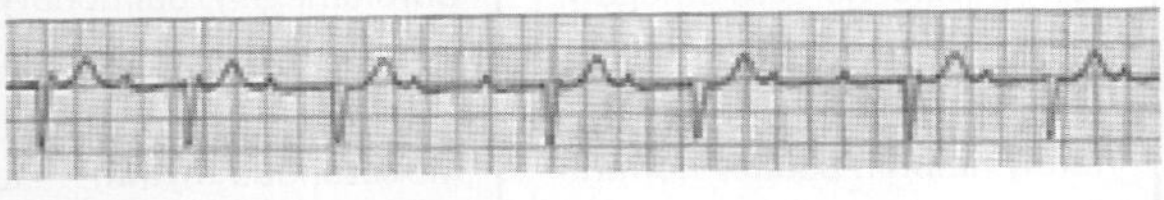

Figure 7.11 Complete heart block. Note atrioventricular dissociation.

  » Indications for permanent pacemaker insertion: HR <55/min (infant) or <50/min (above infancy), wide QRS complex escape rhythm, ventricular dysfunction, complex PVCs, abrupt ventricular pauses, symptomatic bradycardia.

Tachyarrhythmias

Supraventricular tachycardia (SVT) is an umbrella term used to categorise any tachyarrhythmia arising above the level of bundle of His, including atrial and atrioventricular tachycardias.

Paroxysmal Supraventricular Tachycardia (SVT)

- Most common significant arrhythmia in childhood. Starts and stops abruptly.
- Tachycardia from accessory pathway (AV re-entrant SVT) is the most common SVT seen in infancy and early childhood. AV nodal re-entrant SVT becomes more common in later childhood and adolescence.
- Due to re-entrant mechanism involving the AV node.
- ECG characteristics:
  - » Regular fixed-rate tachycardia, typically narrow complex (exceptions include aberrancy, antidromic conduction, pre-existing bundle branch block).
  - » P waves may be hidden, or retrograde.
  - » Wolff–Parkinson–White: Diagnosed when the accessory pathway is evident on ECG as a shortened PR interval, with slurred upstroke of the QRS complex (delta wave).
- SVT may be difficult to differentiate from sinus tachycardia. See Table 7.5 for general guidelines that may help to distinguish between them.

Table 7.5 General Guidelines that Distinguish Sinus Tachycardia from Supraventricular Tachycardia (SVT)

	Sinus Tachycardia	Supraventricular Tachycardia
Rate	<180/min	>220/min
History	Consistent with volume loss, fever, infection	Non-specific — irritability, poor feeding, tachypnoea, sweating, pallor
Physical Examination	Consistent with dehydration, fever, sepsis, bloodloss Clear lungs (creps in chest infection) No hepatomegaly	Poor perfusion Signs of heart failure Fine crepitations in lungs Hepatomegaly
CXR	Non-specific, no cardiomegaly, normal, or, e.g. pneumonia as source of fever/sepsis	Cardiomegaly, pulmonary congestion or oedema
ECG	Rarely helpful, usually normal	Monotonous rhythm — fairly fixed rate despite changes in activity. Sudden termination/initiation. Terminate with heart block

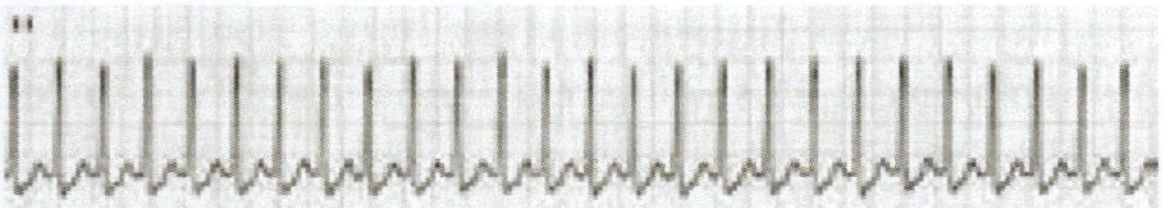

Figure 7.12 Supraventricular tachycardia in an infant. Note the monotony of the rhythm. P waves not evident; they are actually in the terminal part of the QRS complexes (the pseudo-Q waves).

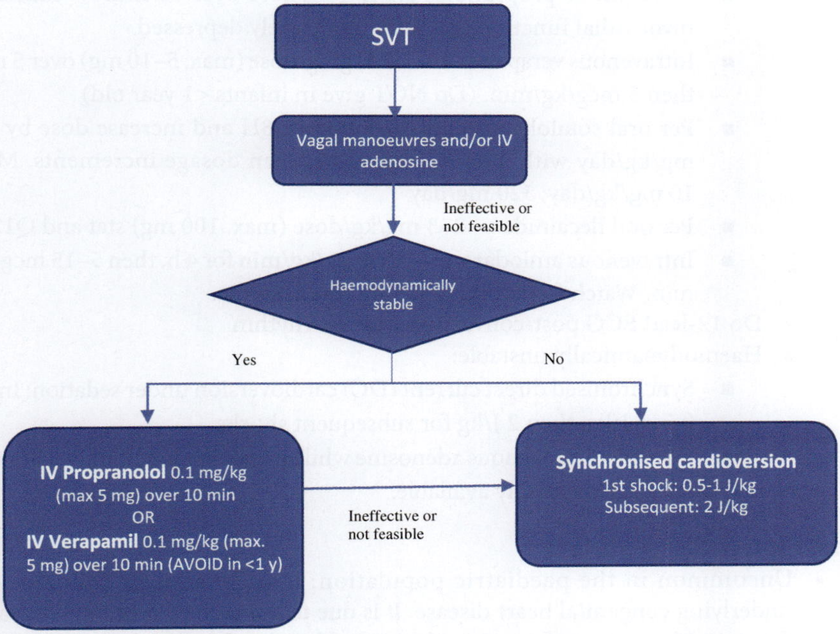

Figure 7.13 Acute SVT management.

- Symptoms:
  - » Infancy — may be non-specific: Irritability, poor feeding, incessant crying. Up to 50% may present in heart failure.
  - » Older children/adolescents — palpitations, chest pain, abdominal pain.
- Management:
  - » Acute: (See summary in Figure 7.13):
  - » Haemodynamically stable:
    - ■ Vagal manoeuvres
    - ■ Adenosine: First dose: 0.1 mg/kg (max. 6 mg), second and subsequent doses: 0.2 mg/kg (max. 12 mg). Give as rapid IV bolus via large proximal vein, followed by 5–10 ml normal saline rapid bolus.

- Run ECG on continuous manual mode (leads I, aVF, V2) as adenosine is being given. This will give diagnostic information on the mechanism of the SVT.

» If SVT persists: Call cardiologist.

» Re-evaluate whether this is SVT (AVRT/AVNRT), vs. sinus tachycardia, or other tachyarrhythmias that do not respond to adenosine, e.g. atrial tachycardia, junctional tachycardia, fascicular VT.

» Other anti-arrhythmic medications include:

- Intravenous propranolol 0.1 mg/kg/dose over 10 min — caution if myocardial function is at least moderately depressed.
- Intravenous verapamil 0.1–0.2 mg/kg/dose (max. 5–10 mg) over 5 min, then 5 mcg/kg/min. (Do NOT give in infants <1 year old)
- Per oral sotalol start at 2 mg/kg/day Q8H and increase dose by 1–2 mg/kg/day with 3 days interval between dosage increments. Max.: 10 mg/kg/day; 320 mg/day
- Per oral flecainide — 2–3 mg/kg/dose (max. 100 mg) stat and Q12H
- Intravenous amiodarone — 25 mcg/kg/min for 4 h, then 5–15 mcg/kg/min. Watch for hypotension and bradycardia.

» Do 12-lead ECG post-conversion to sinus rhythm

» Haemodynamically unstable:

- Synchronised direct current (DC) cardioversion under sedation: Initial 0.5–1 J/kg, then 2 J/kg for subsequent shocks.
- Consider intravenous adenosine while preparing for cardioversion and if IV access readily available.

Atrial Flutter

- Uncommon in the paediatric population. Usually seen in children with underlying congenital heart disease. It is due to a macro re-entrant pathway in the atria. May account for up to one-third of foetal tachyarrhythmias. In infants, the prognosis is good once rhythm has converted back to sinus, and recurrence is rare.
- ECG characteristics:
  » Narrow complex tachycardia, ventricular rhythm may be regular or irregular.

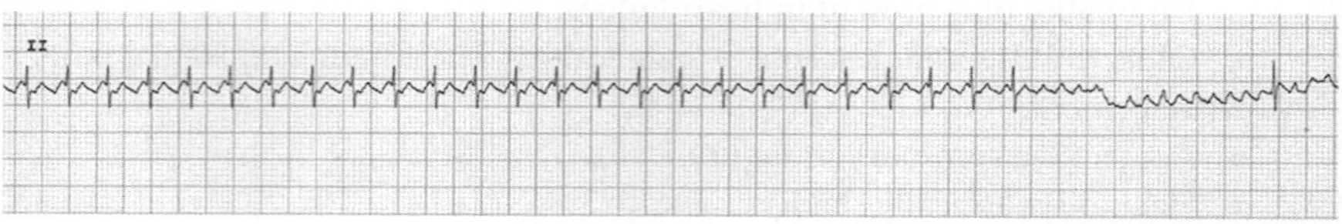

Figure 7.14 Atrial flutter in an infant. Regular, narrow complex tachycardia, rate 200/min. 'Saw tooth' inverted flutter waves seen in lead II, rate 400/min, indicating 2:1 AV conduction block. Adenosine was given, unmasking the flutter waves. Note that flutter waves do not return to isoelectric point.

» 'Saw tooth' inverted flutter waves seen in leads II, III, aVF, with loss of isoelectric baseline.
» Atrial rate ranges from 300 to 600/min; ventricular rate is slower and depends on the degree of AV conduction block. (E.g. 2:1 block when atrial rate is 300/min means a ventricular rate of 150/min.)

- Causes: Congenital heart disease (e.g. Ebstein anomaly, atrioventricular septal defect), post-cardiac surgeries, especially when atrial scars are created (e.g. Mustard, Senning, Fontan, TAPVD repair), cardiomyopathies, hyperthyroidism, muscular dystrophy.
- Management:

» Unstable — synchronised cardioversion: Initial 0.5–1 J/kg, subsequent shocks 2 J/kg
» Stable:

  - Rate control: IV beta blockers, IV Verapamil (avoid in infants <1 year old), IV amiodarone
  - Rhythm control: Rapid atrial pacing — especially in post-op cases where there are pacing wires. Set pacemaker to RAP mode. AAI pacing; set atrial rate higher than the flutter rate by 10–15%.
  - Synchronised cardioversion.

» Note: Adenosine does NOT treat atrial flutter. It slows down AV conduction and may unmask flutter waves.
» Anticoagulation therapy due to higher risk of thromboembolic events
» Flutter ≥ 48 hours or unknown duration: Warfarin 3 weeks before and 4 weeks after.
» Flutter < 48 hours, low risk of thromboembolism: Anticoagulation for DC cardioversion only.
» If immediate cardioversion is needed: Start anticoagulation → Transoesophageal Echocardiography (TEE) → may continue anticoagulation 4 weeks after.

Focal Atrial Tachycardia

- A form of atrial tachycardia due to a single ectopic focus originating from the atrium.
- Uncommon in paediatric population and may be paroxysmal or sustained.
- May be difficult to differentiate from sinus tachycardia or AV re-entrant tachycardias.

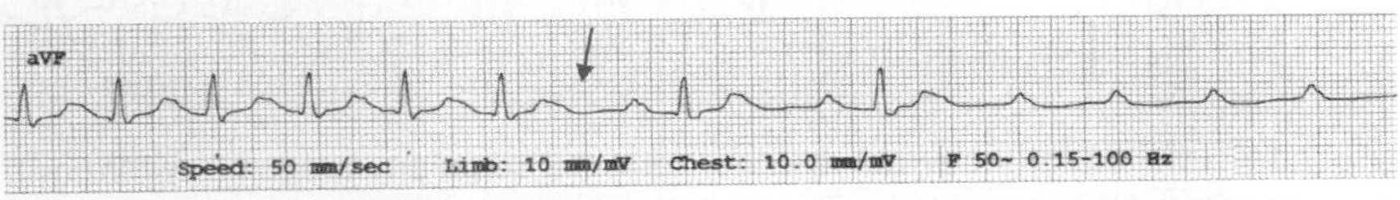

Figure 7.15 Focal atrial tachycardia. This is a slow, regular narrow complex tachycardia of around 100/min. IV adenosine was given where the arrowhead points. Uniform P waves can be seen thereafter, indicating this is not a AV re-entrant tachycardia.

- ECG characteristics:
  - » Narrow complex tachycardia, atrial rate >100/min.
  - » P wave morphology differs from sinus P wave morphology — compare with previous ECGs if possible.
  - » May have 'warm-up' or 'cool down' phenomenon: Tachycardia gradually speeds up at onset and slows down at termination.
- Causes: Congenital heart disease, post-cardiac surgery, hypoxia, pulmonary disease, stimulants, metabolic disturbances
- Management:
  - » Rate control with IV beta blockers or calcium channel blockers.
  - » IV Esmolol infusion 0.05 mg/kg/min, up to 0.2 mg/kg/min. Watch for hypotension. Typically given up to 48 h.
  - » IV Propranolol 0.1 mg/kg (max. 5 mg) over 10 min, then 0.1–0.3 mg/kg (max. 5–15 mg) Q6–8H
  - » IV Amiodarone 5 mg/kg (max. 300 mg) over 60 min (loading dose); infusion 5–15 mcg/kg/min
  - » *Avoid catecholamines* where possible.

Multifocal Atrial Tachycardia (MAT)

- A rapid, irregular atrial rhythm caused by multiple ectopic foci in the atria.
- Rare in infant and paediatric population, occurs in <1% of paediatric SVT.
- ECG characteristics:
  - » At least 3 distinct P wave morphologies in the same lead.
  - » Irregularly irregular PP, PR and RR intervals
  - » Tachycardia for age, HR >100/min
- Causes: Associated with severe pulmonary disease, congenital heart disease, metabolic disturbances, drugs, RASopathies
- Management:
  - » Treat underlying causes/diseases.
  - » Correct electrolyte abnormalities.
  - » Pharmacological treatment include beta blockers, calcium channel blockers, amiodarone.

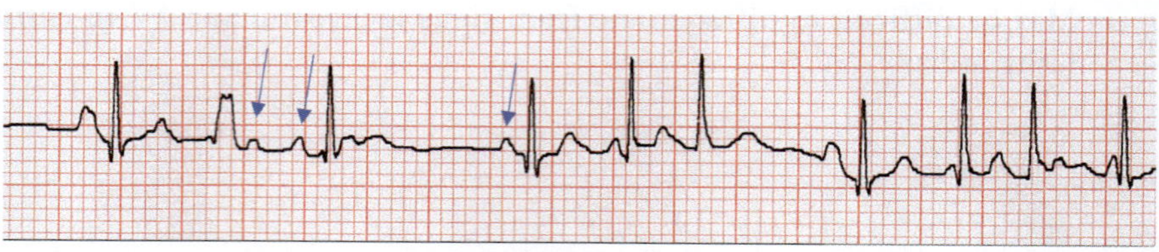

Figure 7.16 Multiatrial focal tachycardia. Note the irregularly irregular rhythm, with a rate ranging from 180 to 270/min. The arrowheads show at least three different P wave morphologies.

Ventricular Tachycardia (VT)

- Wide complex tachycardia originating in the ventricles.
- Can be haemodynamically unstable and potentially life-threatening.
- In children, a wide complex tachycardia should be treated as VT until proven otherwise.
- Sustained VT: Haemodynamic compromise requiring intervention, or duration >30 s. Non-sustained VT: ≥3 consecutive ventricular complexes, spontaneously abort <30 s.
- ECG characteristics:
  - » Wide QRS complex (for age), HR >100/min
  - » Complete AV dissociation, ventricular rate faster than atrial rate
  - » Presence of capture beats or fusion beats, extreme (northwest) axis deviation, positive or negative concordance throughout chest leads V1-6
- Differentials include: SVT with aberrancy, SVT with pre-existing bundle branch block, antidromic SVT.
- Causes: Congenital heart disease, post-cardiac surgery, myocardial ischaemia, myocarditis, cardiomyopathy, long QT syndrome, metabolic disturbances
- Management (as per APLS):
  - » Correct any treatable causes.
  - » Pulseless VT should be managed as VF; defibrillate with 4 J/kg.
  - » Unstable: Synchronised DC cardioversion: 0.5–1 J/kg (first shock), 2 J/kg (subsequent).
  - » Stable: IV Amiodarone 5 mg/kg (max. 300 mg) over 60 min (loading dose); may repeat up to three times (15 mg/kg). 5–15 mcg/kg/min maintenance infusion.
  - » Watch for hypotension. Standby Calcium chloride infusion.
  - » IV Lignocaine 1 mg/kg (bolus). May repeat in 10–15 min for 2 doses. Maintenance level: 1.5–5.0 mg/L
  - » IV Magnesium 50 mg/kg (max. 2 g) may be given for Torsades de Pointes.

Post-Operative Arrhythmia

- Common arrhythmias seen in post-cardiac surgery patients include AV block, SVT and junctional ectopic tachycardia.
- Many patients come out of the operating theatre with atrial and ventricular pacing wires.

Atrial ECG Study

- Connect all ECG leads as usual except for V2 lead (or any chest lead that is running on the rhythm strip).
- Connect V2 lead to the atrial pacing wire.
- The P waves are recorded as sharp, tall spikes on the V2 tracing.
- This helps identify P waves during a tachycardia and demonstrates the association between P and QRS complex.

Junctional Ectopic Tachycardia (JET)

- This is a transient arrhythmia and usually resolves within 24–72 hours post-operatively. However, it may compromise cardiac output in patients.
- Higher risk in cardiac surgeries close to the AV node.
- Due to abnormal automaticity of tissues at the AV node — His bundle complex
- ECG characteristics:
  - » Narrow complex tachycardia.
  - » Atrioventricular dissociation, ventricular rate higher than atrial rate.
  - » Retrograde P waves may be seen — atrial ECG can be performed to identify the relationship of P and QRS.
- Management:
  - » Inform Cardiology — echocardiography may be performed to rule out effusion and check function.
  - » Ensure adequate sedation.
  - » Aim normothermia, can cool to 34–36°C if still in JET.
  - » Correct electrolyte abnormalities, hypovolaemia, anaemia.
  - » Wean off catecholaminergic agents if possible.
  - » Medications:
    - ▪ Intravenous dexmedetomidine: 0.2–1 mcg/kg/h. Higher infusion rate of 3 mcg/kg/h reported to be useful for conversion of JET to sinus rhythm. Reserve loading only for extreme situation. Loading dose: IV 1 mcg/kg over 15 min. Main side effects are hypotension and bradycardia (including complete heart block)
    - ▪ Intravenous amiodarone: 25 mcg/kg/min (= loading over 4 h), then maintenance infusion 5–15 mcg/kg/min; alternatively, intravenous boluses of 1 mg/kg over 10 min (max. 5 mg/kg over 60 min), then maintenance infusion 5–15 mcg/kg/min; alternatively, loading dose: IV 5 mg/kg over 10 min (repeat once if needed), followed by maintenance infusion: 5–15 mcg/kg/min for 48–72 hours. Watch for hypotension and bradycardia. Ensure that calcium chloride is available by the bedside.
    - ▪ *Atrial or AV sequential pacing* may be started to restore synchrony once the JET rate is reduced. This modality cannot be used if JET rates are ≥170–180/min since pacing at higher rates will compromise diastolic filling.

Bibliography

1. Vetter V. (2000) Arrhythmias. In: Moller JH, Hoffman JIE (eds.) *Pediatric Cardiovascular Medicine.* Philadelphia, PA: Churchill Livingstone, pp. 844–869.
2. Case CL. (1999) Diagnosis and treatment of pediatric arrhythmias. *Pediatr Clin North Am* **46**(2):347–354.
3. Khan IA. (2002) Long QT syndrome: Diagnosis and management. *Am Heart J* **143**(1):7–14.
4. Laird WP, Snyder CS, Kertesz NJ, *et al.* (2003) Use of intravenous amiodarone for post-operative junctional ectopic tachycardia in children. *Pediatr Cardiol* **24**(2):133–137.
5. Plumpton K, Justo R, Haas N. (2005) Amiodarone for post-operative junctional ectopic tachycardia. *Cardiol Young* **15**(1):13–18.

6. Chrysostomou C, Beerman L, Shiderly D, *et al.* (2008 Nov) Dexmedetomidine: A novel drug for the treatment of atrial and junctional tachyarrhythmias during the perioperative period for congenital cardiac surgery: A preliminary study. *Anesth Analg* **107**(5):1514–1522.
7. LeRiger M, Naguib A, Gallantowicz M, Tobias JD. (2012) Dexmedetomidine controls junctional ectopic tachycardia during Tetralogy of Fallot repair in an infant. *Ann Card Anaesth* **15**(3):224–228.
8. Park MK, Guntheroth WG. (2006) *How to Read Paediatric ECGs, 4th ed.* Elsevier.
9. Page RL, Joglar JA, Caldwell MA, *et al.* (2015) ACC/AHA/HRS Guideline for the management of adult patients with supraventricular tachycardia: A report of the American college of cardiology/American heart association task force on clinical practice guidelines and the heart rhythm society. *J Am Coll Cardiol* **67**:e27–e115.

CHAPTER 27

Cardiomyopathy and Heart Failure

Zhang Zhewei, Dyan; Sreekanthan Sundararaghavan

Introduction

Heart failure in children (aged 0 to 18 years) can be defined broadly as the failure of the heart to supply blood to either systemic or pulmonary circulation at an appropriate rate of flow or to receive venous return at an appropriate filling pressure, resulting in adverse effects on the heart, circulation and patient. As paediatric heart failure is a relatively uncommon condition, most practitioners in primary care or emergency departments have little practical experience with its presentation or management in children. The clinical manifestations might be dissimilar to those of adults and quite variable. Because 87% of cases of new-onset heart failure only reach a diagnosis when the patient is in a state of severe decompensation, and <50% of children who present with symptomatic heart failure survive beyond 5 years without heart transplantation, early diagnosis and effective treatment remain significant challenges that should be addressed.

Causes

Heart failure can occur in children as a consequence of varied causes, including cardiac (Table 7.6) and non-cardiac causes.

- Heart failure due to cardiac causes include congenital cardiac malformations and primary cardiomyopathies.
- Congenital cardiac malformations typically present with heart failure early in life, resulting from abnormal chamber morphology, valvular function or circulatory connections.
- Primary cardiomyopathies, which result from disorders affecting the myocardium, may be apparent at birth, but usually manifests later in infancy, childhood or during adult life.
- Non-cardiac causes include anaemia, hypothyroidism and systemic lupus erythematosus, which typically occurs later in childhood.
- Right heart failure due to pulmonary hypertension can be due to diverse diseases, predominantly that of idiopathic pulmonary arterial hypertension, developmental lung disease or in association with congenital heart diseases in the paediatric population. Onset can occur at any age.
- Primary cardiomyopathies are the main cause of heart failure in children with a structurally normal heart, and the incidence of heart failure varies amongst the

Table 7.6 Causes of Heart Failure Classified Based on the Principle Fundamental Disturbance in Myocardial Function

- Pre-load:
  - » Volume overload:
    - Left-to-right shunts: VSD, ASD, AVSD, PDA, Arterio Venous (AV) fistula, etc.
    - Valvular regurgitation
    - Complex heart defects with unrestricted pulmonary flow, e.g. TGA, TAPVD
    - Anaemia
    - Iatrogenic
  - » Diastolic under-filling:
    - Pericardial effusion
    - Restrictive cardiomyopathy
    - Constrictive pericarditis
- Afterload (Pressure overload):
  - » Congenital: Coarctation of aorta, aortic stenosis, LV or RV outflow obstruction
  - » Systemic hypertension
  - » Cor pulmonale
  - » Idiopathic Pulmonary Hypertension
- Intrinsic contractility dysfunction:
  - » Myocarditis
  - » Cardiomyopathies:
    - Idiopathic
    - Post-chemotherapy
    - Inborn Errors of Metabolism (IEM), e.g. Pompe's disease
    - Metabolic, e.g. hypothyroidism
  - » Coronary abnormalities:
    - Anomalous origin of coronary artery, e.g.anomalous left coronary artery from the pulmonary artery
    - Kawasaki Disease (KD)
    - Post-cardiac surgery
    - Myocardial contusion
    - Neoplasia: Myxoma, leukaemic infiltration
- Arrhythmias:
  - » Bradyarrhythmia: Complete heart block
  - » Tachyarrhythmia: SVT, PJRT, JET
  - » Conduction abnormalities: Electromechanical dyssynchrony

ASD: atrial septal defect; AVSD: atrioventricular septal defect; JET: junctional ectopic tachycardia; LV: left ventricle; PDA: patent ductus arteriosus; PJRT: permanent junctional reciprocating tachycardia; RV: right ventricle; SVT: supraventricular tachycardia; TAPVD: total anomalous pulmonary venous drainage; TGA: transposition of great arteries; VSD: ventricular septal defect

morphological types of heart failure. Dilated cardiomyopathy (DCM) is the most common myopathic process leading to heart failure in children.

- The causes of cardiomyopathies (Table 7.7) are diverse and may arise from genetic abnormalities often involving sarcomeric and structural proteins or can be secondary to an acquired disease (e.g. myocarditis) or toxic exposure (e.g.

anthracycline toxicity). It is important to note that all known diagnoses account for only approximately 35% of patients, with the remainder being idiopathic.

- In cardiomyopathy, the basis for heart failure is usually reduced systolic function of the left ventricle, although associated diastolic dysfunction is increasingly

Table 7.7 Cardiomyopathies in Children

Characteristics	Dilated Cardiomyopathy (DCM)	Hypertrophic Cardiomyopathy (HCM)	Restrictive Cardiomyopathy (RCM)
Epidemiology	60% idiopathic, 30% familial. Secondary to myocarditis, toxins, myopathies, arrhythmia, inborn errors of metabolism, autoimmune diseases	Autosomal-dominant (30–60%); mutations in sarcomeric or structural proteins; can be due to malformation syndromes or metabolic disorders	Rare in children; can be idiopathic or secondary to systemic disease (e.g. scleroderma, metabolic disease, irradiation)
Structural abnormalities	Dilated, poorly contractile ventricle	Hypertrophied ventricular wall — asymmetric or concentric	Dilated atriums
Pathophysiology	Dilated poorly contractile ventricle leading to congestion and poor systemic perfusion	Stiff hypertrophied ventricle with poor filling; LVOTO due to ventricular septal thickening or systolic anterior motion of anterior mitral leaflet subendocardial ischaemia due to severe hypertrophy	Non-compliant (restrictive) ventricle results in poor filling (i.e. diastolic dysfunction)
Associated lesions	Mitral regurgitation	LVOTO	
Clinical features	Dyspnoea, orthopnoea, poor exercise tolerance, 90% present with CHF, gallop, hepatomegaly	Exercise intolerance syncope, chest pain, ejection systolic murmur at left sternal border. May present with sudden death.	Dyspnoea, orthopnoea, poor exercise tolerance, chest pain, CHF, gallop, hepatomegaly, arrhythmia
Chest X-ray (CXR) findings	Cardiomegaly, pulmonary plethora, pulmonary oedema	Usually minimal	Dilated atria, increased pulmonary vascular markings
ECG findings	Sinus tachycardia, non-specific ST-T changes, low voltage, LVH	LVH, ST-T changes, abnormal Q waves	Right atrial enlargement, left atrial enlargement, ST changes, arrhythmia
Treatment	Management of CHF (diuretics, ACE inhibitors, β-blockers). Consider heart transplantation if end-stage	Activity restriction, β-blockers, myectomy for severe LVOTO, implantable cardioverter defibrillator	Management of CHF, arrhythmia; ± implantable cardioverter defibrillator; ± anticoagulation; heart transplantation
Long-term complications	Progressive heart failure, sudden death	Arrhythmia, worsening LVOTO, sudden death	Arrhythmia, sudden death

ACE: angiotensin converting enzyme; CHF: congestive heart failure; LVH: left ventricular hypertrophy; LVOTO: left ventricular outflow tract obstruction recognised as an important contributing factor in the pathophysiology of heart failure in children.

The age of onset of cardiac failure can also serve as a guide to the differential diagnosis of the underlying aetiology (Table 7.8)

Table 7.8 Age-Related Time of Presentation

- **Foetus**
  - Arrhythmias — SVT, heart block
  - Severe anaemia
  - Large arteriovenous malformation
- **Premature neonates**
  - PDA
  - Fluid overload
  - Tachyarrhythmias — SVT
- **Infants**
  - Congenital heart defects are the most common. Usual age at presentation of failure:
    - First week — HLHS, critical aortic stenosis, large AV fistula, TAPVD
    - Second week — coarctation of aorta, other duct-dependent lesions
    - Fourth to eighth week — Large left-to-right shunts
  - Coronary abnormalities: Anomalous left coronary artery from pulmonary artery
  - Cardiomyopathies
  - Myocarditis
  - Tachyarrhythmias — SVT
- **Older children**
  - Congenital heart defects — first presentation of CHF after 1 yr of age uncommon
  - Myocarditis
  - Cardiomyopathies

HLHS: hypoplastic left heart syndrome; PDA: patent ductus arteriosus; SVT: supraventricular tachycardia; TAPVD: total anomalous pulmonary venous drainage

Clinical Features

Symptoms of heart failure in children may be similar regardless of the underlying aetiology, but physical signs might be more specific. Systemic manifestations are mediated by sympathetic and central neurological pathways, activated in response to pulmonary congestion and/or decreased systemic perfusion. Clinical features of heart failure unique to children are:

- Possible coexistence of structural congenital heart lesions, with simultaneous pulmonary over-circulation and systemic under-perfusion (when two circulations are linked in parallel by an intracardiac shunt or a patent ductus arteriosus).
- A change in symptom complexes over time from infancy through adolescence. In infants and young children, these are primarily respiratory and feeding difficulties (which are similar to the metabolic demands of physical exertion seen in older children).
- Symptoms of isolated right heart failure in children may be non-specific and varied in presentation.

History

See Table 7.9 for the typical features of heart failure in children, categorised as common and less common. The New York Heart Association (NYHA) classification of functional class is best suited to quantify changes in functional capacity in patients with established chronic heart failure. The Modified Ross classification (Table 7.10) has been applied to younger children for the same purpose.

Table 7.9. Symptoms Characteristic of Heart Failure in Children

Symptoms Characteristic of Heart Failure in Children		
	Common	**Less Common**
Infants and young children	• Tachypnoea • Feeding difficulty (reflux, vomiting, feeding refusal) • Diaphoresis • Pallor	• Cyanosis • Palpitations • Syncope • Facial oedema • Dependent oedema • Ascites
Older children and adolescents	• Fatigue • Effort intolerance • Dyspnoea • Orthopnoea • Abdominal pain • Nausea • Vomiting	• Palpitations • Chest pain • Dependent oedema • Ascites

Table 7.10 The Modified Ross Classification

Classification of Symptomatic Severity in Paediatric Heart Failure	
Class of Symptoms	**Symptoms Noted on History**
I	Asymptomatic
II	Infants: Mild tachypnoea or diaphoresis with feeding; no growth failure Older children: Dyspnoea on moderate exertion
III	Infants: Marked tachypnoea or diaphoresis with feeding; growth failure Older children: Dyspnoea on mild or minimal exertion
IV	Tachypnoea, diaphoresis or respiratory distress at rest

Clinical Examination

The cardinal signs of cardiac failure are cardiomegaly, tachycardia, tachypnoea and hepatomegaly. Poor feeding and chest retractions also feature prominently in the younger infants. The signs and symptoms of heart failure are related to three factors: impaired myocardial function with decreased systemic perfusion, pulmonary congestion and systemic venous congestion.

Signs of Impaired Myocardial Function

- Cardiomegaly
  - » A fairly consistent sign of impaired cardiac function, secondary to ventricular dilatation and/or hypertrophy.
  - » May be absent in early stages, especially with myocarditis, arrhythmias, restrictive disorders and pulmonary venous obstruction.
- Tachycardia
  - » Persistently raised heart rate >160/min in infants and >100/min in older children.
  - » Consider supraventricular tachycardia (SVT) if heart rate >220/min in infants and >180/min in older children.
- S3 and/or S4 (gallop rhythm)
- Poor peripheral perfusion — cool extremities, pallor
- Changes in arterial pulse
  - » Weak peripheral pulses
  - » Bounding pulses in PDA, large AV fistula, high output failure
  - » Pulsus paradoxus — accentuation of the normal fall in blood pressure on inspiration. Seen in cardiac tamponade. Can be detected by palpation of the peripheral pulses or by looking at the waveform on the pulse oximeter or invasive blood pressure monitor.
  - » Pulsus alternans — alternating strong and weak beats with a constant beat-to-beat interval.
- Failure to thrive
- Signs of sympathetic overdrive, e.g. diaphoresis, peripheral vasoconstriction, irritability.

Signs of Pulmonary Congestion

- Dyspnoea, tachypnoea and chest retractions
  - » Major presenting manifestations of cardiac failure in infants. Fairly early signs
  - » Result in poor feeding — inability to or taking longer to finish feeds (>30 minutes), increasing symptoms during and after feeds.
- Cough — a chronic, hacking cough
- Crepitations
- Rhonchi
  - » May be present in left ventricular failure.
  - » This, together with cough and crepitations, may make differentiation from bronchiolitis, pneumonia or asthma difficult. Superimposed pulmonary infections can and do occur in patients with congenital heart defects.
  - » Factors that should bring up the possibility of heart failure: Prior history of significant cardiac defect or heart failure, chronicity of symptoms, absence of fever, failure to respond to treatment, cardiomegaly, hepatomegaly.

Signs of Systemic Venous Congestion

- Hepatomegaly
  - » Most consistent sign of systemic venous congestion.
  - » Can be tender, especially if congestion is severe or acute and older children can present with vomiting and abdominal pain mimicking gastritis or an acute abdomen.
- Increased neck vein distension and pulsation
  - » Difficult to observe in infants.
- Peripheral oedema — an infrequent finding in children. Consider right heart failure when this occurs in isolation.

Investigations

Diagnostic testing is always indicated in children with suspected heart failure. The child presenting with symptoms and signs of heart failure requires urgent assessment to establish the diagnosis, rapidly determine their haemodynamic status and identify any reversible causes of heart failure. See Figure 7.17 for a simplified diagnostic approach to cardiomyopathy.

- **Chest radiography (CXR)**
  - » Chest radiography is indicated as the first-line investigation in children with suspected heart failure.
  - » Findings: Cardiomegaly, pulmonary plethora, pulmonary oedema

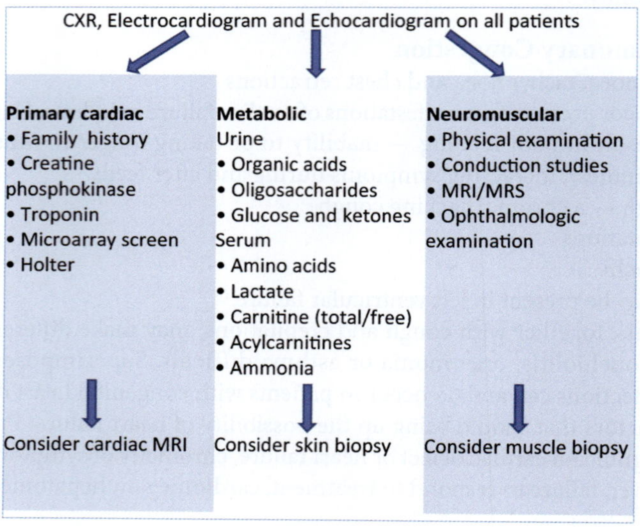

Figure 7.17 Simplified diagnostic approach to cardiomyopathy.

MRI: magnetic resonance imaging; MRS: magnetic resonance spectroscopy

- **Electrocardiography (ECG)**
  - » All patients should have 12-lead ECG performed at the time of presentation with heart failure, to exclude features of congenital or ischaemic heart disease, arrhythmia and pre-excitation.
  - » Findings: Sinus tachycardia, axis deviation, P pulmonale, non-specific T-wave and ST segment changes, LV or RV hypertrophy, first-degree heart block
  - » Specific ECG features for the underlying cardiac defect might be present. A specific arrhythmic cause of heart failure might be identified, such as incessant tachycardia (usually ectopic atrial tachycardia), atrioventricular block or ventricular pre-excitation.
- **Echocardiography**
  - » Delineate underlying structural defect(s)
  - » Assess cardiac chamber dilatation and hypertrophy
  - » Demonstrate decreased myocardial contractility and cardiac function
  - » Determine response to therapy
- **Biochemical and routine laboratory testing**
  - » Blood gas:
    - ■ Acidosis (usually metabolic, mixed metabolic and respiratory in severe pulmonary oedema)
    - ■ Slight decrease in PaO_2 in patients with left-to-right shunt lesions (due to pulmonary congestion, intrapulmonary right-to-left shunting and ventilation-perfusion mismatch); marked hypoxaemia in patients with underlying cyanotic heart defects.
    - ■ Infants with mild and moderate heart failure tend to have a respiratory alkalosis (lower than normal $PaCO_2$). However in severe heart failure or if there is a co-existing lung disorder (e.g. pneumonia), the $PaCO_2$ may be increased.
    - ■ Useful to guide need for further respiratory support (e.g. CPAP or intubation and ventilation)
  - » Urea, electrolytes and creatinine
    - ■ Hyponatraemia reflects increased water retention; hypochloraemia and increase in bicarbonate occurs secondary to diuretic use; potassium levels may be elevated due to cation shift from the intracellular stores; hypokalaemia from the use of loop diuretics.
    - ■ As a baseline prior to commencing treatment and a measure of renal perfusion.
  - » Liver function test (LFT)
    - ■ An evaluation of liver end-organ perfusion/injury owing to low cardiac output
  - » Full blood count (FBC)
    - ■ Findings: Anaemia, abnormal RBC indices may indicate haemoglobinopathies. Cyclic neutropenia occurs in males with Barth syndrome.

- » Erythrocyte sedimentation rate (ESR)
  - ■ Indicates inflammatory disorder/infection.
- **Biomarkers**
  - » Natriuretic peptide biomarkers
    - ■ Brain natriuretic peptide (BNP) or amino terminal (NT-proBNP)are established as a valuable aid to the identification of cardiac disease failure in children presenting with non-specific respiratory symptoms and to evaluate the degree of heart failure severity and treatment response.
    - ■ Serial BNP or NT-proBNP measurements can be used in children to guide therapeutic intervention or to monitor heart failure status.
  - » Cardiac troponins
    - ■ Cardiac troponins are likely to be more elevated in heart failure resulting from acute myocarditis.
    - ■ Troponins can be elevated in cardiomyopathy with increasing levels correlating with severity.
- **Infection markers in suspected myocarditis**
  - » Blood for PCR (parvovirus, adenovirus, Epstein–Barr Virus, Cytomegalovirus, Herpes Simplex Virus, Human Herpesvirus (HHV) 6–8, Influenza A & B, mycoplasma)
  - » Nasopharyngeal/tracheal aspirate/swab for parvovirus, respiratory viruses
  - » Stool/rectal swab for viral PCR (coxsackievirus, echovirus)
- **Metabolic and genetic testing**
  - » Early and accurate identification of a metabolic or genetic aetiology for heart failure may allow for life-saving disease-specific management, identify family members at risk and provide guidance for reproductive counselling.
  - » Primary screening investigations for metabolic disorders include plasma lactate, pyruvate, ammonia, plasma amino acids, acylcarnitine profile, urine amino acids, urine organic acids, urine mucopolysaccharide screen (glycosaminoglycans).
  - » Subspecialty consultation with genetic and/or metabolic services is recommended to guide further testing such as muscle biopsy or specific gene testing, molecular or cytogenetic testing.
- **Family assessment**
  - » A detailed family history with pedigree (3 generations) is important in establishing familial cardiomyopathy. Excluding familial cardiomyopathy is crucial, especially when the presentation is in the foetus or newborn.
  - » Perform ECG and echocardiography in all first-degree relatives.

Management

In the acute management of heart failure, the patients can be thought of as having symptoms related to fluid overload, systemic under-perfusion or both (Figure 7.18).

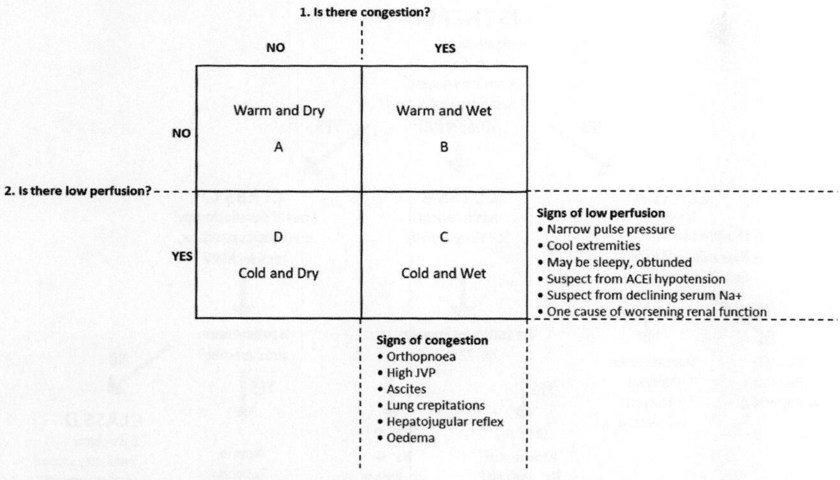

Figure 7.18 Patterns of presentation recognised in acute decompensated heart failure.
Redrawn and modified from Stevenson LW, *et al.* (2002) Treatment of congestive heart failure. *JAMA*; **287**:2209–2210.

The early management of children with heart failure should address these problems. It is important to note that indiscriminate administration of intravenous fluid resuscitation is contraindicated and will worsen the condition of children with heart failure symptoms.

See Figure 7.19 for an approach to the management of acute decompensated heart failure (ADHF) and Figure 7.20 for guidance to the introduction of oral maintenance therapy in chronic heart failure.

Treat the Underlying Cause of the Heart Failure, If Possible

- Surgery or transcatheter therapy for structural heart defect, after stabilisation.
- Pericardiocentesis for pericardial effusion.
- Adenosine, other anti-arrhythmic agents or cardioversion for arrhythmias causing heart failure.

General Measures

- Bed rest, limit activities.
- Nurse propped up or sitting up.
- Thermo-neutral environment; control fever.
- Tube feeding in small infants.
- Fluid restriction is necessary in admitted patients, especially if dilutional hyponatraemia is present or in overtly fluid-overloaded patients.
- Sedation may be used with caution in view of risk of respiratory depression, under supervised settings. Oral chloral hydrate 10–20 mg/kg/dose, 6–8 hourly/

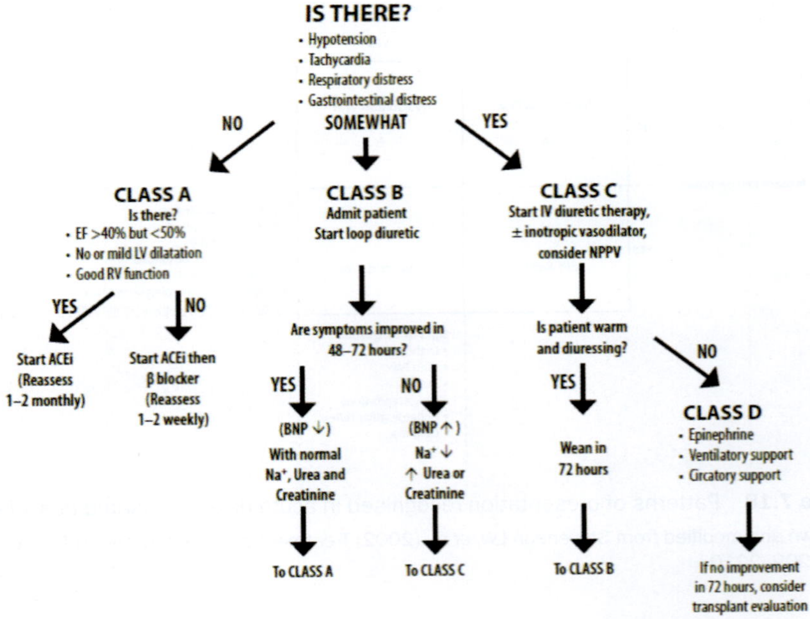

Figure 7.19 Simplified algorithm for heart failure management.

ACEi: angiotensin-converting enzyme inhibitor; BNP: brain natriuretic peptide; EF: ejection fraction; IV: intravenous; LV: left ventricular; NPPV: non-invasive positive pressure ventilation; RV: right ventricular

Redrawn and modified from Kantor PF, *et al.* (2013) Presentation, diagnosis, and medical management of heart failure in children: Canadian Cardiovascular Society Guidelines. *Can J Cardiology*; **29**: 1535–1552.

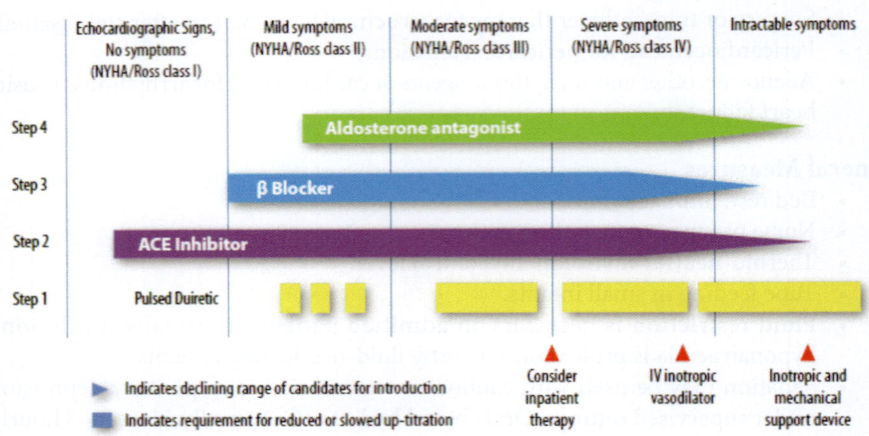

Figure 7.20 Stepwise introduction of medical therapy in heart failure.

Redrawn and modified from Kantor PF, *et al.* (2013) Presentation, diagnosis and medical management of heart failure in children: Canadian Cardiovascular Society Guidelines. *Can J Cardiology* **29**:1535–1552.

as needed. In older patients, IV morphine infusion 10–20 mcg/kg/h can be considered.

- Correct any negative inotropic factors, e.g. acidosis, hypoglycaemia, hypocalcaemia and anaemia.
- Oxygen — caution in patients with left-to-right shunt (e.g. VSD); Oxygen causes pulmonary vasodilatation and thus increases the shunt, aggravating pulmonary congestion and pulmonary oedema.
- Non-invasive ventilatory support with CPAP or mechanical ventilation, if necessary.

Diuretics

- Frusemide IV/PO 1 mg/kg/dose, 6–12 hourly (max. dose 20–40 mg/dose in patient with normal renal function). In selected patients, continuous IV infusion at 0.1–1.0 mg/kg/h.
- Spironolactone as an adjunct (mineralocorticoid receptor antagonist), and a potassium-sparing diuretic PO 1 mg/kg/dose (max. 25 mg) 8–12 hourly.
- Monitor urine output and serum electrolytes.

Inotropic Agents

- Milrinone
  - » A phosphodiesterase III inhibitor that is both a vasodilator and an inotropic agent. Useful in situations in which both these effects are desirable, e.g. post-cardiac surgery, myocarditis.
  - » IV infusion 0.25–0.75 mcg/kg/min.
  - » First choice agent for ADHF requiring moderate inotropic support
- Dobutamine
  - » A β-adrenergic receptor agonist.
  - » Lower doses promote renal vasodilation.
  - » Higher doses discouraged, as they promote tachycardia.

Angiotensin-Converting Enzyme Inhibitors (ACEi)

- The use of ACEi therapy is indicated in children with heart failure due to primary heart muscle disease of the systemic left ventricle.
- Contraindicated in patients with left-to-right shunts.
- In advanced heart failure, ACEi therapy introduction should occur after stabilisation of heart failure symptoms with diuretics and simultaneous to inotropic support withdrawal.
- Captopril (0.1 mg/kg/dose, 8 hourly) is the typical first choice for most infants and enalapril (0.1 mg/kg/dose, 12 hourly) being an appropriate choice for those older than 2 years.
- Up-titration can proceed safely over 3–10 days in most inpatients and can be more gradual in outpatients. Target dose of captopril is 3 mg/kg/day and enalapril 0.5 mg/kg/dose.

Beta-Adrenergic Receptor Antagonist

- Benefits of beta blockers in the treatment of adults with heart failure demonstrated in >20 randomised controlled trials. Only few uncontrolled studies indicating benefits in children.
- Contraindication: Decompensated heart failure, heart block, bradycardia, asthma.
- Caution: Reduced heart function during initial stages of therapy, hypotension, bradycardia.
- Carvedilol is the first choice for most children with normal systolic blood pressure; start at PO 0.1 mg/kg/dose (max. 3.125 mg) 12 hourly. If tolerated, double the dose every 1–2 weeks to max. of 0.4–0.6 mg/kg/dose (adult 12.5–25 mg) 12 hourly.
- Metoprolol is the usual choice for children with reduced systolic blood pressure; for patients <50 kg, start at PO 0.5 mg/kg/day 12 hourly, doubling 2 weekly to a max. of 4 mg/kg/day; for patients>50 kg, start at 12.5 mg/dose 12 hourly, doubling 2 weekly to a max. of 100 mg 12 hourly.

Newer Therapeutic Options

- Levosimendan
  - » A calcium sensitising agent. Both an inotropic agent and peripheral vasodilator that helps in afterload reduction without increasing myocardial oxygen consumption.
  - » Limited studies in paediatric population for heart failure. Some positive effect has been shown in intra-operative settings post-cardiopulmonary bypass.
  - » Consider if unresponsive to traditional inotropic therapy. Used mostly as potential rescue strategy to avoid mechanical circulatory support.
- Sacubitril/Valsartan (Entresto®)
  - » Improvement in cardiovascular outcomes demonstrated in chronic heart failure management in the adult population.
  - » In the ongoing PANORAMA-HF trial (at the time of writing), preliminary results show a reduction in NT-proBNP in the treatment of symptomatic heart failure with systemic left ventricular systolic dysfunction in paediatric patients beyond 1 year of age. Long-term efficacy in the paediatric population remains to be evaluated.
  - » Not to be taken within 36 hours of taking an ACE-inhibitor.

Options for Intractable Heart Failure

- Options available in selected patients include extracorporeal membrane oxygenation (ECMO), ventricular assist devices (VAD) and referral for heart transplant assessment. Intra-aortic balloon pump (IAPB) has been used in young adults.

Bibliography

1. Chang AC, Towbin JA. (2006) *Heart Failure in Children and Young Adults: From Molecular Mechanisms to Medical and Surgical Strategies*. Sanders Elsevier.

2. Kantor PF, Lougheed J, Dancea A, *et al.* (2013) Presentation, diagnosis, and medical management of heart failure in children: Canadian Cardiovascular Society guidelines. *Can J Cardiol* **29**:1535–1552.
3. Kantor PF, Mertens LL. (2010). Heart failure in children. Part I: Clinical evaluation, diagnostic testing, and initial medical management. *Eur J Pediatr* **169**:269–279.
4. Maron BJ, Towbin JA, Thiene G, *et al.* (2006). Contemporary definitions and classification of the cardiomyopathies: An American Heart Association Scientific Statement from the Council on Clinical Cardiology, Heart Failure and Transplantation Committee; Quality of Care and Outcomes Research and Functional Genomics and Translational Biology Interdisciplinary Working Groups; and Council on Epidemiology and Prevention. *Circulation* **113**:1807–1816.
5. Abman SH, Hansmann G, Archer SL, *et al.* (2015) Pediatric pulmonary hypertension. Guidelines from the American Heart Association and American Thoracic Society. *Circulation* **132**:2037–2099.
6. Silvetti S, Silvani P, Azzolini ML, *et al.* (2015) Systemic review on levosimendan in paediatric patients. *Curr Vasc Pharmacol* **13**:128–133.
7. McMurray JJ, Packer M, Desai AS, *et al.* (2014) Angiotensin-Neprilysin inhibition versus Enalapril in heart failure. *N Eng J Med* **371**:993–1004.

CHAPTER 28

Infective Endocarditis

Tan Teng Hong

Definition

Infective endocarditis (IE) is the inflammation of the valvular or mural endocardium caused by microorganisms (bacteria or fungi) involving either the heart or the great vessels (i.e. endarteritis — infection of the lining of blood vessels); the pathology also may include abscess formation.

At Risk Patients

- Congenital heart disease (CHD)
  - >90% of IE cases occur in individuals who have heart disease, usually congenital
  - Post-operative cardiac surgery
    - Cardiac surgery itself is an important risk factor for IE.
    - Highest risk in children who had repair or palliation of cyanotic CHD.
    - Incidence of IE in the first post-operative month is low for most defects and increases with time after surgery.
    - When prosthetic valves or conduits are used in surgical repairs, the risk for IE is high even in the immediate (first 2 weeks) post-operative period.
    - Corrective surgery for isolated ventricular septal defect (VSD), secundum atrial septal defect (ASD) or patent ductus arteriosus (PDA) with documentation of no residual leak, risk for IE is the same as for the general population, 6 months after surgery.
- Degenerative or rheumatic heart disease
- Normal hearts with
  - Central indwelling venous catheters
  - *Staphylococcus aureus* bacteraemia
  - Intravenous drug abuse

Patients with congenital or acquired immunodeficiencies are not at higher risk for IE.

Causative Organisms

- Most common organisms are gram-positive cocci — Viridans group streptococci, staphylococci and enterococci.
- Less commonly, gram-negative bacilli — HACEK group (*Haemophilus* species, *Actinobacillus actinomycetemcomitans*, *Cardiobacterium hominis*, *Eikenella corrodens* and *Kingella* species).
- IE associated with indwelling central catheters, prosthetic valves or materials — *S. aureus*, coagulase-negative staphylococci.
- Newborn infants — *S. aureus*, coagulase-negative staphylococci, Candida species, *group B streptococcus* and *Streptococcus pneumoniae*.
- Fungi — the most common fungus is *Candida*, followed by *Aspergillus*.

Clinical Features

Due to four underlying phenomena:

1. Bacteraemia (or fungaemia) — fever, myalgia, arthralgia, malaise.
2. Valvulitis — new heart murmur or change in murmur, congestive heart failure (CHF).
3. Embolic phenomenon — petechiae, hepatosplenomegaly, splinter haemorrhages, Janeway lesions (painless haemorrhagic lesions on palms and soles), Osler nodes (painful lesions at fingertips), pulmonary emboli, mycotic aneurysm, intracranial haemorrhage and conjunctival haemorrhages.
4. Immunologic responses — glomerulonephritis, Osler nodes, Roth's spots.

Presentation

- Indolent (subacute bacterial endocarditis)
  - » Prolonged low-grade fever
  - » Variety of somatic complaints, including fatigue, weakness, arthralgias, myalgias, weight loss, rigors and diaphoresis
- Fulminant (acute bacterial endocarditis)
  - » High, spiking fever
  - » Rapidly changing symptoms
  - » Acutely ill
- Cardiac signs are variable (see Table 7.11):
  - » Valvular destruction, regurgitant murmurs
  - » Cyanotic CHD in a child who has undergone a systemic-pulmonary shunt procedure may present with declining systemic oxygen saturation, reflecting a graft infection with obstruction of flow.
  - » Patients with right-sided, catheter-related infection may have few or no specific cardiovascular signs but may present with primarily pulmonary symptoms and signs related to septic pulmonary embolisation.

Table 7.11 Presenting Signs in Children with Infective Endocarditis

Sign	%
Fever	99
Petechiae	21
Changing murmur	21
Dental caries	14
Hepatosplenomegaly	14
Congestive heart failure	9
Splenomegaly	7
Splinter haemorrhages	5
Retinal haemorrhages (Roth spots)	5
Osler nodes	4
Arthritis	3

Investigations

- Blood Cultures
  - » The likelihood of culturing the causative organism is directly related to the volume of blood obtained (1–3 ml in infants; 5–7 ml in older children).
  - » It is not necessary to time blood sampling with fever because bacteraemia in IE is usually continuous.
  - » Three blood cultures are obtained by separate venepunctures on the first day, and if there is no growth by the second day of incubation, two more should be obtained.
  - » In patients who are not acutely ill and whose blood cultures are still negative, draw three aerobic blood cultures over the first day and hold antibiotics; if cultures are negative after 24 hours, draw two cultures and incubate for 2 weeks.
  - » For patients with acute IE, three separate venepunctures for blood cultures, with 1 hour separating the first and the last, before administering empiric antibiotics.
  - » Request forms for the blood cultures should indicate that IE is suspected to ensure that the laboratory will incubate the cultures for at least 2 weeks.
  - » If fastidious or unusual organisms are suspected, the microbiology laboratory should be consulted.
  - » Culture of arterial blood is not more useful than venepuncture.
  - » In a stable patient suspected to have IE and treated with antibiotics for <4 days but with no prior blood culture, stopping the antibiotic before taking blood cultures can be considered.

- Miscellaneous Laboratory Tests
  - » Anaemia — can be due to haemolysis or anaemia of chronic disease
  - » Leukocytosis — not a consistent feature of IE
  - » Elevated acute-phase reactants, e.g., ESR, CRP
  - » Renal/urine: Haematuria, red blood cell casts, proteinuria and renal insufficiency, immune complex glomerulonephritis
- Transthoracic Echocardiography (TTE)
  - » Findings:
    - ■ Identify vegetations (hallmark)
    - ■ Determine the site and extent of infection
    - ■ Baseline evaluation of ventricular performance and cardiac chamber dimension
    - ■ Monitor serial cardiac function
    - ■ Pericardial effusion or myocardial abscess
  - » Inadequate in some circumstances:
    - ■ Obese or very muscular adolescent
    - ■ Post-cardiac surgery patients — presence of compromised respiratory function or pulmonary hyperinflation
    - ■ Patients with poor echogenicity
    - ■ Complex cardiac anatomy
    - ■ Absence of vegetations on echocardiography does not rule out IE
    - ■ Conversely, an echogenic mass can represent a sterile thrombus, sterile prosthetic material or normal anatomic variation rather than an infected vegetation.
- Transoesophageal Echocardiography (TEE)
  - » TTE is usually adequate in children and may not need transoesophageal echocardiogram.
  - » TEE should be reserved for those who have poor echo windows, in whom prosthetic valves cause 'shadowing' and TTE view appears normal despite a high index of suspicion for IE.

Diagnosis

The utility of the Modified Duke Criteria (Table 7.12) in diagnosing IE in paediatric patients has been established.

Management

Acute management: Antibiotics (Table 7.13), treatment of CHF, cardiac surgery if severe valvular regurgitation, aortic root abscess, large vegetation or embolic phenomena.

Long-term management: Management of residual lesions or sequelae.

Table 7.12 Modified Duke Criteria for the Diagnosis of Infective Endocarditis

Major Criteria

1. Blood culture positive for IE
   a. Typical microorganisms consistent with IE from two separate blood cultures:
      - Viridans streptococci, *Streptococcus bovi*, HACEK group; OR
      - Community-acquired *Staphylococcus aureus* or enterococci, in the absence of a primary focus; OR
   b. Microorganisms consistent with IE from persistently positive blood cultures, defined as follows:
      - At least two positive cultures of blood samples drawn >12 hr apart; OR
      - All of 3 or a majority of ≥4 separate cultures of blood (with first and last sample drawn ≥1 hr apart)
   c. Single culture positive for *Coxiella burnetii*, or antiphase I IgG antibody titre >1:800
2. Evidence of endocardial involvement on echocardiogram
   a. Echocardiogram positive for IE (TEE recommended in patients with prosthetic valves, rated at least 'possible IE' by clinical criteria, or complicated IE [paravalvular abscess]; TTE as first test in other patients), defined as follows:
      - Oscillating intracardiac mass on valve or supporting structures, in the path of regurgitant jets, or on implanted material in the absence of an alternative anatomic explanation; OR
      - Abscess; OR
      - New partial dehiscence of prosthetic valve
   b. New valvular regurgitation (worsening or changing of pre-existing murmur not sufficient)

Minor Criteria

- Predisposition, predisposing heart condition or IV drug use
- Fever, temperature ≥38°C
- Vascular phenomenon: Major arterial emboli, septic pulmonary infarcts, mycotic aneurysm, intracranial haemorrhage, conjunctival haemorrhage, Janeway lesion
- Immunologic phenomenon: Glomerulonephritis, Osler nodes, Roth spots, rheumatoid factor
- Microbiological evidence: Positive blood culture that does not meet major criteria or serologic evidence of active infection with organism consistent with IE
- Echocardiographic minor criteria eliminated

Definite IE

Pathological Criteria

- Microorganisms demonstrated by culture or histologic examination of vegetation, vegetation that has embolised, or intracardiac abscess; OR
- Pathologic lesions; vegetation or intracardiac abscess confirmed by histologic examination showing active IE

Clinical Criteria

- Two major criteria; OR
- One major and three minor criteria; OR
- Five minor criteria

Possible IE

- One major and one minor criterion; OR
- Three minor criteria

Rejected

- Firm alternative diagnosis; OR
- Resolution of symptoms with antibiotic therapy for ≤4 d; OR
- No pathologic evidence of IE at surgery or autopsy, with antibiotic therapy for ≤4 d; OR
  Does not meet criteria for possible IE, as above

Table 7.13 Antimicrobial Guidelines for Paediatric Infective Endocarditis

Infection	Usual Organisms	Suggested Therapy: First-Line Therapy	Suggested Therapy: Alternative Therapy (if severe penicillin allergy)	What to Do If 'Cultures Negative & Patient Better'	Duration (days)	Remarks
Native valve (community acquired) **Prosthetic devices/valve (>1 yr post-implant)**	Streptococci (viridans & other nutritional variants), *S. aureus* (more common in neonates, IV drug users, presence of indwelling catheters), Enterococci, HACEK organisms	(IV Amoxicillin/Clav 120 mg/kg/d (Amox: 100 mg/kg/d) Q8H PLUS IV Gentamicin 3 mg/kg/d Q8H) WITH/WITHOUT PO Rifampicin 20 mg/kg/d Q8–12H (if prosthetic device)	(IV Vancomycin 60 mg/kg/d Q6H PLUS IV Gentamicin 3 mg/kg/d Q8H) WITH/WITHOUT PO Rifampicin 20 mg/kg/d Q8-12H (if prosthetic device)	Continue IV antibiotics at least 4 wk. Stop Vancomycin (if used) if no evidence of resistant Staph. or enterococci.	**Native valve:** 4 w; (2 w Genta if uncomplicated endocarditis with penicillin sensitive isolates with MIC ≤0.1 mg/L) **Prosthetic valve:** ≥6 w (2 w Genta if uncomplicated endocarditis with penicillin sensitive isolates with MIC ≤0.1 mg/L)	Inform laboratory if unusual organisms suspected. 2 w regimen not recommended if clinical symptoms >3 mth, extracardiac focus of infection, intracardiac abscess, mycotic aneurysm. Enterococci inherently resistant to cephalosporins despite *in vitro* testing. Refer ID for treatment of complicated, drug-resistant endocarditis (any organism). Note: Beta-lactams clinically superior to glycopeptides for beta-lactam-sensitive organisms.
Nosocomial (in presence of vascular cannulae) **Prosthetic devices/valve (≤1 yr post-implant)**	As Above & CoNS, uncommonly Candida, GBS, *S. pneumoniae*	(IV Piperacillin/Tazo. (Pip) 300 mg/kg/d Q8H PLUS IV Clindamycin 40 mg/kg/d Q6H) WITH/WITHOUT PO Rifampicin 20 mg/kg/d Q8–12H (if prosthetic device)	(IV Vancomycin 60 mg/kg/d Q6H PLUS IV Ciprofloxacin 30 mg/kg/d Q8H) WITH/WITHOUT PO Rifampicin 20 mg/kg/d Q8-12H (if prosthetic device)	Continue IV antibiotics at least 4–6 wk. Stop Vancomycin (if used) if no evidence of resistant Staph. or enterococci.	Nosocomial/prosthetic valve: ≥6 w	See above. Use Ciprofloxacin with caution in G6PD deficiency. If G6PD deficient, consider Meropenem (1% cross-reactivity in penicillin allergy).

(*Continued*)

Table 7.13 (*Continued*)

Infection	Usual Organisms	Suggested Therapy: First-Line Therapy	Suggested Therapy: Alternative Therapy (if severe penicillin allergy)	What to Do If 'Cultures Negative & Patient Better'	Duration (days)	Remarks
Pre-exposure Prophylaxis (see Table 7.14: 'Antibiotic Prophylaxis for Infective Endocarditis')	Streptococci (viridans & other nutritional variants), *S. aureus*, Enterococci	PO Amoxicillin 50 mg/kg/dose (max. 2 g) (preferred) OR IV Ampicillin 50 mg/kg/dose (preferred if unable to tolerate PO) OR PO Cephalexin 50 mg/kg/dose (max. 2 g)* OR IV Cefazolin 50 mg/kg/dose* *if intolerant to Amox/Ampi but not allergic	IV/PO Clindamycin 20 mg/kg/dose OR PO Clarithromycin 15 mg/kg/dose	N.A.	1 dose	For oral prophylactic antibiotics (e.g. dental/minor procedures), give 1 hr before surgery. For IV prophylactic antibiotics (major procedures), to give 30 min before surgery

General Principles

- Prolonged course of intravenous therapy for at least 4 weeks duration or 3 weeks afebrile.
- Consider 6 weeks antibiotics if:
  - » Prosthetic valve IE
  - » Highly virulent organisms (e.g. *S. aureus*)
  - » Relative antibiotic resistance of organism
- Dual or more antibiotics for synergistic effect.
- Outpatient antibiotic therapy can be considered in uncomplicated cases on a case-by-case basis, after the initial hospital treatment.

Surgery

- Decisions regarding surgery in patients with IE should be individualised, with input from both the cardiologist and the cardiothoracic surgeon.
- There is limited information concerning the effects of surgical timing on the outcomes in children, but some authors have suggested excellent results with surgical intervention during the active phase of infection.
- If a patient with IE is receiving long-term oral anticoagulation, warfarin therapy should be discontinued and replaced by heparin immediately after the diagnosis of IE has been established in the event that surgical intervention is required.

Indications for Surgical Intervention

- Most common indication — severe valvular insufficiency
- Progressive cardiac failure (usually due to valvular regurgitation)
- Persistent bacteraemia after 1–2 weeks of appropriate antibiotic therapy
- Perivalvular extension of infection/abscess formation
- Valve dehiscence, perforation, rupture or fistula
- Fungal endocarditis
- Prosthetic valve IE (particularly early prosthetic valve IE, that is, <12 months after valve replacement)
- Ruptured sinus of Valsalva or ventricular septum
- Significant embolic events
- Especially when the aortic or mitral valve is involved, that is, left-sided vegetations
- Soft indications — anterior mitral valve vegetation (particularly with size >10 mm), or persistent vegetation after systemic embolisation, or an increase in vegetation size despite appropriate antimicrobial therapy
- Patients may eventually require surgical intervention for chronic valvular stenosis or regurgitation caused by previous IE
- IE related to a haemodynamically trivial VSD should potentially be considered for surgical repair following successful treatment of the infection.

Table 7.14 Antibiotic Prophylaxis for Prevention of Infective Endocarditis

	Cardiac Conditions	Types of Procedures	
Recommended	• Prosthetic cardiac valve or prosthetic material used for cardiac valve repair • Previous infective endocarditis • Certain congenital heart disease (CHD) » Unrepaired cyanotic CHD » Cyanotic CHD with palliative shunts and/or conduits » Complex intracardiac repair of CHD » Repaired congenital heart defect with prosthetic material or device, whether placed by surgery or by catheter intervention, during the first 6 mth after the procedure. » Repaired CHD with residual defects at the site or adjacent to the site of a prosthetic patch or prosthetic device (which inhibit endothelialisation), by cardiac surgery or percutaneous technique. • Cardiac transplantation recipients who develop cardiac valvulopathy	• Dental procedures » All dental procedures requiring manipulation of the gingival or periapical region of the teeth or perforation of the oral mucosa. • Respiratory tract procedures » Invasive procedure of the respiratory tract that involves incision or biopsy of the respiratory mucosa, such as tonsillectomy and adenoidectomy. » Invasive procedure to treat an established infection, such as drainage of an abscess or empyema. • Procedures involving infected skin, skin structure or musculoskeletal tissue.	
Reasonable	• Left-sided valvular lesions » Aortic stenosis » Aortic regurgitation » Mitral stenosis » Mitral regurgitation • Patients who have previously received antibiotic prophylaxis, and who would like to continue having it, despite the rationale for the change in policy being fully explained (even though lesions may not be part of the list of cardiac conditions listed above)	• As Above	
Not Recommended	• Any other form of CHD except for the conditions listed in 'Recommended'	• Dental procedures » Routine anaesthetic injections through non-infected tissue » Treatment of superficial caries » Placement of removable prosthodontic or orthodontic appliances » Removal of sutures » Dental X-rays » Shedding of deciduous/primary teeth » Trauma to the lips or oral mucosa • Respiratory tract » Endotracheal intubation » Bronchoscopy » Tympanostomy tube insertion	• Gastrointestinal or genitourinary tract procedures (unless there is an established infection) • Skin and soft tissue — any procedure on non-infected tissue • Others » Cardiac catheterisation, including balloon angioplasty » Implanted cardiac pacemakers, implanted defibrillators and coronary stents » Incision or biopsy of surgically scrubbed skin » Circumcision » Vaginal or Caesarean delivery

Prognosis

Mortality

- Estimated ~11–17%

Complications of IE

- Congestive heart failure (~7%, secondary to severe valvular regurgitation)
- Embolic events: cerebral (stroke ~8%), pulmonary (~10%), renal, coronary, gastrointestinal tract
- Periannular extension of abscess
- Arrhythmias (~8%), heart block
- Prosthetic device dysfunction
- Valvular dehiscence
- Graft or shunt occlusion
- Persistent bacteraemia or fungaemia
- Metastatic infection: renal abscess (~3%), osteomyelitis (1%)
- Mycotic aneurysms
- Glomerulonephritis or renal failure

Prophylaxis

The most recent revision of the American Heart Association (AHA) guidelines on infective endocarditis prophylaxis occurred in 2015 (see Table 7.14). The new guidelines suggested to shift the disproportionately large focus on antibiotic prophylaxis to an emphasis on oral hygiene, and that prophylaxis should be targeted at conditions that are associated with the highest probability of adverse outcomes from infective endocarditis.

Conclusions

Even though IE is a rare diagnosis in childhood, a high index of suspicion in persistently febrile patients is necessary, especially in the context of congenital heart disease.

Bibliography

1. Martin JM, Neches WH, Wald ER. (1997) Infective endocarditis: 35 years of experience at a children's hospital. *Clin Infect Dis* **24:**669–675.
2. Li JS, Sexton DJ, Mick N, *et al.* (2000) Proposed modifications to the Duke criteria for the diagnosis of infective endocarditis. *Clin Infect Dis* **30**:633–638.
3. TissieresP, Gervaix A, Beghetti M, Jaeggi ET. (2003) Value and limitations of the von Reyn, Duke and Modified Duke Criteria for the diagnosis of infective endocarditis in children. *Pediatrics* **112:**e467–e471.
4. Ferrieri P, Gewitz MH, Gerber MA, *et al.* (2002) Unique features of infective endocarditis in childhood. *Circulation* **105**:2115–2126.
5. Baddour LM, Wilson WR, Bayer AS, *et al.* (2005) Infective endocarditis: Diagnosis, antimicrobial therapy, and management of complications: A statement for healthcare professionals from the Committee on Rheumatic Fever, Endocarditis, and Kawasaki Disease, Council on Cardiovascular Disease in the Young, and the Councils on Clinical Cardiology, Stroke, and Cardiovascular Surgery and Anesthesia, American

Heart Association: Endorsed by the Infectious Diseases Society of America. *Circulation* **111**:e394–e434.
6. Shamszad P, Khan MS, Rossano JW, *et al.* (2013) Early surgical therapy of infective endocarditis in children: A 15-year experience. *J Thorac Cardiovasc Surg* 146:506–511.
7. Baltimore RS, *et al.* (2015) Infective endocarditis in childhood. 2015 update: A scientific statement from the American Heart Association. *Circulation* **132**:1487–1515.

CHAPTER 29

Kawasaki Disease

Kotecha Monika Kantilal; Choo Tze Liang, Jonathan

Introduction

Kawasaki disease (KD) is an acute febrile systemic inflammatory/vasculitic disease of unknown aetiology, affecting predominantly children younger than 5 years. It was first described by Dr Tomisaku Kawasaki in 1967 and is now considered to be the commonest form of acquired heart disease in developed countries.

In Singapore, the incidence is estimated at 51.4 per 100,000 children younger than 5 years old per year (KKH and NUH databases, 2012). This incidence is one of the highest outside Japan, and very similar to that of Hong Kong and Taiwan. At KK Women's and Children's Hospital (KKH), we see an average of about 100 to 120 new cases a year. The incidence of KD appears to be increasing due to overall improved recognition and a more frequent diagnosis of incomplete KD.

Aetiology

The aetiology and pathogenesis of KD remain largely unknown. Acute systemic vasculitis in KD shows inflammatory cells infiltrate the affected tissues. Infectious triggers for KD are reported in several studies. Several genome-wide association studies have identified the variants of ITPKC, FCGR 2A, BLK, and CD40 genes conferring susceptibility to KD. Other determinants, such as the climate, air currents and environmental factors have been studied. However, these studies have provided inconsistent results.

Diagnosis

There is no specific diagnostic test for KD. KD is diagnosed clinically using the criteria originally described by Dr Kawasaki and modified by the AHA Committee on Rheumatic Fever, Endocarditis and Kawasaki Disease. Laboratory tests may be used to support a diagnosis of KD. In case of suspected KD, hospitalisation is recommended to perform a thorough evaluation and to confirm diagnosis.

Diagnostic Criteria

Fever persistent for at least 5 days† and with the presence of at least four of the five following clinical features‡:

- Rash — polymorphous exanthem. The rash may be accentuated in the perineum where it is often associated with local desquamation. Redness or induration at the BCG vaccination scar may be present. The rash in KD is never vesicular or bullous.

- Bilateral conjunctivitis — painless hyperaemia, non-suppurative and usually sparing the limbus of the eye. Anterior uveitis seen on slit lamp examination strongly supports the diagnosis of KD in the first week of illness.
- Changes in lips and oral mucosa — erythema and cracking of lips, strawberry tongue, diffuse injection of oral and pharyngeal mucosa. Exudative pharyngitis and ulcerative intraoral lesions are not features typical of KD.
- Cervical lymphadenopathy (≥1.5cm in diameter) — unilateral or bilateral, usually the former. Generalised lymphadenopathy is not a feature of KD.
- Changes in extremities — acute: Erythema and oedema of hands and feet. convalescent: Skin desquamation of the tips of the fingers and toes (late sign).

† In the presence of classic features, the diagnosis of complete KD can be made by an experienced physician before 5 days of fever.

‡ Patients with fever and less than four other principal signs can be diagnosed as incomplete KD (see below).

Other Significant Clinical Findings

- Cardiovascular: Pericarditis, myocarditis, endocarditis, arrhythmia, angina pectoris, signs of cardiac failure or shock
- Respiratory: Cough, rhinorrhoea
- Skin and Joints
  - » Late (1–2 months): Beau's lines-transverse groove across the nail bed
  - » Arthralgia and arthritis
- Neurological
  - » Striking irritability, inconsolable crying
  - » Facial palsy, sensorineural hearing loss or other mononeuritis (rare)
  - » Aseptic meningitis — mononuclear pleocytosis in the CSF
  - » Encephalopathy, seizures
- Gastrointestinal
  - » Diarrhoea, vomiting, abdominal pain
  - » Hepatitis
  - » Hydrops of the gallbladder
  - » Acute pancreatitis, cholestatic jaundice
  - » Retropharyngeal phlegmon
  - » Paralytic ileus
- Renal
  - » Sterile pyuria is common — urethral origin
  - » Occasional proteinuria
  - » Urethritis
  - » Testicular swelling
- Vascular:
  - » Aneurysms of peripheral arteries, e.g. axillary, or femoral (rare)

- » Raynaud's phenomenon
- » Peripheral gangrene

Investigations

- Haematological
  - » Full blood count (FBC) — increase white blood cells, maximal elevation of polymorphonuclear cells. Normocytic normochromic anaemia. Thrombocytosis, typically in the 2nd and 3rd week, normalisation in 4–8 weeks.
  - » Inflammatory parameters — elevated erythrocyte sedimentation rate (ESR), slow normalisation. Elevated C-reactive protein (CRP), fast normalisation.
  - » Liver function tests (LFT) — increase in alanine amino transaminases, gamma-glutamyl transpeptidase, bilirubin. Hypoalbuminemia in more severe and prolonged illness.
  - » Urea, creatinine, electrolytes (Renal panel) — hyponatraemia.
  - » Anti-streptolysin-O titre (ASOT)
  - » Cardiac enzymes and troponin — may be elevated if myocarditis/ coronary ischaemia with thrombosis.
- Urinalysis and culture sensitivity — urine white blood cells more than 10/high powered field (sterile pyuria).
- Cerebrospinal fluid examination — aseptic meningitis (normal glucose/proteins, white blood cells 125,000–300,000/mm^3)
- Chest radiograph — cardiomegaly, pulmonary infiltrates, pulmonary nodule
- Electrocardiogram: Prolonged PR interval, nonspecific ST and T wave changes, arrhythmias, abnormal T wave changes, abnormal Q waves, low voltages
- Echocardiogram — 2D Echocardiogram is performed at day 14 of illness. Early 2D echocardiogram (before 14 days) may be performed as per the algorithm below. However, a normal echocardiogram does not exclude the diagnosis of KD as coronary artery changes rarely develop in the early phase.
  - » 2D echocardiogram may show coronary artery changes, mitral regurgitation/ aortic and tricuspid regurgitation or pericardial effusion in the acute phase. Aortic dilation may be seen in a later phase.
  - » Classification of coronary artery aneurysms in the acute phase (day 14 or earlier) of Kawasaki disease:
    - ▪ Dilation: Z-score: ≥2 to <2.5
    - ▪ Small aneurysm: Z-score ≥2.5 to <5
    - ▪ Medium aneurysm: Z-score ≥5 to <10
    - ▪ Giant aneurysm: Z-score ≥10 or aneurysm showing an internal diameter ≥8 mm (in children ≥5 years).
- Other imaging modalities like Magnetic Resonance Imaging (MRI) of the vascular tree or coronary angiography or Computed Tomography (CT) may be performed in selected patients.

The following investigations are recommended in all patients with KD: FBC, CRP, ESR (note ESR cannot be used for trending after IVIG administration), Renal panel, LFT, ASOT, Urinalysis and culture, COVID-19 swab (in context of current pandemic), *ECG (to be done before discharge).*

Incomplete Kawasaki Disease

When the clinical presentation is suggestive of KD but does not meet the full criteria, the diagnosis of incomplete KD requires further supportive investigations (Figure 7.21).

One should consider incomplete KD in:

- A child with fever for ≥5 days with 2 or 3 of the principal clinical features.
- Infants under 6 months of age with prolonged fever and irritability.
- Infants with prolonged fever and aseptic meningitis.
- Infants or children with prolonged fever and unexplained lymphadenitis, retro tonsillar collection or shock.

Incomplete KD can present a significant diagnostic dilemma; however, once the diagnosis is made, the treatment for incomplete KD is similar to complete KD. Infants and adolescents who present with an incomplete picture may be at a higher risk for cardiac complications since treatment may be delayed.

Kawasaki disease shock syndrome (KDSS) presents with haemodynamic instability, including hypotension or clinical signs of inadequate perfusion. Patients with KDSS are likely to have lymphadenopathy, coronary involvement and less identifiable foci in comparison to patients with toxic shock syndrome.

Differential Diagnosis

The differential diagnosis in a child with possible KD, presenting with conjunctivitis and rash together with prolonged fever include:

- Infectious:
  - » Streptococcal and staphylococcal toxin-mediated diseases (scarlet fever, toxic shock syndrome)
  - » Measles, adenovirus infection and other viral infections
  - » With epidemiologic risk factors:
    - ▪ Leptospirosis
    - ▪ Yersinia pseudotuberculosis infection (rare)
    - ▪ Rickettsia infection (rare in Singapore)
- Non-infectious:
  - » Drug reactions, Stevens–Johnson syndrome
  - » Macrophage activating syndrome
  - » Autoimmune or immune complex diseases — Systemic Lupus Erythematosus (SLE), Juvenile Rheumatoid Arthritis (JRA), polyarteritis nodosa, Reiter's syndrome, Behçet's disease, inflammatory bowel disease, post-infectious

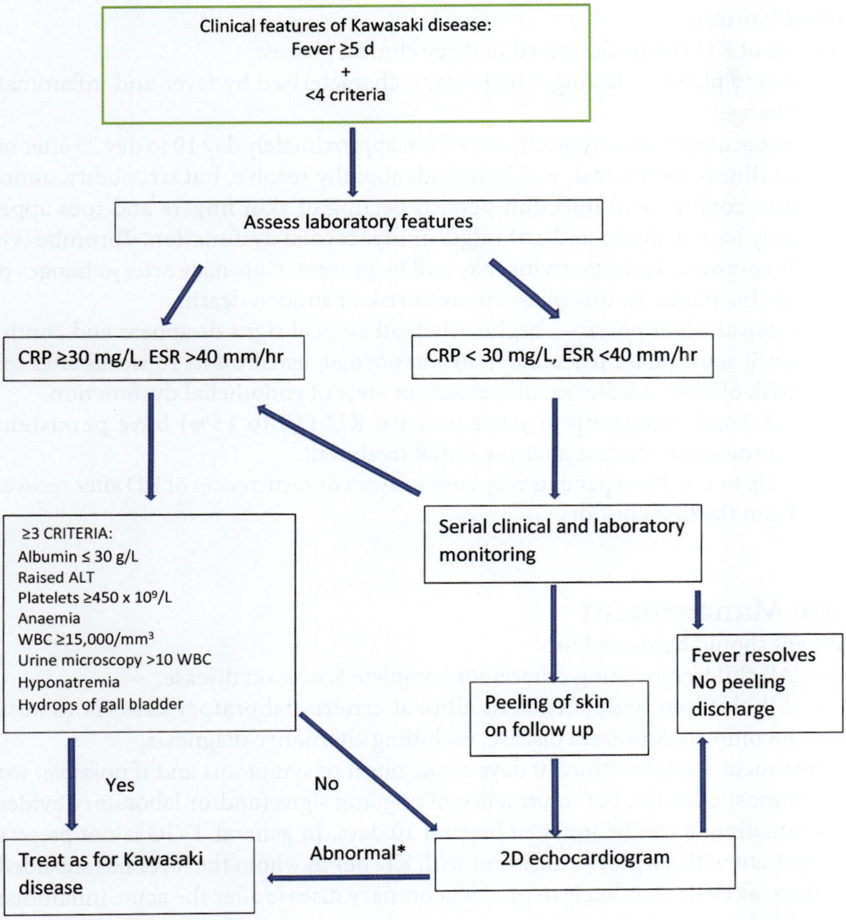

Figure 7.21. Flowchart for diagnosis of Incomplete Kawasaki disease. (Modified from AHA 2017 guideline form management of KD).

*Echocardiography is considered ABNORMAL for purposes of this algorithm if any of the three conditions are met:

- Z-score of left anterior descending coronary artery or right coronary artery ≥2.5;
- Coronary artery aneurysm is observed; or
- ≥3 other suggestive features exist, including decreased left ventricular function, mitral regurgitation, pericardial effusion, or Z-scores in left anterior descending coronary artery or right coronary artery of 2 to 2.5.

Clinical Course

The course of KD can be described in three clinical phases:

- Acute phase — lasting 7 to 14 days, characterised by fever and inflammatory changes.
- Subacute phase — typically lasts from approximately day 10 to day 25 after onset of illness. Fever, rash and lymphadenopathy resolve, but irritability, anorexia and conjunctival injection persist. Peeling of skin fingers and toes appears; may have arthritis and arthralgia or myocardial dysfunction. Thrombocytosis is common. Conjunctivitis may still be present. Coronary artery changes peak in this phase. In this phase, there is risk of sudden death.
- Convalescent phase — begins when all clinical signs disappear and continues until acute phase reactants return to normal, usually 4 to 10 weeks after onset. Risk of acute cardiovascular events in view of endothelial dysfunction.

  A small subgroup of patients with KD (10 to 15%) have persistent or recrudescent disease after the initial treatment.

  Up to 1 to 3% of patients may have relapses or recurrences of KD after recovering from the first episode.

Acute Management

Treatment should be started for:

- All children meeting criteria for complete Kawasaki disease.
- All children with sufficient clinical criteria/laboratory criteria to suspect incomplete Kawasaki disease, excluding alternative diagnosis.

Treatment started within 10 days of the onset of symptoms and if possible, within 7 days, is most effective, but in presence of ongoing signs (and/or laboratory evidence) of inflammation, it can be initiated beyond 10 days. In general, IVIG is not prescribed for the patient with a history consistent with KD but in whom the fever has subsided for many days, as IVIG is unlikely to prevent coronary disease after the acute inflammation has subsided.

First-line Treatment

- **Intravenous immunoglobulin (IVIG)**

  Intravenous immunoglobulin is the primary treatment for patients with KD. Giving IVIG in the acute phase reduces the risk of coronary aneurysms by at least 3 to 5 fold. Note: IVIG reduces the risk but does NOT completely prevent development of coronary abnormalities. Dose: 2 g/kg as a single infusion. Infuse over 8 to 12 hours; start at a very low infusion rate and increase gradually. The infusion rate can be ordered as 0.5 ml/kg/h × 15 min, then 1.0 ml/kg/h × 15 min, then 2.0 ml/kg/h × 15 min, then 4.0 ml/kg/h till completion.

  » Monitoring during infusion
  Temperature, pulse and respiration (TPR), BP Q5min × 3, then
  TPR, BP Q10min × 3, then
  TPR, BP Q15min × 3, then
  TPR, BP Q30min × 3, then

TPR, BP hourly till completion

The infusion site should also be monitored for extravasation during treatment.

» Complications and side effects include chills and rigors, hypotension, drug reactions including anaphylaxis, infections (blood product from pooled donors), aseptic meningitis, haemolytic anaemia (oral steroids may be required for Coombs positive haemolytic anaemia), abnormal liver function tests including jaundice, acute renal failure, thrombocytopenia, pulmonary oedema.

Second-line Treatment

In approximately 10% of patients with KD, there is persistent or recrudescent of fever more than 36 hours after completion of initial IVIG infusion. The following options can be considered in such cases of IVIG failure/resistance as first line therapy:

- Repeat infusion of IVIG 2 g/kg over 10 to 12 hours can be administered.
- Intravenous **Methylprednisolone** 15–30 mg/kg/day for 1–3 days with or without tapering steroids. Side effects are bradycardia, hypertension, hyperglycaemia and hypothermia. During administration, a close monitoring of vital signs, ECG and blood pressure is required.
- **Oral prednisolone** 2 mg/kg/day till defervescence, weaning over 2 to 3 week period.

More studies are required to establish the role of steroids as an adjunct in primary treatment or as rescue for KD patients with refractory or recrudescent KD.

Other Options if Second IVIG/Steroids Fail

- Infliximab
- Cyclosporine
- Cyclophosphamide

Antiplatelet Medications

- **Aspirin**

Aspirin is used for its anti-inflammatory and anti-pyretic effects in the acute phase, in a moderate to high dose, till they subside. Subsequently in the subacute and convalescent phases, the dose of aspirin is reduced to an antiplatelet dose. Low dose aspirin after the acute phase is probably more important when the risk of coronary artery thrombosis is higher; established coronary vasculitis occurs concomitantly with marked thrombocytosis and a hypercoagulable state.

Some studies show that anti-inflammatory doses of aspirin have no added benefit over and above the anti-inflammatory effect of IVIG. Therefore, it may be reasonable to use only antiplatelet low-dose (3–5 mg/kg/day) aspirin. Should a patient present late when acute inflammation has subsided, low dose aspirin can be started.

Aspirin therapy can be stopped after 6 to 8 weeks if the latest echocardiogram shows normal coronary arteries. In patients with persistent coronary abnormalities, aspirin is continued long term.

  - » Dose: Acute phase — moderate dose (30–50 mg/kg/day) to high dose (80–100 mg/kg/day) until afebrile
  - » Subacute/convalescent phase — low dose 3–5 mg/kg/day (antiplatelet dose) as a single dose with meal.
  - » Complications of aspirin therapy — allergy, gastritis, gastrointestinal bleeding, chronic salicylism and Reye's syndrome.
- **Clopidogrel:**
  Clopidogrel is an alternative to patients who are resistant/allergic to aspirin. It is also given as an antiplatelet drug instead of aspirin in those with transaminitis. Clopidogrel can be converted back to aspirin when transaminitis resolves. In children who have contracted varicella while on aspirin or intending to have varicella vaccination, clopidogrel can be replaced for aspirin for 6 weeks. In children who have influenza with acute KD, clopidogrel can be also used instead of aspirin. Clopidogrel is also used as a dual anti-platelet agent (together with aspirin) for moderate aneurysms and as triple therapy for giant aneurysm with thrombosis.
  - » Dose: 0.2 mg/kg/day in children <24 months and 1 mg/kg/day in children >24 months as a single dose.
  - » Side effects: Thrombotic thrombocytopenic purpura, agranulocytosis and severe liver dysfunction may appear early. Others are toxic epidermal necrolysis, gastric ulcer.
- **Dipyridamole**
  Alternative to aspirin if taking ibuprofen/resistant/allergic to aspirin/risk of Reye syndrome.

Anticoagulation/thrombolysis (in Consultation with Cardiologist/ Haematologist):

- **Low molecular weight heparin (LMWH)/heparin** is initiated for rapidly expanding coronary artery aneurysms or large/giant aneurysms (>8 mm or Z-score of ≥10). This is **dual therapy** with low dose aspirin (antiplatelet). Refer to institutional anticoagulation guidelines for titration and target levels.
- For near occlusive/occlusive thrombus, to consider thrombolysis with **recombinant tissue plasminogen activator** or use of glycoprotein IIb/IIIa inhibitor, such as the monoclonal antibody abciximab as per the managing cardiologist's discretion.
- Subsequently for large/giant aneurysms coronary artery with thrombosis, **triple therapy** with aspirin and clopidogrel (2nd antiplatelet) and LMWH/**Warfarin** is recommended. Target INR when on warfarin is 2 to 3.

Supportive Measures

- Maintain fluid balance closely.
- Non-steroidal anti-inflammatory drugs can antagonise the antiplatelet effects of aspirin and is hence avoided.
- Consider need for lansoprazole/omeprazole if high dose aspirin or steroids are given.

- Statins, beta blockers and angiotensin converting enzyme inhibitors may be considered in patients post-thrombolysis on cardiologist's discretion.

Follow-Up of Patients with Kawasaki Disease

Long-term management is aimed at prevention of thrombosis and early detection of thrombosis or stenosis when they occur. This is dependent on the degree of coronary artery involvement and subsequent resolution.

Table 7.15 Long-term Follow up Duration, Cardiac Investigations and Required Medications, According to Coronary Artery Risk

Classification of Risk		KKH Guidelines		
Coronary artery description		Follow-up interval (from disease onset)	Anti-platelet / anti-coagulation	ECG, 2D echocardiogram
1	**No abnormality at any point (Z-score <2)**	• 2 wk, 2 mth, then at 6 mth to 1 yr. • Consider discharge after 6 mth to 1 yr appointment	• Low dose aspirin for 2 mth (from disease onset)	• 2 wk, 2 mth, then at 6 mth to 1 yr.
2	**Dilation only (Z-score 2 to <2.5)**	• 2 wk, 2 mth, 6 mth, 1 yr. • Then annual follow-up if persistent dilatation • Consider discharge at 1 yr or after two normal 2DE, whichever is later	• Low dose aspirin • Stop when 2DE shows normal coronary arteries	• 2 wk, 2 mth, 6 mth, 1 yr. • Subsequently annually till discharge
3	**Small aneurysm**	• 2 wk, 2 mth, 6 mth, 1 yr; subsequently	• Low dose aspirin • Stop when 2DE shows normal coronary arteries.	• 2 wk, 2 mth, 6 mth, 1 yr; Then
3(a)	**Z-score ≥ 2.5 to <5 and not regressing**	Annual follow-up. Transition to adult cardiology service at 17 yr old		Annually
3(b)	**Z-score ≥ 2.5 to <3 and saccular or fusiform, or Z-score ≥3 to <5 then decreased to normal**	Every 2 years. Transition to adult cardiology service at 17 years old		Every 2 years
3(c)	**Z-score ≥2.5 to <3, uniformly dilated which regresses to normal**	Consider discharge at 1 years. Or after two normal 2DE, whichever is later. Recommend review at 5–6 years of age or before primary school		Every 2 years till two normal 2DE. Before primary school or 5–6 years of age

(Continued)

Table 7.15 (*Continued*)

Classification of Risk		KKH Guidelines		
Coronary artery description		Follow-up interval (from disease onset)	Anti-platelet / anti-coagulation	ECG, 2D echocardiogram
4	**Medium aneurysm (Z-score ≥5 to <10)**	• 2 wk, 2 mth, 6 mth, 1 yr (may review at closer intervals at cardiologist discretion) and subsequent long-term follow-up as below. • All transition to adult cardiology service at 17 years old.		2 wk, 2 mth, 6 mth, 1 yr (may review at closer intervals at cardiologist's discretion) and subsequent long-term follow-up as below.
4(a)	**Persistent medium aneurysm**	Every 6 months	Long-term low dose aspirin second anti-platelet (e.g. Clopidogrel)	Every 6 months
4(b)	**Regressed to small aneurysm or regresses to dilation**	Every 12 months	Lifelong aspirin. If on dual antiplatelet, switch to single antiplatelet after CT angiogram.	Every 12 months
4(c)	**Regressed to normal**	Every 2 years	Lifelong aspirin. If on dual antiplatelet, switch to single antiplatelet after CT angiogram	Every 2 years
5	**Giant aneurysm (Z score ≥10 or ≥8 mm)**	• 2 wk, 1 mth, monthly till 6 mth (earlier review as per cardiologist discretion and subsequent long-term management as below: • All will transition to adult cardiology service at 17 years old.	• Long-term low dose aspirin + LMWH/Warfarin • If there is thrombosis, consider aspirin + LMWH/ warfarin+ second anti-platelet, to consider thrombolysis as per cardiologist discretion. • Consider referring to haematologist. • Consider CT angiogram evaluation before change in medication. • To monitor in 3 months after stopping anticoagulation.	2 wk, 1 mth, monthly till 6 mth (earlier review as per cardiologist discretion and subsequent long-term management as below:

Table 7.15 (*Continued*)

Classification of Risk		KKH Guidelines		
Coronary artery description		**Follow-up interval (from disease onset)**	**Anti-platelet / anti-coagulation**	**ECG, 2D echocardiogram**
5(a)	**Persistent giant aneurysm**	Every month (if on enoxaparin) or every 3–4 months (if on warfarin). May review at closer intervals at cardiologist's discretion.	As above.	Every month (if on enoxaparin) or every 3–4 months (if on warfarin).
5(b)	**Regressed to medium aneurysm**	Every 6 months when off warfarin/LMWH.	Consider switch to dual anti-platelets.	Every 6 months when off warfarin/LMWH.
5(c)	**Regressed to small aneurysm**	Every 12 months when off warfarin/low molecular weight heparin.	Consider switch to 1 anti-platelet and continue lifelong.	Every 12 months when off warfarin/LMWH.
5(d)	**Regressed to normal**	2 years, then every 2 years.	Consider switch to 1 anti-platelet and continue lifelong.	2 years, then every 2 years.

*Z-scores are based on Kobayashi Z score: Calculator of Z-scores. http://kwsd.info

Other Measures

- Consider repeating FBC, LFT and CRP during follow up.
- All inactivated vaccines, rotavirus, oral typhoid, intranasal anti-flu, BCG vaccines and yellow fever vaccine may be administered at any time after administration of IVIG in KD patients.
- The MMR, Varicella and MMRV vaccines should be delayed for 11 months after the administration of IVIG in KD patients to avoid a reduced immune response as a result of the specific high antibody titre against the antigens contained in IVIG.
- Varicella-zoster vaccines and annual influenza vaccine are recommended for children on aspirin.
- No restriction in physical activities is recommended for children with normal coronary arteries post-KD. However, competitive sports, endurance training and strenuous exercise is discouraged for those with abnormal coronary arteries. Contact sports are contraindicated in children on anticoagulation.
- The need for further advanced cardiac imaging, for example, CT imaging of coronary arteries or cardiac MRI and stress electrocardiography/echocardiography is dependent on the coronary arterial risk and will be determined by the managing cardiologist.
- General measures to lower cardiovascular risk (such as lipid lowering, control of hypertension, smoking cessation) and support for patients and their families to pursue a healthy lifestyle (healthy diet, exercise and maintain ideal body weight) need to be emphasised. A lipid profile may be considered every 5 years.
- The use of statins in children >8 years can be considered; however, there are no guidelines for target lipid levels for children with KD.

Bibliography

1. Brogan P, Burns JC, Cornish J, *et al.* (2020) Kawasaki disease writing group, on behalf of the Royal College of Paediatrics and Child Health, and the British Cardiovascular Society. Lifetime cardiovascular management of patients with previous Kawasaki disease. *Heart* **106**(6):411–420.
2. McCrindle BW, Rowley AH, Newburger JW, *et al.* (2017) American Heart Association Rheumatic Fever, Endocarditis and Kawasaki Disease Committee of the Council on Cardiovascular Disease in the Young; Council on Cardiovascular and Stroke Nursing; Council on Cardiovascular Surgery and Anesthesia; and Council on Epidemiology and Prevention. Diagnosis, Treatment, and Long-term Management of Kawasaki Disease: A scientific statement for health professionals from the American Heart Association. *Circulation* **135**(17):e927–e999.
3. Fukazawa R, Kobayashi J, Ayusawa M, *et al.* (2020) Japanese Circulation Society joint working group. JCS/JSCS 2020 guideline on diagnosis and management of cardiovascular sequelae in Kawasaki disease. *Circ J* 84(8):1348–1407.
4. Phuong LK, Chen KY, Burgner DP, Curtis N. (2020) What paediatricians need to know about the updated 2017 American Heart Association Kawasaki disease guideline. *Arch Dis Child* **105**(1):10–12.
5. Liu YC, Lin MT, Wang JK, Wu MH. (2018) State-of-the-art acute phase management of Kawasaki disease after 2017 scientific statement from the American Heart Association. *Pediatr Neonatol* **59**(6):543–552.
6. Marchesi A, Tarisside Jacobis I, Rigante D, *et al.* (2018) Kawasaki disease: Guidelines of the Italian Society of Pediatrics, part I-definition, epidemiology, etiopathogenesis, clinical expression and management of the acute phase. *Ital J Pediatr* **44**(1):102.
7. Marchesi A, Tarisside Jacobis I, Rigante D, *et al.* (2018) Kawasaki disease: Guidelines of Italian Society of Pediatrics, part II – treatment of resistant forms and cardiovascular complications, follow-up, lifestyle and prevention of cardiovascular risks. *Ital J Pediatr* **44**(1):103.

SECTION 8

CHILD DEVELOPMENT

CHAPTER 30

Normal Child Development

Tan Hui Yin, Jessica; Rachana Koura

Introduction

The first years of development are crucial for lifelong learning and development. Milestones follow predictable courses, and later developmental skills build on previous ones achieved. Developmental screening should be done at every visit and a good understanding of normal development is crucial for the paediatrician to be able to recognise delayed/abnormal development promptly, for which early intervention would be beneficial. Studies show that beginning intervention earlier in a child's developmental course leads to improved outcomes and can improve engagement of a family in the child's developmental progress.

Parental concerns regarding development should always be addressed as early detection of delays can be picked up and acted upon. Conversely, just because a parent has no concerns does not mean that developmental issues do not exist. Using the tables provided below helps to provide a framework for assessing developmental milestones.

Children with abnormal development should be reviewed by a developmental paediatrician. Pre-schoolers with abnormal development should be referred to the Child Development Unit (CDU) at KKH or NUH. Primary school-aged children over 6 years should be referred to Child and Adolescent Mental Wellness Service (CAMWS) in KKH or the Child Guidance Clinic run by the Institute of Mental Health (IMH) for concerns of attention deficit disorder with or without hyperactivity or other mental health issues. School-going children should be referred to the educational psychologists at the Ministry of Education (MOE) if they require learning needs assessment and to the Dyslexia Association of Singapore for concerns of dyslexia.

Terminology

- **Developmental screening** — Developmental screening refers to the use of a standardised test to identify asymptomatic children who are at risk for a developmental disorder; children who screen positive should undergo a developmental–behavioural evaluation.
- **Developmental surveillance** — Developmental surveillance is the process through which children who have developmental delay or are at risk for developmental delay are identified. Developmental surveillance occurs at preventive care visits and consists of eliciting parental concerns, identifying risk

factors, monitoring development and collaborating with other providers and professionals.

Benefits of Surveillance and Screening

The combination of surveillance and screening for developmental — behavioural problems in children increases early identification, enabling earlier intervention, which is associated with improved outcome.

The response to developmental–behavioural interventions is greatest in early childhood. Children who are identified after school entry miss the opportunity to participate in early developmental or early childhood services. Children with undetected developmental delays are at increased risk for social and emotional problems, early school problems and school failure.

Approach to Developmental Screening

History

Developmental History

- Milestones achieved in each of the main developmental areas and current level of functioning within each domain
  - » Gross motor — Movements using large muscles
  - » Fine motor — Movements using the hands and smaller muscles, often involving skills of daily living
  - » Speech/language — Receptive and expressive communication, speech and non-verbal communication
  - » Social-emotional and behavioural — Eye contact, joint attention, communicative intent, social appropriateness, attachment, play and interaction with others
  - » Cognitive — Reasoning, memory and problem-solving skills
- Any developmental regression
- Atypical development, e.g. perseverations/obsessions/compulsions, rigidity and poor task transitioning, motor mannerisms, sensory issues, idiosyncratic language (echolalia, self-commentary, neologisms)
- Behaviour in different settings, e.g. home vs. school, any concerns from school teachers
- School performance, e.g. academic, behaviour, socialisation skills with peers, reports from teachers

Antenatal and Neonatal History

- Gestational age (e.g. prematurity and corrected age)
- Birth weight

- APGAR Score
- Perinatal events
- Cord thyroid-stimulating hormone level
- Inborn Errors of Metabolism (IEM) screen
- Intrauterine infection/maternal serology
- Maternal medical history — e.g. thyroid disorder/drug abuse

Past medical History

- Chronic medical illness
- Co-morbid conditions, e.g. anxiety, depression, low self-esteem, self-harm, aggression
- Significant head injury/meningitis/seizures
- Otitis media
- Hearing or visual impairment

Dietary and Sleep Habits

- Fussy eaters/poor intake
- Screen time
- Obstructive sleep apnoea, poor sleep

Drug History

- Various drugs can affect behaviour (e.g. steroids, beta-adrenergic receptor agonists, anticonvulsants, montelukast, methylxanthines)

Social History

- Recent stressors, family dynamics, main caregiver(s), spoken language at home
- Environmental deprivation, domestic violence, child abuse, financial difficulty

Family History

- Consanguinity
- Any developmental disorders, hearing impairment, seizures, neurological disorders, genetic/metabolic disorders, psychiatric illness

Clinical Examination

- Assess systematically each of the main developmental areas (see Table 8.1)
- Growth parameters (weight, height, occipital-frontal circumference (OFC)) — review health booklet to look at growth trend
- Any dysmorphic features/neurocutaneous stigmata
- Systems examination
- Full neurological examination (tone, reflexes, gait, cranial nerves, cerebellar) and examination of spine, hips
- Behavioural observations during consult

Investigations

Investigations should only be done when clinically indicated.

Prematurity

The following guidelines apply to children born prematurely:

(i) For pre-term infants born *before 35 weeks*, it is recommended that hospital specialists or private paediatricians follow them up for growth monitoring and developmental screenings for the first 2 years of life, instead of at primary care. Clinicians should use the corrected age (i.e. chronological age minus the number of weeks the child was born early, taking 40 weeks as full term), for their growth monitoring and developmental screenings for the first 24 months.

(ii) For infants born between 35 and 37 weeks, growth monitoring should also be conducted using the corrected age till 24 months. However, developmental screening for infants born at or after 35 weeks should be based on chronological age.

Developmental Domains

The main domains of development are:

1. Gross motor
2. Vision and fine motor
3. Hearing and speech and language
4. Personal social
5. Cognitive ability

- **Normal:** The normal milestones by age refer to the 50th percentile norms by which 50% of children have achieved them.
- **Red flags (RF):** RF refer to the 90th percentile cut off by which 90% of children have achieved them. The presence of 'red flags' is an indication of delay with a need for further evaluation.
- Assess the child by testing one domain first and finding the threshold between what the child can and cannot do.
- For each domain, the child's developmental level is determined by the highest level task achieved and the next level that was not achieved (i.e. if a child uses 2-word phrase but not a 3-word phrase then their speech level is at a 2-year level and less than a 3-year level).
- At any point in time of a child's development, if they lose skills they once had (regression), this is a 'red flag' and immediate referral for further evaluation should be made promptly.

Table 8.1 Domains of Developmental Milestones (Birth to 6 years)

Age	Gross Motor	Fine Motor/Visual	Hearing/Speech and Language (Receptive vs. Expressive)	Personal/Social/Behavioural/Self-care	Cognition/Problem solving	Red Flags (*Developmental regression at any age is a red flag)
Birth	Marked head lag on pulling up Primitive reflexes present (Moro, Stepping, ATNR)	Barely fixates/follows (but can turn eyes towards large and diffuse objects) Grasp reflex present	Alerts/startles to sudden loud sounds Cries when hungry or uncomfortable	Sleeps and feeds Calms down when comforted	N.A.	Floppy baby No response to sudden loud sounds
4–6 wk	Moderate head lag Head in line with body on ventral suspension Prone — attempts to lift the head Turns head when supine	Fixates and follows object from side to midline (90°) Hands fisted near face	Quietens to mother's voice Startles to sounds/voices Coos	Regards face Beginning to have social smile (smiles in response to caregiver)	Face regard	Floppy baby Lack of face regard / lack of fixation
3 mth	Mild head lag (by 4 mth: little or no head lag) Holds head at 45–90° in ventral suspension Props up on forearm in prone position Rolls to side (Rolls prone to supine at 4 mth, supine to prone 5 mth)	Fixes and follows from side to side (180°) Hands un-fisted Grasp objects Hands regard (Watches movements of own hands)	Turns head to sounds at ear level Coos and laughs	Smiles spontaneously Excites at toy or familiar pleasant situations, e.g. feeding, bathing	Regards toy Reaches for face	Does not fix and follow No response to sounds Does not coo or make sounds No social smile

6 mth	Rolls over in both directions (prone to supine and vice versa) Prone — Head up 90°, props up on hands with arms extended Sits (rounded back) with support/tripods Bears weight on legs when held in standing position, might bounce	Fixes on small object (e.g. regards a raisin) Reaches for objects Transfers objects (from one hand to another)	Turns head to sounds out of sight Non-specific, monosyllabic babbling (e.g. ba, ga, ma) Makes sounds to show joy and displeasure (e.g. laughs, squeals)	Stranger anxiety Responds to own name (7 mth) Smiles and vocalises at mirror image Shows affection for caregiver	Looks around at things nearby Bring things to mouth	Unable to roll over Significant head lag by 5 mth Does not reach out for objects No babbling Lack of turning towards voices No smiling/laughing/ expression
9–10 mth	Sits without support Crawls Pulls to stand Stands with support Cruises (walks holding on to furniture, usually at 10–12 mth	Immature pincer grasp Bangs two cubes held in hands	Locates sounds well Says 'papa', 'mama' non-specifically Understands 'no' and 'bye'	Claps hands Waves bye-bye Plays peek-a-boo Makes eye contact with familiar people Wary of strangers Holds own bottle Finger feeds	Looks for a fallen object (object permanence)	Inability to sit without support Does not transfer objects No response to name Absence of back and forth smiles and vocalisation during interaction/play
12 mth	Stands without support Walks with one hand held May shuffle on buttock and hand	Mature pincer grasp Casts objects	**Expressive:** Calls 'papa', 'mama' specifically, and says 2–3 other words with meaning (15 mth) **Receptive:** Obeys one-step command with gesture	Points to indicate wants (proto-imperative pointing) Joint attention Imitates actions/ gestures Plays with cause and effect toys Drink from a cup	Explores things in different ways (e.g. shaking, banging, throwing) Enjoys putting objects in and out of boxes	Does not stand/bears weight on legs when support No immature pincer grasp No babbling, pointing or use of gestures No eye contact with familiar people

(Continued)

Table 8.1 (*Continued*)

Age	Gross/Fine	Fine Motor	Language/Communication	Social/Emotional	Cognition (Problem solving, Learning, Thinking	Red Flags
18 mth	Walks independently Stoops and recover Walks up stairs with one hand held	Scribbles spontaneously Builds a tower with 3 blocks Turns 2–3 pages at a time	**Expressive:** Says ~10 single words with meaning **Receptive:** Follows one-step command without gesture	Points to express interest (proto-declarative pointing) Parallel play Pretend play Copies simple actions and words Eats with a spoon Shows affection to familiar people	Points to 2–3 body parts Points to 2–3 objects when named	Not walking independently Hand dominance less than 18 mth old No single words Not pointing for needs or to express interest/no joint attention
2–2.5 yr	Runs well Jumps with 2 feet off the ground Walks up and down stairs, 2 feet per step Kicks ball forward Throws ball overhand (usually at 2.5 yr of age)	Hand dominance (noted by 2 yr but firmly established by 3–4 yr) Copies a vertical line (Horizontal line at 2.5 yr) Builds a tower of 6 cubes Turns pages one at a time	**Expressive:** Knows ~50 words Says 2–3 word phrases **Receptive:** Follow two-step commands Points to things in a book	Parallel play Throws temper tantrums Shows defiance Some independence Mimicry (copies others)	Points to 4–6 body parts Names 2 pictures	Inability to walk steadily Unable to scribble Does not copy actions/words No use of spontaneous (non-echoed/non initiated) 2 word phrases Does not follow one-step command Poor eye contact
3 yr	Walks up and down stairs with alternate feet Pedals tricycle Stands on 1 foot for 3 sec	Hand dominance (noted by 2 yr but firmly established by 3–4 yr) Copies circle Copies cross (3.5 yr) Awkward tripod grasp of pencil Builds tower of 9 cubes	**Expressive:** Knows ~250 words Says 3–4 word phrase Knows name, age and gender Asking questions — what, who, where Names a friend Holds conversation using 2–3 sentences	Group/interactive play Dresses and undresses with help Toilet trained Shows a wide range of emotions	Names 2–3 colours Matches colours and identifies shapes Imaginative play	Does not run/jump Frequent falling or difficulty with stairs Does not copy a vertical line Does not follow 2-step command No 3-word phrase

		Imitates construction of bridge of 3 cubes Threads beads well Cuts along a straight line	Talks well enough for strangers to understand most of the time **Receptive:** Follows 3-step command			Solitary play No pretend play
4 yr	Hops on 1 foot Has skills in ball games (throwing, catching, bouncing) Balances on either foot for at least 5 sec	Copies a square Dynamic tripod grasp of pencil Builds a tower of 12 blocks Colours within the lines Draws a person with 2–4 body parts besides head Cuts 5-inch circle	**Expressive:** Speaks grammatically and clearly Uses pronouns (I, you), plurals and prepositions (on, in, under) Knows ~ 1000 words and can easily compose sentences consisting 4–5 words Ask questions — why, how, when **Receptive:** Follows more complex instructions (at least 3 steps) Name things when actions are described (e.g. it's something you read — book)	Imaginative play alone and with other children Cooperates with other children Dresses with minimal help, and attends to own toilet needs Buttons clothes Washes hands and face Brushes teeth alone Has a preferred friend	Knows 4 colours Rote count 1–10 Copies some capital letters Recalls parts of a story Understands concepts of time (yesterday, today, tomorrow) Understands concepts of 'same' and 'different'	Can't jump Unable to copy circle Does not follow 3-step commands Speaks unclearly Does not answer simple questions Inability to use pronouns Ignores other children or doesn't respond to people outside the family
5 yr	Stands on 1 foot for 10 sec Skips Rides a bicycle Heel-to-toe walking Enjoys climbing, swings and slides	Copies triangle Draw a person with 6–8 body parts besides head Able to cut out a square shape	**Expressive:** Speaks clearly/fluently with long descriptions Tells a simple story using full sentences (with clear beginning, middle and end) Sings songs and recites nursery rhymes	Has a group of friends and is capable of choosing friends Aware of gender Bathes, dresses and undresses independently	Names 5–10 colours Recognises and can write some numbers and letters	Does not copy a square Speech is unclear Cannot give first and last name Inability to recognise letters, numbers, colours

(Continued)

Table 8.1 (*Continued*)

Age	Gross/Fine	Fine Motor	Language/Communication	Social/Emotional	Cognition (Problem solving, Learning, Thinking)	Red Flags
	Running, broad jump 2–3 feet Jumps backwards Hops on 1 foot 15 times		Uses future tense (e.g. Father will be here) Knows address/phone number ~2000 words vocabulary and can speak a sentence of >5 words **Receptive:** Can follow rules Understand complex instructions Enjoys riddles and jokes	Self-grooms independently (e.g. brushes teeth, combing hair) Uses a fork and spoon Able to distinguish fantasy from reality	Knows opposite, right and left on self Knows function of things used every day (e.g. money, food, objects)	Doesn't show a wide range of emotions Shows extreme behaviour (unusually fearful, aggressive, shy or sad) Difficulties in activities of daily living (e.g. toileting, dressing, self-grooming, eating) Difficulties in fine motor activities (e.g. cutting with scissors, writing) Unable to differentiate between fantasy and reality
6 yr	Walks backward heel-toe Tandem walk Able to jump rope	Copies a diamond Draws an 8- to 10-part person besides head Writes first name Writes A-Z entirely in lower case Writes 1–20 Able to cut out complex shapes	**Expressive:** Speaks in complete sentences with 6–8 words Describes events in order Knows days of the week **Receptive:** Asks what an unfamiliar word means Understands adjectives (e.g. busy, long, thin) Responds to 'why' questions	Enjoys school Wants to be liked and accepted by friends Strong gender affinity (preference to have friends of same sex) Apologises for mistakes	Identify numbers 1–20 Rote count 1–20 Can count fingers Simple addition and subtraction Names letters/numerals out of order Spells and reads Defines simple words	Does not skip or hop on one foot/clumsy Does not write name Handwriting not legible Unable to understand concepts of 1–20 Unable to express self Unable to tell emotions in others No friends Unable to retell stories with clear beginning, middle and end Unable to do basic reading and writing

Bibliography

1. Scharf RJ, Scharf GJ. (2016) Developmental milestones. Annemarie Stroustrup. *Pediatr Rev* **37**(1):25–38.
2. Centers for Disease Control and Prevention. (nd) Developmental milestones. www.cdc.gov/ActEarly
3. Lipkin PH, Macias MM. (2020) Promoting optimal development: Identifying infants and young children with developmental disorders through developmental surveillance and screening. Council on Children with Disabilities, Section on Development and Beavioral Pediatrics. *Pediatrics* **145**(1).
4. Aites J, Schonwald A. (2020) Developmental–behavioral surveillance and screening in primary care.
5. Ministry of Health Singapore (2020) Guidance on childhood developmental screening. Circular No. 183, Annex A.
6. Guevara JP, Gerdes M, Localio R, *et al.* (2013) Effectiveness of developmental screening in an urban setting. *Pediatrics* **131**(1):30.
7. Schonwald A, Huntington N, Chan E, *et al.* (2009) Routine developmental screening implemented in urban primary care settings: More evidence of feasibility and effectiveness. *Pediatrics* **123**(2):660.
8. Hix-Small H, Marks K, Squires J, Nickel R. (2007) Impact of implementing developmental screening at 12 and 24 months in a pediatric practice. *Pediatrics* **120**(2):381.
9. van Agt HM, van der Stege HA, de Ridder-Sluiter H, *et al.* (2007) A cluster-randomized trial of screening for language delay in toddlers: Effects on school performance and language development at age 8. *Pediatrics* **120**(6):1317.
10. Palfrey JS, Hauser-Cram P, Bronson MB, *et al.* (2005) The brookline early education project: A 25-year follow-up study of a family-centered early health and development intervention. *Pediatrics* **116**(1):144.

CHAPTER 31

Developmental Disorders

Lourdes Mary Daniel; Wong Chui Mae

Patterns of Abnormal Development

- **Developmental Delay:**
  - » Development follows the normal sequence but is delayed.
  - » May be a specific or global developmental delay.
- **Developmental Disorder:**
  - » Development does not follow the normal pattern and is aberrant or bizarre, e.g. persistence of primitive reflexes, atypical developmental profiles (e.g. a child with autism who has language skills, but is unable to use it for social interaction and communication).
- **Developmental Arrest or Regression:**
  - » A period of normal development is followed by a failure to acquire new skills or loss of previously established skills.
  - » This may signify a serious underlying condition, e.g. neurodegenerative/ metabolic disorder, Landau–Kleffner Syndrome, Rett Syndrome.

An Approach to Developmental and Behavioural Disorders

A detailed history and physical examination are invaluable. Specialised investigations play only a minor role in the evaluation process.

History

Developmental and Behavioural History

- Gross and fine motor milestones
- Language milestones — Receptive, expressive and non-verbal
- Current functioning in each developmental domain
- Speech — Articulation, phonology and fluency
- Social-emotional awareness, e.g. eye contact, joint attention, communicative intent, social appropriateness, response to family members vs. strangers, etc.
- Play (Parten's social play stage, pretend play abilities)
- Behaviour in different settings, e.g. home vs. school
- Developmental regression

- School performance, e.g. academics (including reading and handwriting) behaviour, socialisation skills with peers
- Atypical development, e.g. perseverations/obsessions/compulsions, rigidity and poor task transitioning, motor mannerisms, sensory issues, idiosyncratic language (echolalia, odd prosody, self-commentary, neologisms), etc.
- Reports from professionals working with the child, e.g. external therapists, teachers
- Co-morbid conditions, e.g. anxiety, depression, low self-esteem, self-harm, aggression
- Activities of daily living
- Early temperament in infancy, e.g. social responsiveness, feeding, sleeping, crying
- Dietary and sleep habits, e.g. nutritional deficiencies, growth problems, fussy feeding, obstructive sleep apnoea, poor sleep

Antenatal and Neonatal History

- APGAR scores, prematurity, perinatal events, intrauterine infection, neonatal screening results (hearing, thyroid stimulating hormone, metabolic screening), maternal drugs, alcohol intake

Medical History

- Chronic medical illness, seizures including absence seizures (staring spells), otitis media, significant head injury, unexplained febrile illnesses, hearing or visual impairment, etc.

Drug History

- Drugs (e.g. steroids, beta-adrenergic receptor agonists, methylxanthines, anticonvulsants) that can affect behaviour

Social History

- Recent stressors, family dynamics, main caregiver(s), spoken language at home, environmental deprivation, exposure to adverse childhood experiences (e.g. exposure to domestic violence, parental incarceration or drug abuse, child abuse, etc.), financial difficulty

Family History

- Consanguinity, developmental delays or disorders, including autism and attention-deficit/hyperactivity disorder (ADHD), hearing impairment, seizures, neurological disorders, genetic/metabolic disorders, psychiatric illnesses

Clinical Examination

- Growth parameters — Weight, height, occipito-frontal circumference (OFC)
- Dysmorphic features
- Neurocutaneous stigmata

- Examination of systems
- Full neurological examination (tone, reflexes, gait, cranial nerves, cerebellar signs)
- Spine, hips
- Demonstration of current development, including reading, numeracy and handwriting, at appropriate ages
- Observations including behaviour, interaction and play

Investigations

Investigations should only be done when clinically indicated. Some investigations that could be considered include:

- Hearing assessment (probably the most useful and essential in any child with language delay)
- Visual assessment
- Thyroid function test (especially in global developmental delay with growth problems)
- Muscle enzymes, urea/electrolytes/glucose, calcium/magnesium
- Inborn Errors of Metabolism (IEM) study or metabolic screen
- Karyotyping, chromosomal microarray analysis, Fragile X analysis
- TORCH screen (in children under 2 years)
- Neuroimaging (Ultrasound/CT/MRI head)
- Electroencephalogram (EEG)

Red Flags that Warrant Refferal

1. Developmental regression at any age*
2. Not meeting the 90th centile developmental milestones in the child health booklet
3. Persistently low tone or floppiness*
4. Asymmetry of movements or other features suggestive of cerebral palsy, such as increased muscle tone*
5. Concerns about vision: lack of fixing and following from 6 weeks onwards**
6. Concerns about hearing: no response to sounds^
7. No social smile by 3 months
8. Unable to roll and reach out for objects at 6 months
9. Unable to walk independently at 18 months
10. No babbling, pointing or use of gestures by 12 months
11. No imitation of actions or words at 2 years
12. No use of spontaneous (non-echoed/non initiated) phrases by 24 months
13. Persistent tiptoe gait

14. OFC above the 97th centile/less than 3rd centile, which cannot be explained by a familial pattern or if the OFC has crossed two centiles (up or down)*

*Refer to general paediatrician/paediatric neurologist

**Refer to an Ophthalmology clinic

^Refer to an Otolaryngology clinic

Some Specific Conditions

Speech and Language Delay

Speech and language are components of communication. All children presenting with a language delay should be screened for autistic features and have a hearing test performed.

- Language is a system of symbolic representation used to communicate meanings, feelings, ideas and intentions.
  - Receptive language (language processing) refers to auditory processing and comprehension of language.
  - Expressive language (language production) refers to non-verbal gestures, vocabulary, phrase length, semantics (appropriate use of single words, phrases and sentences), and syntax (arrangements of words in sentences, clauses and phrases).
  - Pragmatic language refers to the appropriate use of verbal and non-verbal language in a given situation.
- Speech is the expression of language in the verbal mode.
  - Speech disorders include phonological and articulation difficulties and dysfluency (e.g. stuttering).
- Children frequently present with one of the following:
  - Expressive language delay
  - Mixed receptive-expressive language delay
  - Phonological delay/dysfluency
- Management and prognosis of speech and language delay:
  - 70–80% of children with isolated expressive language delay do well with Speech and Language Therapy (SLT) and achieve normal language abilities, especially if detected early.
  - Children with mixed language delays show slower response to SLT, especially if there is an underlying cause such as Autism Spectrum Disorder (ASD). These children may need ongoing SLT support during primary school years.
  - Children with phonological delay or dysfluency tend to also improve with SLT. For children with associated tongue-tie (ankyloglossia), a frenotomy may not be indicated unless there is limited improvement with SLT input.
  - Speech and Language intervention can also be provided as part of the Individualised Education Plan for children in an Early Intervention Programme.

Autism Spectrum Disorder (ASD)

The core clinical features of ASD comprise persistent deficits in social communication and social interaction, with restricted and repetitive patterns of behaviour, including sensory issues. ASD has an incidence of approximately 1 in 100 children and is four times more common in boys than girls. The risk of autism in a sibling of an autistic child is 10–20%.

Characteristics

Persistent Deficits in Social Communication and Social Interaction

1. Deficits in social–emotional reciprocity
2. Deficits in non-verbal communicative behaviours used for social interaction
3. Deficits in developing, maintaining and understanding relationships

Restricted, Repetitive Patterns of Behaviour

1. Stereotyped or repetitive motor movements, use of objects or speech.
2. Insistence on sameness, inflexible adherence to routines or ritualised patterns of behaviour.
3. Highly restricted, fixated interests.
4. Hyper- or hypo-reactivity to sensory input or unusual interest in sensory aspects of the environment.

M-CHAT

The Modified Checklist for Autism in Toddlers (M-CHAT) is a validated screening tool to identify toddlers at risk for ASD who may warrant an early developmental assessment (https://m-chat.org/). It should only be used for children aged 16–30 months. If the child's score is 3 or more, the child should be referred for further evaluation.

Diagnosis and Management

The diagnosis of ASD is made following a detailed autism-specific interview, observation of the child in the clinic setting, information obtained from the preschool or school, and a direct assessment using formal structured assessment tools.

Interventions for ASD include Speech and Language therapy, Occupational therapy, Structured Teaching, Picture Exchange Communication System (PECS), Applied Behaviour Analysis (ABA), etc. Preschool children with suspected or confirmed ASD can be referred to the Early Intervention Programme for Infants and Children (EIPIC). Medication has no place in the regular management of ASD except in certain children who have concurrent ADHD or severe behavioural difficulties. Various diets (gluten-free, casein-free), biomedical therapies and nutritional supplements have not been found to make a difference in well-conducted randomised controlled trials.

Attention-Deficit/Hyperactivity Disorder (ADHD)

The diagnosis of ADHD is based primarily on reports of characteristic inattention and hyperactivity/impulsivity behaviours from various observers, occurring in different settings, over an extended period of time (at least 6 months). The symptoms should result in impairment in social and academic functioning in two or more settings (e.g. at home and at school) and should also be present before the age of 12. However, when considering a diagnosis of ADHD, it is important to remember that inattention, hyperactivity and impulsivity are common till 4 years of age.

ADHD has an estimated incidence of 1 in 10–20 children, but there is a concern of over-diagnosis. Often, other factors may result in a young child behaving as though they have ADHD, but once these are addressed, the child's behaviour may return to normal. These factors include poor sleep, lack of a structure in the household, deprivation, language delay, learning disability, hearing impairment, a major life event (parents divorcing, family bereavement), thyroid disease or subclinical seizures.

Behavioural Features of ADHD Include

- Inattention, e.g. the child is easily distracted, is careless or forgetful, fails to complete tasks, does not follow through on instructions, has difficulty organising tasks, loses things necessary for activities, does not listen when spoken to directly, etc.
- Hyperactivity, e.g. the child fidgets, will not sit still, runs or climbs excessively in inappropriate situations, has difficulty engaging in leisure activities quietly, is often 'on the go', talks excessively, etc.
- Impulsivity, e.g. the child blurts out answers before questions have been completed, has difficulty waiting for turns, often interrupts or is intrusive, etc.

ADHD has Three Sub-classifications

- Combined type (inattentive/hyperactive/impulsive): Children with this type of ADHD show all three behaviours. This is the most common form of ADHD.
- Predominantly hyperactive/impulsive type: Children show both hyperactive and impulsive behaviour, but for the most part, they are able to pay attention.
- Predominantly inattentive type (formerly known as attention-deficit disorder {ADD}): These children are not overly hyperactive. They do not disrupt the classroom or other activities, so their symptoms might not be noticed. This subtype often affects girls rather than boys.

Diagnosis and Management

- A child or adolescent should meet the DSM-5 criteria for ADHD before being given the diagnosis, with impairment in more than one major setting (i.e. social, academic or occupational) with information obtained primarily from reports of parents/guardians, teachers, other school personnel and health clinicians who are involved in the care of the child. Alternative causes of the behaviours should be excluded.
- Comorbid disorders must be screened for, including emotional or behavioural conditions (e.g. anxiety, depression, etc.), developmental conditions (e.g. learning and language disorders, ASD) and physical conditions (e.g. sleep apnoea and tics).
- In the preschool child, DSM-based rating scales should be used to obtain information.

- There are several rating scales and questionnaires that can be useful for assessment. These include the Vanderbilt and Du Paul ADHD rating scales (for core ADHD symptoms) and the Child Behaviour Checklist.
- In preschool children, behavioural therapy (both at home and in the classroom) is the first-line treatment. Methylphenidate should only be considered if a child shows limited response to behavioural therapy with ongoing impairment in the child's function.
- In primary school children, medications (both stimulant and non-stimulant) can be prescribed at doses that can achieve maximum effect with minimum side effects. But it is still highly recommended that it be used concurrently with behavioural therapy. The school should also be involved in the treatment plan.
- In secondary school children, treatment would be the same as for primary school children but should be undertaken with the assent of the adolescent.

Global Developmental Delay (GDD)

Global developmental delay is defined as significant delay in two or more major domains of development (gross motor or fine motor skills, language, cognition, personal and social, activities of daily living) in a child younger than 5 years.

Causes

In up to half of cases, the cause is not known. The common causes of GDD are:

- Genetic conditions, e.g., Down syndrome, Fragile X syndrome, Di George syndrome, Klinefelter's syndrome, neurofibromatosis, Williams syndrome, Angelman syndrome and Prader–Willi syndrome. Congenital hypothyroidism, phenylketonuria (PKU), other inborn errors of metabolism and other less common syndromes should also be considered.
- Antenatal or perinatal complications, e.g. foetal alcohol syndrome, congenital infections, neonatal encephalopathy
- Prematurity
- Severe refractory epilepsy
- Acquired brain injury, e.g. from trauma, meningitis, encephalitis, heavy metal poisoning
- Visual or hearing loss
- Environmental causes, e.g. severe under-stimulation, maltreatment, malnutrition
- Children with ASD often have co-existing GDD, but their primary diagnosis would still be ASD. Conversely, some children with severe GDD or intellectual delay may behave as though they have ASD (with stereotypical or repetitive behaviours) and careful delineation of the correct diagnosis must be made.

Diagnosis and Management

Children with GDD need to be referred for the appropriate therapies in the delayed domains of development (e.g. Speech, Physio, Occupational or Educational therapy, psychological support). As they often need help from more than one allied health professional, most children with GDD benefit from early referral to the EIPIC centres in Singapore. The developmental paediatrician would also screen the child for any underlying cause, perform the relevant investigations, and treat the cause, if found.

If the GDD persists, some children may require cognitive testing (IQ testing) or other school readiness assessments prior to primary school entry to guide appropriate school placement and determine the need for support in mainstream school.

Developmental Coordination Disorder (DCD)

Children with developmental coordination disorder have difficulties with motor coordination, which presents differently according to the age of the child. Their coordinated motor skills are substantially below that expected for the age of the child and the opportunities for learning. They may have the following difficulties:

- Problems with sucking and swallowing during the first year of life
- Delays in sitting up, crawling and walking
- Gross motor incoordination (e.g. jumping, hopping or standing on one foot)
- Fine motor incoordination (e.g. writing, using scissors, tying shoelaces, buttoning)
- Clumsiness

In addition to the physical impairments, DCD is often associated with problems with memory and task-sequencing. This typically results in difficulty remembering instructions, difficulty organising one's time and remembering deadlines, increased propensity to lose things or problems carrying out tasks which require remembering several steps in sequence (such as cooking). Children with DCD are also at risk of low self-esteem.

However, DCD rarely occurs alone — it often co-exists with dyslexia, ADHD and language impairment.

Diagnosis and Management

The diagnosis is made by synthesis of the developmental and medical history, physical and neurological examination, reports from school and appropriate psychometric assessment, usually by an occupational therapist. The symptoms must begin in the early developmental period. There must be significant impact of the child's condition on his/her day-to-day activities such as the child's performance in school, activities at play, or other activities of daily living. Also, the child's problems with motor coordination cannot result from general medical conditions, such as muscular dystrophy, and cannot result directly from having intellectual disability.

Physical education and perceptual motor training are the best interventions for DCD. Using a computer to take notes may help children who have trouble writing. The non-motor problems associated with DCD would require a more structured learning environment. Co-existing developmental problems need to be screened for and appropriate assessment and intervention provided as needed.

Dyslexia

Dyslexia is a type of specific learning difficulty identifiable as a neurodevelopmental disorder. It primarily affects the skills involved in accurate and fluent reading and spelling.

Characteristic features of dyslexia are difficulties in phonological awareness (the ability to hear, identify and manipulate the units of sounds in speech), verbal memory (the ability to remember what is read and heard) and processing speed (the speed of performing simple mental operations). Co-occurring difficulties may be seen in aspects of language, motor coordination, mental calculation, concentration and personal organisation, but these are not, by themselves, markers of dyslexia. It is also a comorbidity of ADHD.

Symptoms of dyslexia can include difficulties in:

- Reading (e.g. reading below age level, hesitant or effortful reading, difficulty in recognising familiar or high frequency words, skipping words or lines, complaining of words or lines of text on a page seeming to move, even with normal standard eye examinations, etc.)
- Comprehension (e.g. difficulty remembering, understanding or extracting important points from text passages)
- Spelling (e.g. spelling below age level, spelling the same word in several different ways, confusing similar sounding words, ['one' and 'won'], reversing letter sequences ['was' and 'saw'], etc.)

In addition, children with dyslexia can also show difficulties in:

- Writing (e.g. messy/badly organised work, difficulty copying, having poor writing skills compared to oral skills, being unable to write down a word even when the letters are dictated, etc.)
- Short-term and/or verbal working memory (e.g. being able to learn and understand how to do a task, but requiring frequent reminders before remembering to do it, having difficulty remembering multiple-step instructions, having excellent long-term memory for movies, experiences, locations and faces, but poor memory for sequences or unfamiliar facts and information)
- Sequencing (e.g. difficulty in reciting the alphabet/numbers, months of the year, days of the week or remembering/executing a list of instructions, not being able to give a good verbal account of events in their correct order)
- Time/Mathematics (e.g. difficulties in telling and managing time, counting, doing calculations using mathematical signs {=, -, < }, doing mathematical word problems despite having ability in mathematical numerical operations, mental calculations)

Diagnosis and Management

The diagnosis of dyslexia should be made through a comprehensive psycho-educational assessment using standardised tests. Longitudinal progress monitoring data measuring response to intervention can also be used. Comorbidities should be actively sought for, so that holistic management can be planned. Early signs of learning difficulties may appear in the preschool years (e.g. difficulty learning names of letters or counting objects), but dyslexia can only be diagnosed reliably after starting formal education.

Children with dyslexia will benefit from educational support during their school years. The two main providers of dyslexia intervention are the Ministry of Education (MOE) that runs the School Dyslexia Remediation Program in Primary 3 and Primary 4, and the Dyslexia Association of Singapore, which has an intervention program starting in Primary 1. MOE also runs a Learning Support Programme in every school for children in Primary 1–2 with literacy delay (including dyslexia). Intervention is also provided by some social service agencies and by trained dyslexia teachers in the private sector.

Common Concomitant Problems in Children with Special Needs and their Families

- Visual and hearing impairment — minimise any impairment to optimise the child's learning.
- Epilepsy — ensure appropriateness and compliance of treatment.
- Orthopaedic problems — physiotherapy and aids to optimise posture and mobility, prevention or reduction of skeletal deformity may help to maximise ability and function.
- Chest infections — provide good parental education about symptoms and easy access to medical care.
- Feeding problems — oromotor incoordination, gastroesophageal reflux and tube feeding need to be managed.
- Bladder and bowel problems— enuresis, encopresis, constipation may affect the functional ability of the child.
- Behavioural and psychiatric concerns — these may need behavioural support, psychiatric assessment or medication.
- Social issues — parents and the home environment need to be supported through referrals to social workers, counsellors and community support organisations.
- Emotional or mental health concerns in the parents — counselling or psychiatric support may be needed.

Transition to the Next Level of Education

Transition points (from preschool to mainstream primary or special school and from primary to secondary school) are important milestones in the journey of the child with developmental, behavioural or learning difficulties and need to be managed according to the needs of the child. Decisions on appropriate school placements, deferment and identifying parental preferences may be necessary. The need for support in school should be determined and communicated to the school, with parental consent. When children transit from EIPIC to a mainstream school, reassessment of the child may be needed to understand the ongoing therapy needs of the child.

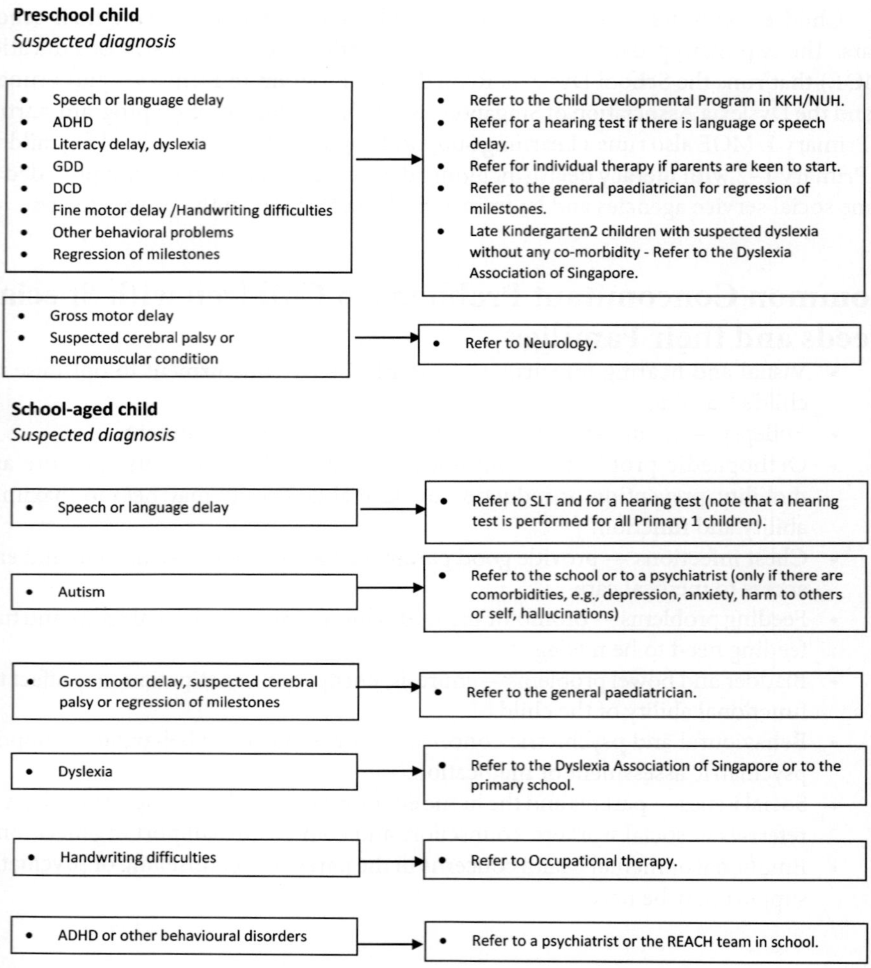

Figure 8.1 Guideline for referral to Child Development Unit (CDU)/Other agencies.
KKH: KK Women's and Children's Hospital; NUH: National University Hospital

Bibliography

1. Sharma A. (2011) Developmental examination: Birth to 5 years. *Arch Dis Child Educ Pract Ed* **96**:162.
2. Horridge KA. (2011) Assessment and investigation of the child with disordered development. *Arch Dis Child Educ Pract Ed* **96**:9.
3. McDonald LAB, Rennie AC. (2011) Investigating developmental delay/impairment. *Paediatr Child Health* **21**:443.
4. Subcommittee on Children and Adolescents with Attention-Deficit/Hyperactive Disorder. (2019) Clinical practice guideline for the diagnosis, evaluation, and treatment of attention-deficit/hyperactivity disorder in children and adolescents. *Pediatrics* **144**(4):e20192528.

5. Kliegman RM, Stanton BF, Behrman RE. (2011) *Nelson Textbook of Pediatrics, 19th ed.* Philadelphia, PA: Elsevier/Saunders.
6. Illingworth RS. (nd) The development of the infant and young child (normal and abnormal).
7. Lim HC, Chan T, Yoong T. (1994) Standardisation and adaptation of the Denver Developmental Screening Test (DDST) and Denver II for use in Singapore children. *Sing Med J* **35**(2):156–160.
8. American Psychiatric Association. (2013) *Desk Reference to the Diagnostic Criteria from DSM-5.* Washington, DC: American Psychiatric Publishing.
9. Aylward GP. (1994) *Practitioner's Guide to Developmental and Psychological Testing.* New York, NY: Plenum Publishing Corporation.
10. Parker S, Zuckerman B. (1995) *A Handbook for Primary Care: Behavioral and Developmental Pediatrics.* Boston, MA: Little, Brown and Company.

SECTION 9

CHILD PROTECTION

CHAPTER 32

Child Abuse and Neglect

Wong Choong Yi, Peter

What is Child Abuse?

'Child abuse' or 'child maltreatment', as defined by the World Health Organization (WHO),

1. includes all types of physical and/or emotional ill-treatment, sexual abuse, neglect, negligence and commercial or other exploitation,
2. which results in actual or potential harm to the child's health, survival, development or dignity,
3. in the context of a relationship of responsibility, trust or power.

Child abuse may involve actions and words that are harmful, or the **absence** of expected actions or words that are protective or nurturing (neglect). Actions may be abusive, whether or not there is **intention** to cause harm: the definition hinges instead on whether harm occurs or may potentially occur. Perpetrators of abuse are persons in a position of responsibility or power over the child or whom the child trusts (a parent, hired caregiver, teacher, etc.).

Public and professional opinions contribute to determining whether an act is regarded as abusive. For example, as public opinion shifts, a growing list of countries have prohibited the corporal punishment of children (including caning and spanking). An evidence-based approach is helpful: what has reliable research shown about benefits and harms to a child arising from any given practice?

The Scale of the Problem

A 2018 systematic review reported that 12.0% and 27.0% of girls and boys, respectively, in Europe have experienced physical abuse, as compared to 50.8% and 60.2% of girls and boys, respectively, in Africa. Reasons for the wide variation include differing cultural beliefs and laws. UNICEF estimates that about three-quarters of all children between the ages of 2 and 4, or around 300 million children worldwide, are regularly subjected to violent discipline by their caregivers. Worldwide, 1 in 5 women and 1 in 13 men report having been sexually abused before the age of 18. The vast majority of child abuse cases worldwide are undetected.

Consequences of Child Abuse

Child abuse and neglect is a significant cause of childhood injuries, disabilities and death.

Apart from causing immediate physical injuries, child abuse in its various forms also gives rise to problems in growth, development, physical health and psychological well-being. Sexual abuse may cause sexually transmitted infections and unintended pregnancies. The impact of child abuse may be long-term, lifelong or even inter-generational: victims may in turn be abusive towards future children in their care.

Adverse Childhood Experiences

Adverse childhood experiences (ACEs) are events or circumstances in the first 18 years of life that are stressful or potentially traumatic:

Abuse — 1. physical abuse, 2. emotional abuse, 3. sexual abuse
Neglect — 4. physical neglect, 5. emotional neglect
Household instability — 6. parental separation or divorce, 7. intimate partner violence against the mother, 8. mental illness in a household member, 9. substance abuse by a household member, 10. incarceration of a household member

The first 5 categories are various forms of child abuse and neglect, and the other 5 frequently co-occur with child abuse and neglect.

ACEs are associated with:

1. Problems **in childhood and adolescence**, such as developmental delay, failure to thrive, recurrent infections, asthma and obesity.
2. Higher rates **in adult life subsequently** of anxiety, depression, suicide attempts, alcoholism, drug abuse, unsafe sex, coronary artery disease, asthma, diabetes, arthritis, autoimmune disease, cerebrovascular disease, cancer and early death.
3. Poorer outcomes in education, employment and income.

The association of ACEs with organic diseases and early death may be accounted for by a combination of neuroendocrine responses to stress, epigenetic changes (DNA methylation and telomere shortening), reprogramming of immune regulatory systems, neurodevelopmental disruption and the impact of risk behaviours.

Victims of child abuse are thus at increased risk of myriad health problems, lifelong disadvantages and shorter life expectancy. Halting abuse and preventing further ACEs will add years to life and life to years for these children.

Physical Child Abuse: Overview

Physical child abuse may cause various injuries, including bruises, burns, fractures and traumatic brain injury. However, physically abused children may also present without any physical injuries.

The term 'non-accidental injury' (NAI) may be used to refer to a physical injury resulting from child abuse. It is not always an 'intentional injury': for example, a parent may have meant to discipline and not injure the child.

Table 9.1 Red Flags in History

Features in the History that are Concerning for Child Abuse — 6 Ds
1. No, inadequate or vague explanation for a serious injury: '**Don't know how** he was injured'
2. Medically implausible explanation given for the injury: **Don't see how** that mechanism could cause this injury
3. Explanation given is discordant with the **Developmental age** of the child
4. Discordant explanations from **Different witnesses**
5. Discordant explanations from the same witness at **Different times**
6. **Delay** in seeking medical attention despite the child being in pain or distress

Recognising possible physical child abuse requires careful history taking and thorough physical examination, paired with knowledge about what findings are concerning for abuse.

Physical child abuse is often an ongoing process, with recurrence of abuse in up to 70% of cases. A quarter of abused infants have, at previous medical encounters, presented with **sentinel injuries** (most commonly bruises, intra-oral injuries and fractures), which are injuries observed by medical professionals but not initially recognised to be abusive in nature. Recognising and reporting abusive injuries at the first instance may save an infant or child from further, even fatal, abuse.

When an injured child is brought to medical attention, where possible, obtain an account from both the child and the parent/responsible caregiver. Ask them to describe in detail the events surrounding each injury, allowing them to provide an account without interruptions, before asking clarifying questions.

Good documentation practices include clearly recording who gave the account(s), whether the parent was present when a child gave an account, any change in the accounts given over time (instead of just 'correcting' the record), and appropriate use of verbatim quotations (e.g. when a child refers to an action or a body part with colloquial terms).

Red flags in the history include inadequate, implausible or inconsistent accounts of the mechanism of injury and delay in presentation.

An injury attributed to a sibling or a pet is concerning. An incidental injury, noticed when a child presents for another complaint, should also receive due consideration. Recurring injuries attributed to accidents should prompt enquiry about any unsafe circumstances or environments.

When abuse is suspected, examination must include undressing the child to look for other injuries, paying particular attention to the scalp, ears, neck, palms, soles, trunk, buttocks and genitalia, and also examining for intra-oral injuries (e.g. a torn lip frenulum or bruising of oral mucosa).

Physical Child Abuse: Bruises

Bruises are the most common type of injury caused by physical child abuse. However, most bruises in children are accidental, not abusive. Differentiating abusive from accidental

Table 9.2 Features of Bruises that are Concerning for Abuse

Age/mobility of the child	• Bruising in an infant aged <9 mth: 'bruising before cruising' • Or, 'TEN4' rule: » bruising on the Torso, Ear or Neck in a child aged ≤4 yr » any bruising in an infant aged ≤4 mth • Bruising in a child who is not independently mobile (e.g. due to cerebral palsy)
Pattern of bruising	• **Clustering** of bruises • Multiple bruises of **similar shape and size** • Multiple bruises at different stages of healing • Imprints/bruises resembling the shape of an object (e.g. clothes hanger, belt, teeth) • 'Tram track' paired linear bruises (from a rod-shaped object) • Bilateral circumferential bruises on the wrists and ankles (signs of ligature)
Location of bruises	• Bruises away from bony prominences • Bruises on the face, ears, neck, abdomen, back and buttocks

bruises requires careful consideration of explanations given by caregivers, witnesses and the verbal child; of the child's age and mobility; and of features such as the location (Figures 9.1 and 9.2), shape, number and pattern of the bruises. When there is uncertainty, underlying medical conditions (such as haemophilia) may need to be excluded as the reason for bruises.

It is NOT possible for physicians to reliably estimate the **age of a bruise** based on colour or the presence of swelling or tenderness.

Evaluation for bleeding disorders with a full blood count and coagulation studies may be necessary in a child with unexplained bruising or bruises attributed to abuse. These tests may however be omitted where a diagnosis of abuse is clear from accounts obtained and the bruising pattern and where features of bleeding disorders are absent.

Physical Child Abuse: Fractures

Fractures are the second most common type of injury caused by physical child abuse, after bruises. Most fractures in children are accidental, but the younger the child, the higher the possibility that a fracture is caused by abuse.

Whilst certain fracture types are highly concerning for child abuse, no one fracture type is exclusively caused by either abuse or by accidents (see Table 9.3). Whether the explanation offered is congruent with the fracture sustained is important. A single linear skull fracture in a toddler 'punched by his brother' would be more concerning for abuse than multiple rib fractures in a toddler with a crushing chest injury from a road traffic accident.

Classic metaphyseal lesions (CMLs), also described as 'metaphyseal corner fractures' or 'bucket-handle fractures', occur almost exclusively in infants and toddlers under 2 years old. CMLs are planar fractures through the subphyseal metaphyses (next to growth plates) at the ends of long bones. They may be caused by traction, torsion or shear forces generated by to-and-fro shaking or by pulling or twisting of the infant's limbs.

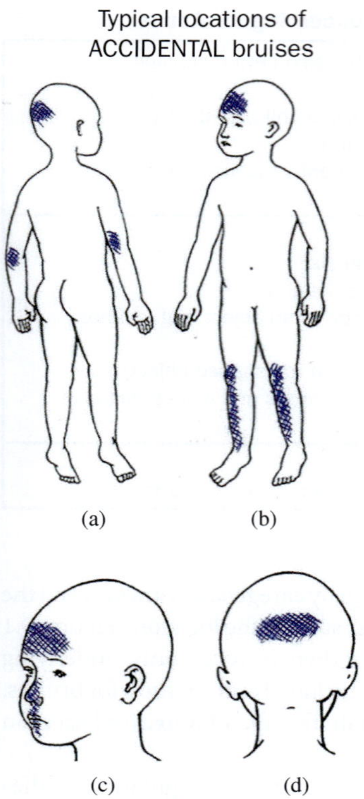

Figure 9.1 Typical locations of accidental bruises in children.

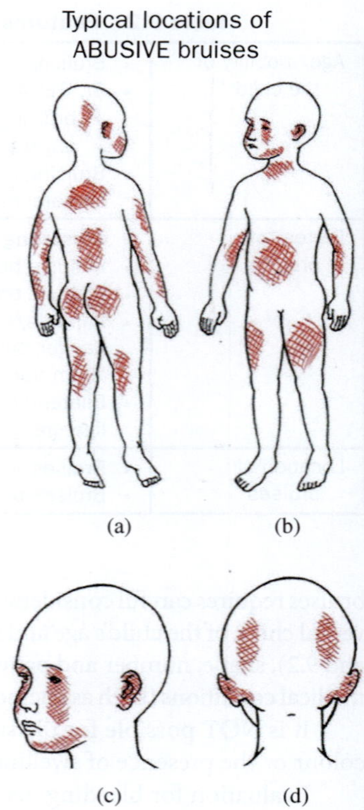

Figure 9.2 Typical locations of bruising in child abuse.

Diagrams drawn with reference to Maguire S, Mann M (2013). Body diagram template courtesy of Dr Terence Donald, University of Adelaide.

Osteogenesis imperfecta, osteopenia of prematurity, vitamin D deficiency rickets, renal bone disease and other medical conditions may present with multiple or recurrent fractures. These conditions can usually be differentiated from child abuse on the basis of clinical and radiological features and laboratory investigations as needed.

A **skeletal survey** is a series of radiographs that collectively show all the bones of the body, performed to look for clinically unsuspected (occult) fractures (see Table 9.4).

Physical Child Abuse: Thermal Injuries

Thermal injuries are found in about 10% of abused children. Two-thirds of abusive thermal injuries are scalds. Second most common are burns inflicted by contact with hot objects, such as a clothes iron, heated cutlery, hair curler/straightener, or cigarettes. Whilst most scalds in childhood are accidental, abuse or neglect account for more than 10% of childhood scalds.

Table 9.3 Radiological Findings that are Concerning for Abuse in Infants and Toddlers

Very concerning (strong statistical association with abuse)	• Classic metaphyseal lesions • Rib fractures (especially posteromedial) • Scapular fractures • Sternal fractures • Spinous process fractures
Moderately concerning	• Epiphyseal separations • Digital fractures • Vertebral body fractures and subluxations • Complex skull fractures • Multiple fractures (especially if bilateral) • Fractures of different ages
Slightly concerning (weak statistical association with abuse)	• Clavicle fractures • Long bone shaft fractures • Linear skull fractures • Subperiosteal new bone formation

Table 9.4 Indications for Obtaining a Skeletal Survey

- All children <2 yr old with obvious abusive injuries
- All children <2 yr old with suspicious injuries, including:
  - » bruises in non-ambulatory infants
  - » oral injuries in non-ambulatory infants
  - » injuries inconsistent with history provided
- Infants and young toddlers with unexplained intracranial injuries (including haemorrhage and hypoxic-ischaemic injury)
- Infants with unexplained, unexpected sudden death (consult with coroner first)
- An abused child's sibling/household member who is <2 yr old
- A twin of an abused infant or toddler

Accidental scalds are most commonly caused by spills when a child pulls a container of hot liquid off a table top or stove; most often scalding the face, neck or upper body. Typically, the margins are irregular, with splash patterns or flow lines, variable burn depth across scalded areas, and asymmetrical distribution (Figures 9.3 and 9.4).

In contrast, **intentional scalds**, which are most commonly caused by **forced immersion** into hot water, often produce clear proximal margins or 'tidal lines', 'glove' or 'stocking' scalds of one or more limbs, uniform scald depth, symmetrical distribution on both sides of the body, and skin fold sparing. Intentional scalds most often occur on the lower body without head or neck involvement. The most commonly affected areas are the legs, buttocks, genitals and perineum (Figures 9.5 and 9.6).

Abusive contact burns inflicted with a **hot object** tend to have sharper demarcations than accidental contact burns, and are more likely to affect multiple sites, often the face and sometimes the back of a child's body. These abusive burns often clearly reflect the shape of the causative object. In contrast, accidental contact burns tend to be single, and usually occur on the palms or the front of a child's body.

Examples of accidental scalds

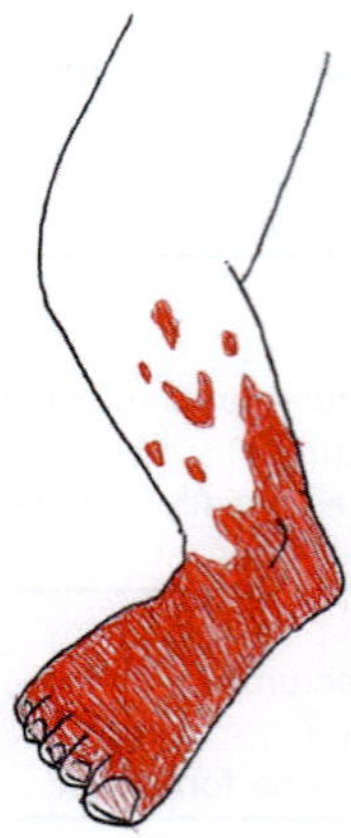

Figure 9.3 Scalding of uneven depth, irregular margins and splash marks on only one limb of a child who has accidentally stepped into a basin of hot water and quickly withdrew his foot in pain.

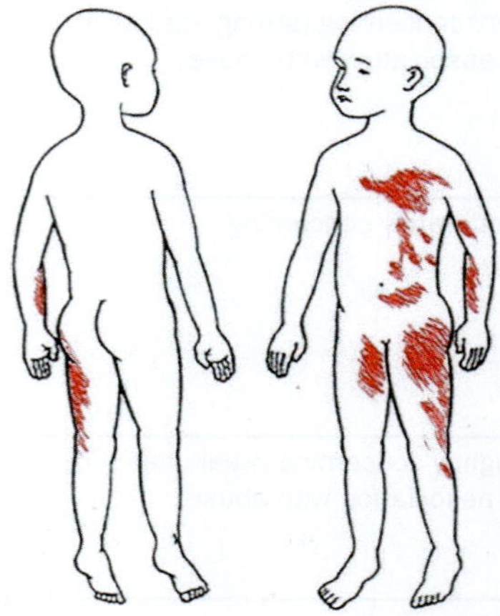

Figure 9.4 Scalding of uneven depth, irregular margins and asymmetrical distribution, with a pattern caused by wet clothing clinging to skin, and flow lines, in a child who has accidentally spilled hot soup onto himself/herself.

Diagrams drawn to show scalding patterns in the author's patients.
Body diagram template in Figure 9.4 courtesy of Dr Terence Donald, University of Adelaide.

Examples of abusive scalds

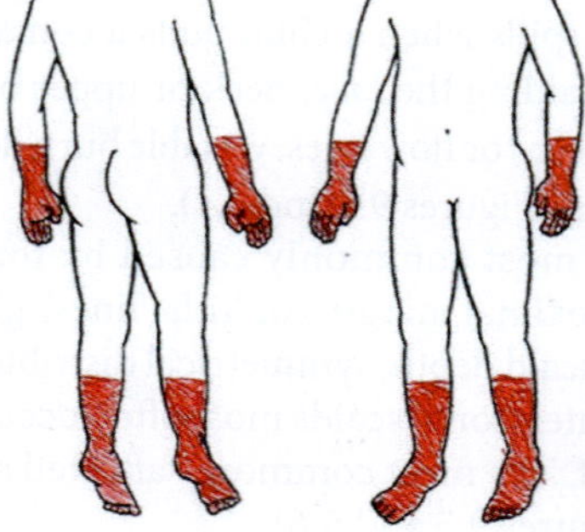

Figure 9.5 Symmetrical 'glove and stocking' scalds from forced immersion into hot water, with uniform scald depth, sharp 'tidal line' proximal margins and absence of splash marks.

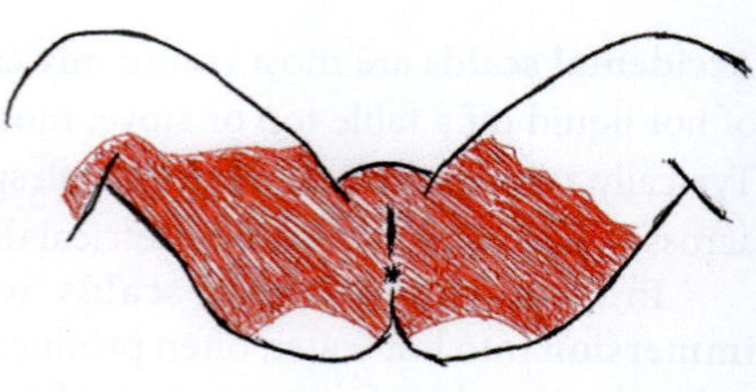

Figure 9.6 Scald pattern with central sparing of buttocks in an infant suspected to have been forcibly immersed into a bathtub of hot water (the spared buttock areas having been pressed against the relatively cooler bathtub surface). The employed caregiver claimed that it was accidental: she was unaware that the water was too hot. (Drawing of author's patient).

Body diagram template in Figure 9.5 courtesy of Dr Terence Donald, University of Adelaide.

Abuse inflicted with a **lighted cigarette** typically causes **sharply demarcated circular burns** around 1 cm in diameter, often multiple and uniform, sometimes on parts of the body normally covered by clothing. Bullous impetigo is an important differential diagnosis. In contrast, accidental contact with a lighted cigarette tends to cause single, more superficial, less sharply demarcated and non-circular burns, on usually unclothed areas.

Physical Child Abuse: Abusive Head Trauma

Abusive Head Injury, or Abusive Head Trauma (AHT), is the foremost cause of death from child abuse.

AHT refers to a constellation of injuries to the head and its contents (including the brain and eyes) caused by the directed application of force to an infant or young child. The forces involved may include acceleration/deceleration forces (such as is caused by shaking), blunt force trauma, penetrating trauma and asphyxiation. The injuries often include a 'triad' of subdural haemorrhage (SDH), cerebral oedema and retinal haemorrhages. The absence of this triad does not exclude AHT.

The term 'Shaken Baby Syndrome' is often used in media to refer to AHT, but should be avoided in medical communication and documentation, as it presumes the specific and seldom proven mechanism of shaking.

Infants and toddlers with AHT often present with non-specific symptoms: drowsiness, irritability, poor feeding or vomiting. Up to 50% present with seizures. In most cases, a history of trauma is denied, or the explanation given is incongruous with the presentation. Scalp haematomas and externally visible injuries are often absent. Increased head circumference and signs of raised intracranial pressure (e.g. bulging fontanelles) may be present.

Neuroimaging may reveal acute or chronic subdural haemorrhage/haemorrhages (in >70% of cases), subarachnoid haemorrhage, cerebral ischaemia, cerebral oedema or diffuse axonal injury. Skull fractures may be absent. Complex skull fractures occur more often in AHT compared to non-abusive head trauma, whereas the opposite is true for linear skull fractures.

Evaluation by an ophthalmologist reveals retinal haemorrhages in up to 85% of cases. Retinal haemorrhages are strongly associated with AHT (odds ratio of 28 favouring abuse over non-abuse, in a 2012 meta-analysis by Piteau *et al*). Skeletal survey often reveals associated metaphyseal fractures and rib fractures.

Mortality in AHT ranges from 11% to 35%, and 45% to 90% of survivors have permanent neurological sequelae: most commonly, visual deficits, hearing impairment and cognitive impairment.

Child Sexual Abuse

Although they overlap, **sexual assault** and **sexual abuse** are not exactly the same thing.

Sexual assault has taken place when a person has been involved in a sexual act **without his or her consent**. From a legal point of view, a child *cannot* consent to a sexual act. Engaging in sexual activity with a person **under 16 years of age** is a criminal offence in Singapore, even if the child agreed to the activity. Accordingly, the police may refer anyone under 16 years old, who may have engaged in sexual intercourse, to the paediatric hospital for forensic evaluation. On our part, medical professionals have a legal obligation to notify the police if we suspect that any patient under 16 years old has participated in sexual activity (even if it was consensual and between two young persons of the same age).

Sexual abuse refers to a child or young person being **exploited** for sexual gratification. Often, the perpetrator is someone who has authority or influence over the victim, or who has the victim's trust (e.g. a parent, sibling, relative, teacher or sports coach) or someone regarded by the victim as a romantic partner, but who is significantly older than the victim. Nine out of ten perpetrators are male.

The perpetrator may have engaged in **sexual grooming**, e.g. by giving gifts, showing favour, providing emotional support, encouraging interest in sexual acts, or persuading the child or young person that such acts are normal or loving.

Whilst touching or penetrative sex may be involved, sexual abuse does not always entail physical contact. Indecent exposure, showing pornography, recording or asking for indecent images or videos, and exchanging messages of a sexual nature ('sexting') with a young person, are also forms of sexual abuse.

Sexual abuse may come to be suspected or uncovered through:

- Disclosure to a family member, friend, teacher or school counsellor.
- Disclosure to a medical professional during clinical encounters.
- Diagnosis of a sexually transmitted infection.
- Diagnosis of pregnancy.
- Discovery of concerning communication, photographs or recordings on electronic devices or social media.
- Developmentally inappropriate sexual behaviours observed by a parent or professional.

Non-leading, open-ended questions are appropriate when asking a child or adolescent about possible sexual abuse. Prompt referral, even if the abuse was not recent, is necessary. A child's first detailed account of abuse is often the most forensically intact and should ideally be obtained by trained interviewers. Repeating the account may be distressing. Thus, many victims of intra-familial sexual abuse in Singapore are now interviewed jointly by the police, Child Protective Service and a paediatrician.

In Singapore, **forensic examination** for suspected sexual assault or sexual abuse in children and young persons is performed by gynaecologists for female victims and paediatric surgeons for male victims.

The forensic examination includes head-to-toe examination for injuries, anogenital examination and the obtaining of forensic specimens depending on the timing and type of sexual contact. Swabs from body surfaces and cavities may be obtained to test for semen, spermatozoa and DNA. Blood and urine samples for toxicology are obtained if drug-facilitated sexual assault is suspected.

This forensic examination is time-sensitive: after sexual intercourse, semen is rarely present in the oral cavity beyond 6 hours, anorectal cavity beyond 24 hours and vaginal cavity beyond 72 hours. Unfortunately, many victims present to medical care long after abuse has taken place. When forensic examination takes place more than 3 to 5 days after sexual intercourse, the collection of forensic specimens may reasonably be omitted. Normal forensic examination does not rule out sexual assault or sexual abuse.

Regardless of time since the alleged sexual abuse/assault, the victim should be tested for sexually transmitted infections (STIs). Locally, these tests comprise serology for HIV, Hepatitis B, Hepatitis C and *Treponema pallidum*; first-catch urine for *Chlamydia trachomatis* and *Neisseria gonorrhoeae* PCR; vaginal swab DNA hybridisation probe test (VP3) for *Candida, Gardnerella vaginalis* and *Trichomonas vaginalis*, and occasionally cultures where appropriate.

After specimen collection for STI tests, post-exposure prophylaxis for HIV and Hepatitis B, as well as presumptive antibiotic therapy for *Neisseria gonorrhoeae, Chlamydia trachomatis* and *Trichomonas vaginalis* (usually IM ceftriaxone, PO azithromycin and PO metronidazole) are offered if indicated, based on risk assessment.

For adolescent females presenting acutely after a sexual assault, the gynaecologist may offer emergency contraception, after first testing for pregnancy.

In cases where the alleged perpetrator is a household member, it is urgent and important to consider the safety and suitability of the victim remaining at home. Even if the alleged perpetrator has been taken into police custody, there are other concerns, such as how interaction with family members may affect the integrity of forensic history. Immediate removal of the victim from the household for the time being is usually necessary.

Victims often benefit from psychologists' assessment and support. Medical follow-up usually involves repeat serological tests for HIV and Hepatitis C (also Hepatitis B if the victim is non-immune), up to the end of a 6-month window period from the last sexual contact.

Emotional Abuse

Emotional abuse is also known as psychological abuse or psychological maltreatment.

Amongst all the types of child abuse, emotional abuse is probably the most prevalent, most under-reported, most difficult to assess and least understood. Emotional abuse often goes undetected, even though it is seldom deliberately hidden, as sexual abuse is. When witnessed, it may not be recognised.

Emotional abuse is characterised by a **repeated pattern** of behaviour by a parent or caregiver that causes a child to feel unwanted or unloved or that is detrimental to the child's well-being, including his or her development and socialisation. These harmful behaviours include:

- **Spurning:** e.g. rejecting the child's bids for attention, excluding the child from family activities, ridiculing, humiliating, scapegoating, belittling, denigrating (including calling a child 'stupid').
- **Terrorising:** e.g. threatening physical harm, threatening deprivation of basic needs, threatening abandonment, damaging the child's loved possessions, making unreasonable demands.
- **Isolating:** e.g. confining a child within a room or within the home, depriving the child of social interactions.
- **Emotional unresponsiveness:** e.g. withholding affection, withholding praise.
- **Corrupting/exploiting:** e.g. encouraging or reinforcing misbehaviour, demanding behaviour inappropriate for the developmental age, using the child to meet the parent's emotional needs.

Isolated incidents of these behaviours do not necessarily constitute emotional abuse, but it is possible for a single incident (e.g. of severe terrorising) to cause great harm to a child.

Emotional abuse may occur on its own, or alongside physical abuse, sexual abuse or neglect. On the other hand, physical abuse, sexual abuse or neglect seldom occur without an accompanying element of emotional abuse. In all forms of child abuse, the greatest harm is often psychological harm, and the harm may not be intended.

Children with intellectual disabilities are at higher risk of emotional abuse, as are children living in households where there is family conflict, custody disputes, intimate partner violence, mental health problems or substance abuse.

Children and adolescents who have been emotionally abused are more likely to have anxiety, depression and eating disorders. They may manifest maladaptive behaviours, developmental delay, poor academic performance or social difficulties. They may also present with somatic symptoms such as headache, chest pain and abdominal pain.

Observations concerning for emotional abuse include:

- A child with behaviour that is attention-seeking, anti-social, aggressive or oppositional.
- A child who seems withdrawn, unconfident or insecure.
- A child who has poor emotional regulation.
- A child who is age-inappropriately responsible.
- A child who uses age-inappropriate language, including swear words.
- A child who deliberately annoys or hurts others or is cruel to animals.
- A child who seems wary or fearful of his or her parent.
- A young child who does not seem affectionate toward his or her parent.
- A young child who is overly affectionate to strangers.
- A parent who displays negativity or hostility towards the child.

Besides enquiring about the experiences of such a child, there is also a need to explore parental expectations and parenting difficulties faced. The boundary between suboptimal parenting and emotional abuse is difficult to define. Rather than applying a label of 'emotional abuse', it is more helpful for physicians and other professionals to:

- Describe specific harmful actions or words and explain how these are harmful.
- Encourage and enable modification of parenting behaviours, e.g. by referring for parenting skills training.

- Plan with the parents for the child's safety and well-being going forward.

In emotional abuse, the need for protection is usually less immediately pressing than in sexual abuse and physical abuse. Nevertheless, referral to the Child Protective Service may still be needed, especially if emotionally abusive behaviours persist. Clear evidence of harm is not a prerequisite for referral.

Paediatricians have a unique opportunity to prevent the emotional abuse of children, by proactively discussing approaches to parenting, helping parents to understand children's needs and normal behaviours at each stage of development and pointing parents to useful parenting resources.

Neglect

Child neglect has occurred when a parent or caregiver has the means to, but does not, provide for the development of the child in any of these spheres: health, education, emotional development, nutrition, shelter and safe living conditions (definition adapted from the WHO). Examples of neglect include failure to provide a child with adequate food, clothing, supervision, medical care or opportunities to attend school.

The prevalence of child neglect worldwide has been estimated at 16–40%. Unlike victims of physical or sexual abuse, victims of neglect are not often brought to hospital for forensic evaluation. They may nevertheless require medical assessment and interventions, whether in primary care (e.g. to catch up with missed vaccinations) or by specialists (e.g. for associated failure to thrive or developmental delay).

Referral to the Child Protective Service may be necessary if a child has suffered serious accidental injury, is severely malnourished or significantly delayed in development due to suspected neglect, or if the parent consistently does not meet the child's basic needs.

Removal of a child from the home environment/admission to hospital as a place of safety may be necessary, such as when home conditions are eminently unsafe, or when caregivers are remanded for drug offences or incapacitated by intoxication or mental health issues.

Table 9.5 Some Alerting Features for Child Neglect

- Malnutrition/faltering growth due to inadequate or inappropriate diet
- Persistently poor hygiene/persistent infestation with head lice or scabies
- Poor school attendance without valid explanation
- Missed vaccinations/non-compliance to medications
- Recurrent accidental injuries due to lack of supervision or unsafe living environment

Adapted from WHO guidelines for the health sector response to child maltreatment, 2019

Bibliography

1. Ministry of Social and Family Development (2021) *Protecting the Safety and Well-being of Children.* Singapore: Ministry of Social and Family Development. https://www.msf.gov.sg/policies/Strong-and-Stable-Families/Nurturing-and-Protecting-the-Young/Child-Protection-Welfare/Pages/Protecting-Children.aspx
2. Gilgoff R, Singh L, Koita K, *et al.* (2020) Adverse childhood experiences, outcomes, and interventions. *Pediatr Clin N Am* **67**(2):259–273.

3. World Health Organization (2019) WHO guidelines for the health sector response to child maltreatment, Geneva, Switzerland. https://www.who.int/publications/i/item/who-guidelines-for-the-health-sector-response-to-child-maltreatment
4. Christian CW. (2015) Committee on child abuse and neglect, American Academy of Pediatrics. The evaluation of suspected child physical abuse. *Pediatrics* **135**(5):e1337–e1354. Erratum in: *Pediatrics* **136**(3):583.
5. Maguire S, Mann M. (2013) Systematic reviews of bruising in relation to child abuse-what have we learnt: An overview of review updates. *Evid Based Child Health* **8**(2):255–263.
6. Kemp AM, Jones S, Lawson Z, Maguire SA. (2014) Patterns of burns and scalds in children. *Arch Dis Child* **99**(4):316–321.
7. Flaherty EG, Perez-Rossello JM, Levine MA, Hennrikus WL. (2014) American Academy of Pediatrics, Committee on Child Abuse and Neglect; Section on Radiology, American Academy of Pediatrics; Section on Endocrinology, American Academy of Pediatrics; Section on Orthopaedics, American Academy of Pediatrics; Society for Pediatric Radiology. Evaluating children with fractures for child physical abuse. *Pediatrics* **133**(2):e477–e489.
8. Maiese A, Iannaccone F, Scatena A, *et al.* (2021) Pediatric abusive head trauma: A systematic review. *Diagnostics* **11**(4):734.
9. Chiesa A, Goldson E. (2017) Child sexual abuse. *Pediatr Rev* **38**(3):105–118.
10. Kellogg N. (2005) American Academy of Pediatrics, Committee on Child Abuse and Neglect. The evaluation of sexual abuse in children. *Pediatrics* **116**(2):506–512.
11. Kimber M, MacMillan HL. (2017) Child psychological abuse. *Pediatr Rev* **38**(10):496–498.

SECTION 10

DERMATOLOGY

CHAPTER 33

Rashes

Ho Pui Yoong, Valerie; Koh Jean Aan, Mark

The key to establishing an accurate diagnosis and subsequent management of skin disorders in children is through a **focused clinical history and examination**.

History

Pertinent key points to obtain on history include:

- Age of onset (congenital or acquired)
- Duration of the rash
- Distribution of the rash
- Progression of the rash
- Recent new oral medications or topical contactants in the last 2 months
  - » Severe cutaneous adverse drug eruptions like drug reaction with eosinophilia and systemic symptoms (DRESS) are delayed hypersensitivity reactions and have a latency period of 2 weeks to 2 months
  - » Topical applications of contactants can cause acute contact dermatitis
- Family history of skin conditions, similar acute eruptions or autoimmune conditions
  - » e.g. atopic dermatitis runs in families with a strong atopy history
  - » e.g. infestations like scabies and fungal infections can spread within close family contacts
- Contact history: Other affected family members, pets
- Travel history
- Vaccination history
- Associated fever, systemic symptoms like arthralgia, mucous membrane involvement and constitutional symptoms like loss of weight and lethargy

Clinical Examination

It is important to ascertain the following during clinical examination:

- General appearance of the child, vital signs and presence of fever
- Morphology and distribution of the rashes and presence of secondary changes (see Tables 10.1 and 10.2)
  - » Accurate morphological description of the rash will help to narrow down the differential diagnoses or clinch the diagnosis

- Mucous membrane involvement and presence of Nikolsky sign (epidermal sloughing from gentle shearing pressure)
- Examine the nails, hair and teeth
- Systemic examination, e.g. hepatosplenomegaly, lymphadenopathy and arthritis

Table 10.1 Primary Morphology of Rashes

Primary Lesions	Definition
Macule	Flat, non-palpable lesion ≤1 cm in diameter
Patch	Flat, non-palpable lesion >1 cm in diameter
Papule	Elevated palpable solid lesion ≤1 cm in diameter
Plaque	Elevated palpable solid lesion >1 cm in diameter
Nodule	Elevated, rounded palpable solid lesion >1 cm in diameter and usually located primarily in the dermis and/or subcutis
Vesicle	Blister ≤1 cm (containing clear, serous or haemorrhagic fluid)
Bulla	Blister >1 cm (containing clear, serous or haemorrhagic fluid)
Pustule	A circumscribed lesion containing pus
Petechiae	Small (<3 mm) non-blanching haemorrhages
Purpura	Larger (>3 mm) non-blanching haemorrhages
Weal/Urticaria	A transient elevation of the skin due to dermal oedema, usually pale centrally with an erythematous rim

Table 10.2 Secondary Changes

Secondary Changes	Definition
Crust	Dried serum, blood or pus on the surface of the skin
Scale	A visible accumulation of keratin, forming a flat plate or flake
Erosion	A loss of either a portion of or the entire epidermis
Excoriation	A loss of the epidermis and a portion of the dermis, usually due to scratching or an injury (often linear)
Ulcer	Full-thickness loss of the epidermis and a portion of the dermis

Clinical Pearls

In general, rash in the absence of fever or other systemic symptoms tend to be benign.

'Red flags' that require prompt attention include:

- Association with fever/prolonged fever, systemic symptoms like arthralgia ± unwell child
  - » Serious systemic bacterial infections: Meningococcemia, staphylococcal scalded skin syndrome (SSSS)
  - » Drug eruptions: DRESS, Stevens–Johnson syndrome (SJS) and toxic epidermal necrolysis (TEN)

   - » Vasculitic/rheumatologic conditions: Kawasaki disease, systemic onset juvenile idiopathic arthritis (SoJIA), systemic lupus erythematosus
   - » Malignancy: Acute lymphocytic leukaemia
- Mucocutaneous involvement (oral, conjunctival, anogenital) may signify a delayed hypersensitivity cutaneous drug eruption like SJS and TEN
- Wheals or urticarial rash with angioedema, respiratory distress, wheezing and hypotension may signify acute anaphylaxis and needs urgent management

Clinically, a rash may be broadly classified as **macular/maculopapular**, **papular**, **vesiculobullous**, **pustular**, **urticaria** or **petechial/purpuric**. These rashes may co-exist or evolve from one form to another. Diagnosis should be focused on the exclusion of emergent or life-threatening conditions that require prompt intervention.

Please refer to the attached algorithms.

When to Refer Urgently to the Dermatologist

- Diagnostic dilemmas that may warrant a skin biopsy
- Index of suspicion for a severe cutaneous adverse reaction to drugs like DRESS, SJS and TEN
- Concerns for atypical presentations of serious systemic infections in the immunocompromised population and very young children
- Concerns for autoimmune conditions, in which concurrent rheumatological opinion should also be sought if needed
- Complex or complicated dermatological conditions (genodermatoses or vascular anomalies) that require specialised or multi-disciplinary care

Bibliography

1. Nast A, Griffiths CE, Hay R, *et al.* (2016) The 2016 International League of Dermatological Societies' revised glossary for the description of cutaneous lesions. *Br J Dermatol* **174**(6):1351–1358.
2. Manoharan KS, Ramasamy K, Heinz P. (2017) Rash with fever in children: A clinical approach. *Paediatr Child Health* **27**(4):196–201.
3. Muzumdar S, Rothe MJ, Grant-Kels JM. (2019) The rash with macula papules and fever in children. *Clin Dermatol* **37**(2):119–128.

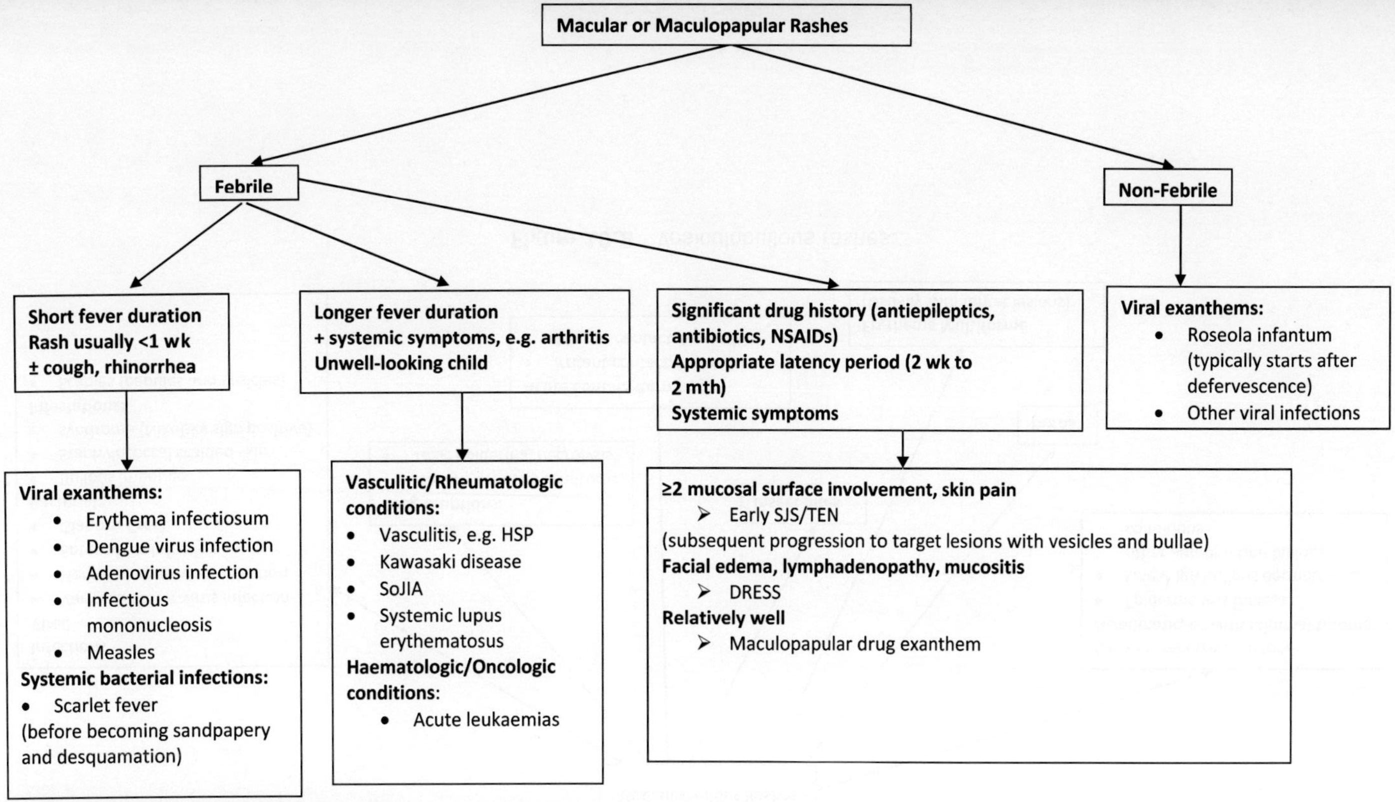

NAIDs : nonsteroidal anti-inflammatory drugs
SoJIA : systemic onset juvenile idiopathic arthritis
SJS: Stevens–Johnson syndrome
TEN: toxic epidermal necrolysis
DRESS: drug reaction with eosinophilia and systemic symptoms;
HSP: Henoch–Schonlein Purpura

Figure 10.1 Maculopapular rashes.

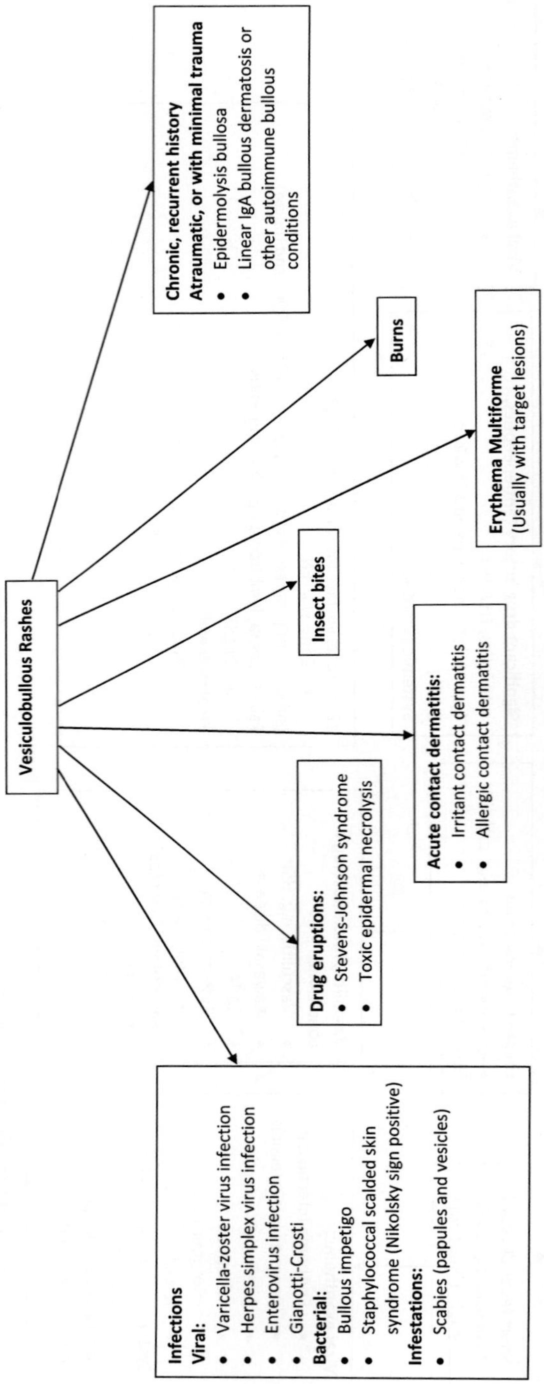

Figure 10.2 Vesiculobullous rashes.

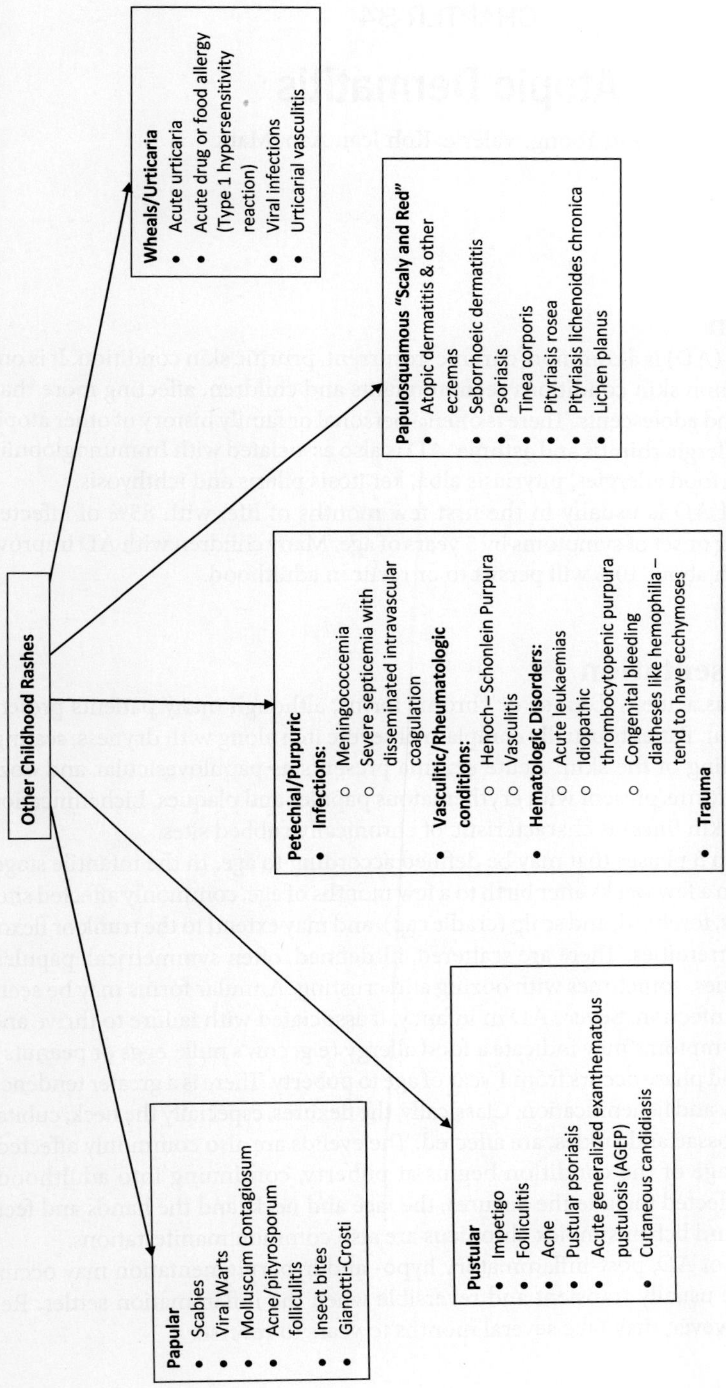

Figure 10.3 Other childhood rashes.

CHAPTER 34

Atopic Dermatitis

Ho Pui Yoong, Valerie; Koh Jean Aan, Mark

Introduction

Atopic dermatitis (AD) is a common, chronic, recurrent, pruritic skin condition. It is one of the most common skin conditions seen in infants and children, affecting more than 20% of children and adolescents. There is often a personal or family history of other atopic conditions, like allergic rhinitis and asthma. AD is also associated with Immunoglobulin E (IgE)-mediated food allergies, pityriasis alba, keratosis pilaris and ichthyosis.

The onset of AD is usually in the first few months of life, with 85% of affected individuals having onset of symptoms by 5 years of age. Many children with AD improve with age, although about 10% will persist to or recur in adulthood.

Clinical Presentation

AD may present as acute, subacute, or chronic forms, although many patients present with a combination. Patients usually complain of severe itch along with dryness, scaling, oozing, and swelling of the skin. Acute eczema presents as papulovesicular and oozy lesions. Subacute forms present with erythematous papules and plaques. Lichenification (accentuation of skin lines) is characteristic of chronically rubbed sites.

There are also 3 phases that may be defined according to age. In the infantile stage, which occurs from a few weeks after birth to a few months of age, commonly affected sites include the cheeks, forehead, and scalp (cradle cap), and may extend to the trunk or flexor surfaces of the extremities. There are scattered, ill-defined, often symmetrical, papules, patches, and plaques, sometimes with oozing and crusting. Annular forms may be seen, mimicking tinea infection. Severe AD in infancy, if associated with failure to thrive and gastrointestinal symptoms may indicate a food allergy (e.g. cow's milk, eggs or peanuts).

The childhood phase occurs from 1 year of age to puberty. There is a greater tendency towards chronicity and lichenification. Classically, the flexures, especially the neck, cubital fossae, popliteal fossae and ankles, are affected. The eyelids are also commonly affected.

The adult stage of the condition begins at puberty, continuing into adulthood. Common areas affected include the flexures, the face and neck, and the hands and feet. Prurigo nodules and lichen simplex chronicus are also common manifestations.

In all phases of AD, post-inflammatory hypo- and hyperpigmentation may occur. These changes are usually transient and reversible when the inflammation settles. Re-pigmentation, however, may take several months to years to reverse.

Treatment

Dry Skin Care

- Daily baths with cool or luke-warm water, for 5-10 minutes is ideal. A mild soap or soap substitute should be used during showers or baths.
- After patting dry, moisturisers should be applied immediately. Creams and ointments are more effective than lotions. The 'best moisturiser' is one that the child and parent will use frequently, which works for the patient and is affordable. Moisturisers should be applied at least 2 to 3 times daily, with applications more frequent during exacerbations.
- The frequent daily use of moisturisers, even during times of quiescence of disease, should be emphasised to patients and parents.

Avoid Irritants/Allergens

- Common triggers of eczema include changes in climate, sweating, dusty environments, harsh soaps, cigarette smoke, and chemicals. Carpets, pets and soft toys should be avoided as they are common sources of house dust mites. Soft, loose cotton clothing is recommended. Food allergy as a cause of eczema is controversial. It may play a role in some infants with severe eczema. Allergen-specific IgE or skin prick tests should be ordered only after consultation with a paediatric allergist or dermatologist.

Topical Corticosteroids

- Topical corticosteroids (TCS) are the mainstay of treatment of AD. Complications of TCS use can be minimised with appropriate and safe use. TCS should be applied just before the application of moisturisers. In general, ointments are more moisturising, afford better penetration, more efficacious and less irritating than creams and lotions. Creams are less potent than ointments but are more cosmetically elegant. Lotions are used for scalp application.
- The recommended guidelines for use of TCS are:
  - Low-potency TCS (e.g. 1% hydrocortisone cream, 0.025% betamethasone valerate cream, 0.05% desonide) are recommended for the face, flexures and genitalia for all ages.
  - Mid-potency TCS (e.g. 0.1% betamethasone valerate cream, mometasone furoate cream) are recommended for thicker plaques on the trunk and limbs of children.
  - High-potency TCS (e.g. betamethasone diproprionate) are reserved for stubborn, severely lichenified eczematous plaques, and should be ordered only by paediatric dermatologists.
- Patients should be advised to use TCS twice daily and to stop applications once the eruptions are not itchy, red or bumpy. After 2 weeks, if the rash does not improve, patients should be reviewed.
- The use of oral corticosteroids should only be reserved for severe exacerbations of AD (e.g. prednisolone 0.5 mg/kg/day, in tailing doses over 10-14 days).

Topical Calcineurin Inhibitors

- Topical calcineurin inhibitors (TCI), tacrolimus ointment (Protopic) and pimecrolimus cream (Elidel) are non-steroidal anti-inflammatory medications used for the treatment of eczema. Tacrolimus may be used in patients with moderate to severe AD and pimecrolimus in patients with mild AD. They are recommended to be used twice daily over affected areas. Common side effects include irritation and burning. Similar to TCS, TCI should be applied until the skin is not itchy, red or bumpy.

Treatment of Infections

- *Staphylococcus aureus* is a common coloniser of the skin of patients with AD and can lead to infective flares. Anti-staphylococcal antibiotics should be prescribed during exacerbations of disease (e.g. 50 mg/kg/day TDS or cloxacillin 50 mg/kg/day QDS or erythromycin 50 mg/kg/day QDS for 1 to 2 weeks). Skin swabs should be sent for bacterial culture. Adjunctive therapies, including potassium permanganate soaks and a TCS/antibiotic combination (e.g. fucicort or 0.1% betamethasone/vioform), can be applied to the oozy lesions.
- If eczema herpeticum is suspected, systemic acyclovir, either oral or intravenous, can be started. Herpes simplex virus polymerase chain reaction swab should be sent from a blister or erosion to confirm the diagnosis.

Oral Anti-histamines and other Anti-itch Measures

- Sedative anti-histamines (e.g. hydroxyzine or chlorpheniramine) before bedtime may help lessen scratching during sleep. Non-sedating anti-histamines have minimal effect on itch in AD. Other anti-itch topicals can also be recommended (e.g. Suu Balm, Suu Balm Kids, Kidsclin Mousse, Awemed Spray). Application of fridge-chilled moisturisers can also help to relief the itch. Avoid calamine lotion as it is very drying and can worsen AD.

Wet-wrap Treatment

- The use of wet-wrap therapy has shown good effect in patients with acute flares of eczema. It can also be used for patients with thick, lichenified plaques of eczema (e.g. lichen simplex chronicus). It is best to initiate wet-wraps as inpatient treatment.

When To Refer To A Paediatric Dematologist

- Moderate to severe AD.
- Patients with frequent, recurrent flares of AD, especially if recurrent bacterial infections or eczema herpeticum.
- Patients with reduced quality of life secondary to AD or if there are other psychosocial problems that are associated with AD.
- Patients with suspected complications of AD treatment (e.g. from corticosteroid use) or patients with poor compliance or understanding of AD treatment.

Bibliography

1. Cheok S, Yee F, Song Ma JY, *et al*. (2018) Prevalence and descriptive epidemiology of atopic dermatitis and its impact on quality of life in Singapore. *Br J Dermatol* **178**(1):276–277.
2. Tay YK, Chan YC, Chandran NS, *et al.* (2016) Guidelines for the management of atopic dermatitis in Singapore. *Ann Acad Med Sing* **45**(10):439–450.
3. Wollenberg A, Barbarot S, Bieber T, *et al.* (2018) Consensus-based European guidelines for treatment of atopic eczema (atopic dermatitis) in adults and children: Part I. *J Eur Acad Dermatol Venereol* **32**(5):657–682.

SECTION 11

ENDOCRINOLOGY

CHAPTER 35

Adrenal Insufficiency

Aravind Venkatesh; Chan Wei Keong, Daniel; Chin Xinyi;
Lek Ngee; Rashida Farhad Vasanwala; Yap Kok Peng, Fabian

Introduction

Glucocorticoids are important in carbohydrate, protein and fat metabolism and also play an integral part in the stress response. Mineralocorticoids deal with water retention as well as sodium and electrolyte balance. Glucocorticoid replacement is required in *all forms* of adrenal insufficiency, while mineralocorticoids are *only* required in primary adrenal insufficiency.

Acute adrenal insufficiency (adrenal crisis) in children is a medical emergency.

Suspect acute adrenal insufficiency in any:

- **Unwell child known to have adrenal insufficiency who has an intercurrent illness,**
- **Child withdrawing from steroid therapy, and**
- **Child with fluid unresponsive shock.**

Causes

- Primary adrenal insufficiency
  - » Congenital adrenal hyperplasia
  - » Adrenal hypoplasia congenita
  - » Adrenoleukodystrophy
  - » Adrenal damage or removal
  - » Autoimmune adrenalitis
- Secondary adrenal insufficiency
  - » Hypothalamic/Pituitary damage or tumours
  - » Cranial irradiation
  - » Withdrawal from chronic steroid therapy causing adrenocorticotropic hormone (ACTH) suppression

Clinical and Biochemical Features

- Acute manifestations include:
  - » Hypotension and shock (from loss of vasomotor tone)
  - » Hypoglycaemia (from low liver glucose output)
- Subacute/Chronic manifestations include:

- » Hyperpigmentation (from chronic ACTH exposure in primary adrenal insufficiency)
  - » Lethargy, weakness and tiredness (from electrolyte changes)
  - » Loss of appetite and weight loss (from anorexia and volume depletion)
- Biochemical features
  - » Hyponatraemia ± hyperkalaemia (from aldosterone deficiency)
  - » Hypoglycaemia (from cortisol deficiency)
  - » Raised urea ± creatinine (from dehydration)
  - » Raised plasma renin activity (from volume depletion) and serum ACTH (in primary adrenal insufficiency)
  - » Inadequate cortisol response to Synacthen stimulation

Investigations

In any severely ill child who may be presenting with features of suspected adrenal insufficiency for the first time, take samples for: serum electrolytes (Na/K), glucose, cortisol, 17-OH progesterone, ACTH, plasma renin and aldosterone before administering glucocorticoids.

Management

Adrenal Crisis

- **Fluid Management**
  - » Resuscitate with intravenous (IV) normal saline bolus 20 ml/kg if hypotensive, in shock or poorly perfused.
  - » Repeat IV normal saline bolus 10 ml/kg, if needed.
- **Hyperkalaemia**
  - » Manage severe hyperkalaemia urgently, if needed.
- **Hydrocortisone Replacement**
  - » Administer IV or intramuscular hydrocortisone (100 mg/m^2 body surface area [BSA]) IMMEDIATELY. [BSA guide: 3-year-old 0.5 m^2 (50 mg), 8-year-old 1 m^2 (100 mg), adult 1.7 m^2 (150–200 mg)]
  - » Continue stress doses of IV hydrocortisone 100 mg/m^2/day in 4–6 divided doses until the clinical condition stabilises.
- **Hypoglycaemia Management**
  - » Administer 10% dextrose **2 ml/kg** as a slow bolus if blood glucose is low.
  - » Subsequently, provide adequate dextrose (5%) in the maintenance drip (0.9% normal saline), withholding potassium until the serum potassium is normal.
- **Consult Paediatric Endocrinologist**

Replacement Therapy

- **Hydrocortisone**
  - » Hydrocortisone is the preferred glucocorticoid option.

» The replacement hydrocortisone dose in primary adrenal insufficiency is 12–15 mg/m^2/day. Requirements are higher (3–4 times) during stress to the body (febrile illness, injury, surgery, anaesthesia).
» The replacement hydrocortisone dose in secondary adrenal insufficiency due to ACTH deficiency is usually less than the above doses at about 8–10 mg/m^2/day.

- **Mineralocorticoid**
  » The replacement fludrocortisone dose in primary adrenal disease is 0.05–0.2 mg/day (NOTE: Absolute dose and not per body weight or surface area). Dose adjustments are based on serum electrolytes, blood pressure and plasma renin activity.

Glucocorticoid Cover for Intercurrent Illness

- Children with, or who are at risk of, adrenal insufficiency **must be given increased** replacement hydrocortisone doses for stress according to the following guidelines:
  » Moderately unwell and/or temperature 38–39°C: give **two to three times** the usual dose of hydrocortisone.
  » More unwell and/or temperature >39°C: give **three to four times** the usual dose of hydrocortisone.
  » If the dose is vomited within 30 minutes of ingestion, **repeat the dose.**
  » If the dose is vomited again, bring the child to Children's Emergency.
  » For gastroenteritis or diarrhoea: Give **four times** the usual dose of hydrocortisone.
  » When the stress is over, return to routine dosing regimen without tapering.

Peri-operative Glucocorticoid Cover

- **Major surgery**
  » At induction of anaesthesia give IV hydrocortisone 100 mg/m^2.
  » Then continue IV hydrocortisone 100 mg/m^2/day in 4–6 hourly doses intra and post-operatively for 24–48 hours.
  » Hydrocortisone doses are weaned down depending on the post-operative recovery.
- **Minor surgery**
  » At induction of anaesthesia give IV hydrocortisone 100 mg/m^2.
  » Then give three to four times the usual dose of oral hydrocortisone for 24 hours.

Bibliography

1. Bornstein SR, Allolio B, Arlt W, *et al.* (2016) Diagnosis and treatment of primary adrenal insufficiency: An endocrine society clinical practice guideline. *J Clin Endocrinol Metab* **101**(2):364–389.
2. Miller BS, Spencer SP, Geffner ME, *et al.* (2020) Emergency management of adrenal insufficiency in children: Advocating for treatment options in outpatient and field settings. *J Investig Med* **68**(1):16–25.

CHAPTER 36

Hypoglycaemia

Chin Xinyi; Chan Wei Keong, Daniel; Aravind Venkatesh;
Lek Ngee; Rashida Farhad Vasanwala; Yap Kok Peng, Fabian

Definition

What constitutes low blood glucose (BG), i.e. hypoglycaemia, depends on the clinical context, epidemiological norms, long-term neurological outcome or threshold for neuroendocrine counter-regulatory response. Autonomic effects and hypoglycaemia awareness occur at BG of 3 mmol/L. As such, recurrent BG <3 mmol/L (<3.5 mmol/L if symptomatic) warrants further investigation. (The definition for hypoglycaemia for diabetic patients is BG <4.0 mmol/L.)

Normal responses to hypoglycaemia include:

- Hormonal: Suppressed insulin, and raised growth hormone (GH), glucagon and cortisol levels.
- Metabolic: Fat catabolism to produce ketones as an alternative metabolic fuel.

Causes

Inadequate responses to a drop in BP lead to hypoglycaemia. See Table 11.1 for causes of hypoglycaemia.

History

- Symptoms of hypoglycaemia
  - » Palpitations, tremor, anxiety, sweating, hunger, paraesthesia
  - » Severe hypoglycaemia: Lethargy, irritability, uncharacteristic behaviour, hypothermia, confusion, coma, seizures
  - » Neonate <48 hours: Apnoea, hypotonia, jitteriness, poor feeding, high pitched cry
- Past history
  - » Birth history (Birth weight, gestation, maternal gestational diabetes mellitus
  - » Neonatal history of hypoglycaemia
  - » Episodes suggestive of hypoglycaemia (undiagnosed seizure disorder)
  - » Previous gastric surgery, fundoplication (postprandial hypoglycaemia)
- Dietary history
  - » Milk products (galactosaemia)
  - » Fructose, e.g. juices (hereditary fructose intolerance)

Table 11.1 Causes of Hypoglycaemia

• Poor/low substrate: » Inadequate feeding » Gastrointestinal losses » Intrauterine growth restriction/ Prematurity/Donor twin » Thin child with poor glycogen stores	• Hyperinsulinaemic hypoglycaemia » Transient: Infant of diabetic mother, excessive maternal intravenous glucose, perinatal asphyxia » Congenital: ABCC8/NCNJ11/GCK » Islet cell adenoma » Beckwith–Wiedemann syndrome » Dumping syndrome
• Increased glucose utilisation: » Sepsis, shock, hypothermia, or asphyxia » Polycythaemia, hyperviscosity or fever	• Drug-induced » Sulphonylurea/insulin/beta-blocker/ salicylates/alcohol
• Inborn errors of metabolism » Defects in hepatic glycogen release/ storage (Glycogen storage disease) » Defects in gluconeogenesis » Carnitine metabolism » Fatty acid oxidation » Defects in ketone body synthesis/ utilisation » Others: Congenital disorder of glycosylation, organic acidaemias, hereditary fructose intolerance	• Accelerated starvation (also known as idiopathic ketotic hypoglycaemia) is a diagnosis of exclusion

   - » Protein (amino acid or organic acid disorders, hyperinsulinism-hyperammonaemia syndrome)
- Relationship to mealtime
   - » Short fast 2–3 hours: Glycogen storage disease
   - » Long fast 8–12 hours: Disorder of gluconeogenesis
   - » Postprandial: Dumping syndrome
- Intercurrent illness with poor feeding
- Increased glucose requirements, e.g. sepsis, trauma
- Suggestion of cortisol insufficiency (recurrent abdominal pain, anorexia, weight loss, poor growth)
- History of drug or toxin ingestion
- Family history
   - » Consanguinity
   - » Unexplained infant deaths (inborn errors of metabolism [IEM])
   - » Hormonal deficiencies and hyperinsulinism

Clinical Examination

- Macrosomia (Beckwith–Wiedemann syndrome)
- Dysmorphic features

- Features of endocrinopathy
  - » Hypopituitarism (midline defects, micropenis, undescended testes, growth failure)
  - » Skin hyperpigmentation (primary adrenal insufficiency)
  - » Ambiguous genitalia (congenital adrenal hyperplasia)
- Hepato- or hepatosplenomegaly and/or hypotonia (IEM)
- Blood pressure

Investigations

- Obtain blood and urine samples **at the time of hypoglycaemia** (critical sample) AND **before any glucose load is given** (if this is not possible, always treat the patient first and do not send any critical sample to the lab)
  - » Hormonal — Insulin, C-peptide, cortisol and GH
  - » Metabolic
    - ■ 1st line: Glucose, ketones, plasma acylcarnitine, free fatty acid, lactate
    - ■ 2nd line: Plasma ammonia, amino acid, urine organic acid
- Estimate the glucose utilisation needs from the intravenous (IV) glucose infusion rate:
  - » Glucose infusion rate >10 mg/kg/min is usually due to hyperinsulinism.
  - » Glucose infusion rate <10 mg/kg/min is due to other causes of hypoglycaemia.
- A fasting study that might induce hypoglycaemia (to be done under close medical supervision).
- Further tests may be needed to define:
  - » Hormonal abnormality
  - » Hepatic enzyme function

Table 11.2 Interpretation of Laboratory Results

High Ketones, High Free Fatty Acid, Acidaemia	Low Ketones, No Acidaemia	
	Low Free Fatty Acid	High Free Fatty Acid
• Ketotic hypoglycaemia • Disorder of gluconeogenesis (high lactate) • Glycogenoses • Cortisol/Growth hormone deficiencies	• Hyperinsulinism	• Fatty acid oxidation defects • Carnitine deficiency

Treatment

- Obtain critical samples before corrective measures (if possible).
- Aim to restore BG >3.5 mmol/L through normal nutritional intake.
- If asymptomatic, offer:
  - » Dose of Rapilose (Glucose 40% oral gel): Buccal 0.5 mg/kg
  - » Oral glucose 15 g or 150 ml juice

   - Followed by a carbohydrate serving
- If symptomatic, administer IV glucose:
   - Slow bolus 2 ml/kg of 10% dextrose over 2–5 min
   - Maintenance IV dextrose at 4–8 mg/kg/min
   - The rate must be adjusted to achieve and maintain BG >3.5 mmol/L
- Recheck BG 15–30 minutes after each corrective measure
- If hypoglycaemia recurs after Rapilose, give IV 10% dextrose bolus 2 ml/kg and commence IV dextrose drip.
- If hypoglycaemia recurs after IV dextrose bolus, repeat IV 10% dextrose bolus and increase the IV glucose infusion rate.
- For recalcitrant cases, refer to endocrine to consider the use of:
   - Intramuscular/IV/Subcutaneous glucagon 0.5 mg (<3 years old); 1 mg (> 3 years old).
   - Glucagon can be used as a continuous IV infusion at 5–20 μg/kg/h in severe ongoing hyperinsulinism
   - IV hydrocortisone 3–5 mg/kg/day
- Definitive therapy is based on specific aetiology of the hypoglycaemic disorder:
   - Nutritional therapy
   - Avoidance of prolonged fast
   - Hyperinsulinism:
      - Oral diazoxide 3–15 mg/kg/day Q6–12H
      - Chlorothiazide in conjunction with diazoxide
      - Somatostatins — Safety issues in its use
      - Total or sub-total pancreatectomy

Bibliography

1. Langdon DR. (2014) Hypoglycemia in the toddler and child. In: *Pediatric Endocrinology, 4th ed.*
2. Hussain K. (2011) Hypoglyceamia in infants and children. In: *Diagnostics of Endocrine Function in Children and Aolescents, 4th ed.*
3. Thornton PS, Stanley CA, De Leon DD, *et al.* (2015) Recommendations from the pediatric endocrine society for evaluation and management of persistent hypoglycemia in neonates, infants, and children. *J Pediatr* **167**(2):238–245.

CHAPTER 37

Hyperglycaemia

Aravind Venkatesh; Chan Wei Keong, Daniel; Chin Xinyi;
Lek Ngee; Rashida Farhad Vasanwala; Yap Kok Peng, Fabian

Introduction

Hyperglycaemia refers to high blood glucose (BG). In the fasted state, people without diabetes maintain BG level between 4 and 6 mmol/L. A person whose BG is consistently above 7mmol/L has hyperglycaemia. Symptoms of hyperglycaemia (increased passage of urine and thirst) may not be noticeable until BG levels remain consistently above 15 mmol/L. **Hyperglycaemia may be transient or persistent, asymptomatic or symptomatic. It may or may not indicate that the person has diabetes mellitus (DM).**

Causes

- DM
- Stress hyperglycaemia
  - » Febrile child
  - » Critically ill child
  - » Dehydrated child
- Medication induced, e.g. steroids
- Other endocrine cases
  - » Thyrotoxicosis
  - » Cushing syndrome/disease
  - » Phaeochromocytoma

Diabetes Mellitus

DM can present as early as the neonatal period. Neonatal DM can be temporary or permanent. In pre-pubertal patients, the most likely diagnosis is Type 1 DM associated with autoimmune destruction of pancreatic beta cells. In the pubertal and post-pubertal age group, both Type 1 and Type 2 DM, as well as Maturity Onset Diabetes in the Young (MODY) can occur. Both Type 1 and Type 2 patients can present with diabetic ketoacidosis (DKA). Antibody tests, presenting clinical features, insulin, C-peptide and family history may help differentiate the two.

Impaired Glucose Tolerance (IGT) and Type 2 DM may be asymptomatic. It should be looked for in a child who is overweight or obese, has a family history of DM or gestational diabetes, intrauterine growth restriction or is large for gestational age, acanthosis nigricans, hypertension for age and obstructive sleep apnoea. An oral glucose tolerance test (OGTT) may be useful.

Workup of a Child with Hyperglycaemia

- Determine the clinical context to identify if immediate action is needed.
- Take a complete history, focusing on the following and the timing of the events:
  - » Polyuria and thirst
  - » Weight loss and appetite
  - » Energy levels
  - » Nausea, vomiting and abdominal pain
- Examine for Kussmaul breathing (for clinical acidosis) and quantify the degree of dehydration.
- Determine the neurological state (which will be affected in more acidotic states).
- Check blood or urine for ketones.
- Check blood for urea, creatinine, glucose and electrolytes.
- Check the capillary blood gas.

Further Workup of a Child with Suspected Diabetes Mellitus

- Assess and investigate to classify the aetiology of diabetes.
  - » Take a full family history
    - Autoimmune conditions
    - Metabolic conditions
  - » Examine for signs of insulin resistance
    - Acanthosis nigricans (hyperinsulinism)
    - Skin tags (hyperinsulinism)
  - » Examine for autoimmune conditions
    - Goitre
    - Vitiligo
    - Mucocutaneous candidiasis
  - » Examine for features of metabolic syndrome
    - High Body Mass Index
    - Hypertension
    - Hirsutism in females
  - » Determine the pubertal stage
  - » Obtain blood samples for:
    - Glutamic acid decarboxylase (GAD) antibodies/islet cell antibodies (ICA)
    - Fasting glucose, fasting lipids, fasting insulin, C-peptide and HbA1c

Table 11.3 Practical Issues and Responses

Issue	Question/Action	Practice Points	
Diagnosis	Does the hyperglycaemic child have diabetes mellitus (DM)? Test • Fasting blood glucose (BG) • Oral glucose tolerance test (OGTT)	Existing diagnostic criteria for DM are: • Symptoms of diabetes AND • Random BG ≥11.1 mmol/L OR • Fasting BG ≥7.0 mmol/L (no caloric intake for at least 8 hr) OR • 2-hr post glucose load BG ≥11.1 mmol/L during an OGTT (glucose 1.75 g/kg body weight, max 75g) Asymptomatic or mildly symptomatic children with equivocal hyperglycaemia may have 'pre-diabetes' and need retesting on another day.	
Classification of diabetes	Does the hyperglycaemic child have insulin deficiency or resistance? Test • Fasting BG • Fasting lipids • Fasting insulin and C-peptide • Blood ketones • HbA1c • Glutamic acid decarboxylase antibodies • Islet cell antibodies	Type 1 diabetes mellitus (T1DM): • Diabetic ketoacidosis (DKA) at presentation is common • Family history (FH) of autoimmune conditions, including T1DM, thyroid disease, vitiligo and celiac disease • Immune- mediated (autoantibody positive)	Type 2 diabetes mellitus (T2DM): • DKA at presentation is uncommon • FH of obesity, T2DM, raised triglycerides and hypertension • Acanthosis nigricans • Autoantibody negative
		Classification may not be obvious. Early diagnosis of T1DM is mandatory as it may be life-saving. Refer suspected diabetes early, where possible on the same day.	
Therapy	How severe is the insulin deficiency?	See Table 11.4 for management of hyperglycaemia in children and adolescents.	

Management

The clinical presentation of a child with newly diagnosed or known to have diabetes depends on the degree of insulin deficiency and metabolic compensation.

Varying degrees of insulin deficiency are reflected by the insulin deficiency pyramid score (IDPS, 0 being the most severe) and corresponding symptoms and biochemical markers are mapped into the insulin deficiency pyramid (See Table 11.4). These indicators help define the clinical context and appropriate management.

Diabetic Ketoacidosis

DKA is the leading cause of morbidity and mortality in children and adolescents with Type 1 DM. DKA may also occur in patients with Type 2 DM.

Suspect DKA if:

- Dehydration
- Tachycardia
- Tachypnoea
- Deep sighing respiration
- Breath smells of acetone
- Nausea and/or vomiting
- Abdominal pain
- Blurry vision
- Confusion
- Drowsiness
- Decrease in the level of consciousness and eventually loss of consciousness

Criteria for DKA are:

- Hyperglycaemia (BG >11 mmol/L)
- Metabolic acidosis (pH <7.3, HCO_3 <15 mmol/L)
- Blood ketones >1.5 mmol/L or urine ketones 2+ and higher

Upon diagnosis, note the **goals, principles and complications of DKA treatment.** Then refer to Figure 11.1 for the workflow for the management of DKA.

Goals of treatment are:

- Correction of acidosis and reversal of ketosis
- Gradual, smooth correction of dehydration
- Restoration of BG to near normal
- Avoid complications of therapy (hypokalaemia)
- Identify and treat precipitating illness

Key principles of management are:

- To recognise differences in the severity of DKA
- Provide sufficient fluid correction based on severity of DKA
- To correct dehydration over 48–72 hours
- To maintain sufficient insulin dose (adding dextrose if needed) until acidosis (HCO_3 >15 mmol/L) is reversed
- To assess neurological and biochemical status frequently during insulin infusion

Complications of DKA are:

- Cerebral oedema
  - » Risk factors: Age <5 years, elevated serum urea, severe acidosis, severe hypocapnia

Table 11.4 Management of Hyperglycaemia in Children and Adolescents

Management of Hyperglycaemia in Children and Adolescents																			
1 Assess Symptoms Look/ask specifically for each of these symptoms									2 Assess Biochemistry Test blood ketones, renal panel and arterial blood gas in all children with high blood glucose							3 Establish the Clinical Context Determine the IDPS		4 Decide Appropriate Action Integrate context, implication and action needed	
Description	Reduced Sensorium	Kussmaul Breathing	Dehydration	Nausea, Abdominal Pain	Weight Loss	Increased Thirst	Increased Passing of Urine	Insulin Deficiency Pyramid Score (IDPS)	Raised Blood Glucose	Raised Blood Ketones	Low Bicarbonate	Raised Urea Creatinine	Low Corrected Sodium	Low Partial Pressure CO_2	pH <7				
	S	KB	D	NAP	Wt	Th	PU	Score	BG	BK	BC	UCr	Na	$PaCO_2$	pH		Implications	What's Needed	Action
High BG								10	↑BG							Asymptomatic high BG	May/may not be diabetes	Diagnostic testing	OGTT
							↑PU	9	↑BG							Symptomatic high BG	Meets criteria for diagnosis of diabetes; type is unclear Low risk of DKA, therefore insulin therapy not urgent	Classification Appropriate therapy	Early referral
						↑Th	↑PU	8	↑BG										
					↓Wt	↑Th	↑PU	7	↑BG										
Ketosis					↓Wt	↑Th	↑PU	6	↑BG	↑BK						Early decompensation	High risk of progression to DKA Urgent insulin Rx needed	Insulin	Consult Endocrine
				↑NAP	↓Wt	↑Th	↑PU	5	↑BG	↑BK									
Acidosis			D	↑NAP	↓Wt	↑Th	↑PU	4	↑BG	↑BK	↓BC					Early diabetic ketoacidosis (DKA)	Metabolic emergency!	Fluids Insulin	DKA workflow
			D	↑NAP	↓Wt	↑Th	↑PU	3	↑BG	↑BK	↓BC	↑UCr							
		KB	D	↑NAP	↓Wt	↑Th	↑PU	2	↑BG	↑BK	↓BC	↑UCr	↓Na			Moderate DKA			
	↓S	KB	D	↑NAP	↓Wt	↑Th	↑PU	1	↑BG	↑BK	↓BC	↑UCr	↓Na	↓$PaCO_2$		Severe DKA			
	↓S	KB	D	↑NAP	↓Wt	↑Th	↑PU	0	↑BG	↑BK	↓BC	↑UCr	↓Na	↓$PaCO_2$	pH <7				

- Hypokalaemia
- Hypoglycaemia
- Inadequate rehydration
- Venous thromboembolic disease

Practice Points

- **Inform the paediatric endocrinologist of all patients with DKA.**
- **Resuscitation**
  - » Bolus fluid as needed.
  - » All moderate to severe DKA patients should be kept 'nil by mouth'.
- **Fluid therapy**
  - » Hydrate intravenously over 48 hours.
  - » Correct for 5–10% dehydration (dehydration is rarely above 10%).
  - » For children and young people who are clinically dehydrated but not in shock:
    - ▪ Give an initial intravenous (IV) bolus of 10 ml/kg 0.9% normal saline over 30 minutes.
    - ▪ Only consider giving a second bolus after discussion with a senior if needed to improve tissue perfusion and only after reassessing their clinical status.
    - ▪ When calculating the total fluid replacements, subtract these initial bolus volumes from the total fluid deficit.
  - » For children and young people who have signs of shock (weak thread pulse, hypotension):
    - ▪ Give an initial IV bolus of 20 ml/kg 0.9% normal saline as soon as possible.
    - ▪ When calculating the total fluid requirement, do not subtract this fluid bolus from the total fluids.
  - » Use 0.9% NaCl as the initial fluid for the first 12 hours.
  - » Replace ongoing fluid losses such as vomiting or excess diuresis only if significant.
- **Ongoing fluid prescription**
  - » There is usually some deficit in body sodium (Na) and potassium at DKA presentation.
  - » Always determine corrected Na levels, as high glucose causes pseudohyponatraemia.
  - » Falling corrected serum Na during DKA therapy may indicate excessive rehydration.
  - » Rehydrate over 72 hours if corrected Na >150 mmol/L.
  - » After 12 hours, consider switching to 0.45% sodium chloride if plasma Na level is stable or increasing.
  - » Add 5% dextrose once glucose level falls below 14 mmol/L.
  - » If necessary, use 10% dextrose to maintain glucose between 5 and 11 mmol/L, until ketoacidosis resolves.

- **Insulin therapy**
  - » Start insulin therapy 1 hour after initiating fluid therapy.
  - » Prepare insulin infusion by adding 50 units (0.5 ml) of soluble insulin (Actrapid) to 49.5 ml of 0.9% normal saline in a 50 ml syringe pump to produce an insulin concentration of 1 units/ml.
  - » Commence insulin infusion at 0.1 units/kg/h; consider using 0.05 units/kg/h for children <5 years.
  - » Consider reducing to 0.05 units/kg/h if the rate of fall of BG exceeds 5 mmol/L per hour or when the acidosis is corrected (pH >7.3, HCO_3 >15 mmol/L).
  - » Mild DKA can be managed with subcutaneous (SC) insulin — please consult the paediatric endocrinologist.
- **Potassium replacement**
  - » If the patient is hypokalaemic at presentation, start potassium replacement at the time of initial volume expansion, before starting insulin therapy. Otherwise, start concurrent with insulin. If the patient is hyperkalaemic, defer potassium therapy until urine output is documented.
  - » Starting potassium concentration should be 40 mmol/L. Subsequently, base it on potassium measurements.
  - » Potassium phosphate may be used together with potassium chloride (half and half) as administration of potassium chloride alone contributes to the risk of hyperchloraemic metabolic acidosis. Do not use potassium phosphate alone as it may precipitate hypocalcaemia.
- **Acidosis and bicarbonate therapy**
  - » Adequate hydration and insulin therapy will reverse even severe acidosis.
  - » Bicarbonate therapy is rarely required and may increase risk of cerebral oedema.

Table 11.5 Important Formulae

	Formula/Fluid	Additional Instructions
Maintenance fluid	First 10 kg: 100 ml/kg; Next 10–20 kg: add 50 ml/kg; Above 20 kg: add 20 ml/kg	Males: max 2500 ml/day Females: max 2000 ml/day
Fluid requirement	48 hr' maintenance fluids + volume deficit	Give over 48 hr Give over 72 hr if corrected Na >150 mmol/L
Fluid deficit (ml)	% Dehydration x body weight (kg) x 1,000	5–7% if mild or moderate, 8–10% if severe
Initial fluid choice	0.9% NaCl with 20 mmol KCl to each bag of 500 ml	Given for at least 12 hr
Subsequent fluid	0.45% NaCl with 20 mmol KCl to each bag of 500 ml	
Corrected Na (mmol/L)	Measured Na + 0.4 (blood glucose - 5.5 mmol/L)	Estimate: add 1 mmol/L Na for every 3 mmol/L glucose >5.5 mmol/L

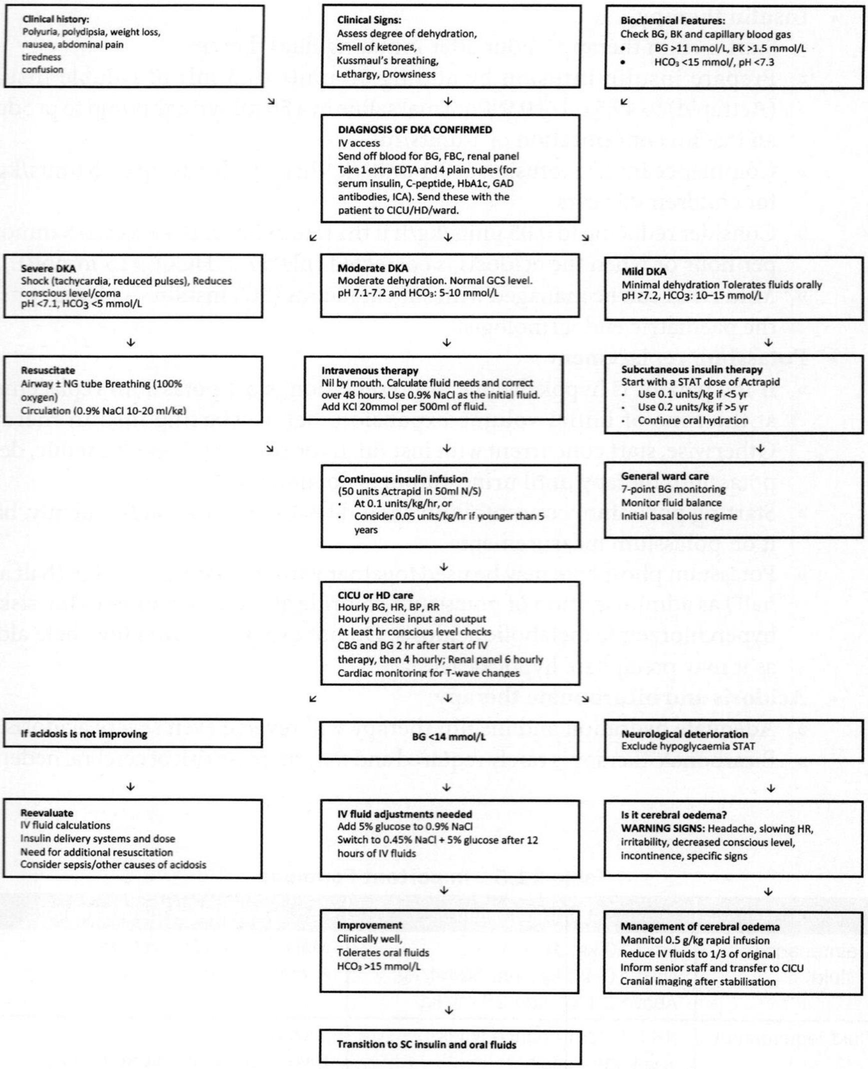

Figure 11.1 Workflow for the management of diabetic ketoacidosis.

BG: Blood glucose; FBC: Full blood count; BK: Blood ketone; BP: Blood pressure; CBG: Capillary blood gas; CICU: Children's Intensive Care Unit; GAD: glutamic acid decarboxylase; GCS: Glasgow Coma Scale; HD: High Dependency Unit; ICA: islet cell antibodies; IV: intravenous; HR: Heart rate; NG: Nasogastric; N/S: Normal saline; RR: Respiratory rate.

   - » Bicarbonate therapy should only be considered in the rare patient with life-threatening hyperkalaemia or to improve cardiac contractility in patients who are severely acidotic (arterial pH <6.9) with circulatory failure despite fluid replacement.
   - » **Bicarbonate should never be given without prior discussion with a senior doctor.**
- **Transition to SC insulin and oral fluids (this should be done after discussion with the paediatric endocrinologist)**
   - » Children with pH >7.3, HCO_3 >15 mmol/L and blood ketones <1 mmol/L can be transitioned to SC insulin if they are ready and able to eat and drink.
   - » 30 minutes after SC insulin is administered, stop IV insulin ± fluids.

Bibliography

1. International Society for Pediatric and Adolescent Diabetes. (2018) ISPAD clinical practice consensus guidelines 2018. https://www.ispad.org/page/ISPADGuidelines2018
2. National Institute for Health and Care Excellence. (2015) Guideline for Diabetes (type 1 and type 2) in children and young people: Diagnosis and management. https://www.nice.org.uk/guidance/ng18

CHAPTER 38

Normal Puberty and Disorders of Puberty

Aravind Venkatesh; Chan Wei Keong, Daniel; Chin Xinyi;
Lek Ngee; Rashida Farhad Vasanwala; Yap Kok Peng, Fabian

Introduction

Puberty is a process of physical transformation of the child into a sexually functional adult.

- Puberty is a **process**, meaning a series of related events and not a single event.
- The process is **sequential**, meaning there is an order to the process of normal puberty.
- There is **substantial variation** in the onset, tempo and hence duration of normal puberty.
- The **outcomes** of normal puberty are:
  - Attainment of adult height and reproductive competence.
- Disorders of puberty can therefore be categorised into:
  - Disorders of **timing** — Precocious or delayed onset of puberty.
  - Disorders of **tempo and duration** — Rapid or poor progress/arrest of puberty.
  - Disorders of **sequence** — Also known as pseudo-puberty.

Normal Female Puberty

The physical changes of normal female puberty are primarily the result of rising levels of ovarian oestrogen.

- Breast development is typically the first sign, which may begin as early as 7–8 years old or as late as 13 years old.
- Breast development is followed by height acceleration, change in body fat distribution and vaginal discharge.
- Vaginal discharge is initially random, then becomes cyclical and precedes menstruation.
- Menarche typically occurs 2–3 years after the onset of breast development.
- Menarche is the penultimate event of normal puberty.
- The final event of normal female puberty is epiphyseal fusion and commonly occurs 1–2 years after menarche.

The appearance of pubic and/or axillary hair is mediated by adrenal and ovarian androgens and is dependent on genetic factors, race, ethnicity as well as body fat mass. Sexual hair development typically occurs 1–1.5 years following onset of breast development.

Normal Male Puberty

The physical changes of normal male puberty are primarily the result of rising levels of testicular androgens.

- Testicular enlargement (≥4 ml) represents the onset of normal male puberty which may occur as early as 9 years old or as late as 14 years old.
- As the testicular volume increases, the scrotal skin becomes progressively thinner, the penile length and girth increase, the glans penis becomes obvious and pubic hair growth begins.
- Muscle mass acquisition is followed by height acceleration.
- Voice changes occur late as a result of chronic androgen stimulated changes to the voice box structure.

Like females, the appearance of pubic and/or axillary hair is variably influenced by genetic, race and ethnicity factors.

Adrenarche

Adrenarche is the onset of adrenal gland production of sex hormones, mainly adrenal androgens, responsible for the following changes in both sexes:

- Pubic hair
- Oily skin
- Oily hair
- Body odour

Premature adrenarche is when these changes begin early, i.e. before the age of 8 years for girls and 9 years for boys. While this may be physiological in some children, an evaluation should be done.

Hirsutism and Hypertrichosis

Hirsutism is the excessive growth of thick or dark hair in sex-hormone-dependent areas while **hypertrichosis** is the increase in hair growth anywhere on the body in males and females.

Table 11.6 Guidelines for Referral to a Paediatric Endocrinologist

Refer disorders of TIMING: • Girls with breast development before the age of 7 yr. • Girls with both breast development and pubic/axillary hair development before the age of 8 yr. • Girls with no evidence of breast development by the age of 13 yr. • Boys with testicular volumes of ≥4 ml before the age of 9 yr. • Boys with testicular volumes of ≤4 ml by the age of 14 yr. Note: Early normal puberty is not precocious puberty and care should be taken not to 'medicalise' an otherwise normal condition.
Refer disorders of SEQUENCE: • Girls with pubic/axillary hair development and no evidence of breast development. • Girls with vaginal discharge or menstruation and no evidence of breast development. • Boys with pubic/axillary hair development and testicular volumes of ≤4 ml. Note: Pseudo-precocious puberty may be pathological and needs to be evaluated.
Refer disorders of TEMPO: • Girls with breast development who fail to menstruate by the age of 15 yr. • Girls who start breast development when they are ≤120 cm tall. • Any child whose pubertal development fails to progress along the expected trajectory (pubertal arrest). Note: The duration from onset of breast development to menstruation is typically 2–3 yr.

Determining the Pubertal Stage

Pubertal stage is determined by a combination of visual inspection and palpation.

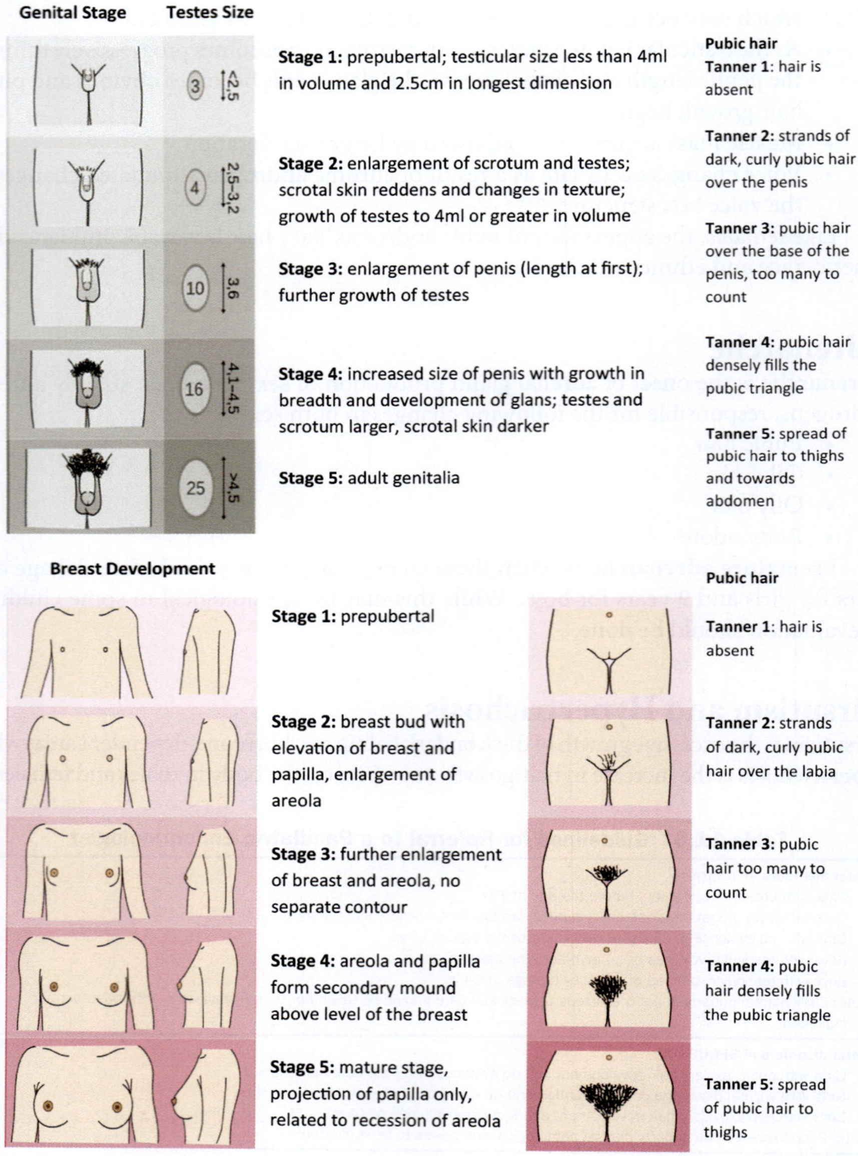

Figure 11.2 Pubertal development.

Bibliography

1. Bordini B, Rosenfield RL. (2011) Normal pubertal development: Part 1: the endocrine basis of puberty. *Pediatr Rev* **32**(6):223–229.
2. Bordini B, Rosenfield RL. (2011) Normal pubertal development: Part 2: clinical aspects of puberty. *Pediatr Rev* **32**(7):281–292.
3. Dorn LD, Biro FM. (2011) Puberty and it's measurement: A decade in review. *J Res Adolesc* **21**(1):180–195.

CHAPTER 39

Obesity

Chin Xinyi; Chew Chu Shan, Elaine; Chan Wei Keong, Daniel; Aravind Venkatesh; Lek Ngee; Rashida Farhad Vasanwala; Yap Kok Peng, Fabian

Introduction

Obesity has become a worldwide epidemic resulting in significant health problems and costs, for both the individual and the society. Childhood obesity tends to track into adulthood and is an early risk factor for adult morbidity and mortality. As such, the prevention and treatment of obesity should be a paediatric goal.

Definition

Obesity refers to having excess body fat and is commonly defined in terms of Body Mass Index (BMI) >97th percentile for age and gender. Increased morbidity and mortality associated with obesity can vary for different racial, ethnic and socioeconomic groups, as well as between individuals. Children with BMIs in the 90–97th percentile can also be at risk of developing obesity-related morbidities.

Pathogenesis and Aetiology

The pathogenesis of obesity is often multi-factorial — genetic, biological, psychological, sociocultural, and environmental (intra- and extra-uterine) — and affects both ends of the energy balance equation. See Table 11.7 for some causes of obesity.

Workup

History

- Birth and antenatal history, including birth weight, presence of maternal gestational diabetes
- Previous growth/weights (in particular the onset of weight gain)
- Detailed dietary intake
- Physical activity, screen time
- Symptoms suggestive of secondary causes of obesity (see Table 11.7)
- Symptoms suggestive of co-morbidities (see Table 11.8)

Table 11.7 Causes of Childhood Obesity

Primary Obesity • Exogenous Obesity	**Central Nervous System (CNS) Disorders** • Hypothalamic tumours • Infection, inflammation, ischaemia • Previous CNS surgery
Endocrine Disorders • Cushing Syndrome • Hypothyroidism • Growth Hormone deficiency • Hyperinsulinaemia	**Miscellaneous** • Drugs (e.g. Risperidone, tricyclic antidepressants, corticosteroids)
Genetic Syndromes • Prader–Willi Syndrome • Bardet–Biedl Syndrome • Down Syndrome • Pseudohypoparathyroidism • Klinefelter Syndrome • Alstrom Syndrome	**Monogenic (Rare)** • Mutations in: » Leptin » Leptin receptor » Pro-opiomelanocortin (POMC) » Prohormone convertase 1 » Melanocortin receptor (MC4R and MC3R)

Table 11.8 Co-morbidities and Complications of Obesity

Cardiovascular • Dyslipidaemia • Hypertension • Arteriosclerosis	**Neurological** • Pseudotumour cerebri
Endocrine • Insulin resistance, hyperinsulinism • Impaired glucose tolerance • Type 2 Diabetes Mellitus • Polycystic ovary syndrome, absent/ irregular menses	**Orthopaedic** • Blount disease • Slipped upper femoral epiphysis • Spondylolisthesis • Long-term osteoarthritis
Respiratory • Obstructive sleep apnea • Pickwickian syndrome • Restrictive lung disease • Asthma	**Gastrointestinal** • Gallbladder disease • Non-alcoholic fatty liver disease • Gastroesophageal reflux
Dermatology • Skin tags • Acanthosis nigricans	**Psychological** • Depression • Disordered eating • Low self-esteem • Poor quality of life

- Drug history, e.g. steroids, herbal supplements, traditional cures
- Family history of obesity ± co-morbidities
- Social history including assessment of caregivers' involvement in daily routine, i.e. meals, physical activity

- Psychosocial history, including issues of self-esteem, depression, risk for disordered eating

Clinical Examination

- Accurate height and weight, calculate BMI
- Growth charts:
  - » Children with exogenous obesity from over-nutrition are usually tall for age with good growth velocity.
  - » Children with underlying pathology tend to be short for age with poor growth velocity.
  - » Reducing height velocity associated with increasing weight is suggestive of an endocrine cause.
- Pattern of obesity: Central or generalised
- Dysmorphic features
- Signs of endocrinopathy: Cushingoid features, i.e. moon face, acne, hirsutism, truncal obesity, violaceous striae and hypertension.
- Signs of hypothyroidism
- Pubertal assessment
  - » Hypogonadism may suggest a syndromic cause, e.g. Prader–Willi syndrome (PWS), Bardet–Biedl syndrome, Alstrom syndrome
- Acanthosis nigricans, skin tags
- Blood pressure
- Assessment of other complications of obesity as guided by clinical history

Investigations

- To identify:
  - » Causes of obesity
  - » Consequences arising from obesity
- Based on clinical assessment, investigations may include:
  - » Liver function test
  - » Thyroid function test
  - » Lipid profile
  - » Fasting glucose, insulin and oral glucose tolerance test
  - » LH, FSH, oestradiol, androgens, sex hormone binding globulin (if suspicious for polycystic ovary syndrome)
  - » Serum cortisol levels (if suspicious for Cushing syndrome)
  - » Genetic testing

Management

Children with lower degree of obesity and without any obesity-related complications can be managed in a primary care setting. Emphasis is placed on age-appropriate gradual weight loss and/or weight maintenance.

Management of children on exogenous obesity include:

- Dietary intervention

- Physical activity intervention
- Family intervention
- Assessment for complications and co-morbidities
- Regular follow-up with the primary care team

Referral Guidelines

- Guidelines for referral to the Weight Management Clinic in our institution:
  - » Patients older than 6 years (i.e. primary school age and above) who are:
    - BMI >97th percentile
    - BMI >90th percentile AND have the following co-morbidities: Obstructive sleep apnoea and hypopnoea syndrome, Type 2 Diabetes mellitus, essential hypertension, hypercholesterolaemia
- Guidelines for referral to a paediatric endocrinologist:
  - » Obesity with an early onset younger than 6 years.
  - » Obesity with short stature

Bibliography

1. Schneider MB, Brill SR. (2005) Obesity in children and adolescents. *Pediatr Rev* **26**(5):155–162.
2. National Institute for Health and Clinical Excellence (2014) Obesity: The prevention, identification, assessment and management. https://www.nice.org.uk/guidance/cg189
3. Kipping RR, Jago R, Lawlor DA. (2008) Obesity in children. Part 2: Prevention and management. *BMJ* **337**:a1848.
4. Health Promotion Board and Ministry of Health Singapore. (2016) HPB-MOH clinical practice guidelines 1. https://www.moh.gov.sg/docs/librariesprovider4/guidelines/obesity-cpg_summary.pdf

CHAPTER 40

Thyroid Disorders

Chan Wei Keong, Daniel; Chin Xinyi; Aravind Venkatesh; Lek Ngee;
Rashida Farhad Vasanwala; Yap Kok Peng, Fabian

Hyperthyroidism in Children

Hyperthyroidism refers to thyroid gland overactivity leading to excess thyroid hormone synthesis. The most common cause of thyrotoxicosis in childhood is Graves' Disease.

Clinical Features

- **Suspect hyperthyroidism** when the patient reports clusters of the following:
  - Palpitations
  - Difficulty in sleeping
  - Heat intolerance
  - Muscle fatigue
  - Unintentional weight loss or difficulty gaining weight, despite increased food intake
  - Restlessness/emotional lability
    - There may be feedback about a child having poor concentration and a deterioration in school performance.
  - Increased bowel motility/frequency — diarrhoea

Clinical Examination

- Examine for clinical signs of:
  - **Goitre**
    - Usually smooth, symmetrical and diffuse
    - A bruit may be found on auscultation of the thyroid gland.
  - **Signs of excessive sympathetic activity**
    - Sweaty palms
    - Fine hand tremors
    - Tachycardia with increased pulse volume indicative of a hyperdynamic circulation. An irregularly irregular pulse may be present if complicated by atrial fibrillation (rare in children).
    - Hyperreflexia
    - Proximal muscle weakness

» **Eye signs and other autoimmune features**
  - Proptosis, lid lag and exophthalmos may be present, which is associated with Graves' disease. This may be complicated by exposure keratopathy.
  - Vitiligo

Investigations

- Send blood investigations for:
  - » Free thyroxine (fT4)
  - » Thyroid stimulating hormone (TSH)
  - » Thyroid antibodies (usually thyroid receptor antibodies [TrAb] and thyroid peroxidase antibodies [TPOAb])
- Further evaluation may include:
  - » Thyroid ultrasound (US)
  - » Random blood glucose level

Management

- Refer early to a paediatric endocrinologist for further evaluation and management, especially in severe thyrotoxicosis, which can cause life-threatening thyrotoxic crisis or thyroid storm.
- Consult a paediatric ophthalmologist if eye signs are severe on clinical examination.
- Therapy:
  - » **Reduce thyroid hormone synthesis** — Anti-thyroid drug (ATD) treatment with carbimazole is a common first-line treatment. The recommended starting dose for carbimazole is 0.5–1 mg/kg/day in two divided doses. Inform patients of uncommon but potentially serious side effects of ATDs, including agranulocytosis, skin rashes, arthralgia and hepatotoxicity.
  - » **Control the symptoms of sympathetic overdrive** — Beta-blockers (propranolol) are often used as an adjunct to treatment in the first few weeks for symptom control. The recommended starting dose for propranolol is 0.5–1 mg/kg/day in two divided doses.
  - » **Consider alternative therapy** for patients who relapse or are refractory to first-line therapy with ATDs. Alternative modalities such as radioactive iodine or thyroidectomy may be offered.

Acquired Hypothyroidism in Children

Hypothyroidism can result in significant detrimental effects on the child's health, growth and development. Hence, prompt diagnosis and treatment are important for improved outcomes.

Clinical Features

- **Suspect hypothyroidism** when the patient reports clusters of the following:
  - » Lethargy, low energy levels

    - This can adversely affect a child's school work and academic performance.
  - Cold intolerance
  - Constipation
  - Muscle ache and pains
  - Faltering height growth — may present with short stature due to delay in skeletal maturation.
  - Dry skin
  - Neurological symptoms or manifestations of other pituitary hormone deficiencies may be present in a patient with central hypothyroidism.

Clinical Examination

- Examine for clinical signs of:
  - Bradycardia
  - Goitre
  - Myxoedema
  - Slow relaxing deep tendon reflexes
  - Hair loss and thinning may be noted
  - Patients may appear apparently obese/overweight due to reduced metabolic rate and faltering height.
  - Pericardial/pleural effusions may be present in severe presentations.

Investigations

- **Avoid ordering thyroid function test (TFT) for patients who have been acutely unwell/ill**, as an abnormal thyroid function test may reflect non-thyroidal illness syndrome (NTIS) (previously also known as 'sick euthyroid syndrome'). If in doubt, consult a paediatric endocrinologist before ordering.
- **Always interpret TFT in the clinical context** to determine if hypothyroidism is central (rarely)/primary in origin (much more common):
  - Low fT4, raised TSH: Suggests primary hypothyroidism.
  - Low fT4, low TSH: Suggests central hypothyroidism.
  - Low fT4, normal TSH: May be central hypothyroidism. Consult endocrine.
  - Normal fT4, raised TSH: Suggests subclinical hypothyroidism.
- **Further evaluation** for primary hypothyroidism includes:
  - TPOAb is associated with Hashimoto's thyroiditis, a common cause of autoimmune hypothyroidism.
  - Thyroid US looking for signs of thyroiditis
- **Further evaluation** for central hypothyroidism includes:
  - Testing for deficiencies in other pituitary hormones
  - Performing Magnetic Resonance Imaging of the pituitary gland, if indicated

Management

- **Start levothyroxine (LT4) replacement** for patients diagnosed with hypothyroidism. Treatment may be lifelong, and regular follow-up of growth and dose adjustment is required.

- Patients with Hashimoto's thyroiditis may have a transient hyperthyroid phase or Hashitoxicosis. They may require treatment as per hyperthyroidism during this period. However, with time, the child is likely to develop hypothyroidism and require LT4 replacement accordingly.

Hypothyroidism in Newborn

Ensure that all newborn babies are screened for congenital hypothyroidism.

A newborn baby can still have congenital hypothyroidism even if the screening result is normal. **Early recognition** is critical and **timely treatment** must be instituted to reduce the risk of developing neurodevelopmental delay.

Clinical Features

- Ask for history of:
  - » Poor feeding
  - » Lethargy
  - » Detailed birth history, including cord TSH, neonatal jaundice requiring phototherapy
  - » Family history of thyroid disorders, including maternal history of hyperthyroidism requiring ATDs

Clinical Examination

- Examine for signs of:
  - » Coarse facies
  - » Protruding tongue
  - » Jaundice
  - » Abdominal distension
  - » Umbilical hernia
  - » Goitre
  - » Lingual thyroid

Investigations

- **Suspect congenital hypothyroidism if** screening cord TSH >20 mIU/L.
- **Confirm congenital hypothyroidism by** obtaining venous blood samples for TFT (fT4/TSH) after 72 hours of life (Day 4) if the baby has an abnormal cord TSH.
- **Perform imaging**, with either a thyroid US or scintigraphy using Technetium (^{99m}Tc). However, imaging should never be allowed to delay the initiation of treatment.

Management

- **Commence LT4 replacement** as soon as the diagnosis is confirmed, ideally within 2 weeks after birth. Aim to normalise TSH levels within 2 weeks after initiation of treatment.

- Follow-up and monitor closely, with regular TFTs and assessment of the child's growth and developmental milestones. The physician who follows up the baby through childhood and adolescence must be adequately trained and experienced in the management of patients with congenital hypothyroidism.

Bibliography

1. van Trotsenburg P, Stoupa A, Léger J, *et al.* (2021) Congenital hypothyroidism: A 2020–2021 consensus guidelines update-an ENDO-European reference network initiative endorsed by the European Society for Pediatric Endocrinology and the European Society for Endocrinology. *Thyroid* **31**(3):387–419.
2. Bauer AJ, Wassner AJ. (2019) Thyroid hormone therapy in congenital hypothyroidism and pediatric hypothyroidism. *Endocrine* **66**(1):51–62.
3. Wassner AJ. (2017) Pediatric hypothyroidism: Diagnosis and treatment. *Paediatr Drugs* **19**(4):291–301.
4. Hanley P, Lord K, Bauer AJ. (2016) Thyroid disorders in children and adolescents: A review. *JAMA Pediatr* **170**(10):1008–1019.
5. Srinivasan S, Misra M. (2015). Hyperthyroidism in children. *Pediatr Rev* **36**(6):239–248.
6. Kaplowitz PB, Vaidyanathan P. (2020) Update on pediatric hyperthyroidism. *Curr Opin Endocrinol Diabetes Obes* **27**(1):70–76.

CHAPTER 41

Disorders of Calcium Metabolism

Chan Wei Keong, Daniel; Chin Xinyi; Aravind Venkatesh; Lek Ngee; Rashida Farhad Vasanwala; Yap Kok Peng, Fabian

Introduction

Normal reference ranges for serum calcium levels are adjusted according to age and corrected according to serum albumin levels.

$$\text{Adjusted Calcium} = \text{Total Calcium} + 0.02\,(40 - [\text{Alb}])$$

[Alb] : Plasma albumin in g/L

The total adjusted serum calcium levels normally range between 2.3 and 2.6 mmol/L. When the pH is 7.35–7.45, ionised calcium constitutes approximately 50% of the total calcium and is normally maintained between 1.1 and 1.3 mmol/L. The threshold for parathyroid hormone (PTH) secretion is when ionic calcium starts falling below 1.0 mmol/L.

Hypocalcaemia

The patient with hypocalcaemia usually remains asymptomatic unless plasma concentrations of ionised calcium fall below 1.0 mmol/L and drop rapidly.

Causes

Neonatal Hypocalcaemia

- Maternal factors (vitamin D deficiency, hyperparathyroidism, pre-eclampsia, diabetes — pre-existing or gestational)
- Placental factors (placental insufficiency, calcium transporter defects)
- Neonatal factors (low birth weight, prematurity, perinatal hypoxia, intrauterine growth restriction/small for gestational age, neonatal sepsis or stress)
- High phosphate load — from total parental nutrition or high phosphate milk formula
- Inadequate calcium supply — oral or parenteral
- Hypoparathyroidism — transient versus permanent

Hypocalcaemia with Low PTH

- Abnormal parathyroid gland development or defects in PTH synthesis (e.g. DiGeorge syndrome, autosomal recessive hypoparathyroidism, HDR [hypoparathyroidism, sensorineural deafness and renal disease] syndrome)

- Postsurgical, radiation, infiltrative process of the parathyroid gland
- Hypomagnesaemia

Hypocalcaemia with Inappropriately Normal PTH

- Abnormal calcium sensing receptor, e.g. Familial hypercalciuric hypocalcaemia
- Familial hypocalcaemia (Autosomal-dominant)
- Hypoparathyroidism is also a consideration (causes as per 'Hypocalcaemia with low PTH')

Hypocalcaemia with High PTH

- Vitamin D related
  - » Vitamin D deficiency — dietary insufficiency, poor intestinal absorption, inadequate sun exposure
  - » Vitamin D metabolism defects — vitamin D dependent rickets, liver/renal dysfunction, vitamin D resistance
- Increased calcium consumption — tumour lysis syndrome, pancreatitis, hungry bone syndrome, intravenous (IV) infusions containing citrate (some forms of continuous renal replacement therapies, massive blood transfusions)
- End-organ resistance to PTH — pseudohypoparathyroidism

Clinical Features

- Muscle cramps and twitching
- Carpopedal spasms
- Seizures — which can be focal or generalised
- In neonates/infants, they can present with non-specific symptoms like apnoea and/or stridor
- Chronic untreated hypocalcaemia can result in cardiomyopathy (especially from vitamin D deficiency)

Clinical Examination

- Chvostek sign (twitching of the ipsilateral facial muscles on tapping on the face, just below the zygomatic bone)
- Trousseau sign (trigger of a carpopedal spasm from inflation of the blood pressure cuff)
- Dysmorphic features if hypocalcaemia is related to underlying genetic condition, such as DiGeorge syndrome, pseudohypoparathyroidism

First-Line Investigations

- Point of care tests — Electrocardiogram (ECG) to look for prolonged QT interval, blood gas to look for ionic calcium levels and alkalosis.
- Critical samples should include:
  - » Renal panel

  - » Total adjusted serum calcium
  - » Serum magnesium
  - » Serum phosphate
  - » Serum Alkaline phosphatase
  - » Serum intact PTH
  - » Serum 25-hydroxyvitamin D
  - » Urine calcium, magnesium, phosphate and creatinine levels
  - » Urinary calcium/creatinine ratio
- Blood and urine samples should always be **paired**, and whenever possible, taken before administering any treatment.

Management

Acutely Symptomatic Patients

- To obtain critical samples and correct with IV 10% calcium gluconate 0.5 ml/kg over 10 minutes diluted with saline. Treatment of the patient must **never** be delayed in order to collect the samples.
  Note: Ensure good venous access
  This must be followed by calcium replacement either enterally or parenterally, providing 50–70 mg/kg/day of elemental calcium (monitor IV site closely for tissue necrosis).
  Note: Calcium Gluconate 1 ml = 9 mg elemental calcium.
- In persistent symptomatic hypocalcaemia, calcitriol can be used to normalise calcium levels faster in addition to oral or parenteral calcium replacement.
  Note: Calcitriol is available as oral capsules 0.25 mcg or 0.5 mcg.
- It is important to correct low serum magnesium as well, if present.

Asymptomatic Patients and Post-Correction of Symptomatic Hypocalcaemia

- Treatment depends on the underlying aetiology:
  - » Vitamin D supplementation: Cholecalciferol (D3), Alfacalcidol (1α Vitamin D3), or Calcitriol (1,25 Vitamin D3), depending on the aetiology of hypocalcaemia
  - » Calcium supplementation: Oral (PO) Calcium Lactogluconate, PO Calcium Carbonate. Starting elemental dose of calcium ranges from 50 to 70 mg/kg/day.
  - » *Note: Different calcium preparations have varied content of elemental calcium, please check with pharmacist before prescribing.*

After achieving normocalcaemia, it is important for patients on long-term calcium and vitamin D replacement to be monitored for iatrogenic hypercalcaemia, hypercalciuria, nephrocalcinosis and renal insufficiency.

Table 11.9 Calcium and Phosphate Preparations

Calcium Preparations	Content	Amount	Elemental Calcium (mg)	Elemental Calcium (mmol)
Injections				
Calcium Chloride 10% (6.8 mmol/10 ml) Injection	Calcium chloride	6.8 mmol/10 ml 1000 mg/10 ml	27 mg/ml	0.68 mmol/ml
Calcium Gluconate 10% (2.25 mmol/10 ml) Injection	Calcium gluconate	940 mg/10 ml	9 mg/ml	0.23 mmol/ml
Oral Tablets				
Calcium 600 mg (Caltrate®) (Calcium Carbonate 1.5 g) Tablet	Calcium carbonate	1.5 g	600 mg/ tablet	15 mmol/ tablet
Calcium Acetate 667 mg Tablet	Calcium acetate	667 mg	167 mg/ tablet	4.2 mmol/ tablet
Calcium Carbonate 623 mg Tablet	Calcium carbonate	625 mg	250 mg/ tablet	6.3 mmol/ tablet
Calcium Carbonate 450 mg, Vitamin D 200 Units Tablet	Calcium carbonate Vitamin D_3	450 mg 200 IU	180 mg/ tablet	4.5 mmol/ tablet
Oral Suspension/Syrup				
Lactogluconate Syrup	Calcium Lactogluconate	300 mg/15 ml	20 mg/ml	0.5 mmol/ ml
Phosphate Preparations	**Content**	**Amount**	**Elemental Phosphorus (mg)**	**Elemental Phosphate (mmol)**
Injections (can also be given orally)				
Potassium Dihydrogen Phosphate 10 mmol/10 ml Injection	Potassium (K^+) Phosphate	10 mmol/10 ml 10 mmol/10 ml	31 mg/ml	1 mmol/ml
Sodium Glycerophosphate (Phosphate 20 mmol/20 ml) Injection	Sodium (Na^+) Phosphate	40 mmol/20 ml 20 mmol/20 ml	31 mg/ml	1 mmol/ml
Oral Tablets				
Phosphorus 500mg Effervescent Tablet	<u>Per tablet contains</u>: Phosphate Potassium Sodium	 16.1 mmol 3.1 mmol 20.4 mmol	500 mg/ tablet	16.1 mmol/ tablet

Table 11.9 (*Continued*)

Phosphate Preparations	Content	Amount	Elemental Phosphorus (mg)	Elemental Phosphate (mmol)
Oral Suspension/Syrup				
Fleet/Phospho-soda oral solution (45 ml) *As phosphate replacement, requires 1:10 dilution with water before administering	Per ml contains: Phosphate Sodium	 4.15 mmol 4.82 mmol	128.7 mg/ml	4.15 mmol/ml
Sodium Phosphate (Phosphate 0.52 mmol/ml) solution	Per ml contains: Phosphate Sodium	 0.52 mmol 0.85 mmol	16.1 mg/ml	0.52 mmol/ml

Note: Approximate percentages of elemental calcium are as follows:
a. Calcium acetate (25%)
b. Calcium carbonate (40%)
c. Calcium chloride (27.3%)
d. Calcium citrate (21%)
e. Calcium glubionate (6.5%)
f. Calcium gluconate (9%)
g. Calcium glycerophosphate (19%)
h. Calcium hypophosphite (23.6%)
i. Calcium lactate (13%)
j. Calcium pantothenate (8.4%)
k. Calcium phosphate, dibasic (23%)
l. Calcium phosphate, tribasic (38%)

Hypercalcaemia

Patients with mild hypercalcaemia are usually asymptomatic. However, as adjusted calcium concentrations rise above 3.0 mmol/L, they may start experiencing symptoms of hypercalcemia.

Mechanisms of Hypercalcaemia

- Increased PTH secretion (inappropriate for the serum calcium levels)
- Increased 1,25(OH)$_2$ Vitamin D$_3$ synthesis
- Increased bone resorption
- Abnormal set point of Calcium Sensing Receptor
- Increased PTH-related peptide secretion

Causes of Childhood Hypercalcaemia

- Primary and tertiary hyperparathyroidism
- Familial benign hypercalcaemia
- Williams Syndrome
- Idiopathic infantile hypercalcaemia
- Vitamin D toxicity
- Hypercalcaemia of malignancy
- Immobilisation
- Granulomatous disorders
- Subcutaneous fat necrosis

Clinical Features

'Painful bones, renal stones, abdominal groans, psychic moans'

- Vomiting, constipation
- Failure to thrive
- Muscle hypotonia, lethargy
- Loss of appetite
- Abdominal pain
- Polyuria, polydipsia, dehydration
- If complicated by nephrolithiasis/nephrocalcinosis, patient may experience dysuria, haematuria and other lower urinary tract symptoms.
- Neuropsychiatric disturbances — altered mental state, confusion.

Clinical Examination

- Hypotension, arrhythmia, shortened QT interval
- Confused state, abnormal Glasgow Coma Scale (GCS)
- Hypotonia, hyporeflexia
- Dry mucous membranes, reduced skin turgor, cool peripheries
- Abdominal tenderness, if complicated by pancreatitis, peptic ulcer disease
- Abdominal masses, organomegaly or lymphadenopathy may be present if there is underlying malignancy
- A neck nodule may be present if hypercalcemia is due to a parathyroid adenoma
- Dysmorphic features if related to underlying genetic syndrome, such as Williams syndrome.

First-Line Investigations

- ECG to look for shortened QT interval
- Adjusted serum calcium
- Serum magnesium
- Serum phosphate
- Serum alkaline phosphatase
- Serum intact PTH
- Serum 25-hydroxyvitamin D
- Paired urine calcium, magnesium, phosphate and creatinine levels
- Urinary calcium/creatinine ratio
- Renal ultrasound — to look for nephrocalcinosis, nephrolithiasis, especially in long-standing hypercalcaemia

Follow-Up Investigations

- Hand X-ray for phalangeal erosions
- Serum calcium of parents
- Sestamibi scan/neck ultrasound
- Search for malignancy, e.g. bone marrow aspirate
- Genetic analysis for MEN 1

Management

- Management involves treating the underlying aetiology.
- A symptomatic patient with total serum calcium level more than 3 mmol/L with an increasing trend should be initiated with hyperhydration, at 1.5 to 2 times the daily maintenance fluid requirement. Fluid balance must be strictly monitored, and forced diuresis with a loop diuretic (frusemide) must be judiciously instituted as necessary.
- Renal function must be monitored as there is potential risk of acute renal failure.
- Most patients should respond to hyperhydration and forced diuresis; consult a paediatric endocrinologist for other therapeutic options such as:
  - Bisphosphonates
  - Calcitonin
  - Steroids

Bibliography

1. Stokes VJ, Nielsen MF, Hannan FM, Thakker RV. (2017) Hypercalcemic disorders in children. *J Bone Miner Res* **32**(11):2157–2170.
2. Lietman SA, Germain-Lee EL, Levine MA. (2010) Hypercalcemia in children and adolescents. *Curr Opin Pediatr* **22**(4):508–515.
3. Dawrant J, Pacaud D. (2007) Pediatric hypocalcemia: Making the diagnosis. *CMAJ* **177**(12):1494–1497.
4. Davies JH, Shaw NJ. (2012) Investigation and management of hypercalcaemia in children. *Arch Dis Child* **97**(6):533–538.
5. Zhou P, Markowitz M. (2009) Hypocalcemia in infants and children. *Pediatr Rev* **30**(5):190–192.
6. Vuralli D. (2019) Clinical approach to hypocalcemia in newborn period and infancy: Who should be treated? *Int J Pediatr* **9**:4318075.
7. Allgrove J, Cheung M. (2019) The parathyroid and disorders of calcium and bone metabolism. In: Dattani MT, Brook CG (eds.) *Brook's Clinical Pediatric Endocrinology, 7th ed.* Wiley-Blackwell, pp. 409–479.

CHAPTER 42

Diabetes Insipidus

Chan Wei Keong, Daniel; Chin Xinyi; Aravind Venkatesh; Lek Ngee;
Rashida Farhad Vasanwala; Yap Kok Peng, Fabian

Introduction

Diabetes insipidus (DI) is characterised by primary polyuria due to the lack of anti-diuretic hormone (ADH) or ADH action.

- Polyuria must first be objectively assessed by means of strict intake/output charting.
- Polyuria refers to urine output in excess of 4–5 ml/kg/h (up to 6 ml/kg/h for neonates at birth).

Note that urinary frequency, incontinence and enuresis must be distinguished from polyuria:

- *Urinary frequency* refers to the increased occurrence of usually voluntary episodes of micturition compared to normal; however, it may be either large or small volumes of urine each time. Hence, frequency does not equate a polyuric state.
- *Incontinence* refers to the inability to retain urine voluntarily, leading to leakage of urine. It may be mistaken for increased urinary frequency.
- *Enuresis* refers to involuntary episodes of micturition in children older than 6 years , leading to bedwetting.

Table 11.10 Causes of Diabetes Insipidus

Type	Cranial Diabetes Insipidus	Nephrogenic Diabetes Insipidus
Familial	• Familial Neurohypophyseal Diabetes Insipidus (FNDI) — Autosomal Dominant • DIDMOAD or Wolfram syndrome	• X-linked Nephrogenic Diabetes Insipidus • Autosomal recessive Nephrogenic Diabetes Insipidus
Acquired	• Trauma (head injury, neurosurgery) • Tumours (craniopharyngioma, germinoma, glioma) • Infections (meningoencephalitis, congenital CMV/toxoplasmosis) • Granulomatous disease (tuberculosis, sarcoidosis, histiocytosis) • Hypoxic brain injury • Vascular malformations	• Chronic renal disease • Post-obstructive uropathy • Osmotic diuresis » Glucose (Diabetes mellitus) » Calcium (Hypercalcaemia) » Mannitol (Drug induced)

CMV: cytomegalovirus; DIDMOAD: diabetes insipidus, diabetes mellitus, optic atrophy and deafness.

Clinical Approach

An accurate history is crucial to differentiate polyuria (increase in frequency and volume), from frequent urination and to exclude other reasons, such as:

- Primary polydipsia/excessive water intake causing secondary polyuria
- Primary monosymptomatic nocturnal enuresis
- Urological issues like overactive bladder, detrusor instability
- Renal pathologies like urinary tract infections, tubulopathies
- Spinal pathologies
- Diabetes mellitus

Basic Investigations for Frequent Urination

- Basic investigations for all children with frequent micturition includes:
  - » Renal panel
  - » Urinalysis (especially specific gravity, glucose)
  - » Urine culture
  - » Urine calcium/creatinine ratio
- If DI is suspected, include **paired** samples for:
  - » Urine osmolality
  - » Serum osmolality
- Based on the clinical presentation, a water-deprivation test (with Desmopressin [DDAVP] trial) may be required in equivocal cases.

Diagnosis of Diabetes Insipidus

- Polyuria (exclude urinary frequency, incontinence and enuresis)
- The consequences of polyuria secondary to DI include:
  - » Excessive thirst
  - » Weight loss
  - » Headache due to dehydration and hypernatremia
- In an appropriate clinical setting, we can usually diagnose DI if there is polyuria for 2 or more consecutive hours, with:
  - » Urine-specific gravity <1.005 and/or urine osmolality <300 mOsm/kg H_2O (before hydration), AND
  - » Elevated serum sodium >145 mmol/L, AND
  - » Serum osmolality nears or exceeds 300 mOsm/kg.
- Note that serum sodium and osmolality may also be within normal ranges if child has an intact thirst mechanism and is allowed free access to fluids.
- In established clinical DI in the absence of renal pathology, Magnetic Resonance Imaging (MRI) of the pituitary gland will be needed to evaluate the hypothalamic-pituitary region for any pathologies, including a space-occupying lesion or congenital anomaly. Evaluation of the other pituitary hormone axes is also required. Absence of a normally placed bright spot in the posterior pituitary on T1-weighted MRI scan is highly suggestive of central DI.

- If further assessment with a water deprivation test is required, consult with a paediatric endocrinologist.

Overnight Water Restriction under Monitoring

(*Note: This must never be performed in children with severe polyuria*)

- No fluids after bedtime and at breakfast.
- Collect sample at 8:00 am to 8:30 am for paired serum and urine osmolality, serum sodium.
- Patients with complete DI may not be able to tolerate overnight fluid restriction. Where desired, patients must be allowed access to water and the water restriction process aborted.
- Those unable to tolerate overnight water restriction may require a formal water deprivation test to be performed by a paediatric endocrinologist.

Water Deprivation Test

- Patient must be closely observed and supervised throughout the test.
- Before the test, the patient is allowed usual fluid intake.
- The biochemistry laboratory must be informed ahead of the test in order to coordinate rapid processing of samples and timely reporting of the results.
- Start the test at 8:00 am in the morning after collecting baseline paired serum and urine osmolality, serum sodium.
- Patient is not allowed to drink water or any fluid after that.
- Timed collection of paired serum and urine osmolality, serum sodium is done at every 1–2 hourly intervals. Patient must be under close surveillance, and this test is discontinued when a set endpoint is met: i) DI is diagnosed or excluded ii) patient is unable to tolerate the test safely.
- Administration of DDAVP could help differentiate central DI from nephrogenic DI.

Treatment of Diabetes Insipidus

- The treatment of central DI hinges on replacing *fluids* and ADH. The former is dependent on functional thirst mechanisms as well as the child's ability or inability (e.g. mental impairment, post-operative states, neonates and infants) to source for and consume fluids independently.
- Anti-diuresis can be achieved *orally* (PO Desmopressin), sublingually (MELT - orally disintegrating lyophilisate tablet), *intranasally* (IN Desmopressin) and where indicated, through injections either *subcutaneously* or *intravenously* (SC/IV Vasopressin).

Bibliography

1. Refardt J. (2020) Diagnosis and differential diagnosis of diabetes insipidus: Update. *Best Pract Res Clin Endocrinol Metab* **34**(5):101398.

2. Nigro N, Grossmann M, Chiang C, Inder WJ. (2018) Polyuria-polydipsia syndrome: A diagnostic challenge. *Intern Med J* **48**(3):244–253.
3. Christ-Crain M, Bichet DG, Fenske WK, *et al.* (2019) Diabetes insipidus. *Nat Rev Dis Primers* **5**(1):54.
4. Dabrowski E, Kadakia R, Zimmerman D. (2016) Diabetes insipidus in infants and children. *Best Pract Res Clin Endocrinol Metab* **30**(2):317–328.
5. Di Iorgi N, Napoli F, Allegri AE, *et al.* (2012) Diabetes insipidus--diagnosis and management. *Horm Res Paediatr* 77(2):69–84.
6. Patti G, Ibba A, Morana G, *et al.* (2020) Central diabetes insipidus in children: Diagnosis and management. *Best Pract Res Clin Endocrinol Metab* **34**(5):101440.
7. Paediatric & Adolescent Endocrinology. (2017) Water deprivation test for suspected diabetes insipidus in children, Yorkshire Regional Centre, Leeds Children's Hospital. http://www.leedsformulary.nhs.uk/docs/24.06.11.WaterDeprivationTest.pdf
8. St. George's University Hospitals. (2021) Water deprivation test. https://www.stgeorges.nhs.uk/wp-content/uploads/2021/06/DIB_WDT_01.pdf
9. Chin X, Teo SW, Lim ST, *et al.* (2022) Desmopressin therapy in children and adults: pharmacological considerations and clinical implications. European Journal of Clinical Pharmacology, **78**(6): 907–917.

SECTION 12

FLUIDS & ELECTROLYTES

CHAPTER 43

Management of Fluids & Electrolytes

Chan Meng Fai, Joel; Leow Hui Min, Esther; Mok Yee Hui; Ng Yong Hong

Management of Fluids

1. Maintenance fluid requirement

- Full-term neonates:
  - » Day 1 – 60 ml/kg/day
  - » Day 2 – 90 ml/kg/day
  - » Day 3 – 120 ml/kg/day
  - » Day 4 – 150 ml/kg/day

  *In a sick neonate (>Day 3 of life), consider restricting intravenous (IV) fluids to 100 to 120 ml/kg/day.

  **IV fluid requirements should be capped at 100 ml/kg/day.
- Child:

Table 12.1 Calculating Maintenance Fluids in Children

<10 kg	100 ml/kg/d Or 4 ml/kg/hr
10–20 kg	1000 ml + 50 ml/kg/d for each kg over 10 kg Or 40 ml/hr plus 2 ml/kg/hr for each kg over 10 kg
>20 kg	1500 ml plus 20 ml/kg/d for each kg over 20 kg Or 60 ml/hr plus 1 ml/kg/hr for each kg over 20 kg

For example: the maintenance fluid requirement of a 35 kg child would be (100 x 10) + (50 x 10) + (20 x 15) = 1800 ml

- Special considerations
  - » Higher fluid requirements: Children who are febrile, under phototherapy, or a radiant warmer, children with ongoing fluid losses (vomiting, diarrhoea, high stoma output, burns).
  - » Lower fluid requirements: Stable post-operative children, children with renal or cardiac failure, children with Syndrome of Inappropriate Anti-Diuretic Hormone (SIADH).
- Choice of IV fluids:
  - » The recommended maintenance fluids for the various age groups are shown in Table 12.2. The choice of fluids should also be based on the ongoing physiological disorder and prevalent electrolyte or glucose abnormality.

Table 12.2 Choice of IV Fluids

Age	Fluid
<1 mth	Dextrose 10% (with appropriate NaCl and KCl)
1–3 mth	Dextrose 5% with 0.45% NaCl
>3 mth	Dextrose 5% with 0.9% NaCl

Table 12.3 Assessment of Hydration Status

	Mild Dehydration (3–5%)	Moderate Dehydration (6–9%)	Severe Dehydration (>10%)
General Condition	Alert, thirsty	Thirsty, restless or lethargic/irritable	Drowsy, floppy, unconscious
Eye	Normal	Sunken	Very sunken and dry
Tears	Present	Absent	Absent
Mouth/Tongue	Moist	Dry	Very dry
Capillary Refill	Normal	Prolonged >2 sec	Prolonged >2 sec
Skin Turgor	Instant recoil	Recoil in >2 sec	Recoil in >2 sec
Skin	Normal	Normal	Cold, clammy, mottled
Fontanelle	Normal	Sunken	Very sunken
Urine	Normal	Reduced amount	Anuria/severe oliguria
Pulse Rate	Normal rate and volume	Rapid and weak	Rapid, feeble
Blood Pressure	Normal	Normal/low	Low/un-recordable
Respiration	Normal	Deep/maybe rapid	Deep and rapid
Weight Loss	3–5%	6–9%	≥ 10%

2. Fluid deficit in dehydrated children

- Children with reduced intravascular fluid status should be assessed early and preferably with a senior doctor.
- Table 12.3 provides a guide to the assessment of the intravascular fluid status of a child. When in doubt, the more severe dehydration status should be used.
- The rate of replacement of fluid deficit depends on the primary pathology and its severity. For example, a slower replacement rate should be used for children with diabetic ketoacidosis and intracranial pathology, due to the risk of cerebral oedema.
- Oral rehydration therapy is discussed in Chapter 51: 'Acute Gastroenteritis'.

Table 12.4 Calculating Fluid Deficit

Body weight x % dehydration = Deficit in Litres • E.g. 10 kg child, 3% dehydration: 10 x 0.03 = 0.3 L = 300 ml deficit Fluid used for rehydration is the same as maintenance fluids. Rehydration should be carried out evenly over at least 24–48 hr. • E.g. 20 kg child, 5% rehydration Maintenance: 1500 ml/d, Deficit: 1000 ml Therefore prescribe 2500 ml/d for first 24 hr, 1500 ml/d thereafter

Management of Electrolytes

1. Introduction

Electrolyte abnormalities are frequently encountered in paediatric practice. When encountering problems with fluid and electrolyte imbalance, it is useful to think about what the expected renal response is to a given situation and evaluate the actual response. This is done by measuring serum and urine parameters:

- Serum: urea, creatinine, sodium (Na), potassium (K), chloride (Cl), calcium (Ca), magnesium (Mg), phosphate (PO_4), osmolality, pH, pCO_2
- Urine: Na, K, Cl, osmolality, creatinine, pH

When considering the appropriate level of care that the patient requires (general ward, high-dependency, intensive care unit), particular attention should also be given to the requirement for:

- Cardiac monitoring
- Haemodynamic monitoring/intervention
- Neurological monitoring: Level of consciousness, seizures
- Frequency of blood sampling and availability of venous access

2. Daily electrolyte requirement

Table 12.5 Daily Electrolyte Requirement

Sodium	2–4 mmol/kg/d
Potassium	1–2 mmol/kg/d
Chloride	2–4 mmol/kg/d
Calcium	0.5–1 mmol/kg/d
Magnesium	0.2–0.4 mmol/kg/d
Phosphate	2 mmol/kg/d

CHAPTER 44

Sodium Disorders

Chan Meng Fai, Joel; Leow Hui Min, Esther; Mok Yee Hui; Ng Yong Hong

Introduction

Sodium (Na) abnormalities are more commonly the result of disruption in fluid homeostasis rather than sodium homeostasis. Assessment of the intravascular volume status and anti-diuretic hormone (ADH) activity (via comparison of serum and urine sodium and osmolality) provides a guide to the underlying pathology.

Hypernatraemia

- Definition: Serum sodium [Na] >150 mmol/L
- Clinical presentation:
  - » Irritability, lethargy, hyper-reflexia, ataxia, seizures, coma
- Assessment:
  - » Refer to Figure 12.1 for a diagnostic approach.
  - » History: Weight changes, intake and output (urinary, gastric, stool), medication history.
  - » Examination: Assess the fluid status
    - ▪ Weight, skin changes (oedema, skin turgor), fontanelle changes, blood pressure, mucous membranes, cardiac gallop.
    - ▪ In hypernatraemic dehydration, the extracellular fluid volume may be preserved, the classic signs of dehydration (sunken eyes and fontanelle, reduced skin turgor, hypotension) may be absent.
  - » Determine the urine volume.
  - » Paired serum and urine osmolality and sodium, serum urea, creatinine and chloride.
- Management
  - » Water deficit (L) = $0.6 \times$ Weight (kg) $\times$ ([Current Na]/140 – 1)
  - » Aim: Decrease of [Na] by no more than 0.5 mmol/L/hour (max. of 8–10 mmol/L/day) due to risk of cerebral oedema.
  - » Hypervolaemia: Restriction and removal of excess Na with loop diuretics and hypotonic fluids.
  - » Hypovolaemia: Give relatively hypo-osmolar fluid.
  - » Treat underlying cause
    - ▪ Vasopressin (DDAVP) for central diabetes insipidus (DI)
    - ▪ Removal of exogenous Na

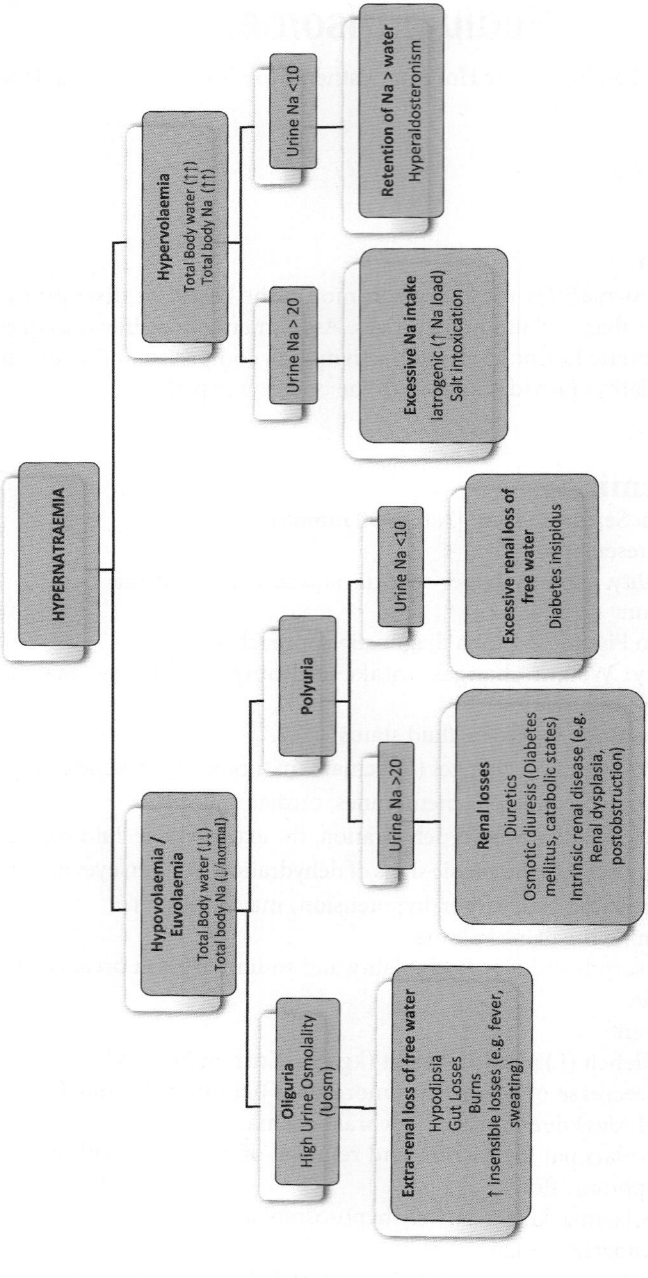

Figure 12.1 Diagnostic approach to hypernatraemia.

(Urine Na in mmol/L)

Hyponatraemia

- Definition: Serum Na <135 mmol/L
  - » Corrected [Na] levels = measured [Na] + 0.3 (glucose – 5.5) mmol/L
- Clinical presentation
  - » Lethargy, weakness, altered sensorium, decreased level of consciousness, seizures, coma
- Assessment
  - » History: changes in weight, intake and output (urinary, gastric, stool), medication history.
  - » Assess the hydration status.
    - ■ Weight, skin changes (oedema, turgor), fontanelle changes, blood pressure, mucous membranes, apex beat, cardiac gallop.
  - » Determine the urine volume.
  - » Investigations:
    - ■ Paired serum and urine: Osmolality (osm), sodium and creatinine
    - ■ Serum urea and chloride
  - » Calculated serum osmolality = (2 × [Na]) + [Glucose] + [Urea]
  - » Calculate the Fractional Excretion of Sodium, FeNa (%) = [(UNa/PNa) / (UCr/PCr)] × 100
    (UNa - urine sodium, PNa - plasma sodium, UCr - urine creatinine, PCr - plasma creatinine)
- Management
  - » Depends on
    - ■ Chronicity of hyponatraemia
    - ■ Severity of symptoms
    - ■ Underlying cause (see Figure 12.2)
      - Hypovolaemia: Sodium and water replacement
      - Euvolaemia: Water restriction
      - Hypervolaemia: Sodium and water restriction, diuretics
  - » Na deficit (mmol) = 0.6 × Weight (kg) × [135 – (current Na)]
  - » Aim: Increase of [Na] by no more than 0.5 mmol/L/h (max. of 12 mmol/L/day) due to risk of central pontine myelinolysis (acute paralysis, dysphagia, dysarthria)
  - » If [Na] ≥120 mmol/L, correct by restriction of free water
  - » If [Na] <120 mmol/L or severely symptomatic (e.g. hyponatraemic seizures)
    - ■ Correct to 125 mmol/L (can be 1–2 mmol/L/hour in the first few hours).
    - ■ Monitor for the resolution of symptoms and rate of rise of [Na] and scale back the speed of correction accordingly.
  - » Drugs used
    - ■ 3% NaCl: 0.5 mmol of Na per ml
      - 2 ml/kg of 3% NaCl increases Na by approximately 1 mmol/L
    - ■ Dextrose 5%/0.45% NaCl or Dextrose 5%/0.9% NaCl: As fluid replacement or maintenance

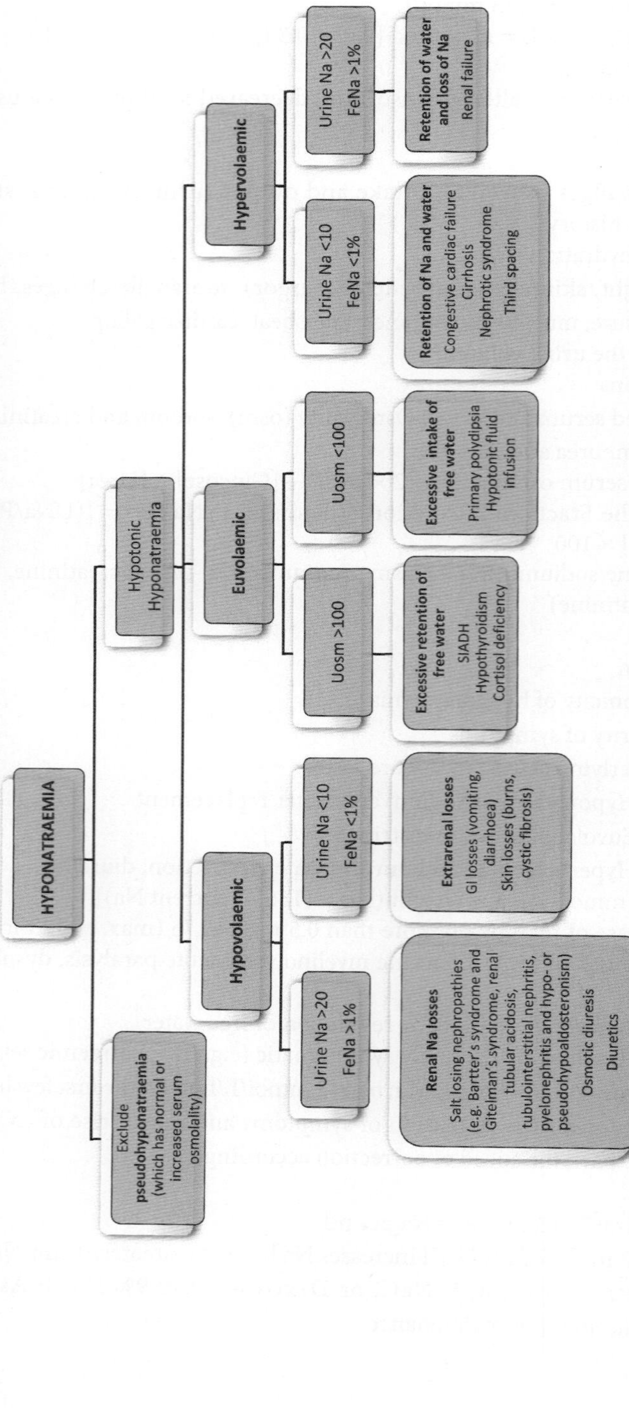

(Urine Na in mmol/L; Urine Osm (Uosm) in mOsm/kg)

Figure 12.2 Diagnostic approach to hyponatraemia.

- 20% NaCl solution: 3.4 mmol of Na per ml
- NaCl tablet (500 mg): 8.5 mmol of Na per tablet
- Na-citrate (Shohl's solution): 1 mmol of Na per ml

Bibliography

1. Moritz ML, Ayus JC. (2002) Disorders of water metabolism in children: Hyponatraemia and hypernatraemia. *Paediatr Rev* **23**(11):371–380.
2. Veis JH. (2021) Evaluation of hyponatraemia. *BMJ Best Pract.*

CHAPTER 45

Potassium Disorders

Chan Meng Fai, Joel; Leow Hui Min, Esther; Mok Yee Hui; Ng Yong Hong

Hyperkalaemia

- Definition:
  - » Serum potassium levels:
    - Neonate: K >6.0 mmol/L
    - Older child: K >5.5 mmol/L
  - » Exclude spurious results (e.g. blood taken from a vein proximal to a drip containing potassium) or haemolysed sample
- Clinical presentation:
  - » Arrhythmia (with palpitations, syncope)
  - » Electrocardiogram (ECG) abnormalities (tall T-waves, depressed ST-segment, decreased R-wave amplitude, prolonged PR, small or absent P-waves, prolonged QRS, sine-wave, ventricular fibrillation). ***Hyperkalaemia with ECG abnormalities is a medical emergency. The ECG changes may not progress in a particular sequence and may not be reflective of the degree of hyperkalaemia.***
  - » Neuromuscular weakness (ascending from the legs to the arms and trunk) or paraesthesia, hyporeflexia
- Causes:
  - » Increased intake: Over-replacement via oral route, IV fluids (containing excessive potassium), massive transfusion
  - » Transcellular movement of potassium: Increased cellular injury (rhabdomyolysis, tumour lysis, haemolysis), metabolic acidosis, insulin-deficiency states
  - » Decreased renal excretion: decreased glomerular filtration rate (in kidney injury), hypoaldosteronism or impaired sensitivity to aldosterone, impaired renin-angiotensin-aldosterone system (congenital adrenal hyperplasia, potassium-sparing diuretics, angiotensin-converting enzyme [ACE] inhibitors)
- Management
  - » Management guidelines are discussed in Table 12.7.
  - » It is crucial to correct the underlying cause of the hyperkalaemia.

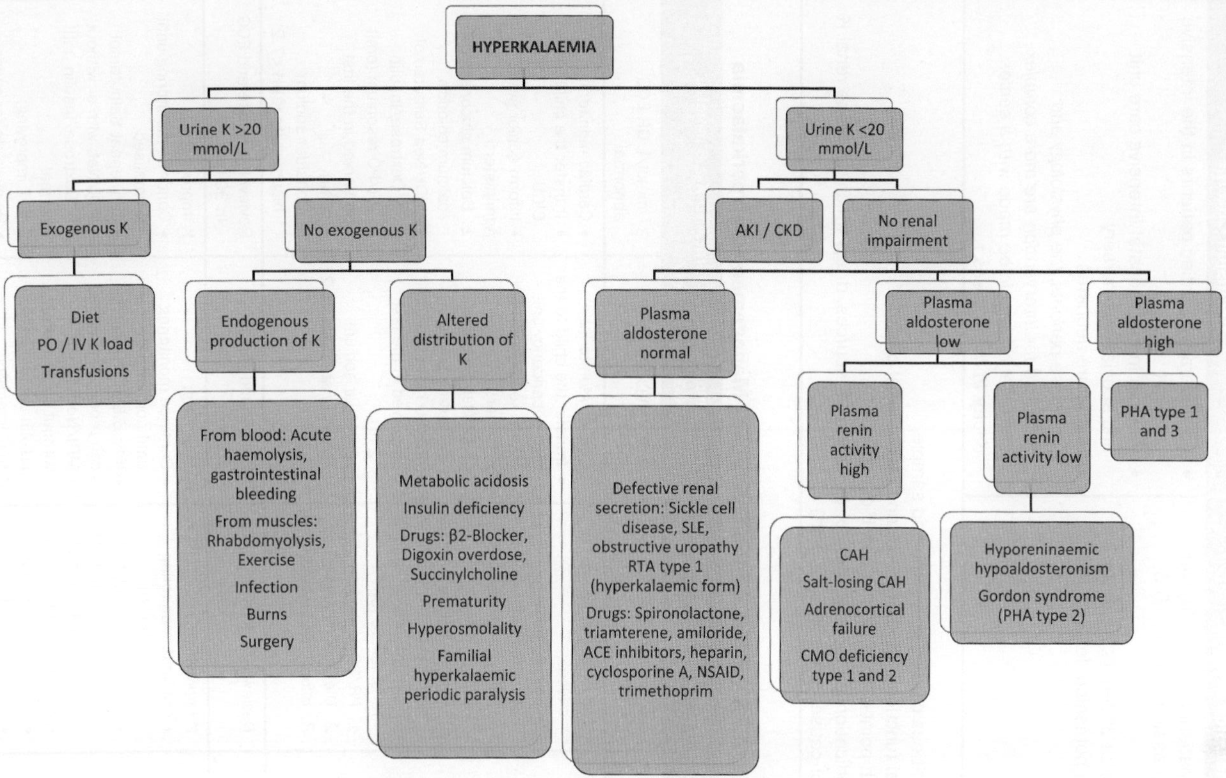

Figure 12.3 Diagnostic approach to hyperkalaemia.

ACE: angiotensin converting enzyme; AKI: acute kidney injury; CAH: congenital adrenal hyperplasia; CKD: chronic kidney disease; CMO: corticosterone methyloxidase; NSAID: non-steroidal anti-inflammatory drugs; PHA: pseudohypoaldosteronism; RTA: renal tubular acidosis; SLE: systemic lupus erythematosus

Table 12.6 In-Patient Emergency Management of Hyperkalaemia in Children and Neonates

Inclusion Criteria	Exclusion Criteria
• Paediatric patient (>1 mth old) with a serum potassium level of ≥5.5 mmol/L • Term neonatal patient (≤1 mth age) with serum potassium level of >6 mmol/L	• Post-operative cardiac patients in the intensive care unit • Patients in the neonatal intensive care unit and special care nursery • Premature neonates *(For these patients, the physiology and threshold for intervention are more complex. Consultation should be made with a senior doctor in these cases.)*
Caution: • Exclude fictitious causes or lysed blood sample • Check renal function if not done so (send urgent renal panel) • Repeat with point-of-care electrolytes if critical • Review medications/infusions (look for exogenous K sources, drugs which decrease renal K excretion or cause transcellular K shift)	

Table 12.7 Algorithm for the Emergency Management of Hyperkalaemia

Age >1 month old AND K ≥5.5 mmol/L, OR Age ≤1 month old, full term AND K ≥ 6 mmol/L Perform electrocardiogram (ECG) immediately			
Potassium level	5.5–6 mmol/L	6.1–6.9 mmol/L	≥7 mmol/L OR ECG abnormal
Initial treatment	If acute and ongoing cause: 1. Salbutamol via metered dose inhaler (MDI) or nebulisation (Neb) 2. Per rectal (PR)/Oral (PO) resonium For patients with chronic renal failure (CRF): 1. PR/PO resonium 2. Diet modification 3. Inform nephrologist	• Cardiac monitoring • Transfer the child to the high dependency unit • Inform senior staff Administer: 1. MDI/Neb Salbutamol 2. IV Dextrose/Insulin 3. PR/PO resonium (omit if served in the last 2 hr) 4. Consider sodium bicarbonate if pH <7.2	• Cardiac monitoring • Transfer the child to the CICU • Inform senior staff Administer: 1. Calcium gluconate OR calcium chloride 2. MDI/Neb Salbutamol 3. IV Dextrose/Insulin 4. PR/PO resonium (omit if served in the last 2 hr) 5. Consider sodium bicarbonate if pH <7.2
Review	Review K in 1 hr	Review K and glucose in 1 hr	Review K, glucose and ECG in 30 min
Further management	K improving: • Continue monitoring until normalised • If K: 5.5–6 mmol/L, can repeat Salbutamol MDI/Neb until normal K NOT improving: • Re-evaluate for cause • If K >6 mmol/L, escalate to the next level of management	K improving: • Continue monitoring until normalised • If K: 5.5–6.9 mmol/L, can repeat Salbutamol MDI/Neb with or without IV Dextrose/ Insulin until normal K NOT improving: • Re-evaluate for cause • If K >6.9 mmol/L, escalate to the next level of management	K improving: • Continue monitoring until normalised • Can repeat Salbutamol MDI/Neb with or without IV Dextrose/Insulin until normal K NOT improving: • Re-evaluate for cause • If ECG changes persist, can repeat Calcium • Consider continuous renal replacement therapy (CRRT)

Table 12.8 Drugs for the Emergency Management of Hyperkalaemia

Drug Name	Dosage and Route	Onset of Action	Duration	Comments
Salbutamol 0.5%	Nebulised with 8 L/gas flow: • <25 kg: 2.5 mg in 4 ml N/S Q1–2H • >25 kg: 5 mg in 4 ml N/S Q1–2H	30–60 min	3–4 hr	May cause tachycardia. May be repeated.
Insulin	IV 0.1 unit/kg/dose (max. 10 units/dose) To take 50 units using insulin syringe and reconstitute to 50 ml in normal saline • Final concentration is **1 unit/ml** ****Administer appropriate dose using diluted solution.****	15–20 min	4–6 hr	1 unit per 5 g of glucose. May cause hypoglycaemia. ****Monitor blood glucose 1 hr after dose**** May be repeated.
Dextrose 10%	IV 5 ml/kg/dose	—	—	To administer with IV insulin.
Sodium resonium (Sodium Polystyrene Sulfonate)	PO 1 g/kg/dose (max. 15–30 g/dose) Q8H PR 1 g/kg/dose (max. 30–60 g/dose) Q2 – 6H (evacuate previous dose before administration)	1–2 hr	4–6 hr	Contraindicated if ileus, recent abdominal surgery, or perforated gut. Contraindicated in neonates with reduced gut motility. May cause nausea, constipation, paralytic ileus or diarrhoea. May be repeated.
10% Calcium gluconate (2.25 mmol/10 ml)	IV 0.5–1 ml/kg/dose over 10 min (max. IV 30 ml/dose)	5–10 min	30–60 min	May cause hypercalcaemia or tissue necrosis. May be repeated if ECG changes persist.
10% Calcium chloride (5.5 mmol/10 ml)	IV 0.2 ml/kg/dose (max. 20 ml) over 10 min ****May use in place of calcium gluconate if fluid restricted****	—	—	May cause hypercalcaemia or tissue necrosis. May be repeated if ECG changes persist.
Sodium bicarbonate 8.4% (1 mmol/ml)	IV 1ml/kg/dose over 10–15 min (max. IV 50 mmol/dose) To dilute with equal parts of water-for-injection to make up 4.2% solution before administration	4–6 hr	4–6 hr	May cause sodium overload/hypertension. May use when evidence of acidaemia present (pH <7.2; serum HCO_3 <15 mEq/L). ****Not to give simultaneously with calcium.****

Comments

1. Salbutamol is a preferred first-line treatment for hyperkalaemia because of the ease of administration, while other treatments are being prepared.
2. Concentrated insulin is a high-alert medication and care should be taken in its dilution and preparation.
3. Salbutamol and insulin are short-term treatments for hyperkalaemia and can be repeated. Efforts should be made in the meantime to identify and treat the underlying cause.

Hypokalaemia

- Definition: Serum K <3.5 mmol/L
- Clinical presentation: Arrhythmia, ECG abnormalities (prolonged PR, ST depression, T-inversion), neuromuscular weakness
- Management:
  - » Correction of hypokalaemia is more crucial in children with cardiac disease or who are on digoxin
  - » Correct deficit on top of providing maintenance potassium. The required maintenance may be higher depending on the underlying pathology (e.g. severe dehydration in DKA, with the expected requirement for IV Insulin)
  - » Correcting hypokalaemia
    - ■ K-Deficit (mmol): (Desired [K] – current [K]) × 0.3 × Weight (kg)
    - ■ Non-urgent replacement:
      - Oral K replacement is the preferred route (due to risk of cardiac arrhythmia with rapid IV administration)
      - Increase maintenance K in the IV drip
    - ■ Urgent replacement: Consider IV replacement in the following cases
      - Severe hypokalaemia K < 2.5 mmol/L
      - Symptomatic: Severe weakness, arrhythmia, post-cardiac surgery
      - Unpredictable enteral absorption: Significant enterocolitis, post-major surgery
    - ■ Concentrated potassium chloride (KCl)
      - Replacement of K deficit over 2 to 3 hours
        - o Peripheral line: Dilute the 7.45% KCl into 0.9% NaCl (maximal concentration of 40 mmol/L)
        - o Central line: Dilute the 7.45% KCl into 0.9% NaCl (maximal concentration of 150 mmol/L)
        - o Maximum rate of 0.4 mmol/kg/hour
      - Replacement should be done under cardiac monitoring and in high dependency, oncology wards or intensive care unit
      - Recheck K level at the end of replacement
      - IV 7.45% KCl should **NEVER** be given undiluted or as bolus
  - » Potassium-containing preparations
    - ■ Oral KCl: 1 ml contains 1.34 mmol of K
    - ■ Oral Span K (600 mg): 8 mmol of K/tablet
    - ■ IV 7.45% KCl: 1 ml contains 1 mmol of K and 1 mmol of Cl
    - ■ KH_2PO_4: 1 ml contains 1 mmol of K and 1 mmol of PO_4

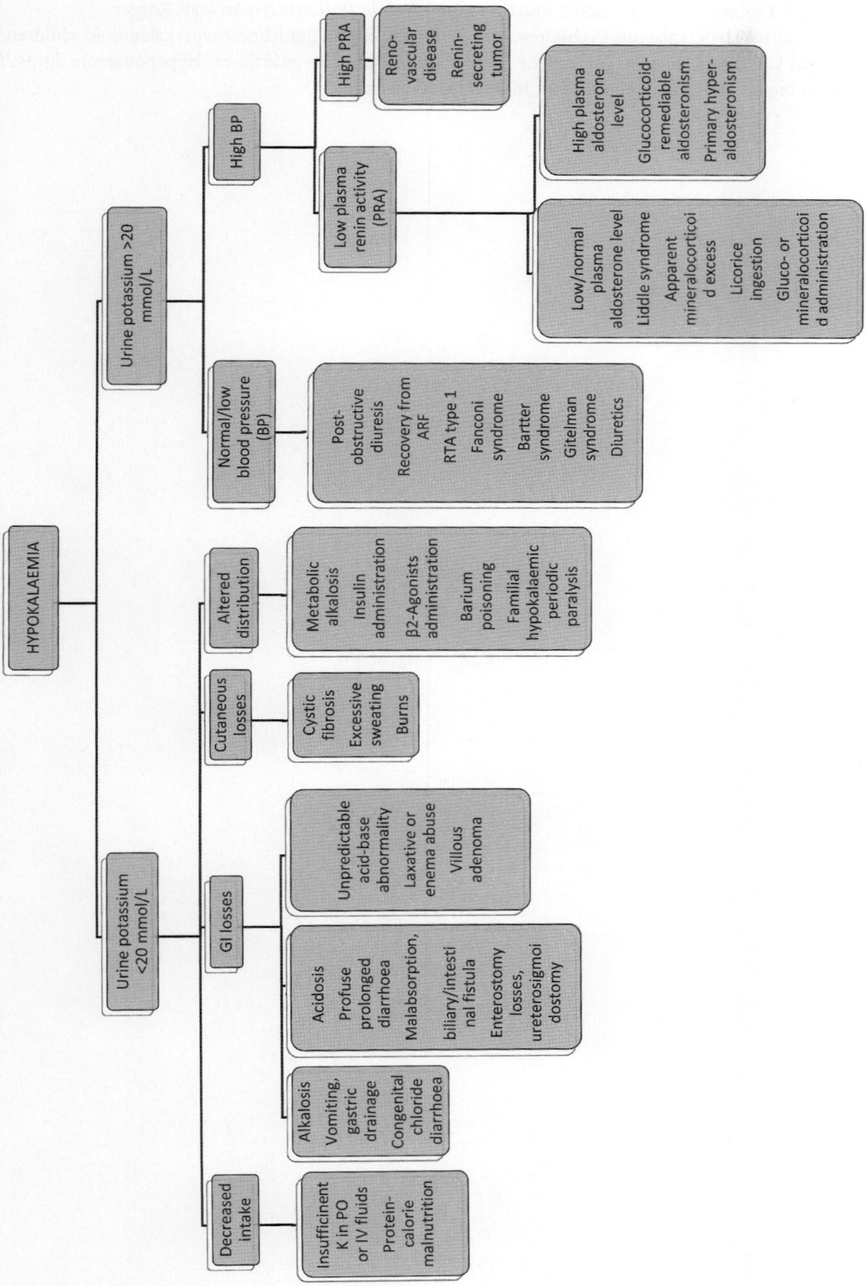

Figure 12.4 Diagnostic approach to hypokalaemia.

Bibliography

1. Zelikovic I, Eisenstein I. (eds.) (2008) *Practical Algorithms in Pediatric Nephrology*. Karger.
2. Starship. (2018) Hyperkalaemia in children. https://starship.org.nz/guidelines/hyperkalemia-in-children/
3. The Royal Children's Hospital Melbourne (2016) Clinical practice guidelines: Hyperkalaemia. https://www.rch.org.au/clinicalguide/guideline_index/Hyperkalaemia/

CHAPTER 46

Acid–Base Disorders

Chan Meng Fai, Joel; Leow Hui Min, Esther; Mok Yee Hui; Ng Yong Hong

Introduction

- A good *clinical evaluation* is essential to guide the workup of acid–base disorders.
  - » History of underlying medical problems (e.g. diabetes, cardiac failure)
  - » Symptomatology: e.g. vomiting, diarrhoea
  - » Vital signs (e.g. shock, hypoxia)
  - » Respiratory status: Rate and depth of breathing (e.g. Kussmaul's respiration)
  - » Neurological status: Level of consciousness
  - » Medication or drug use
- Blood gas: Determine the primary acid–base disorder
  - » Ascertain if there is acidaemia (pH <7.38) or alkalaemia (pH >7.42).
  - » Is this a primary respiratory or metabolic disorder?
  - » Determine the appropriate physiological response to the primary disorder. Hence, evaluate if there is a secondary component to the acid–base disorder. Please refer to Figures 12.5 and 12.6.
- For high-anion gap metabolic acidosis, evaluate:
  - » Osmolal gap = measured serum osmolality – calculated serum osmolality
  - » Calculated serum osmolality = 2[Na] + [glucose] + [Urea]
  - » Osmolal gap of greater than 10 mmol/L suggests the presence of toxic alcohols (ethylene glycol, methanol) or the presence of ketoacidosis or lactic acidosis.

High Anion-gap Metabolic Acidosis (HAGMA)

- Overproduction of acid
  - » Ketoacidosis (diabetic ketoacidosis, starvation)
  - » Lactic acidosis
    - ▪ Type A (hypoxic): Shock, carbon monoxide and cyanide poisoning
    - ▪ Type B (non-hypoxic): Medications (propofol, metformin, isoniazid, salicylates), toxic alcohols (methanol, ethylene glycol)
- Impaired clearance of acid: Severe renal injury, liver failure (lactate clearance)
- Cell lysis: Severe rhabdomyolysis

Normal Anion-gap Metabolic acidosis (NAGMA)

- Loss of bicarbonate
  - » Gastrointestinal (GI) losses: Diarrhoea, stoma losses, fistulae

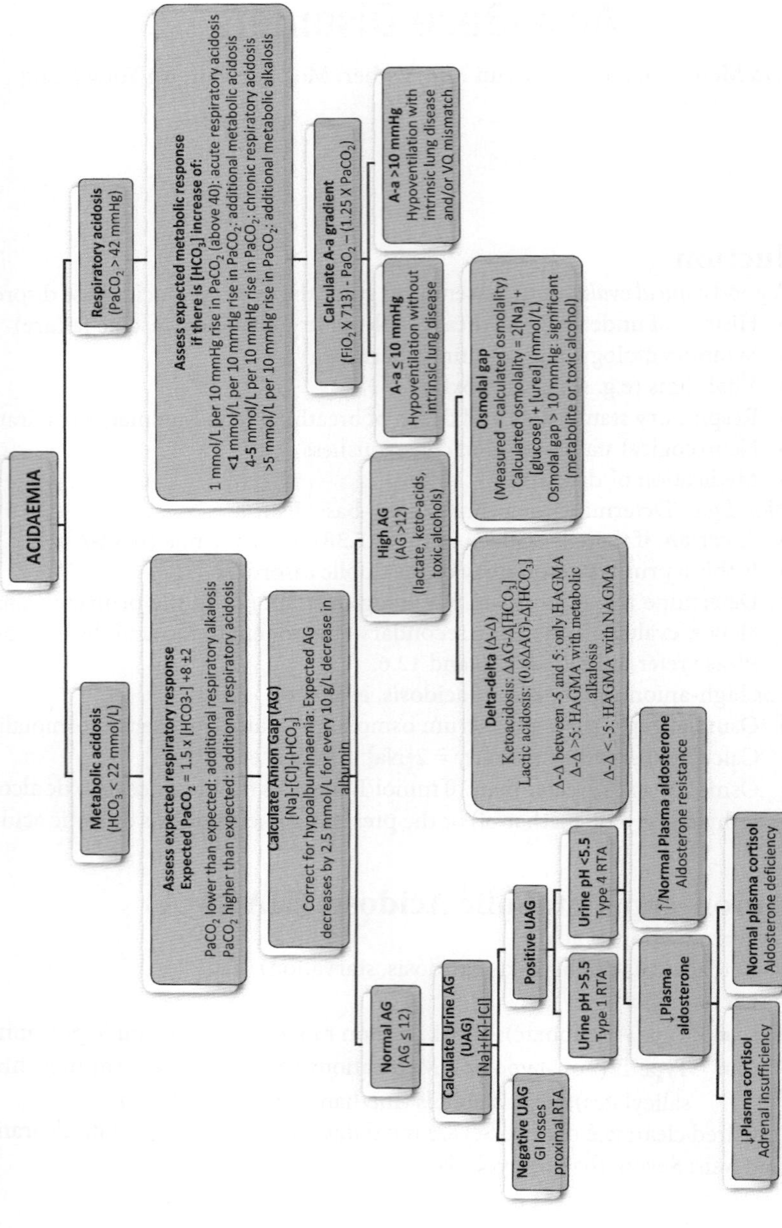

Figure 12.5 Diagnostic approach to acidaemia.

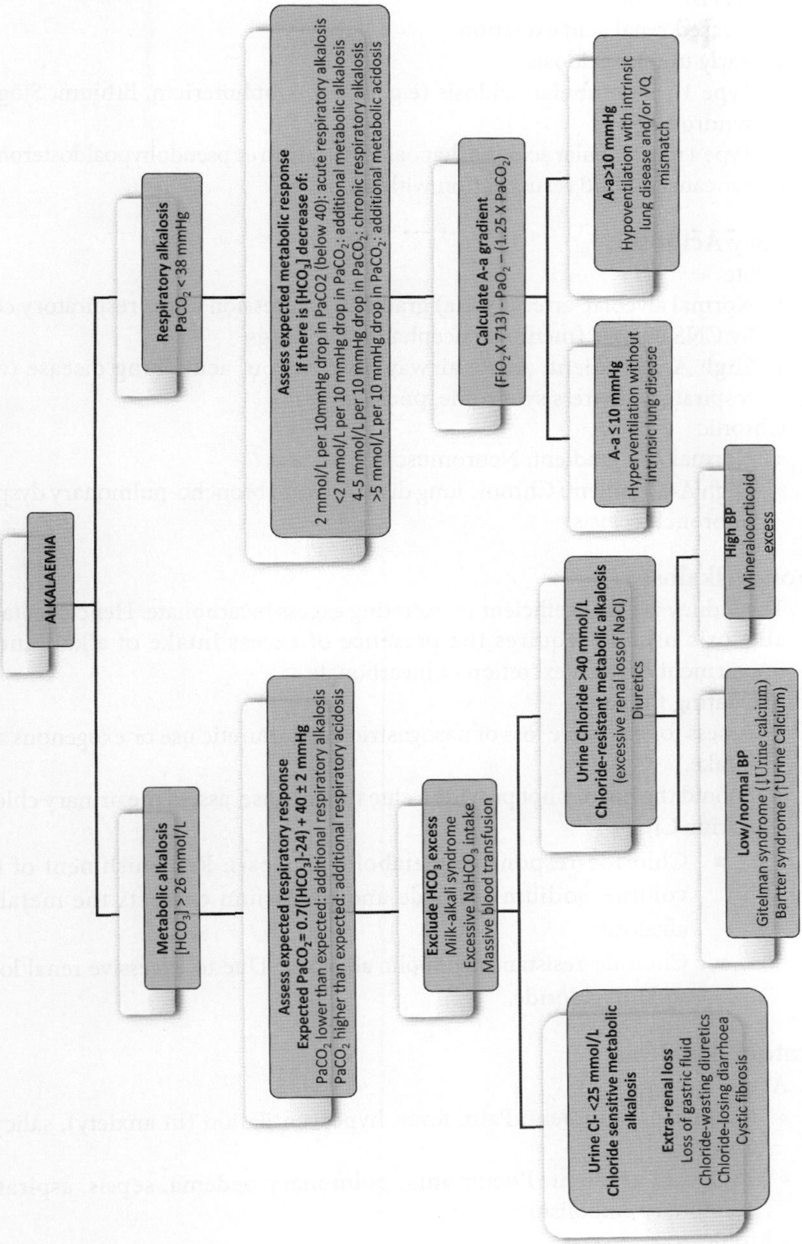

Figure 12.6 Diagnostic approach to alkalaemia.

- » Renal losses: Proximal RTA, medications (ifosfamide, topiramate, acetazolamide)
- Decreased renal acid excretion
  - » Early uremic acidosis
  - » Type 1 renal tubular acidosis (e.g. due to amphotericin, lithium, Sjögren's syndrome)
  - » Type 4 renal tubular acidosis (hypoaldosteronism or pseudohypoaldosteronism)
- Other causes: Fluid resuscitation with saline

Respiratory Acidosis

- Acute
  - » Normal alveolar-arterial (A-a) gradient: Depression of the respiratory centre by CNS disease (meningoencephalitis) or drugs
  - » High A-a gradient: Acute airway obstruction, acute lung disease (acute respiratory distress syndrome, pneumonia)
- Chronic
  - » Normal A-a gradient: Neuromuscular disease
  - » High A-a gradient: Chronic lung disease (from broncho-pulmonary dysplasia or bronchiectasis)

Metabolic Alkalosis

- The kidney is highly efficient in excreting excess bicarbonate. Hence, metabolic alkalosis usually requires the presence of excess intake of alkali and the impairment of renal excretion of bicarbonate.
- Evaluating the cause
  - » Assess for excessive loss of nasogastric fluid, diuretic use or exogenous alkali intake.
  - » Should the history not provide a clue to the cause, assess the urinary chloride (Urine Cl).
    - ▪ Chloride-responsive metabolic alkalosis: Replenishment of fluid volume, sodium chloride and potassium corrects the metabolic alkalosis.
    - ▪ Chloride-resistant metabolic alkalosis: Due to excessive renal loss of sodium chloride.

Respiratory Alkalosis

- Acute
  - » Normal A-a gradient: Pain, fever, hyperventilation (in anxiety), salicylate toxicity
  - » High A-a gradient: Pneumonia, pulmonary oedema, sepsis, aspiration, pulmonary embolism
- Chronic
  - » Normal A-a gradient: Hyperthyroidism
  - » High A-a gradient: Pulmonary embolism
- Treatment of the acid–base disorders will depend on the underlying cause

Bibliography

1. Berend K, de Vries APJ, Gans ROB. (2014) Physiological approach to assessment of acid-base disturbances. *N Eng J Med* **371**:1434–1445.
2. Hsu BS, Lakhani SA, Wilhelm M. (2016). Acid-base disorders. *Pediatr Rev* **37**(9):361–369.
3. Nitu M, Montgomery G, Eigen H. (2011) Acid-base disorders. *Pediatr Rev* **32**(6):240–251.

SECTION 13

GASTROENTEROLOGY

CHAPTER 47

Failure to Thrive

Charanya Rajan; Veena Logarajah

Introduction

Failure to thrive (FTT) in childhood is a state of impaired growth due to inadequate caloric intake, inadequate caloric absorption/retention, or excessive caloric expenditure. In the developed world, it is seen in 5–10% of children. A careful history and physical examination can identify most causes of FTT, thereby avoiding protracted or costly evaluations.

Definition

A child is said to have FTT in the presence of one of the following:

- Weight for age that falls below the 5th percentile on multiple occasions
- Weight deceleration that crosses two major percentile lines on a growth chart

Use of any single indicator has a low positive predictive value, hence the below anthropometric criteria are also helpful to diagnose FTT:

- Length <5th percentile
- Weight <75% of median weight for length
- Weight velocity <5th percentile
- Body mass index <5th percentile

NOTE: Criteria should be met on multiple occasions.

Causes

Most cases of FTT involve inadequate caloric intake caused by behavioural or psychosocial issues. Routine laboratory testing identifies an organic cause of FTT in <1% of children and is not generally recommended. Child neglect or abuse must be considered in all age groups, because children with FTT are four times more likely to be abused than children without FTT.

A practical way to categorise FTT is according to calories (see Table 13.1):

- Inadequate caloric intake
- Inadequate caloric absorption/retention
- Excessive caloric expenditure
- Unclassified (unrelated to calories)

Table 13.1 Differential Diagnosis of Failure to Thrive

Inadequate Caloric Intake	Inadequate Caloric Absorption/ Retention	Excessive Caloric Expenditure	Unclassified
Infant or toddler			
Feeding difficulties	Food allergy	Thyroid disease	SGA
Improper food/formula preparation	GER	Chronic infections	Neglect/abuse
Caregiver depression	Pyloric stenosis	Immunodeficiency	Skeletal dysplasia
Behavioural/ neurological issues	Malabsorption, e.g. Coeliac, CF	Chronic pulmonary disease	Hypopituitarism
Poverty/lack of food availability/cleft lip or palate/airway issues	Inborn error of metabolism	Congenital heart disease	Genetic Russell-Silver, Turner Syndrome
		Chronic liver disease	
		Malignancy	
Child or adolescent			
Mood disorder	Food allergy	Thyroid disease	Constitutional
Eating disorder	Inflammatory bowel disease	Chronic infection or immunodeficiency	Delayed puberty
Drug abuse	Malabsorption, e.g. Coeliac, CF	Chronic pulmonary disease	
	Inborn error of metabolism	Heart disease or failure	
		Malignancy	
		Renal failure, renal tubular acidosis	

Note: In certain conditions there may be an overlap between the categories.

CF and coeliac disease is extremely rare in the Chinese race.

Approach

History

The most important part of the outpatient evaluation of FTT is obtaining an accurate account of:

- Age of onset and growth pattern
- Feeding history
- Dietary intake
- Parent–child interactions
- Review of systems to elicit symptoms of organic causes

In exclusively breast-fed infants, help of a lactation specialist nurse should be sought to ensure proper technique, latch-on, and swallow. In rare cases where intake is uncertain, consider asking breastfeeding mothers to express breastmilk and measure the amount of consumed breast milk. Alternatively, obtaining the weight of an undressed breastfed infant before and after feeding may be considered. For formula-fed infants, apart from the volume of feeds consumed, the correct feed preparation technique should also be checked.

Observing a toddler's eating habits can be helpful in evaluating for picky eating or food refusal. Asking older children and adolescents, together with their parents, to maintain a food journal for 3 days can give the physician a way to measure caloric intake. Particular attention should also be given to chart "loss of calories" via regurgitation and vomiting.

Taking a psychosocial history is essential for detecting parental or patient depression or identifying concerns about the caregiver's intellectual abilities or social circumstances.

Some children who fail to meet normal growth parameters actually demonstrate a normal variant of growth, such as children of small parents who are growing to their full genetic potential but along a lower percentile curve, large-for-gestational-age infants who regress toward the mean ("catch-down growth"), children with constitutional delay in growth or premature infants whose growth parameters are normal when corrected for gestational age.

A review of systems that elicits recurrent infections, respiratory symptoms, developmental delay, vomiting, or diarrhoea may point to an organic cause. In a study on children without obvious organic symptoms elicited on history, 92% were ultimately diagnosed with a behavioural cause of FTT.

Clinical Examination

The first consideration in examining a child with FTT is ensuring accurate measurements. Height (or length), weight, and head circumference should be plotted on an appropriate growth chart over time.

Although most children with FTT will have a normal examination, physicians should be alert for signs of physical abuse or neglect. Physicians should also seek red flag signs or symptoms of medical conditions that might be causing FTT (See Table 13.2).

Table 13.2 Red Flags Signs and Symptoms Suggesting Medical Causes of Failure to Thrive

- Cardiac findings suggesting congenital heart disease (e.g. clubbing, cyanosis, murmur)
- Developmental delay
- Dysmorphic features
- Recurrent or severe respiratory, mucocutaneous, or urinary infection
- Failure to gain weight despite adequate caloric intake
- Organomegaly or lymphadenopathy
- Recurrent vomiting, diarrhoea, or dehydration

Investigations

Routine laboratory testing rarely identifies a cause of FTT and is not generally recommended. However, history or physical examination findings sometimes suggest the need for further testing.

Baseline tests: Consider full blood count, renal panel, liver function test, thyroid function, C-reactive protein, erythrocyte sedimentation rate, urinalysis, urine culture.

If indicated by history, physical examination or initial laboratory testing, consider the following:

- Respiratory — Chest X-ray, sweat test
- Cardiovascular — Echocardiography
- Gastrointestinal Tract — Stool for culture, ova, parasites, analysis for fat globules, elastase and reducing substances, celiac screen
- Endocrine — Bone age, Synacthen test, and growth hormone testing (under specialist supervision)
- Infection and immunology — Tests for human immunodeficiency virus, TORCHES, tuberculosis, complements, immunoglobulins, and allergy
- Genetic and chromosomal — Turner syndrome, etc.

In rare cases, hospitalisation for observed feeding and further investigation may be helpful. Hospitalisation should be considered for the following:

- If the child does not improve with outpatient management
- Suspicion of abuse or neglect exists
- Signs of traumatic injury are present
- Severe psychosocial impairment/stress of the caregiver is evident
- There are signs of serious malnutrition

Management

If a disease or medical condition is identified on history, physical examination, or additional testing, the correct treatment will vary depending on the condition.

If a diagnosis of FTT is made and no medical conditions are suggested on evaluation, appropriate guidance for catch-up growth should be made and age-appropriate nutritional counselling should be provided to parents. Consider early referral to dietitian for suggestion of suitable forms, amount, and frequency of nutrition to allow for meeting daily nutritional requirements and allowing for catch-up growth.

Breastfed infants: Recommend feeding more often. Ensure lactation support. Consider expressed breastmilk to quantify feed volume accurately. **Discuss concentrating or supplementing feeds with milk formula until catch-up growth is achieved.**

Formula-fed infants: Clear instructions on how to make energy-dense formula by concentrating the ratio of formula to water may be helpful.

Toddlers should avoid excessive juice or milk consumption as this interferes with nutrition. Nutritional supplements may be given until catch-up growth is achieved.

Parents may also be instructed to provide calorie-dense foods by adding rice cereal to foods for toddlers, cream sauces, or butter to foods for older children or adolescents.

For children with swallowing difficulties or underlying neurological problems, consider speech therapist assessment of swallowing function. Alternative methods of feeding, e.g. orogastric tube feeding, may be required temporarily in severely malnourished children who are unable to or refuse to take adequate oral feeds.

In those who are severely malnourished, it is important to watch for refeeding syndrome while feeds are being established. Consider monitoring electrolytes (especially serum potassium, magnesium, phosphate) closely for at least 3–5 days and address any electrolyte abnormality promptly.

Close and serial follow-up including evaluation of height (or length) and weight should be performed in the physician's office after intervention to ensure appropriate catch-up growth. Multidisciplinary interventions, including home medical social worker visits, dietetic advice, and psychology inputs should be considered to optimise weight gain, parent–child relationships, and cognitive development. Finally, although medications such as cyproheptadine have been shown to help promote weight gain in children with cancer-related cachexia, they have not been studied in other causes of FTT.

Prognosis and Outcomes

There is consensus that severe, prolonged malnutrition, which is common in developing countries, can negatively affect a child's future growth and cognitive development. Low-birth-weight infants who develop FTT have also demonstrated long-term developmental effects. However, it is unclear from current studies if normal-birth-weight infants who develop FTT and then recover have similar long-term consequences. A systematic review showed that FTT during the first 2 years of life was not associated with a significant reduction in IQ, although some long-term reductions in weight and height were present. Nevertheless, it important to always review the nutritional status of our patients and attempt to optimise them at every encounter.

Bibliography

1. Levy Y, Levy A, Zangen T, *et al.* (2009) Diagnostic clues for identification of nonorganic vs organic causes of food refusal and poor feeding. *J Pediatr Gastroenterol Nutr* **48**(3):355–362.
2. Cole SZ, Lanham JS. (2011) Failure to thrive: An update. *Am Fam Physician* **83**(7):829–834.
3. Kliegman RM, Stanton BF, St. Geme JW, *et al. Nelson Textbook of Pediatrics, 19th ed.*, Chap. 38, pp. 147–149.
4. Panetta F, Magazzu D, Sferlazzas C, *et al.* (2008) Diagnosis on a positive fashion of nonorganic failure to thrive. *Acta Paediatr* **97**(9):1281–1284.
5. Black MM, Dubowitz H, Krishnakumar A, Starr RH Jr. (2007) Early intervention and recovery among children with failure to thrive: Follow-up at age 8. *Pediatrics* **120**(1):59–69.

CHAPTER 48

Recurrent Abdominal Pain

Charanya Rajan; Veena Logarajah

Introduction

Approximately 10–45% of school-aged children experience recurrent abdominal pain (RAP). In most cases, the cause of the symptoms is not attributed to a particular medical condition. Children with RAP are diagnosed with functional abdominal pain disorders (FAPD) when there are no organic causes to explain their symptoms. Only 3–8% of children have an underlying pathology, presenting with RAP associated with alarm features as listed below. A complete history, including a detailed pain history, effect on the daily activities of the child and family, possible psychosocial factors and examination, including growth and pubertal status, are the most important components in evaluating the cause of the abdominal pain.

Definition

Abdominal pain occurring at least four times per month over a period of at least 2 months and severe enough to affect the child's ability to perform daily activities.

Alarm Features Suggestive of Organic Cause

- Family history of inflammatory bowel disease, coeliac disease, peptic ulcer disease
- Persistent right upper or lower quadrant pain
- Dysphagia
- Odynophagia
- Persistent vomiting
- Gastrointestinal blood loss
- Nocturnal diarrhoea or abdominal pain
- Constitutional symptoms, e.g. arthritis, oral ulcers, unexplained fever
- Perirectal disease
- Involuntary weight loss
- Deceleration of linear growth
- Delayed puberty

Table 13.3 Organic Causes of Abdominal Pain

Gastrointestinal Disorders	Non-gastrointestinal Disorders
• Peptic ulcer disease • Infection • Inflammatory bowel disease • Gallbladder disease • Pancreatic disease • Hepatitis • Carbohydrate malabsorption • Surgical disorders • Foreign body • Tumour • Coeliac disease • Eosinophilic gastrointestinal disease	• Recurrent urinary tract infection • Pelvic–ureteric junction obstruction • Nephrolithiasis • Ovarian or uterine disorders • Diabetes mellitus • Respiratory disorders

Functional Abdominal Pain Disorders

FAPD are characterised by recurrent symptoms occurring at least four times a month for at least two months, which is not explained by another medical condition.

FAPD can be further classified according to the Rome IV criteria as:

- Functional dyspepsia
- Irritable bowel syndrome (IBS)
- Abdominal migraine
- Functional abdominal pain — not otherwise specified (FAP–NOS)

Functional Dyspepsia

Dyspepsia refers to pain or discomfort centered in the upper abdomen. This may be characterised by fullness, early satiety, bloating, belching, nausea, retching, or vomiting. Functional dyspepsia is further classified into two subtypes: post-prandial distress syndrome and epigastric pain syndrome.

Diagnostic Criteria

One or more of the following bothersome symptoms for at least 4 days a month:

- Postprandial fullness
- Early satiation
- Epigastric pain or burning not associated with defecation
- After appropriate evaluation, the symptoms cannot be fully explained by another medical condition

Subtype

- Post-prandial distress syndrome includes postprandial fullness or early satiety that prevents finishing a regular meal. Other features include:
  - » Upper abdominal bloating
  - » Post-prandial nausea
  - » Excessive belching

- Epigastric pain syndrome includes epigastric pain or burning severe enough to limit daily activities. The pain is not generalised or localised to other areas and is not relieved by defecation or passing of flatus. Other features include:
  - » Burning pain without a retrosternal component
  - » Pain induced or relieved by meals but may occur during fasting

Assessment

- A detailed symptom history as well as a dietary, psychological, and social history to determine whether symptoms are likely to represent organic disease.
- Physical examination and growth parameters should be normal.

Management

- Avoidance of triggers: Caffeine, spicy or fatty food, non-steroidal anti-inflammatory agents
- Acid suppressive therapy (if pain predominant): Proton-pump inhibitors, H_2 receptor blockers, antacids, low-dose tricyclic antidepressants
- Prokinetic agents (for nausea, bloating, early satiety): Domperidone, cyproheptadine
- Address psychosocial factors
- Gastric electrical stimulation (if refractory to medical treatment)

Indications for Upper Gastrointestinal Endoscopy

- Family history of peptic ulcer disease or *Helicobacter pylori* infection
- Children older than 10 years
- Symptoms persist for more than 6 weeks despite acid suppressants
- Symptoms severe enough to affect activities of daily living including sleep

Irritable Bowel Syndrome

IBS is a disorder of the brain–gut axis and the symptoms may vary depending on which part of the axis is involved. Alterations in gut microbiome are associated with IBS. Increased self-reported stress, anxiety, depression and emotional problems are seen in children with IBS.

Diagnostic Criteria

Must include all of the following:

- Abdominal pain at least 4 days per month for at least 2 months associated with one or more of the following:
  - » Related to defecation
  - » Change in stool frequency
  - » Change in form (appearance) of stool
- Pain does not resolve with resolution of constipation
- After appropriate evaluation, symptoms cannot be fully explained by another medical condition

Assessment

- History fulfilling diagnostic criteria with normal examination and normal growth pattern
- Detailed history to ensure absence of red flags, which may suggest organic pathology
- Explore for any triggering events and psychosocial factors

Management

- Patient education of IBS and reassurance
- Psychotherapy — Coping with stress and dealing with symptoms
- Dietary modifications (low-FODMAP [fermentable oligosaccharides, disaccharides, monosaccharides, and polyols], high-fibre, low-fat, avoid caffeine)
- Symptomatic relief (anti-spasmodics, laxatives)
- Probiotics

Abdominal Migraine

Abdominal migraine is characterised by acute, intense, non-colicky, midline abdominal pain that lasts for hours. It occurs intermittently with long symptom-free periods. Children with abdominal migraine and classic migraine have similar triggers (e.g. stress, fatigue, travel), associated symptoms (e.g. anorexia, nausea, vomiting) and relieving factors (e.g. rest and sleep).

Diagnostic Criteria

Must include two or more episodes of all the following features for at least 6 months:

- Paroxysmal episodes of intense, acute periumbilical, midline or diffuse abdominal pain that lasts for 1 hour or more
- Episodes separated by weeks or months
- Pain interferes with normal activities
- Stereotypical pattern and symptoms in the individual patient
- Associated with two or more of the following:
  - » Anorexia
  - » Nausea
  - » Vomiting
  - » Headache
  - » Photophobia
  - » Pallor
- After appropriate evaluation, symptoms cannot be fully explained by another medical condition

Assessment

Association of non-specific prodromal symptoms (behaviour or mood changes), photophobia and vasomotor symptoms and symptom relief with antimigraine therapy supports the diagnosis of abdominal migraine. Targeted investigations may be considered to exclude other organic causes:

- Abdominal ultrasound to evaluate for abdominal masses, cholelithiasis or renal abnormalities
- Upper gastrointestinal study to rule out malrotation
- Cranial imaging (indicated in those with recurrent headache and vomiting) to rule out space-occupying lesions and raised intracranial pressure

Management

- Avoidance of potential triggers
  - » Diet containing caffeine, amine and nitrite
  - » Prolonged fasting
  - » Altered sleep pattern
  - » Exposure to flickering/glaring lights
- Prophylactic pharmacotherapy
  - » Propranolol
  - » Cyproheptadine
  - » Sumatriptan/Amitriptyline
  - » Pizotifen

Functional Abdominal Pain: Not Otherwise Specified

This term substitutes what used to be known as 'functional abdominal pain' and 'functional abdominal pain syndrome'. There is no clear aetiology elicited for FAP-NOS. There is evidence for association between psychological distress and chronic abdominal pain in children and adolescents. This could be precipitated by stressful life events.

Diagnostic Criteria

Must be fulfilled at least four times per month for at least 2 months, and include all of the following:

- Episodic or continuous abdominal pain that does not occur solely during physiologic events (e.g. menses, eating)
- Insufficient criteria for IBS, functional dyspepsia or abdominal migraine
- After appropriate evaluation, abdominal pain cannot be fully explained by another medical condition

Assessment

It is important to take a detailed symptom and psychosocial history. Physical examination and growth parameters are expected to be normal. There is limited role for laboratory or radiological investigations for the non-specific and extra-intestinal symptoms reported. A limited diagnostic screen may be considered for parental reassurance.

Management

- Reassurance and explanation about pain due to visceral hypersensitivity
- Recording symptoms with pain diary
- Looking at possible psychosocial triggering factors

- Symptomatic relief (e.g. rubbing tummy with oil; analgesia, if more severe pain)
- Consider paediatric pain team referral for complex pain with significant impact on function not improving with usual analgesia

Bibliography

1. Hyams JS, Lorenzo C, Saps M, *et al.* (2016) Functional disorders: Children and adolescents. *Gastroenterology* S0016-5085(16)00181-5.
2. McFerron BA, Waseem S. (2012) Chronic recurrent abdominal pain. *Pediatr Rev* **33**(11):509–517.
3. Plunkett A, Beattie RM. (2005) Recurrent abdominal pain in childhood. *J R Soc Med* **98**(3):101–106.
4. Reust CE, Williams A. (2018) Recurrent abdominal pain in children. *Am Fam Physician* **97**(12):785–793.

CHAPTER 49

Vomiting

Ho Wen Wei, Christopher; Veena Logarajah

Introduction

Vomiting is a common, nonspecific symptom of a range of childhood illnesses, ranging from benign, self-limiting illnesses to severe, life-threatening conditions. Although vomiting can arise from many conditions in the gastrointestinal (GI) tract, it can also be a symptom from a more generalised systemic disorder.

Definition

Vomiting: Forceful oral expulsion of gastric contents, associated with contraction of the abdominal, diaphragmatic and chest wall musculature.

Nausea: The unpleasant sensation of the imminent need to vomit, usually referred to the throat or epigastrium; a sensation that may or may not ultimately lead to the act of vomiting.

Regurgitation: The act by which food is brought back into the mouth without the abdominal and diaphragmatic muscular activity that characterises vomiting.

Causes

Causes of vomiting can be categorised by organ system or age at presentation (see Table 13.4).

Approach

History

- Complete vomiting history: Onset, frequency, time frame, provoking or alleviating factors, characteristics of the vomit (amount, contents).
- Associated symptoms, e.g. fever, abdominal pain, diarrhoea or headache.
- Past medical history includes known or suspected congenital anomalies or diseases, developmental delay, neurologic symptoms or previous abdominal surgery.

Table 13.4 Causes of Vomiting

Gastrointestinal Causes	Non-gastrointestinal Causes
Gastrointestinal obstruction	**Neurologic**
Pyloric stenosis	Hydrocephalus
Malrotation with volvulus	Subdural hematoma
Intussusception	Intracranial haemorrhage
Intestinal duplication, stenosis or atresia	Intracranial mass
Antral or duodenal web	**Infectious**
Hirschsprung disease	Sepsis
Foreign body	Meningitis
Incarcerated hernia	Urinary tract infection
Superior mesenteric artery (SMA) syndrome	Pneumonia
Other gastrointestinal disorders	Otitis media
Gastroenteritis	Hepatitis
Gastroesophageal reflux	**Metabolic/endocrine**
Food protein-induced (e.g. anaphylaxis, food protein-induced enteropathy, food protein-induced enterocolitis syndrome)	Diabetic ketoacidosis Galactosaemia Hereditary fructose intolerance
Peptic ulcer disease	Urea cycle defects
Eosinophilic oesophagitis/gastroenteritis	Amino and organic acidaemias
Gastroparesis	Fatty acid oxidation disorders
Inflammatory bowel disease	Congenital adrenal hyperplasia
Appendicitis	**Cardiac**
Hepatobiliary disease	Heart failure
Pancreatitis	**Renal**
	Obstructive uropathy
	Renal insufficiency
	Toxic ingestion
	Drugs
	Lead
	Others
	Cyclical vomiting syndrome

- Feeding and dietary history, including volume of each feed, type of formula/ breastfeeding, time interval between feeds.
- Growth trajectory.
- Family medical history.
- Prior pharmacological and dietary interventions.
- Presence of alarm features (see Table 13.5).

Clinical Examination

The physical examination should include a general assessment of hydration status, detailed evaluation of the abdomen for signs of obstruction or focal tenderness, as well as a thorough neurologic assessment.

Investigations

Investigations to consider, based upon the history, physical examination and differential diagnosis of the symptoms (see Table 13.6).

Table 13.5 Alarm Features Indicating Need for Prompt Evaluation

Symptoms/signs	Remarks
Significant weight loss/poor growth Lethargy Excessive irritability/pain Onset of regurgitation/vomiting >6 mth and/or increasing/persisting >12–18 mth of age	Systemic infections, metabolic disorders, raised intracranial pressure
Bilious vomiting	Gastrointestinal obstruction, intestinal atresia or mid-gut volvulus or intussusception
Projectile vomiting	Hypertrophic pyloric stenosis (infants up to 2 mth old)
Haematemesis Haematochezia	Gastroesophageal reflux disease-associated, occurring from acid-peptic disease, Mallory–Weiss tear or reflux oesophagitis Bacterial gastroenteritis, inflammatory bowel disease, surgical conditions, allergic proctocolitis
Marked abdominal distension and tenderness/guarding	Indicative of obstruction, dysmotility or anatomic abnormalities
Bulging fontanelle/rapidly increasing head circumference Seizures Early morning vomiting Severe headache History of head trauma Focal neurologic abnormalities Bruising/physical signs of trauma	May suggest raised intracranial pressure due to, e.g. meningitis, intracranial bleed, brain tumour or hydrocephalus

Treatment

For most children with vomiting, no treatment is needed. In children at risk for dehydration and electrolyte abnormalities, the first step in managing vomiting should be clinical stabilisation with emphasis on the correction of fluid deficit and electrolyte abnormalities. Identification and correction of the primary problem is the next most important step.

Gastroesophageal Reflux and Gastroesophageal Reflux Disease

Reported symptoms of infant gastroesophageal reflux disease (GERD) vary widely and may include excessive crying, back arching, regurgitation and irritability, yet many of these symptoms occur in all babies, even those without GERD.

Definitions

Gastroesophageal reflux (GER): The passage of gastric contents into the oesophagus with or without regurgitation and vomiting.

Table 13.6 Investigations for Vomiting

Investigations	Remarks
Renal panel	Acute kidney injury from dehydration Electrolyte abnormalities seen in conditions such as pyloric stenosis, adrenal insufficiency, metabolic diseases
Full blood count	Anaemia may be associated with gastrointestinal obstruction, IBD, gastritis and peptic ulcer disease Leucocytosis is associated with bacterial infections and sepsis
Liver function tests	Elevated AST, ALT, total bilirubin and GGT are seen in liver and gallbladder disease
Amylase, lipase	Elevated in pancreatitis
Plasma amino acids, lactate, ammonia, urine organic acids, urine ketones, blood glucose	If suspecting metabolic disorder
Plain radiograph of the abdomen	If suspecting intestinal obstruction
Upper gastrointestinal contrast studies	If suspecting an anatomic abnormality of the upper gastrointestinal tract
Abdominal ultrasound	If suspecting pyloric stenosis or intussusception
Neuroimaging (CT/MRI)	If suspecting increased intracranial pressure
Endoscopy	If suspecting peptic ulcer disease, eosinophilic oesophagitis, IBD

ALT: alanine transaminase, AST: aspartate transaminase, CT: computed tomography, GGT: gamma-glutamyltransferase, IBD: inflammatory bowel disease, MRI: magnetic resonance imaging.

GERD: When GER leads to troublesome symptoms that affect daily functioning and/or complications, such as poor growth.

Refractory GERD: GERD not responding to optimal treatment after 8 weeks.

Management

Look for alarm features in history and clinical examination as above.

Infants with GER are commonly referred to as 'happy spitters' and do not require any acid suppressant therapy. Instead, reassurance should be provided to the family that physiologic reflux will peak at 4 months of age, and almost always resolves by a year of age. Parental education about the natural course of infantile GER is the key to successful management. Avoid unnecessary treatments of physiologic GER in infants.

Non-pharmacological therapy

- Modify feeding volumes and frequency according to age and weight to avoid overfeeding.
- Continue breastfeeding.

- Consider use of thickened feeds.
- Expressed breast milk can be thickened with commercial thickeners.
- 2- to 4-week trial of extensively hydrolysed protein-based (or amino-acid based) formula in infants suspected of GERD after optimal non-pharmacological treatment has failed.
- Transpyloric/jejunal feedings may be considered in refractory cases of GERD.

Pharmacological therapy

- Healthy infants do not benefit from medications.
- For treatment of typical symptoms (i.e. heartburn, retro-sternal or epigastric pain) in children with GERD, may consider a 4- to 8-week course of proton-pump inhibitors (PPI) or H_2 receptor antagonists (H2RAs).
- PPIs are helpful for treating irritation or injury related to acid exposure, not for reducing the regurgitation/vomiting.
- Domperidone, metoclopramide and other prokinetics are not recommended in the treatment of GERD in infants and children.

Surgery

- Anti-reflux surgery should only be considered in infants with GERD under certain circumstances.

Further Investigations

If symptoms do not improve or recur, additional testing should be considered to determine aetiology of symptoms. An oesophago-gastro-duodenoscopy (OGD) with biopsies and upper GI series can be considered to exclude anatomical abnormalities and exclude other causes by a histology of the biopsies.

OGD is useful:

- In the presence of red flag symptoms (e.g. haematemesis).
- To detect complications of GERD (e.g. strictures, Barrett oesophagus).
- To diagnose conditions that predispose to GERD (e.g. hiatal hernia).
- To diagnose conditions that might mimic GERD (e.g. eosinophilic oesophagitis, infectious oesophagitis)

Other investigations, such as pH-Impedance monitoring, can be considered to correlate persistent troublesome symptoms with acid and non-acid GER events.

Bilious Vomiting

Bilious vomiting in a neonate is concerning for intestinal obstruction and requires urgent attention. It can represent a proximal obstruction such as duodenal atresia, malrotation with volvulus, or a distal obstruction, such as Hirschsprung disease.

The first step in management is decompression with a nasogastric tube. This should be followed by correction of dehydration and any electrolyte abnormalities. An urgent surgical consult should be sought.

An abdominal radiograph can help localise the obstruction. Follow-up with an upper GI contrast study with or without a small-bowel follow-through is often warranted.

Referral for Further Evaluation

If symptoms are persistent or the cause of vomiting is uncertain, a referral should be made to the relevant sub-specialities (paediatric gastroenterologists, neurologists, metabolic team, endocrinologists, surgeons) for further evaluation and management.

Bibliography

1. Rosen R, Vandenplas Y, Singendonk M, *et al.* (2018) Pediatric gastroesophageal reflux clinical practice guidelines: Joint recommendations of the North American Society for Pediatric Gastroenterology, Hepatology, and Nutrition. *J Pediatr Gastroenterol Nutr* **66**(3):516–554.
2. Shields TM, Lightdale JR. (2018) Vomiting in children. *Pediatr Rev* **39**(7):342–358.
3. Di Lorenzo C. (2021) Approach to the infant or child with nausea and vomiting. *UpToDate*. https://www.uptodate.com/contents/approach-to-the-infant-or-child-with-nausea-and-vomiting

CHAPTER 50

Constipation

Goh Suk-Hui, Lynette; Phua Kong Boo

Introduction

Constipation is a common paediatric complaint presenting as a delay or difficulty in passing motion. It accounts for 3% of general paediatric outpatient consults and 25% of paediatric gastroenterology visits. The commonest cause beyond the neonatal period is functional constipation, which is constipation in the absence of any organic pathology.

Diagnostic Criteria of Functional Constipation

Functional constipation is defined, according to the Rome IV criteria, as follows:

Must include 1 month of at least two of the following

- 2 or fewer defecations in the toilet per week in a child of a developmental age of at least 4 years
- History of retentive posturing or excessive volitional stool retention
- History of painful or hard bowel movements
- Presence of a large faecal mass in the rectum
- History of large diameter stools that can obstruct the toilet
- At least one episode per week of incontinence after acquisition of toilet training

After appropriate evaluation, the symptoms cannot be fully explained by another medical condition.

Table 13.7 Differential Diagnosis of Constipation

Hypothyroidism, hypercalcaemia, hypokalaemia*
Cow's milk protein allergy*
Drugs — opiates, anticholinergics, antidepressants, lead poisoning
Botulism/hypotonia
Hypertonia
Hirschsprung disease*
Anorectal malformations — imperforate anus*
Pelvic mass (sacral teratoma)
Spinal cord anomalies, trauma, tethered cord, spina bifida, myelomeningocele*
Encephalopathy*
Abnormal abdominal musculature (prune belly, gastroschisis, Down syndrome)
Pseudo-obstruction (visceral neuropathies, myopathies)
Sexual abuse
Celiac disease*
Cystic fibrosis*
*More likely in the younger child

Table 13.8 Alarm Signs and Symptoms in Constipation

Constipation starting extremely early in life <48 h
Family history of Hirschsprung disease
Ribbon stools
Blood in the stools in the absence of anal fissures
Failure to thrive
Fever
Bilious vomiting
Abnormal thyroid gland
Severe abdominal distension
Perianal fistula
Abnormal position of anus
Absent anal or cremasteric reflex
Decreased lower extremity strength/tone/reflex
Tuft of hair on spine
Sacral dimple
Gluteal cleft deviation
Extreme fear during anal inspection
Anal scar

Pathophysiology

- Passage of hard and painful stool triggers an unpleasant experience and the child becomes fearful.
- Suppression of subsequent urge to defecate by contracting the anal sphincter and gluteal muscle.
- Withholding behaviour (rising on toes, fidgeting, stiffening back and legs) in order to avoid defecation may be seen, which is often mistaken for straining.
- Rectal mucosa absorbs water, making retained stools hard and more difficult to evacuate.
- Gradual increase in rectum size, resulting in impaction of hard stools, overflow incontinence, loss of rectal sensation and eventually loss of urge to defecate.

Evaluation

In most cases, a thorough history and examination is adequate in establishing whether constipation is functional or related to an organic cause requiring further investigations.

History

- Details of bowel history, including frequency and consistency of stools according to the Bristol stool chart (See Figure 13.1)
- Age of onset of constipation and potential trigger factors
- Associated symptoms, e.g. pain, bleeding, soiling, weight loss

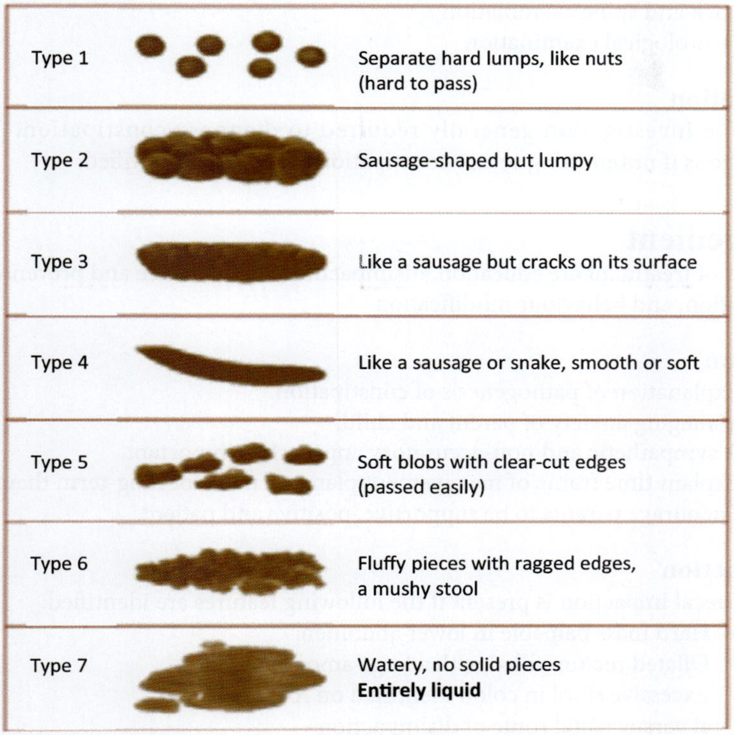

Figure 13.1 Bristol stool chart.

- Age of onset
- Toilet training/toilet habits
- Withholding behaviour
- Dietary history
- Family history
- Previous/current therapy
- Estimate of parent/patient adherence
- Development and school performance
- Psychosocial history
- Psychosocial disruption of child or family

Clinical Examination

- Growth parameters
- Abdomen signs, e.g. distension, faecal masses, organomegaly
- Anal inspection, e.g. position, skin tags, fissures, soiling, perianal erythema
- Rectal examination: Not needed to be done routinely

- Back and spine examination
- Neurological examination

Investigation

No routine investigation generally required to diagnose constipation. Targeted investigations if unremitting severe constipation or red flags identified.

Management

Principles of treatment are education, disimpaction, maintenance and prevention of re-accumulation, and behaviour modification.

Education

- Explanation of pathogenesis of constipation.
- Managing anxiety of parent and child.
- A sympathetic and non-accusatory approach is important.
- Explain time frame of management plan and need for long-term therapy.
- Encourage parents to be supportive, positive and patient.

Disimpaction

- Faecal impaction is present if the following features are identified:
  - » Hard mass palpable in lower abdomen.
  - » Dilated rectum filled with a large amount of stool.
  - » Excessive stool in colon identified on X-ray.
- Oral versus rectal route of disimpaction
  - » Rectal route faster but INVASIVE.
  - » Oral route may have issues with non-compliance.

Maintenance

- Prevention of recurrence of faecal impaction.
- Well-balanced diet, adequate fluid intake.
- Use of medications to achieve regular bowel movements.
- Medication to be tailed down slowly and not stopped abruptly.

Behavioural Modification

- Encourage child to sit on toilet for 5–10 min after meals.
- Advice on proper positioning and foot support.
- Stool diary.
- Rewards system.

Table 13.9 Oral Laxatives

Osmotic Laxatives	Stimulant Laxatives
Lactulose 1–2 ml/kg, 1–2 times daily	Bisacodyl 3–10 yr: 5 mg/d; >10 yr: 5–10 mg/d
Macrogol 1–1.5 g/kg/d for disimpaction; 0.4–0.8 g/kg/d for maintenance	Senna 2–6 yr: 2.5–5 mg once to twice daily; 6–12 yr: 7.5–10 mg/d; >12 yr: 15–20 mg/d

Indications to refer to Specialist Care

- Children in whom aggressive bowel clearance needs to be considered
- Presence of significant behavioural/psychosocial problems impacting on the management
- Failure to respond to a high dose of laxatives
- Persistent soiling despite laxatives
- Structural/physical causes are suspected
- Poor growth/nutritional status
- Presence of anal fissure/rectal prolapse if there is failure to be cured by a reasonable course of laxatives (~3 months)

Bibliography

1. Hyams JS, Di Lorenzo C, Saps M, *et al.* (2016) Functional disorders: Children and adolescents. *Gastroenterology* S0016-5085(16)00181-5.
2. Tabbers MM, Di Lorenzo C, Berger MY, *et al.* (2014) Evaluation and treatment of functional constipation in infants and children: Evidence-based recommendations from ESPGHAN and NASPGHAN. *J Pediatr Gastroenterol Nutr* **58**(2):258–274.
3. Lewis SJ, Heaton KW. (1997) Stool form scale as a useful guide to intestinal transit time. *Scand J Gastroenterol* **32**(9):920–924.

CHAPTER 51

Acute Gastroenteritis

Ho Wen Wei, Christopher; Phua Kong Boo

Introduction

Acute gastroenteritis is defined as a decrease in the consistency of stools (loose or liquid) and/or an increase in the frequency of evacuations (typically >3 in 24 hours), with or without fever or vomiting. Acute diarrhoea typically lasts <7 days and not >14 days. Transmission is usually via faecal–oral route.

In Singapore, rotavirus is the most common pathogen causing gastroenteritis in children. Norovirus is also a leading cause of medically attended gastroenteritis in countries with high rotavirus vaccine coverage. Occasionally, children may have bacteria dysentery or, very rarely, protozoal disease, which may need specific antimicrobial therapy (see Table 13.10).

It is important to establish if there were any foreign travel or contact history. Recent antibiotic ingestion in an unwell child may suggest *Clostridium difficile* infection. Immunocompromised children are at risk of infection with more unusual organisms.

Table 13.10 Infective Causes of Acute Gastroenteritis

Viral	Bacterial	Intestinal Parasites
Rotavirus Calicivirus, e.g. Norovirus Astrovirus	*Salmonella* species *Campylobacter jejuni* *Escherichia coli* *Shigella* species *Yersinia enterocolitica* *Clostridium difficile*	*Giardia lambia* *Entamoeba histolytica* *Cryptosporidium*

Clinical Presentation

- Watery diarrhoea
- Dysentery (more likely in bacterial infection)
- Vomiting
- Fever
- Abdominal cramps
- Dehydration
- Electrolyte imbalance
- Upper respiratory tract signs may be present

Risk Factors for Severe or Persistent Diarrhoea

- Younger age (<6 months)
- Feeding practices — predominant breast feeding reduces the severity of acute gastroenteritis
- Underlying chronic disease/immunodeficiency:
  - » Children with immunodeficiency may have prolonged disease
  - » Children with malnutrition or immunodeficiency are at risk of persistent parasitic diarrhoea
  - » Children with inflammatory bowel disease (IBD) and oncology patients have a higher risk of *C. Difficile*

Differential Diagnoses

There are many possible differential diagnoses, which include other non-gastrointestinal infections, non-infective pathology of the gut or other systemic illnesses. Important differential diagnoses include:

- Surgical causes: Intussusception, appendicitis, partial intestinal obstruction, Hirschsprung associated enterocolitis, toxic megacolon
- Other infections: Urinary tract infection, upper respiratory tract infection, meningitis, staphylococcal toxic shock syndrome
- Haemolytic uremic syndrome
- IBD
- Food intolerance: Excessive fructose or sorbitol, lactose intolerance, food allergy
- Endocrinopathy: Congenital adrenal hyperplasia, hyperthyroidism
- Immunodeficiency
- Drugs/toxins: Antibiotic-associated diarrhoea, laxatives, organophosphates

Approach

A careful history and thorough physical examination is important for diagnosis (see Figure 13.2).

The key issues to address are:

- Evaluation of dehydration
- Rehydration strategies
- Oral refeeding
- Medications

Evaluation of Dehydration

Dehydration can be identified by various clinical parameters (see Table 13.11).

- Prolonged capillary refill time >2 seconds, tachycardia, absence of tears and abnormal respiratory pattern are reliable signs of dehydration.
- An active child with normal capillary refill time and moist mucous membrane is unlikely to have severe dehydration.

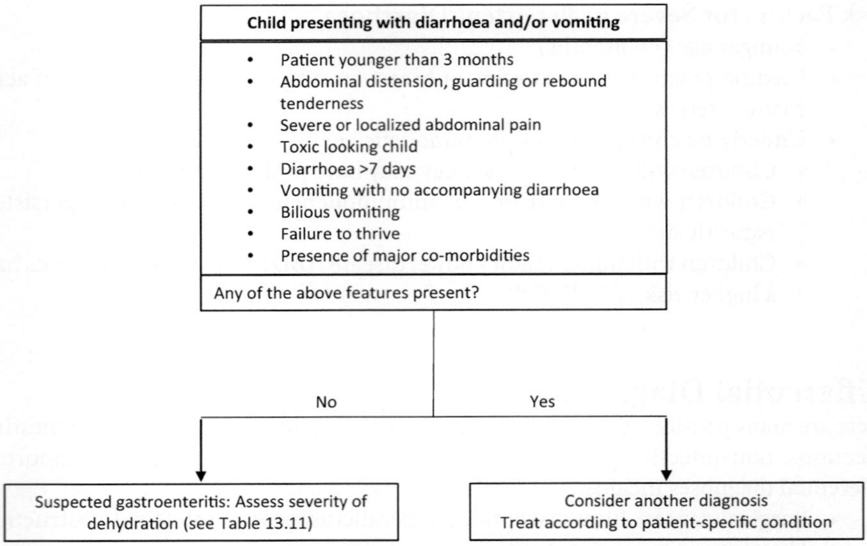

Figure 13.2 Suggested pathway on the management of acute gastroenteritis.

Table 13.11 Assessment of Hydration Status

	Mild Dehydration (3–5%)	Moderate Dehydration (6–9%)	Severe Dehydration (>10%)
General Condition	Alert, thirsty	Thirsty, restless or lethargy/irritable	Drowsy, floppy, unconscious
Eye	Normal	Sunken	Very sunken and dry
Tears	Present	Absent	Absent
Mouth/ Tongue	Moist	Dry	Very dry
Capillary Refill	Normal	Prolonged >2 sec	Prolonged >2 sec
Skin Turgor	Instant recoil	Recoil in >2 sec	Recoil in >2 sec
Skin	Normal	Normal	Cold and clammy, mottled
Fontanelle	Normal	Sunken	Very sunken
Urine	Normal	Reduced amount	Anuria/severe oliguria
Pulse rate	Normal rate and volume	Rapid and weak	Rapid and feeble
Blood Pressure	Normal	Normal/low	Low/unrecordable
Respiration	Normal	Deep/maybe rapid	Deep and rapid
Weight loss	3–5%	6–9%	≥10%

- If unsure which category of dehydration patient falls under, therapy for the more severe category should be used.

Investigations

There is usually **no need** for any investigation if the child is clinically well with normal hydration status.

For patients with moderate or severe dehydration, investigations include:

- Renal panel for electrolytes, urea, creatinine, acid/base status
- Stool culture, stool virology, particularly, rotavirus as indicated
- Septic workup if indicated

Rehydration Strategies (See Figure 13.3)

- Enteral rehydration
  - » Enteral rehydration using oral rehydration solution (ORS) is preferred in children with mild to moderate dehydration (See Table 13.12 for composite of available ORS).
- Intravenous (IV) hydration
  - » IV therapy is indicated if a child has severe dehydration (10%) or is in shock. IV bolus of crystalloid 20 ml/kg (normal saline) should be given. If the patient does not respond to rapid bolus rehydration, consider the possibility of an underlying disorder such as septic shock, toxic shock syndrome, myocarditis, cardiomyopathy or pericarditis. Use of colloids and inotropes should be considered.
  - » In children with moderate dehydration, IV fluids are indicated if the child cannot retain oral liquids due to persistent vomiting. It is also important to correct for fluid deficit (see Table 13.13).

Diet

- Allow usual age-appropriate diet/feeds in child with no or mild dehydration.
- For infants and toddlers, one may supplement with ORS for rehydration.
- If child is not vomiting, give usual milk formula, breast milk or solid foods.
- If requiring IV hydration, early resumption of oral feeding is recommended.
- Avoid fatty or fried foods.
- Limit use of simple sugars (especially fruit juices, carbonated drinks).
- Lactose-free feeds should not be routinely used, but can be considered in cases with prolonged symptoms and secondary lactose intolerance.

Medications

- Most bacterial gastroenteritis **does not need antibiotics** except for bacterial dysentery or protozoal disease. Antibiotics may be indicated for the very young (<3 months old), immunocompromised or septic patients (see Table 13.14).

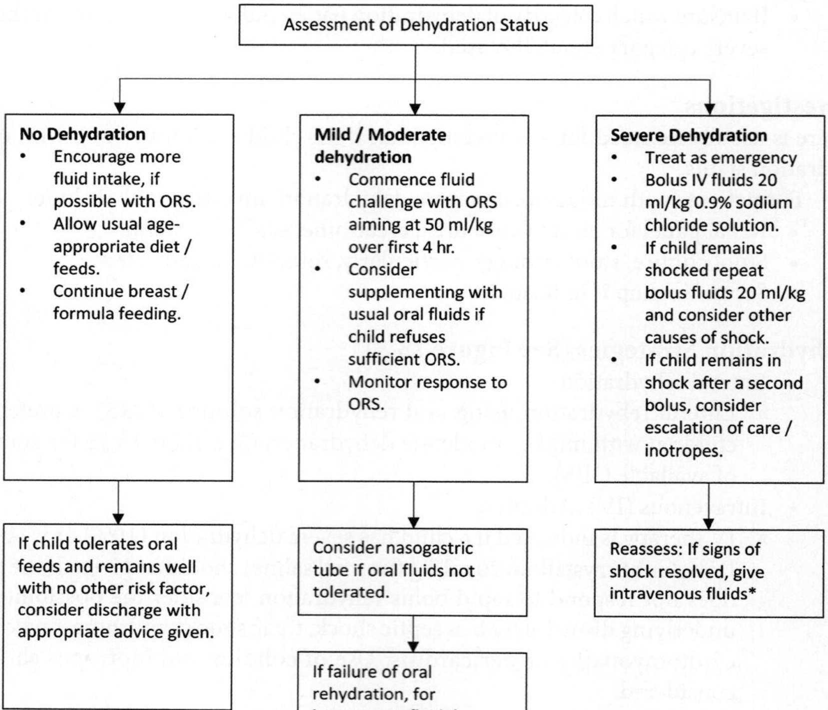

*Intravenous therapy for dehydration

- Standard intravenous fluid orders according to age:
  <1 month old — 10% dextrose + 2–4 mmol/kg/d of sodium
  1 to 3 month old — 5% dextrose + 0.45% sodium chloride
  >3 month old — 5% dextrose + 0.9% sodium chloride
- Measure plasma sodium, potassium, urea, creatinine and glucose at the start.
- Consider intravenous potassium supplementation when serum potassium level is normal or low and child has passed urine.
- During intravenous replacement attempt to introduce ORS early and gradually, if tolerated, stop IV and continue with ORS.

Figure 13.3 Rehydration strategy.

Table 13.12 Composition of Available ORS

Per Litre	*Hydralyte*	WHO Recommendation
Sodium (mmol)	55	75
Potassium (mmol)	20	15–25
Chloride (mmol)	45	50–80
Citrate (mmol)	30	8–12
Dextrose (mmol)	80	75
Osmolality (mOsmol/kg)	~240	245

Table 13.13 Intravenous Fluid Calculation

Calculating Maintenance Fluids in Patients	
<10 kg	100 ml/kg/d or 4 ml/kg/hr
10–20 kg	1000 ml + 50 ml/kg/d for each kg over 10 kg or 40 ml/hr + 2 ml/kg/hr for each kg over 10 kg
>20 kg	1500 ml + 20 ml/kg/d for each kg over 20 kg or 60 ml/hr + 1 ml/kg/hr for each kg over 20 kg
Calculating Fluid Deficit	
Body weight × % dehydration = Deficit in litres — E.g. 10 kg child, 3% dehydration → 10 × 0.03 = 0.3 L = 300 ml deficit Fluid used for rehydration is the same as maintenance fluids. Rehydration should be carried out evenly over at least 24–48 hr *— E.g. (1) 20 kg child, 5% dehydration* *Maintenance: 1500 ml/d, Deficit: 20 × 0.05 = 1 L = 1000 ml* *Therefore, prescribe 2500 ml/d for first 24 hr, 1500 ml/d thereafter* *— E.g. (2) 20 kg child, 10% dehydration* *Maintenance: 1500 ml/d, Deficit: 20 × 0.1 = 2 L = 2000 ml* *To replace the fluid deficit over 48 hr: deficit + 2 d of daily fluid maintenance* *Fluid requirement over 48 hr: 2000 ml + (1500 × 2) ml = 5000 ml over 48 hr* *Therefore prescribe (2000/2) ml + 1500 ml = 2500 ml over 24 hr for 2 d*	

- Trial of ondansetron (oral) at presentation can be considered for management of vomiting, other antiemetics are not recommended.
- Probiotics generally reduce the duration of diarrhoea by approximately one day. Options include Lactobacillus rhamnosus GG (LactoGG®), BioGaia® Oil Drops/Tablets and Vivomixx®.
- Use of adsorbents such as Diosmectite (Smecta) and anti-secretory agents such as Racecadotril may be considered, but evidence of efficacy is poor.
- Antimotility agents such as Lomotil (Diphenoxlylate) or Imodium (loperamide) are potentially harmful and should be avoided.

Table 13.14 Bacterial Pathogens and Recommended Treatments

Pathogen	Indication for Treatment	First-line Therapy	Alternative Therapy	Duration (days)
Shigella	Culture proven dysentery	PO Bactrim (TMP) 10 mg/kg/d Q12H OR IV/IM Ceftriaxone 100 mg/kg/d Q12-24H	PO Azithromycin 20 mg/kg/ dose ×1 (max. 1 g), followed by 10 mg/kg/d Q24H (max. 500 mg)	14 (Ceftriaxone, Bactrim) 7 (Azithromycin) IV to PO switch: after 2d & patient better
Salmonella	High risk children: Age <3 mth, immunodeficiency, toxic looking, haemoglobinopathy, malignancy, chronic GI tract disease.	IV/IM Ceftriaxone 100 mg/kg/d Q12-24H	PO/IV Bactrim (TMP) 10 mg/kg/d Q12H OR PO Azithromycin 10 mg/kg/d Q24H	14 (Ceftriaxone, Bactrim) 7 (Azithromycin) IV to PO switch: after 2d & patient better
Campylobacter	Culture proven dysentery	PO Erythromycin 50 mg/kg/d Q6H OR PO Clarithromycin 15 mg/kg/d Q12H	PO Azithromycin 10 mg/kg/d Q24H	7–10 (Erythromycin, Clarithromycin) 3 (Azithromycin)
Escherichia coli	None	None	—	—

Adapted from KKH Paediatrics Antibiotic Guidelines, Mar 2021 and Whyte LA, *et al.* (2015) Guidelines for the management of acute gastroenteritis in children. Arch Dise Child Educ Pract Ed 100(6).

Bibliography

1. Holliday MA, Segar WE. (1957) The maintenance need for water in parenteral fluid therapy. *Pediatrics* **19**(5):823–832.
2. Sandhu BK; European Society of Pediatric Gastroenterology, Hepatology and Nutrition Working Group on Acute Diarrhoea. (2001) Practical guidelines for the management of gastroenteritis in children. *J Pediatr Gastroenterol Nutr* **33**(2):S36–S39.
3. Elliott EJ. (2007) Acute gastroenteritis in children. *BMJ* **334**(7583):35–40.
4. Whyte LA, Al-Araji RA, McLoughlin LM. (2015) Guidelines for the management of acute gastroenteritis in children in Europe. *Arch Dis Child Educ Pract Ed* **100**(6):308–312.
5. Guarino A, Ashkenazi S, Gendrel D, *et al.* (2014) European Society for Pediatric Gastroenterology, Hepatology and Nutrition/European Society for Pediatric Infectious Disease evidence-based guidelines for the management of acute gastroenteritis in children in Europe: Update 2014. *J Pediatr Gastroenterol Nutr* **59**(1):132–152.

CHAPTER 52

Chronic Diarrhoea

Ng Lay Queen; Phua Kong Boo

Definition

Diarrhoea refers to the passage of excessively liquid or frequent stools with increased water content. This would result in stool output of >10 g/kg/day or >200 g/24 hours. Chronic diarrhoea refers to diarrhoea that has persisted for >2 weeks.

Causes

- Enteric Infections
  - » Bacterial: *Shigella*, *Campylobacter*, *Salmonella*, etc.
  - » Parasitic: *Giardia*, *Cryptosporidium*, *Amoeba*
  - » Viruses: Rotavirus, Adenovirus
- Post-enteritis Syndrome
  - » Common cause of persistent diarrhoea in childhood.
  - » Diagnosis is established on the following grounds:
    - ■ History of an acute gastroenteritis
    - ■ Identification of a specific pathogen if possible
    - ■ History of diarrhoea persisting after 2 weeks
  - » Following gastroenteritis, carbohydrate intolerance may occur, e.g. lactose intolerance. This may lead to osmotic diarrhoea, which usually responds well to the removal of the offending carbohydrate.
- Chronic non-specific diarrhoea (toddler's diarrhoea)
  - » Usually associated with passing large amount of loose, often explosive stools with undigested food particles seen in the stools.
  - » Growth parameters usually normal and child is well otherwise.
  - » Occurs secondary to absorptive capacity of intestine overwhelmed by excessive sugar consumption.
  - » May be associated with high intake of fruit juice or low dietary fat.
- Enteropathies
  - » Cow's Milk or Soy Protein Allergy
    - ■ Common cause of chronic diarrhoea.
    - ■ Symptoms usually occur before 6 months of age.
    - ■ Associated manifestations: Bloody diarrhoea, anaemia, protein losing enteropathy, extraintestinal manifestations of atopy.

- » Inflammatory Bowel Disease (IBD)
    - ■ Chronic autoimmune inflammatory disease of the intestinal tract with rising incidence in paediatric patients.
    - ■ Two major types: Ulcerative colitis and Crohn's disease, depending on the area of gastrointestinal tract involvement.
    - ■ Those diagnosed under 6 years of age are categorised under Very Early Onset (VEO-IBD), with distinct characteristics and frequent overlapping immune deficiencies.
    - ■ Extra-intestinal findings: Joint involvement, uveitis, skin rash (pyoderma gangrenosum/erythema nodosum).
    - ■ Aetiology: Multifactorial (diet, infections, environmental triggers, genetics).
- Immunodeficiency
- Coeliac disease
- Eosinophilic gastrointestinal disease (i.e. eosinophilic enteritis/eosinophilic colitis)
- Intraluminal causes
    - » Bacterial overgrowth
    - » Bile salt deficiency or malabsorption (liver cirrhosis, cholestasis, terminal ileum disease)
    - » Pancreatic insufficiency (cystic fibrosis, Shwachman–Diamond syndrome)
- Congenital disorders
    - » Glucose-galactose malabsorption
    - » Tufting enteropathy
    - » Congenital microvillous syndrome
    - » Deficiency of disaccharidases
    - » Congenital chloride-losing diarrhoea
    - » Congenital sodium-losing diarrhoea
- Surgical causes
    - » Short gut syndrome
    - » Intestinal blind loop — bacterial overgrowth
- Hyperthyroidism
- Acrodermatitis enteropathica
- Intestinal lymphangiectasia
- Abetalipoproteinaemia
- Vasoactive Intestinal Peptide (VIP) producing tumour
- Lymphoma
- Vasculitis — Systemic lupus erythematosus, Henoch-Schonlein purpura
- Drug-induced — Antibiotics, laxatives, etc.

Table 13.15 Pathophysiology

	Mechanism	Characteristics	Stool Osmolar Gap (Formula: 290 – 2 × [(Na+) + (K+)])	Examples
Osmotic Diarrhoea	Occurs secondary to the presence of non-absorbable solutes in the gastrointestinal tract, usually malabsorption of carbohydrates. This will generate an osmotic load causing water to be secreted into the lumen.	Large volume, watery stools Resolves with fasting	>100 mmol/L	Lactose intolerance Laxative use/abuse (lactulose, polyethylene glycol) Lactase deficiency Glucose-galactose malabsorption
Secretory Diarrhoea	Occurs when there is excess of secretion over absorption. It is caused by the activation of intracellular mediators, such as Cyclic Adenosine Monophosphate (cAMP), which stimulate chloride secretion and inhibit neutral coupled sodium chloride absorption.	Large volume, watery stools Persists with fasting	<100 mmol/L	Cholera Enterotoxigenic *Escherichia coli* *Clostridium difficile* Vasoactive peptide
Mucosal injury/insult	Occurs most commonly due to inflammation, leading to decreased absorptive ability.	Blood and mucus often present in stool	Not routinely done	Infectious enteritis, Inflammatory bowel disease or Allergic enterocolitis
Loss of absorptive surface	Occurs due to decreased functional capacity or due to major anatomical abnormalities.	Large volume watery stools	Not routinely done	Short gut syndrome (congenital or acquired), Coeliac disease
Intestinal dysmotility	2 mechanism types: — Increased motility leading to decreased absorption — Decreased motility affecting bacterial stasis	Rapid transit time Slow transit time	Not routinely done	Irritable bowel syndrome, Thyrotoxicosis Small intestine bacterial overgrowth

Approach

A thorough history and complete physical examination are essential in the evaluation of chronic diarrhoea.

History

- Characteristics of stools
  - » Stool frequency, including age/time of onset and duration
  - » Stool volume
  - » Stool appearance and consistency: Watery (osmotic or secretory diarrhoea); greasy (pancreatic insufficiency, cystic fibrosis); presence of blood or mucus (IBD, allergic colitis, infectious)
  - » Nocturnal stooling: likely organic disease
- Pertinent associated symptoms
  - » Abdominal pain, bloating, flatulence
  - » Urgency, tenesmus
  - » Weight loss or loss of appetite
  - » Vomiting
  - » Extraintestinal manifestations: Fever, rashes, joint pains, oral ulcers
- Dietary and medication history
- Past history of bowel surgery
- Family history of bowel disease
- Recurrent infections
- Systemic illness/autoimmune conditions (e.g. hyperthyroidism, vasculitis, etc.)

Clinical Examination

This would include anthropometric measurement taking into context family growth data. Puberty should be assessed in older children.

A complete physical examination is essential, including a nutritional assessment checking subcutaneous fat mass and muscle bulk. Abdominal exam to focus on signs of distention, ascites and organomegaly. Perianal examination should be performed to exclude perianal excoriation, rectal prolapse or perianal signs of Crohn's disease (skin tags, fissures, fistula openings).

Investigations

- Stool tests
  - » Stool calprotectin
  - » Stool culture, gastrointestinal polymerase chain reaction panel, *Clostridium difficile* toxins, stool parasite microscopy, fungal microscopy
  - » Malabsorption workup: Stool pH (carbohydrate malabsorption); stool fat globules, stool elastase (fat malabsorption); stool alpha-1-antitrypsin (protein malabsorption)
- Blood tests
  - » Full blood count and erythrocyte sedimentation rate
  - » Renal panel and serum glucose
  - » Serum albumin and total protein
- Endoscopy and Imaging
  - » Gastroscopy and colonoscopy allows for direct visualisation of the gastrointestinal mucosal lining. It is indicated to rule out mucosal aetiologies such as enteropathies, IBD.

    - » Newer imaging modalities, including Magnetic Resonance Enterography (MRE) and Video Capsule Endoscopy, allow for more comprehensive evaluation of the small intestines.
- Other Investigations to detect specific disease:
    - » Immune status to assess for immunodeficiency
    - » Stool electrolytes and osmolarity
    - » Evaluate for secretory tumour with urine Vanillylmandelic Acid (VMA) and serum VIP
    - » Hydrogen breath test or duodenal fluid to check for bacterial overgrowth
    - » Coeliac disease: Serum IgA levels, Anti-tissue transglutaminase (Ttg) IgA
    - » Sweat test for cystic fibrosis
    - » Serum zinc level

Management

Mainstay of initial management is focused on hydration and evaluation for an aetiology. Dietary modifications and medications (anti-diarrhoeals/anti-motility/anti-microbials) are unique to each case and dependent on the eventual aetiology.

Bibliography

1. Thomas PD, Forbes A, Green J, *et al.* (2003). Guidelines for the investigation of chronic diarrhoea, 2nd edition. *Gut* **52**(5) v1–15.
2. Binder HJ. (2006). Causes of chronic diarrhea. *N Eng J Med* **355**(3):236–239.
3. Zella GC, Israel EJ. (2012) Chronic diarrhea in children. *Pediatr Rev* **33**(5):207–217.
4. Thiagarajah JR, Kamin DS, Acra S, *et al.* (2018). Advances in evaluation of chronic diarrhea in infants. *Gastroenterology* **154**(8):2045–2059.e6.

CHAPTER 53

Prolonged Jaundice

Goh Suk-Hui, Lynette; Chiou Fang Kuan

Prolonged jaundice is defined by hyperbilirubinaemia that persists beyond 14 days of life in a term infant or beyond 21 days of life in a preterm infant.

The following should be performed:

- Inspect stools: Look for pale chalky stools and/or dark urine that stains the nappy.
- Investigations: Direct bilirubin (or liver function test [LFT]), thyroid function test (TFT), full blood count, urine culture
- Check blood group and previous routine metabolic screen

If the patient has pale stools and/or conjugated hyperbilirubinaemia (conjugated fraction >15% or direct bilirubin >20 μmol/L), the patient needs to be referred to the paediatric gastroenterologist as soon as possible.

Unconjugated Hyperbilirubinaemia

The most common cause of prolonged unconjugated jaundice is breast milk jaundice. It peaks around the second week and may persist for up to 3 months. Current guidelines advocate the continuation of breastfeeding. Although cessation of breastfeeding for 1–2 days may be useful in confirming the diagnosis, nursing should be resumed as soon as possible.

Pathological causes of unconjugated hyperbilirubinaemia include hypothyroidism, haemolytic disease (e.g. G6PD deficiency, hereditary spherocytosis) and inherited syndromes such as Crigler–Najjar syndrome and Gilbert Syndrome.

Conjugated Hyperbilirubinaemia

Conjugated hyperbilirubinaemia is **always pathological**. It is defined by conjugated bilirubin fraction >15% or direct bilirubin >20 μmol/L. All infants who present with prolonged jaundice must have their direct bilirubin levels checked and stools inspected.

Important causes of conjugated hyperbilirubinaemia to consider:

- Structural: Biliary atresia (BA), choledochal cyst
- Infections: Intra-uterine infections (TORCH), urinary tract infection, neonatal sepsis
- Metabolic: Inborn errors of metabolism (e.g. galactosaemia, urea cycle defects, tyrosinaemia, neonatal haemochromatosis, alpha-1-antitrypsin deficiency
- Endocrinopathy: Hypothyroidism, hypopituitarism
- Toxic: Drugs, parenteral nutrition

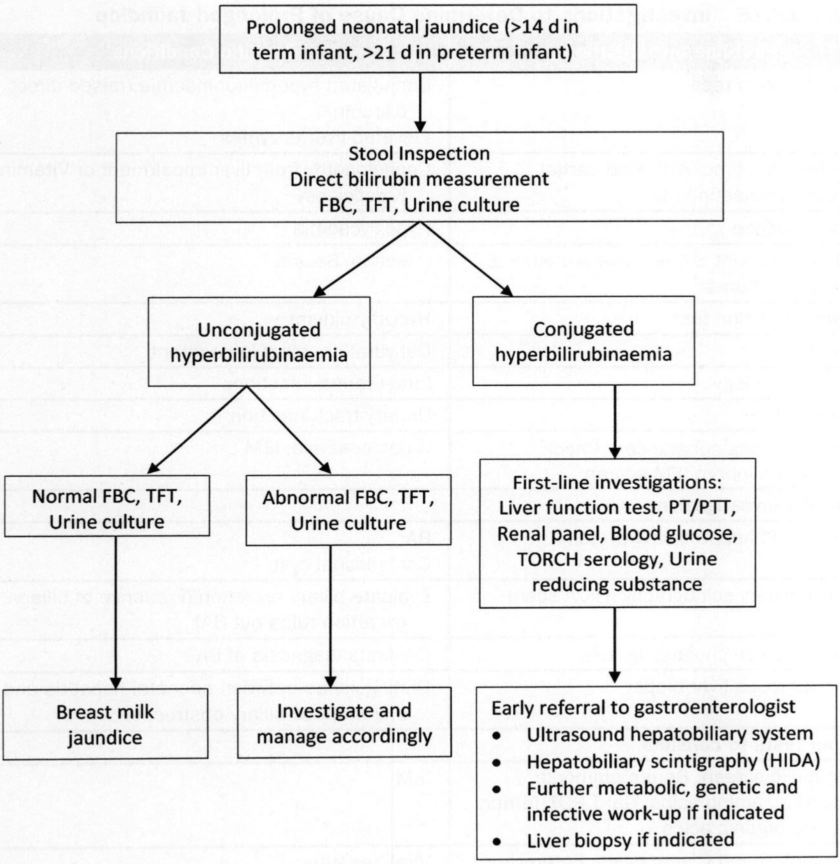

Figure 13.4 Suggest approach to prolonged neonatal jaundice.

FBC: Full blood count; TFT: Thyroid function test; PT/PTT: Prothrombin time/Activated partial thromboplastin time

- Haematologic: Haemophagocytic lymphohistiocytosis (HLH)
- Familial: Alagille syndrome, progressive familiar intrahepatic cholestatic (PFIC) syndromes
- Idiopathic neonatal hepatitis

If conjugated hyperbilirubinaemia is confirmed, the infant should be referred to the gastroenterologist for further evaluation. It is important to rule out BA as early surgical intervention (before 60 days of life) is associated with better outcome.

Biliary Atresia

BA is a rare condition characterised by progressive fibrosis and obliteration of the extra- and intra-hepatic biliary system. The pathogenesis is unknown. Anatomically, BA can be classified into the following types:

Table 13.16 Investigations to Determine Cause of Prolonged Jaundice

First-line Investigations	Specific Conditions
Liver function test	Conjugated hyperbilirubinaemia (raised direct bilirubin) Elevated liver enzymes
Prothrombin time/Activated partial thromboplastin time	Coagulopathy from liver impairment or Vitamin K deficiency
Blood glucose	Hypoglycaemia
Full blood count ± C-reactive protein P ± blood cultures	Infection/Sepsis
Thyroid function test	Hypothyroidism
Renal panel	Dehydration, renal impairment
TORCH serology	Intra-uterine infections
Urine culture	Urinary tract infection
Urine reducing substance + Check previous inborn IEM screen	Galactosaemia, IEM
Specific investigations	
Ultrasound hepatobiliary system	BA Choledochal cyst
Hepatobiliary scintigraphy (HIDA scan)	Evaluate biliary excretion (Presence of biliary excretion rules out BA)
Intraoperative cholangiography	Confirms diagnosis of BA
Percutaneous liver biopsy	Distinguishes between neonatal hepatitis and extrahepatic biliary obstruction
Other tests to consider	
Metabolic screen: Serum ammonia, lactate, amino acids, Gal-1-PUT, ferritin, urine organic acids	IEM
Hepatitis B and C serologies, Enterovirus, Parvovirus, HHV-6	Viral hepatitis
Serum alpha-1-antitrypsin and phenotype	Alpha-1-antitrypsin deficiency
Serum triglyceride, fibrinogen, ferritin	Neonatal haemophagocytic lymphohistiocytosis

IEM: inborn errors of metabolism; BA: biliary atresia

- Type 1: Atresia of the common bile duct
- Type 2: Atresia of the common hepatic duct, common bile duct and gallbladder
- Type 3 (commonest): Atresia of right, left and common hepatic ducts, with the dysplastic gallbladder

The child with BA presents with prolonged jaundice, acholic stools and dark urine. Hepatomegaly is usually present, while splenomegaly is a late sign. Occasionally, infants may present with bleeding due to vitamin K deficiency. LFT will show conjugated hyperbilirubinaemia, associated with raised gamma glutamyl transferase (GGT) and alkaline phosphatase (ALP). Hepatobiliary ultrasonography may demonstrate an enlarged liver and absent or irregularly shaped gallbladder. Hepatobiliary scintigraphy (HIDA scan) following phenobarbitone priming for 3 to 5 days shows good hepatic uptake but absent excretion into the intestine.

The diagnosis is confirmed at surgery with or without cholangiography where the atretic biliary tree is evident. Kasai portoenterostomy is the surgical procedure that aims to re-establish bile drainage into the intestines. Early surgery within 60 days of life is associated with a better outcome in terms of jaundice clearance and native liver survival. Medical management after surgery is focused on prevention and treatment of ascending cholangitis, optimising nutrition and provision of fat-soluble vitamin supplementation. Ursodeoxycholic acid may be effective in encouraging bile drainage. The role of corticosteroids in BA remains controversial as current evidence has been inconclusive.

BA patients will require long-term follow-up to monitor for complications of liver cirrhosis and portal hypertension.

Bibliography

1. National Institute for Health and Care Excellence. (2010) Jaundice in newborn babies under 28 days. Clinical Guideline No. 98. https://www.nice.org.uk/guidance/cg98
2. Lauer BJ, Spector ND. (2011) Hyperbilirubinemia in the newborn. *Pediatr Rev* **32**(8):341–349.
3. Venigalla S, Gourley GR. (2004) Neonatal cholestasis. *Semin Perinatol* **28**(5):348–355.
4. Kelly DA, Davenport M. (2007) Current management of biliary atresia. *Arch Dis Child* **92**(12):1132–1135.

CHAPTER 54

Gastrointestinal Haemorrhage

Ho Wen Wei, Christopher; Chiou Fang Kuan

Introduction

Gastrointestinal (GI) bleeding in paediatrics is a common problem that occurs due to various causes at different ages. The initial approach to all patients with significant GI bleeding is to ensure patient stability, establish adequate oxygen delivery, place intravenous (IV) access, initiate fluid and blood resuscitation, and correct any underlying coagulopathies.

GI bleeds are classified into:

- Upper GI bleeding (UGIB) is defined as blood loss proximal to the ligament of Treitz in the distal duodenum. May present as haematemesis, coffee-ground vomitus, melaena or haematochezia from a rapid transit of blood through the intestinal tract.
- Lower GI bleeding (LGIB) is defined as bleeding distal to the ligament of Treitz. May present as haematochezia or melaena (small bowel).

Table 13.17 Common Causes of Gastrointestinal Bleeding on Age and Location

Age Group	Upper Gastrointestinal Bleeding	Lower Gastrointestinal Bleeding
Neonates	Swallowed maternal blood Gastroesophageal reflux Stress gastritis Medication induced	Swallowed maternal blood Anal fissures Necrotising enterocolitis Haemorrhagic disease of the newborn Malrotation with volvulus Hirschsprung disease
1 mth to 1 yr	Oesophagitis — Due to GERD Gastritis and Gastroduodenal ulcer NSAID-induced ulcer Foreign body ingestion Mallory Weiss tears Oesophageal varices Dieulafoy's lesions (gastric vascular anomaly)	Anal fissures Allergic colitis (cow's milk) Bacterial enteritis Intussusception Meckel's diverticulum Polyps Ischaemic bowel
2 yr and older	Mallory Weiss tears Oesophageal varices Gastritis and Gastroduodenal ulcer Dieulafoy's lesions (gastric vascular anomaly)	Anal Fissures Bacterial enteritis Inflammatory bowel disease Juvenile Polyps and Vascular lesions Henoch-Schonlein Purpura

Aetiologies

Common Causes of GI Bleeding in Neonates

- UGIB
  - Maternal blood ingestion — Apt tests differentiate between maternal and faetal haemoglobin (Hb).
  - Stress gastritis is seen mainly in neonates in the neonatal intensive care unit; drugs like steroids and nonsteroidal anti-inflammatory drugs (NSAIDs) used in their care are often the offending agents. They are rarely of large volume.
- LGIB
  - Anorectal fissures produce bright red blood that streaks the stool and is caused by a tear at the mucocutaneous lining. It is often associated with constipation and is one of the commonest causes of rectal bleeding in all age groups.
  - Necrotising enterocolitis (NEC) usually develops within 10–16 days after birth, most commonly in premature infants, though can present in 13% of term infants. Early symptoms can be non-specific before frank bloody stools appear. Diagnosis is confirmed by the classic finding of pneumatosis intestinalis on an abdominal X-ray.
  - Haemorrhagic disease of the newborn is caused by a deficiency in vitamin K. If there is no improvement within 2 hours of IV vitamin K, work up for coagulopathy and liver disease should be considered. It is also an important cause of UGIB.

Common Causes of GI Bleeding in Children (1 month to 2 years)

- UGIB
  - Oesophagitis secondary to gastroesophageal reflux is seen more commonly in infants with neurodisability.
  - Gastritis causes small and rarely large bleeds and it is usually related to systemic infections or NSAID use.
- LGIB
  - Milk protein allergy causes allergic colitis by an adverse immune reaction to cow's milk and has additional symptoms, including diarrhoea, weight loss, vomiting and irritability.
  - Bacterial enteritis is suspected when LGIB occurs in association with profuse diarrhoea. Recent antibiotic use raises suspicion for antibiotic associated colitis and *Clostridium difficile* colitis.
  - Intussusception is most common in infants ranging from 6 to18 months of age. Symptoms include cramping, abdominal pain, vomiting, a palpable sausage-shaped mass and diarrhoea, followed by red currant jelly stools.
  - Meckel diverticulum occurs in 2% of the population, it presents as a sudden onset of painless bleeding per rectum (PR) consisting of large volumes of altered blood. The bleeding is due to ileal ulceration caused by acid secretion from the ectopic gastric mucosa.

Common Causes of GI Bleeding in Children (2 years and above)

- UGIB
  - » Mallory Weiss tears present as small streaks of coffee-ground contents in the vomitus. It is due to tears in the gastro-oesophageal mucosa secondary to retching or a violent vomiting episode. Majority are self-limiting.
  - » Gastroduodenal ulcers due to *Helicobacter pylori* can present as haematemesis with altered blood or coffee-ground appearance. It should be suspected if there is another affected family member.
  - » Oesophageal and gastric varices are caused by portal hypertension, which occurs when there is increased resistance to blood flow through the portal system. The most common causes of portal hypertension in children are portal vein thrombosis and chronic liver disease due to biliary atresia.
- LGIB
  - » Inflammatory bowel disease (IBD) refers to ulcerative colitis and Crohn's disease, which are chronic diseases that result in inflammation of the intestines. It is the commonest cause of persistent bleeding PR in this age group. Majority of them have systemic symptoms, raised inflammatory markers and anaemia. Refractory anal fissures, especially when associated with skin tags, should alert the physician about the possibility of IBD.
  - » Juvenile polyps are mainly located in the rectum but can also be seen throughout the colon. These are benign hamartomas and sometimes autoamputate. Children present with painless bleeding PR, which often streaks normal stools with fresh blood.

History

- First make sure it is indeed blood!
  - » Elicit a history of foods consumed or drugs used that may give a stool bloody appearance. This list includes certain antibiotics, iron supplements, red liquorice, coloured vegetables, chocolate, flavoured gelatine, etc. If in doubt, a test for occult blood can be done; however, be aware of false positives.
- Ask about acuteness or chronicity of bleeding, colour and quantity of the blood in stools or emesis.
  - » Melaena, rather than bright red blood per rectum, is usually a sign of bleeding that comes from a source proximal to the ligament of Treitz. Blood mixed in stool or dark red blood implies a proximal source with some degree of digestion of the blood. However, massive upper GI bleeding can produce bright red blood PR if GI transit time is rapid.
- Antecedent symptoms like consistency of stool, history of straining, abdominal pain, generalised lethargy, allergies and trauma.
- A history of vomiting, diarrhoea, fever, ill contacts or travel suggests an infectious aetiology. Any history of concurrent illness may predispose to stress gastritis or ulcers.
- Recurrent or forceful vomiting is associated with Mallory Weiss tears.

- Familial history of *Helicobacter pylori* or NSAID/medication use may suggest peptic ulcer disease.
- Ask questions that may reveal underlying, but as yet undiagnosed, organ dysfunction, e.g. recent jaundice, easy bruising and changes in stool colour may signal liver disease.
- Any history of liver disease that may predispose to variceal bleed, e.g. biliary atresia, autoimmune hepatitis, portal vein thrombosis, etc.
- Any family or self-history of clotting disorders, e.g. haemophilia, Von Willebrand disease.
- History of easy bruising or bleeding.
- Epistaxis: Recent or recurrent, which may account for haematemesis.
- Recent medications, particularly NSAIDs/corticosteroids/selective serotonin reuptake inhibitors (SSRIs). Patient on β2 antagonist may have impaired haemodynamic response to hypovolaemia (consider stopping).

Clinical Examination

- Assess vital signs, look for signs of shock such as pallor, heart rate, blood pressure, capillary refill and alertness.
- In the head and neck, look for causes such as epistaxis, nasal polyps and oropharyngeal erosions.
- Examine abdomen for surgical scars and elicit the reason for the surgery.
- Abdominal tenderness, with or without a mass, raises the suspicion of intussusception or ischaemia.
- Hepatomegaly, splenomegaly, jaundice or caput medusa suggest liver disease and portal hypertension.
- Inspection of the perianal area may reveal fissures, fistulas, skin breakdown or evidence of trauma. Gentle digital rectal examination may reveal polyps.
- Looking for evidence of child abuse, such as perianal tearing, tags or irregularities in anal tone and contour, is also important.
- Examination of the skin may reveal evidence of systemic disorders, such as Henoch–Schönlein purpura and Peutz–Jeghers polyposis.

Management of Upper GI Bleed

Initial Assessment

Primary goal is to determine whether the patient requires urgent intervention (e.g. endoscopic, surgical, transfusion) or can undergo delayed endoscopy or even be discharged to outpatient management. Majority of UGIB will stop spontaneously, however, if fresh or active bleeding is confirmed; oesophago-gastro-duodenoscopy (OGD) is used to determine the source of UGIB.

In general, trace or small amounts of blood that is a first-time occurrence are not of emergent concern. Children rarely require an extensive laboratory workup or invasive procedures, and parents can be advised to observe the child at home to see if these situations arise again.

Although numerous factors from the patient history, physical examination and initial tests have been examined for an association with a need for intervention, no single factor is sufficiently predictive of UGIB severity to be used for triage. The most predictive individual factors are:

- Presentation with haematemesis, with signs of hypovolaemia and a Hb <8 g/dL.
- Co-morbidities, e.g. liver disease, cardiac disease, immunodeficiency, malignancy.
- History of aspirin or NSAID use.

Patients who have significant co-morbidities may require admission regardless of the severity of the UGIB.

Investigations

- Full blood count, renal panel, C-reactive protein, liver function test, clotting profile.
- Group and crossmatch.
- Stool for inspection, stool for occult blood (if confirmation of UGIB is needed), stool *H. Pylori* (UGIB).
- Other investigations as clinically indicated.
- Hb should be repeated in 12–24 hours as the initial Hb may be normal.
- An elevated urea in the absence of renal disease may be indicative (although not diagnostic) of UGIB rather than LGIB.

Treatment of Non-variceal Bleed

Stable patients (normal vitals with no signs of significant ongoing GI bleeding):

- Ensure good IV access.
- Keep Nil by mouth (NBM).
- Start IV maintenance fluids.
- Correct any coagulopathy.
- Start IV Omeprazole.
- Sucralfate oral or via nasogastric tube (NGT).
- Consider inserting NGT for monitoring of ongoing UGIB — active aspirate 3–4 hourly.
- Check for risk factors whereby early endoscopy may be indicated (see below, section on Endoscopy).
- Early referral to paediatric gastroenterologist as indicated.

Unstable Patients (abnormal vital signs, ongoing GI bleeding):

- Check airway, breathing, circulation.
- IV access with two large bore cannulas, blood investigations as above.

- Fluid resuscitate. Normal saline may be used until blood products are available.
- Keep NBM.
- Aim for Hb >9 g/dL (Transfusion has to be judicious in patients with portal hypertension).
  [Formula for calculating packed cell transfusion volume (ml) = body weight (kg) × Hb (g/dL) rise (desired Hb – actual Hb) × 3.5
- Aim for platelets $>100 \times 10^9$/L.
- Correct any coagulopathy with vitamin K and/or Fresh frozen plasma (FFP).
- Start IV Esomeprazole.
- Sucralfate oral or via NGT.
- Insert NGT — put on passive drainage and active aspiration 1–3 hourly.
- Urgent referral to paediatric gastroenterologist/hepatologist
- Endoscopy is indicated if there is evidence of active ongoing bleeding. Patient should be stabilised prior to endoscopic procedure.
- Magnetic Resonance Imaging (MRI) or Computed Tomography (CT) Angiography may be indicated if there is rapid bleeding and an endoscopy is unable to identify the source of UGIB.

Treatment of Variceal Bleed

- Urgent referral to paediatric gastroenterologist/hepatologist
- Resuscitate with fluids or blood products if hypovolaemic. The patient should not be over transfused. The target level of Hb should be 10 g/dL in order to avoid rebound rise in the portal pressures.
- Correct coagulopathy with IV vitamin K, FFP and platelet transfusion (if platelets $<60 \times 10^9$/L)
- Placement of a large bore NGT should be considered. This will help identify ongoing bleed and decompress the stomach, reduce possibility of aspiration.
- Antibiotics, antivirals and antifungal therapy should be considered in sick children.
- Specific measures to achieve haemostasis:
  - » IV Esomeprazole
  - » PO Sucralfate, even when child is NBM.
  - » Octreotide — reduces portal flow by an immediate direct splanchnic vaso-constrictive effect and by inhibiting the release of vaso-dilator peptides such as glucagon. It can either be given as an IV bolus or by continuous infusion.
- Gastroscopy should be performed once the child is stable to confirm the site of bleeding.

Pharmacotherapy

Table 13.18 Drugs used for Upper Gastrointestinal Bleeding

Vitamin K	IV 0.3 mg/kg/dose (Max.: 10 mg/dose)
Omeprazole	IV 1 mg/kg/dose BD-TDS (Max.: 40 mg/dose)
Esomeprazole (for 1 mth and above)	IV loading dose 1 mg/kg/dose (Max.: 80 mg), followed by 0.1 mg/kg/hr continuous infusion (Max.: 8 mg/hr)
Sucralfate	PO 1 mth–2 yr old: 250 mg QDS 2–12 yr old: 500 mg QDS >12 yr old: 1 g QDS
Octreotide (for bleeding oesophageal varices) – keep the child NBM (except for certain oral medicines) whilst on octreotide.	IV 1–2 mcg/kg bolus followed by 2–5 mcg/kg/hr Maximum dilution 25 mcg/ml. Stable at room temperature for 48 hr. Compatible with 0.9% saline/TPN. Make 1250 mcg of Octreotide in 50 ml of normal saline, i.e. concentration 25 mcg/ml. Starting dose 3 mcg/kg/hr. Run initially at weight × 0.12 ml/hr = 3 mcg/kg/hr Increase if poor response to: Run at weight × 0.2 ml/hr = 5 mcg/kg/hr Preferable infuse as a single agent, but if necessary, may mix with maintenance or parenteral nutrition.

Endoscopy

After the initial stabilisation of patients with UGIB, upper endoscopy is the preferred diagnostic and therapeutic tool. All patients with significant UGIB should be referred to paediatric gastroenterologist for an endoscopy.

Treatment of peptic ulcers and Dieulafoy lesion can be carried out with adrenaline injection in combination with thermal or mechanical techniques (haemostatic clips). Haemostatic spray has been shown to be an effective treatment as well.

Haemostasis of oesophageal variceal bleeding can be achieved using band ligation, if feasible, or sclerotherapy as an alternative.

Video capsule endoscopy (VCE) is indicated when there is suspected small intestinal bleeding and, in addition, balloon-assisted enteroscopy for therapeutic purposes.

Risk factors whereby early endoscopic intervention may be indicated:

- Significant pre-existing conditions, e.g. chronic liver disease, portal hypertension, previous peptic ulcers
- Large amount of fresh haematemesis (reported/observed)
- Presence of melaena
- Heart Rate >20/min from the mean heart rate for age
- Prolonged Capillary Refill (>2 s)
- First recorded Hb after bleed <10 g/dL
- Hb drop of >2 g/dL
- Need for fluid bolus
- Need for blood transfusion

- Need for other blood products

Surgery

Surgery should be considered in patients with UGIB in the following scenarios:

- Severe, life-threatening haemorrhage not responsive to resuscitative efforts
- Failure of medical therapy and endoscopic haemostasis with persistent recurrent bleeding
- A coexisting reason for surgery (e.g. perforation, obstruction, malignancy)
- Prolonged bleeding, with loss of 50% or more of the patient's blood volume

Management of Lower GI Bleed

General principles of initial assessment and management of patients with substantial LGIB are similar to UGIB (given above). However, urgent colonoscopy is rarely required.

It is very crucial to rule out a surgical cause, as in most of the cases like intussusception, malrotation with volvulus, Meckel's diverticulum and ischaemic gut, children may look surprising well initially. High index of suspicion is required for early detection and this may influence outcome.

History and examination may point towards a particular diagnosis and they are managed accordingly (given below).

- Full blood count, renal panel, liver function test, clotting profile, C-reactive protein, Erythrocyte sedimentation rate, group and crossmatch, stool culture
- In cases of severe LGIB, especially when malaena is present or haemodynamic instability, the source of bleeding may include the upper GI tract.
- Imaging studies like abdominal ultrasound or Meckel's scan may be needed before colonoscopy.
- Colonoscopy can detect several lesions in 80% of cases, including IBD and colonic polyps. Vascular lesions include a wide variety of malformations, including haemangiomas, arteriovenous malformations and vasculitis. If these lesions are located in the colon, colonoscopy may be diagnostic and therapeutic. However, brisk bleeding may obscure the visual field, making localising the bleeding impossible.
- Nuclear scintigraphy (Tc99m labelled red blood cell scan) can be used to detect bleeding at a rate as low as 0.1 ml per minute. This technique is sensitive but less specific than angiography; it may help to localise the general area of bleeding to guide subsequent endoscopy, angiography or surgery.
- MRI or CT Angiography can be used to detect bleeding in patients with ongoing fresh rectal bleeding. However, the bleeding rate must be ≥0.5 ml per minute to detect extravasation into the gut. It offers the advantage of providing treatment, consisting of embolsation and intra-arterial administration of vasoconstrictors.
- When arteriography and nuclear scanning fail to diagnose or localise the cause of bleeding, further options remain, including repeat endoscopy and enteroscopy.
- If all fails, diagnostic laparoscopy and intraoperative endoscopy can be performed.

Management of Specific Conditions Causing Lower GI Bleed

- For neonates with NEC, the standard treatment is aggressive medical resuscitation with bowel rest, antibiotics, total parenteral nutrition and nasogastric decompression. Non-operative management of NEC yields a 70–80% recovery rate, but urgent laparotomy or drain placement is required in neonates where conservative therapy is unsuccessful owing to progressive sepsis, bowel perforation or persistent bleeding.
- The history should also be used as a guide with regard to when stool microbial studies should be ordered. Systemic antibiotics are sometimes needed in an unwell child.
- Treatment for anal fissures consists of administration of stool softeners and topical agents.
- The symptoms of milk protein allergy generally resolve in 48 hours to 2 weeks after withdrawal of the offending milk product or starting hypoallergenic formula.
- If Henoch–Schonlein purpura is suspected and intussusception has been ruled out, a trial of IV steroids can be considered.
- Management of IBD requires referral to paediatric gastroenterologist and involves a combination of immunosuppression as well as anti-inflammatory medications.

Bibliography

1. Paten N, Kay M. (nd) Lower gastrointestinal bleeding in children: Causes and diagnostic approach. *UpToDate*. https://www.uptodate.com/contents/lower-gastrointestinal-bleeding-in-children-causes-and-diagnostic-approach
2. Gilger MA. (2004) Upper gastrointestinal bleeding. In: Walker WA, Goulet O, Kleinman RE, *et al.* (eds.) *Pediatric Gastrointestinal Disease, vol. 1*. Hamilton: BC Decker, pp. 258–265.
3. Owensby S, Taylor K, Wilkins T. (2015) Diagnosis and management of upper gastrointestinal bleeding in children. *J Am Board Fam Med* **28**(1):134–145.
4. Tringali A, Thomson M, Dumonceau JM, *et al.* (2017) Pediatric gastrointestinal endoscopy: European Society of Gastrointestinal Endoscopy (ESGE) and European Society for Paediatric Gastroenterology Hepatology and Nutrition (ESPGHAN) Guideline Executive summary. *Endoscopy* **49**(1):83–91.
5. Thomson MA, Leton N, Belsha D. (2015) Acute upper gastrointestinal bleeding in childhood: Development of the Sheffield scoring system to predict need for endoscopic therapy. *J Pediatr Gastroenterol Nutr* **60**(5):632–636.
6. Romano C, Oliva S, Martellossi S, *et al.* (2017) Pediatric gastrointestinal bleeding: Perspectives from the Italian Society of Pediatric Gastroenterology. *World J Gastroenterol* **23**(8):1328–1337.
7. Ghassemi KA, Jensen DM. (2013) Lower GI bleeding: Epidemiology and management. *Curr Gastroenterol Rep* **15**(7):333.
8. Raphaeli T, Menon R. (2012) Current treatment of lower gastrointestinal hemorrhage. *Clin Colon Rectal Surg* **25**(4):219–227.

CHAPTER 55

Acute Liver Failure

Siti Nur Hanim Buang; Goh Suk-Hui, Lynette;
Tan Wei Wei; Mok Yee Hui; Chiou Fang Kuan

Introduction

Acute liver failure (ALF) in children

- Is associated with multi-organ involvement
- Has a high mortality rate, without transplantation
- Aetiology is age-dependent and varies with geographical location
- Mainstay of management is supportive care

Definition

Severe hepatic dysfunction and hepatocellular necrosis in the absence of chronic liver disease. Extent of hepatic encephalopathy (HE) is variable.

Paediatric Acute Liver Failure (PALF) study group criteria:

1. No known evidence of chronic liver disease
2. Biochemical evidence of acute liver injury
3. Hepatic-based coagulopathy
    a. PT ≥15 s or INR ≥1.5, uncorrectable by vitamin K, in the presence of HE
    b. PT ≥20 s or INR ≥2.0, uncorrectable by vitamin K, regardless of the presence or absence of HE

Aetiologies

- Indeterminate cause, non-Hepatitis A–E
    - » Usually diagnosis of exclusion once other causes are eliminated
    - » Associated with worse prognosis
- Infections
    - » Hepatotrophic viruses, e.g. Hepatitis A–E, Cytomegalovirus, Epstein–Barr virus, Varicella-zoster virus, Herpes simplex virus (esp. neonates can be fatal), Parvovirus (in aplastic anaemia), Echovirus and Coxsackie Virus (esp. neonates)
- Inborn errors of metabolism
- Paracetamol overdose
- Other drugs/Toxins

- Shock
- Miscellaneous
- Autoimmune hepatitis
- Wilson disease

History

Pertinent history to elicit includes:

- Recent prodromal illness (fever, abdominal pain, rashes, 'flu'-like illness)
- Onset of jaundice (late feature)
- Alteration in mental status
- Evidence of bleeding tendency, easy bruising
- Drug ingestion and doses (acetaminophen, anti-Tuberculosis treatment, traditional medication)
- Developmental delay or seizures
- Relevant family history (consanguinity, spontaneous abortions, early infantile death, liver/autoimmune/metabolic diseases)

Clinical Examination

- Bruises
- Hepatomegaly, ascites
- Encephalopathy, signs of raised intracranial pressure (ICP) from cerebral oedema
- Signs that are diagnostic hallmarks of specific conditions, e.g. Kayser–Fleischer ring (Wilson disease)
- Evidence of heart failure (myocarditis, cardiomyopathy)
- Splenomegaly in the presence of persistent fever and characteristic biochemical profile (Haemophagocytic lymphohistiocytosis [HLH])

Table 13.19 Assessment of Encephalopathy for Young Children (birth to age 3 years)

Grade	Clinical	Asterixis/ Reflexes	Neurological Signs
Early (I and II)	Inconsolable crying Sleep reversal / Disturbed sleep rhythm Inattention to task / Mild drowsiness	Unreliable/ normal, or hyperreflexic	Untestable
Mid (III)	Somnolence Stupor Combativeness	Unreliable, or hyperreflexic	Most likely untestable
Late (IV)	Comatose, Arouses with painful stimuli (IVa) No response to painful stimuli (IVb)	Absent	Decerebrate or decorticate

Investigations

A systematic diagnostic workup is paramount to help identify conditions, which have specific directed therapy, like acetaminophen toxicity, tyrosinaemia and autoimmune hepatitis, as well as differentiate patients in whom liver transplantation is contraindicated.

Poor Prognostic Factors

- Age <10 years
- Period of onset of illness prior to liver failure >7 days
- Non-A Non-B hepatitis
- Shrinking liver size
- Renal failure/Hepatorenal syndrome
- Higher grade of encephalopathy
  - » Grade IV: 90% mortality
  - » Grade II–III: 85% mortality
- Acute Respiratory Distress Syndrome

Goals of Management

- Optimal organ systems support
- Anticipation, prevention and treatment of potential complications

Table 13.20 Investigations to Evaluate ALF

First-line Investigations	
General	*Liver synthetic function tests*
FBC, peripheral blood film, GXM	Coagulation profile
Renal panel	Glucose
Calcium, Phosphate, Magnesium	Albumin
Blood gas	Ammonia
Acetaminophen level	Conjugated bilirubin
CRP, ESR	*Tests for liver injury*
Amylase, Lipase	ALT, AST, GGT, ALP, LDH
Second-line Investigations	
Infectious screen	*Metabolic screen*
Blood culture	Serum amino acids, Urine organic acids
Urinalysis and urine culture	Cu, Caeruloplasmin levels
Viral hepatitis serology	Lactate
anti-HAV IgM, HBsAg, anti HBc IgM, anti HEV, anti HCV	*Autoimmune markers*
	ANA, SMA,
HSV serology/PCR	LKM antibodies
EBV serology	Immunoglobulins
HIV serology	*Imaging*
	Abdominal ultrasound

ALP: alkaline phosphatase; ALT: alanine transaminase; ANA: antinuclear antibodies; AST: aspartate aminotransferase; CRP: C-reactive protein; Cu: copper; EBV: ebstein-barr virus; ESR: erythrocyte sedimentation rate; FBC: Full blood count; GGT: gamma-glutamyl transferase; GXM: Group and crossmatch; HAV: hepatitis A virus; HBc: hepatitis B core; HBsAg: hepatitis B surface antigen; HCV: hepatitis C virus; HEV: hepatitis E virus; HIV: human immunodeficiency virus; HSV: herpes simplex virus; LDH: lactate dehydrogenase; LKM: liver-kidney-microsome. SMA: smooth muscule antibody;

- Maximise chances of spontaneous hepatocyte recovery and maintain optimal clinical condition for best post-transplant survival

General Supportive Management

Early identification and immediate initiation of appropriate supportive therapy is crucial to maximise the potential for recovery. After stabilisation, ill-looking patients should be promptly sent to the critical care setting.

Acute Resuscitative Measures

- Assess and support airway and breathing accordingly. Oxygen therapy, if required. Need for definitive airway and ventilation more likely in Grade III–IV HE.
- Obtain venous access for volume resuscitation, if required.
- Consider central venous access for monitoring central venous pressure (CVP) and delivery of high dextrose concentration solution or inotropes.
- High Dependency/Intensive Care Unit admission depending on clinical status. Consider timely transfer to liver transplant centre after stabilisation

General Measures

- Nurse in a quiet environment.
- Monitor vitals (heart rate, respiratory rate, blood pressure), blood parameters (electrolytes, glucose) and neurological status (for presence of encephalopathy) 4 to 6 hourly.

Fluids/Haemodynamics

- Fluid restrict to 2/3 maintenance.
- Avoid fluid overload (can worsen cerebral oedema).
- Use colloid for volume expansion.
- If hypotensive with normal circulating volume (CVP 4 to 8 cmH_20), consider vasoactive drugs (noradrenaline, alpha agonist) in view of low systemic vascular resistance.

Metabolic and Nutrition

- Maintain normoglycaemia (Blood glucose >4 mmol/L). Monitor 1 to 2 hourly initially.
- Consider higher dextrose concentrations if necessary.
- Nasogastric tube insertion for early enteral feeding. Consider total parenteral nutrition if ileus present.
- Provide protein intake of about 1–2 g/kg/day (titrate protein intake based on patient's clinical status)

Renal

- Urinary catheterisation for accurate intake/output monitoring
- Maintain urine output of 1 ml/kg/h. If oliguric, consider

  - » Low cardiac output
  - » Hepatorenal syndrome
  - » Dehydration (low CVP)
- CVP low — colloid challenge 10 ml/kg
- CVP high — Intravenous (IV) frusemide 1–2 mg/kg/dose
- Haemofiltration may be considered for renal failure (continuous veno-venous haemodialysis [CVVHD]) or hyperammonaemia >200 μmol/L

Gastrointestinal

- Gastric acid suppression
  - » Omeprazole (proton-pump inhibitor) IV 1 mg/kg/dose BD
  - » Esomeprazole (proton-pump inhibitor) IV 0.5 mg/kg/dose OD
  - » Note dose adjustment may be needed in severe liver impairment.
- Suppression of ammonia production (by bowel flora)
  - » Oral neomycin 50–100 mg/kg/day Q6H for a maximum of 7 days with or without lactulose. Maximum daily dose: 12 g/day
  - » Oral lactulose 2–4 ml/kg/dose (max.: 30 ml/dose) Q6H (Aim for 3–5 bowel output/day)
  - » Monitor for bowel distension and intravascular depletion. Excessive use increases risk of pneumatosis intestinalis.
- N-acetylcysteine (NAC) infusion
  - » For non-acetaminophen-induced ALF (to discuss with paediatric gastroenterologist), IV NAC infusion 100 mg/kg/day over 24 hours, review after 24 to 48 hours
  - » For acetaminophen-induced ALF, refer to toxicology guidelines

Management of Specific Complications

Hepatic Encephalopathy and Cerebral Oedema

HE is a spectrum of altered cerebral function secondary to hepatic failure. The most serious complication of ALF is cerebral oedema resulting in raised ICP. The risk of cerebral oedema increases with increasing severity of HE.

HE Grade I–II: Minimal risk
HE Grade III: 25–35% risk
HE Grade IV: 65–75% risk

- Elective intubation in patients with:
  - » HE Grade II but agitated
  - » HE Grade III–IV
- Institute neuroprotective measures in the presence of raised ICP to maintain cerebral perfusion pressure (CPP) and oxygenation:
  - » Head elevated to 30°, in neutral position.

- » Maintain normothermia.
- » Keep well sedated (low dose fentanyl preferred because of its short half-life, and its elimination half-life is less affected in liver impairment than morphine.
- » Consider a muscle relaxant. Atracuronium is preferred in liver failure as it undergoes ester hydrolysis and Hofmann elimination and is independent of both liver and renal functions. No dosage adjustment is required in liver failure.
- » Maintain normocarbia pCO_2 35 mmHg and pO_2 80–100 mmHg.
- » Keep Na 145–150 mmol/L with hyperosmolar therapy.
  - Hypertonic saline IV 3% NaCl 4 ml/kg over 30 min.
  - IV Mannitol 0.5–1 g/kg over 30 min. Repeat 6 to 8 hourly, only if good urine output. Keep serum osmolarity <320 mOsmol/kg.
- » Consider ICP monitoring (Correct coagulopathy first).
  - Keep CPP >50 mmHg and ICP <20 mmHg.
  - Consider volume expansion and/or vasopressors.
  - Consider thiopentone for recalcitrant raised ICP.
  - Aim for burst suppression if electroencephalogram monitoring is utilised.

- Exclude other non-hepatic causes of altered mental status
  - » Hypotension
  - » Hypoglycaemia
  - » Hyponatraemia
  - » Seizures
  - » Cerebral oedema (infection, acute renal failure, fluid overload)
  - » Intracranial haemorrhage (urgent computed tomography of the head)
- Contributory factors
  - » Hyperammonaemia: Consider CVVHD for serum ammonia >200 μmol/L
  - » Fluid overload
  - » Metabolic derangements (hypoglycaemia, hyponatraemia)
  - » Hypotension and ischaemia
  - » Alteration in cerebral vascular permeability
  - » Failure of intracellular homeostasis (disrupted neuronal Na-K pump)

Seizures

- May be subtle in children with HE.
- Causes include:
  - » Electrolyte imbalances (hyponatremia, hypomagnesaemia)
  - » Raised ICP
  - » Intracranial haemorrhage
  - » Encephalitis
- Consider intracranial imaging.
- Correct electrolyte imbalances, if any.
- Mannitol or hypertonic saline, if there is suspected cerebral oedema.
- For status epilepticus, first-line treatment with benzodiazepines (diazepam, lorazepam).

- For recurrent seizures, treat with phenobarbitone (loading and maintenance doses).

Coagulopathy and Haemorrhage

- ALF is characterised by reduced synthesis of coagulation factors (II, V, VII, IX, X), accelerated fibrinolysis and impaired hepatic clearance of activated clotting factors and fibrin degradation products.
- Thrombocytopenia with depressed platelet function is tolerated, as long as platelet level >20000 /mm^3 and there is no active bleeding.
- Hypofibrinogenaemia results from both decreased hepatic synthesis and increased catabolism.
- Parenteral Vitamin K is recommended empirically for 3 days
  - » IV 250–300 mcg/kg/day OM (max. 10 mg)
- In the absence of haemorrhage, no prophylaxis fresh frozen plasma (FFP) is recommended, unless discussed with hepatology team, as it
  - » Does not reduce risk of significant bleeding.
  - » Obscures trending of PT as a prognostic marker.
  - » Increases risk of volume overload.
- In the presence of bleeding or in anticipation of an invasive surgical procedure,
  - » Transfuse FFP to achieve INR <1.5.
  - » Keep platelets >50000 /mm^3.
  - » Consider cryoprecipitate if fibrinogen <100 mg/dL.
- Recombinant factor VIIa ([rFVIIa], 40 mcg/kg) can be given when FFP fails to correct INR
  - » Must be administered immediately before a procedure.
  - » Procedure must be performed within 30–60 min (effect persists for >2 hours).
  - » FFP must be given before rFVIIa, if fibrinogen <100 mg/dL.
  - » Plasma exchange can be considered where rFVIIa is contraindicated.

Gastrointestinal Bleeding

Upper gastrointestinal bleeding can be improved with gastric acid suppression with histamine type 2 receptor antagonists.

Ascites

Clinically evident ascites (not common in ALF) occur in less than half of ALF patients. Therapy is not usually indicated, apart from correction of oncotic pressure with IV 20% Albumin (with frusemide) and general fluid management.

Renal Insufficiency

- Ensure urine output 1 ml/kg/h. If oliguric, consider:
  - » Low cardiac output
  - » Intravascular volume depletion with low CVP (Give colloid challenge)
  - » Hepatorenal syndrome
- Can also be precipitated by an overzealous use of diuretics and/or nephrotoxic drugs.

- Hepatorenal syndrome is the most common cause of renal insufficiency in ALF. It is secondary to intense renal vasoconstriction in response to splanchnic vasodilation due to portal hypertension. This can be effectively reversed with vasopressors.
- Institute early haemofiltration if:
  - » Oliguria with fluid overload, in the presence of cerebral oedema
  - » Symptomatic uraemia, intractable hyperkalaemia or metabolic acidosis

Metabolic and Electrolyte Abnormalities

- High risk of hypoglycaemia (approx 40%) due to failure of hepatic gluconeogenesis. Keep blood glucose >4 mmol/L. Monitor 1 to 2 hourly initially. Glucose infusion rates up to 12–15 mg/kg/min may be required. Consider higher dextrose concentration with fluid restriction.
- Metabolic acidosis can be caused by hypoxia, hypovolaemia, sepsis and renal failure. Consider correctable parameters. If refractory, correct with IV sodium bicarbonate if BE >–10 and pH <7.25.
- Avoid metabolic alkalosis and hypokalaemia as this enhances conversion of NH_4 to ammonia, which can cross the blood brain barrier.
- Hyponatraemia, hypokalaemia, hypophosphataemia, hypocalcaemia and hypomagnesaemia are often observed.
- In the absence of hypoxic ischaemic encephalopathy, fluid resuscitation and sodium management should be targeted at maintaining sodium levels at 140–145 mmol/L. Conversely, hypernatraemia may occur due to excessive use of lactulose.
- Alterations in potassium, phosphate, calcium and magnesium should be monitored and corrected as clinically appropriate.
- Hypophosphataemia is postulated to be related to the amount of regenerative liver mass, as phosphate is a substrate for various enzymatic reactions that phosphorylate proteins need during rapid liver regeneration.

Infection Prophylaxis and Surveillance

Susceptibility to infection is a result of impaired host immune defences. Additional risk factors include poor respiratory effort (drowsiness) and the presence of endotracheal tube, urinary catheters, central line. Peritonitis from ascites must also be considered.

- Obtain surveillance cultures (sputum, urine, blood, rectal swab) at presentation and with any evidence of clinical deterioration.
- Empirical antibiotics is recommended where the likelihood of infection is high
  - » Surveillance cultures reveal significant isolates.
  - » Progression of, or advanced stage (grade III/IV) of HE.
  - » Refractory hypotension.
  - » Presence of systemic inflammatory response syndrome (SIRS): Temperature >38°C or <36°C, WCC >12000 or <4000 /mm^3, HR >90/min.
- Consider IV fluconazole prophylaxis for all patients.
- Start empirical IV acyclovir therapy in neonates and infants <6 months.
- Prophylactic antibiotics are not indicated in ALF.

Nutrition

ALF is a catabolic state characterised by a negative nitrogen balance. Patients exhibit increased resting energy expenditure.

- Maintain blood glucose >4 mmol/L.
- Ensure sufficient carbohydrates for energy metabolism.
- Provide protein intake of about 1–2 g/kg/day (titrate protein intake based on patient's clinical status)

Acute Pancreatitis

Is uncommon in ALF, although mildly raised amylase levels may be present. Predisposing factors include shock, viral illness or haemorrhage into/around the pancreas.

- Check amylase/lipase in the presence of abdominal pain and/or hypocalcaemia.
- Treatment is usually supportive.

Adrenal Suppression

Occurs in 60% of adults with ALF.

- Consider diagnosis in fluid refractory, catecholamine-resistant hypotension.
- May need further evaluation with a synacthen test.
- Treat with corticosteroids.

Indications for Liver Transplantation

ACETAMINOPHEN-induced ALF	Non-ACETAMINOPHEN-induced ALF
ABG pH <7.3 ***OR*** Presence of all 3 on the same day: 1. PT >100 sec 2. Creatinine >300 μmol/L 3. Hepatic encephalopathy Grade III/IV	PT >100s, INR >6.5 ***OR*** Presence of 3 of the following: 1. Age <10 yr old, >40 yr old 2. Aetiology of non-A non-B hepatitis 3. Bilirubin > 300 μmol/L 4. PT >50 sec 5. Jaundice to encephalopathy interval of 7 d

Contraindications to Liver Transplantation

- Diseases not cured by transplantation (leukaemia, lymphoproliferative disease, HLH)
- Reye syndrome
- Mitochondrial respiratory chain disorders with neurological involvement
- Uncontrolled multiorgan failure

Usual Causes of Death

- Cerebral oedema or haemorrhage
- Sepsis
- Haemorrhage

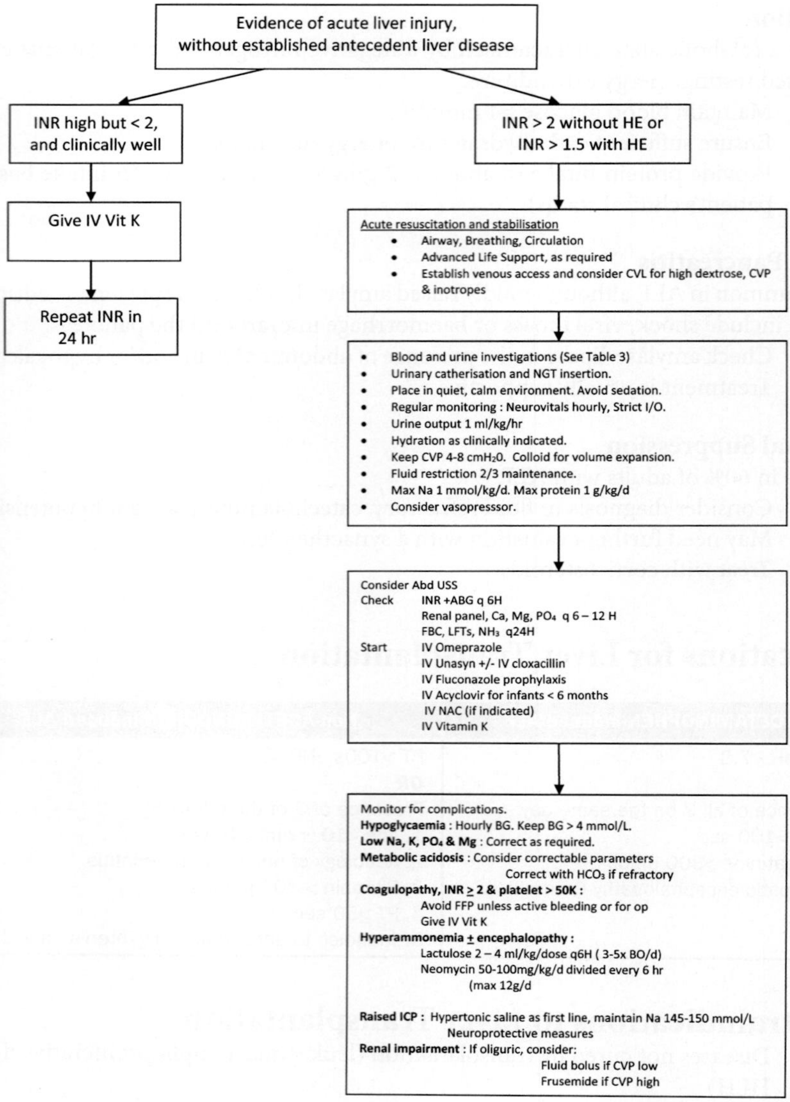

For non-Acetaminophen ALF:
NAC infusion (discuss with Gastro)
IV :100 mg/kg/day for 24 h

For paracetamol-related ALF:
Refer to toxicology guidelines

Figure 13.5 Management of acute liver failure.

ABG: arterial blood gas; ALF: acute liver failure; CVL: central venous line; CVP: central venous pressure; FBC: full blood count; FFP: fresh frozen plasma; HE: hepatic encephalopathy; INR: international normalised ratio; I/O: input/output; IV: intravenous; LFT: liver function test; NAC: N-acetylcysteine; NGT: nasogastric tube; Vit K: Vitamin K.

Bibliography

1. Drey C, Davidson CS. (1970) The management of fulminant hepatic failure. In: Popper H, Schaffner F (eds.) *Progress in Liver Disease*. New York, NY: Grune & Stratton, pp. 282–298.
2. Squires RH Jr, Shneider BL, Bucuvalas J, *et al.* (2006) Acute liver failure in children: The first 348 patients in the pediatric acute liver failure study group. *J Pediatr* **148**(5):652–658.
3. Whitington PF, Alonso AE. (2003) Fulminant hepatitis and acute liver failure. In: Kelly DA (ed.) *Paediatric Liver Disease*. Oxford: Blackwell, pp. 107–126.
4. Stravitz RT, Kramer AH, Davern T, *et al.* (2007) Intensive care of patients with acute liver failure: Recommendations of the U.S. acute liver failure study group. *Crit Care Med* **35**(11):2498–2508.
5. Chiou FK, Logarajah V, Ho CWW, *et al.* (2021) Demographics, aetiology and outcome of paediatric liver failure in Singapore. *Sing Med J.*

CHAPTER 56

Infant Milk Formula Guide

Ng Lay Queen; Phua Kar Yin; Chiou Fang Kuan

Cow's Milk Protein-Based Infant Formula

Most commercially available cow's milk protein-based formulas are made to simulate human milk:

- Standard preparation yields same caloric concentration to human milk (0.67 kcal/ml).
- Composed of carbohydrate (lactose, corn syrup solids), fat (vegetable oils, AHA/DHA) and protein (mix of whey protein and casein protein).
- Most formulas aim for a higher whey protein > casein protein ratio to mimic human milk.
- Additionally, whey-based milk empties more quickly from the stomach while casein-based milk forms curds, which are more slowly digested.
- Other additives include iron fortification, probiotics, prebiotics.

Follow-on milk formula (stage 2 and above) can only be used after 6 months old and is marketed to have higher iron content than infant first milk, different nutrient compositions and flavours.

Soy Formula

- Soy protein-based formula is indicated in infants with galactosaemia, congenital lactase deficiency (rare) and in situations in which a vegetarian diet is preferred.
- It may also be given to previously well infants with transient secondary lactose intolerance following acute gastroenteritis.
- Soy formula is not indicated in infants with cow's milk protein allergy as 10–14% of these infants will also be allergic to soy protein due to cross-reactivity of the protein molecule.

Specialised Formula

There are a variety of indications where specialised formulas (see Table 13.21) may be required for infants. These formulas are commonly recommended for disease-specific conditions and may vary in terms of protein/carbohydrate type, additives and/or caloric counts.

Table 13.21 Summary Table of Specialised Milk Formulas

	Categories of Milk Formulas	Some Examples
Hydrolysed and Elemental formulas Indication: For patients with cow's milk protein allergy or severe intestinal malabsorption.	Partially hydrolysed (large peptides)	Aptamil HA, Enfamil A+ Gentlease, Nan Optipro HA, Peptamen Junior, Similac Total Comfort
	Extensively hydrolysed (small peptides)	Alfare, Aptamil Allerpro, Nutramigen Lipil, Similac Alimentum
	Elemental (Amino acid based)	Comidagen, Comidagen Plus, Neocate LCP
High-calorie, high-protein formulas for infants Indication: Energy-dense formulas for infants with poor growth and infants with cardiac conditions to optimise caloric intake	High calorie (1–1.5 kcal/ml)	Similac Neosure and Enfamil A+ Post-Discharge (0.75 kcal/ml). Infatrini (0.92 kcal/ml)
Nutritionally complete formulas Indication: For patients who depend primarily on milk for their complete nutritional requirements (e.g. tube fed patients)	Nutritionally complete (1–1.5 kcal/ml)	For 1 to 12 yr old: Nutren Junior, Pediasure, S26 Ascenda From 10 yr old onwards: Boost Optimum, Ensure Life HMB, Ensure Plus, Fortisip, Resource Protein
MCT enriched formulas Indication: For use in patients with impaired fat absorption or lymphatic abnormalities (e.g. post-op chylothorax, certain chronic liver diseases)	MCT-enriched	Kanso Lipano
Anti-regurgitation formulas Indication: May help to alleviate symptoms of gastro-oesophageal reflux	Anti-regurgitation (with added thickener: rice starch, carob bean gum)	Enfamil A+ AR, Frisolac Gold AR, Nan AR, Similac RS
Disease-specific specialty formulas	Protein-restricted formula	Renastart, Nepro Lower Protein, Novasource Renal
	Branched chain amino acid enriched formula	Generaid Plus
	Specific amino acid restricted formula	Comida MSUD, Comida HCys, Comida PKU, Glutarex, Nutricia PKU, Propimex, Vitaflow EAA
	Exclusive enteral nutrition formula (Crohn's disease)	Modulen IBD
	Fibre-enriched formula	Fibersource 1.2 HN, Jevity
	Carbohydrate restricted formula	Glucerna Triplecare, Nutren Diabetes

Bibliography

1. Puntis J. (2018) Formula and complementary feeding. In: Beattie M, Dhawan A, Puntis J, *et al.* (eds.) *Oxford Specialist Handbook of Paediatric Gastroenterology, Hepatology and Nutrition, 2nd ed.* New York, NY: Oxford University Press, pp. 47–52.
2. Bhatia J, Greer F; American Academy of Pediatrics Committee on Nutrition. (2008) Use of soy protein-based formulas in infant feeding. *Pediatrics* **121**(5):1062–1068.
3. Chu HP. (2013) Choosing the right milk formula for your paediatric patient. *Ann Acad Med Sing* **42**(6):311–312.
4. NASPGHAN Foundation. (nd) Pediatric enteral nutrition: A comprehensive review https://naspghan.org/files/documents/pdfs/medical-resources/nutrition/Enteral%20Nutrition%20Slide%20Deck%20PDF%20COMPLETE-%20v12Oct2012.pdf

SECTION 14

GENETICS AND METABOLIC

CHAPTER 57

Suspected Genetic Syndrome

Koh Ai Ling; Saumya Shekhar Jamuar; Lai Hwei Meeng, Angeline

Introduction

The presenting features of a child with a suspected genetic syndrome may include:

- Dysmorphic features, referring to physical features, especially facial, not usually found in a child of the same age or ethnic background
- One or more congenital anomalies, e.g. cleft lip/palate or congenital heart disease (CHD)
- Developmental delay or intellectual disability
- Autism spectrum disorder and/or other behavioural problems, e.g. attention deficit hyperactivity disorder (ADHD)
- Disorders of growth: Failure to thrive (FTT), short stature or overgrowth
- Disorder of sexual development
- Unexplained systemic findings

Why is it Important to Make a Genetic Diagnosis?

In most situations, having a diagnosis for a child with suspected genetic syndrome does not mean that there is a specific intervention or treatment. Why, then, should we try to come to a diagnosis? Having a specific diagnosis:

- Makes available all the accumulated knowledge about the condition
- Gives information about the possible complications, allowing early detection, treatment, and possibly prevention of complications
- Gives information about prognosis and risk of recurrence
- Gives families the option to access relevant support groups
- Facilitates participation in research into identification of causative genes and therapeutic options

Clinical Approach

History and physical examination are important in establishing the diagnosis.

History

- Pregnancy
  - » Previous pregnancy losses
  - » Maternal illnesses during the pregnancy, e.g. fever or rash
  - » Exposure to medications, alcohol, cigarette-smoking or recreational drug

   - Results of prenatal tests, e.g. non-invasive prenatal tests (NIPT), ultrasound scans, chorionic villus sampling (CVS), amniocentesis
- Perinatal
   - Details of the birth, including evidence of polyhydramnios, oligohydramnios or fetal distress, gestation at birth, mode of delivery
   - Birth weight, length and head circumference of the baby at birth
   - Condition of the baby soon after birth, including evidence of respiratory distress, feeding problems and neonatal hypoglycaemia
- Developmental
   - Early developmental milestones
   - Developmental regression
   - Formal developmental, hearing or vision assessments
   - Behaviour
   - Sleep patterns, e.g. frequent nocturnal awakening and fragmented sleep in children with Smith–Magenis syndrome
   - Personality, e.g. unique personality characteristics in Williams syndrome
- Medical
   - Thorough list of congenital anomalies present
   - Medical problems, e.g. seizures
- Family
   - A three-generation pedigree, noting consanguinity, miscarriages, stillbirths and deaths of siblings
   - Family history of similar medical condition

Clinical Examination

- Overall appearance (gestalt)
- Facial appearance
   - Shape of head and face
   - Spacing of eyes (hyper- or hypotelorism), length of palpebral fissures, upslanting or downslanting palpebral fissures
   - Size and shape of nose and mouth
   - Shape and position of ears
- Proportion of limbs, joint contractures, joint hypermobility
- Hands and feet: Size, shape, number of digits, nails
- External genitalia
- Skin changes, e.g. hyperpigmented or depigmented lesions
- Birth defects, e.g. cleft lip
- Cardiovascular examination
- Abdominal palpation for organomegaly

Minor Anomalies

- These are defined as physical features present in <5% of the general population, which are of no clinical significance in themselves.
- They may be clues to the underlying diagnosis, especially if >3 are present together.

- They are most common in the face, external ears, hands and feet.
- They may be present as a familial trait. Parents and siblings should be examined before ascribing significance to a particular anomaly.

Objective Measurements

- Height, weight and head circumference.
- Other measurements that should be taken depending on the diagnosis considered, e.g. measuring arm span, upper-to-lower-segment ratios when considering Marfan syndrome.
- There are standard charts for the normal measurements at different ages.

Photographs

- If the child is seen for the first time in late childhood or adolescence, reviewing baby and early childhood photographs may help in making the diagnosis, especially with syndromes in which the dysmorphic features become less apparent with age, e.g. Beckwith–Wiedemann syndrome.
- Photography at the time of clinical assessment, with parental consent, serves as an important part of the medical record. If the child is undiagnosed, the photographs can be shown to fellow geneticists for their opinion.

Making a Clinical Diagnosis

- **Gestalt:** Some diagnoses are made based on the overall appearance of the patient, e.g. the way that most people can recognise a child with Down syndrome.
- **Pattern recognition:** An uncommon malformation or combination of anomalies may point to a particular diagnosis or group of conditions. The next step is to compare the clinical findings and history with those expected in the syndrome being considered. Several textbooks describe many of the syndromes and include photographs that can be used for comparison.
- **Computerised database search:** This may suggest possible diagnoses from thousands of identifiable syndromes that have been reported. An example of such a computerised database is Online Mendelian Inheritance in Man (OMIM). Training and experience are needed to use these databases effectively.

If the diagnosis is uncertain, it would be better to defer assigning a specific diagnosis rather than assigning an incorrect diagnosis because labels, once applied, are hard to remove. An incorrect diagnosis also leads to inappropriate counselling and possible stigmatisation. Using terms such as 'funny-looking kid (FLK)', 'elfin faces' or 'happy puppet' is not acceptable, as they have unfavourable connotations.

Laboratory Investigations

In general, genetic or genomic tests are labour-intensive and expensive. Thus, they should be ordered judiciously.

- Chromosome studies
  - » Standard banded karyotype (Chromosome analysis)

- To be visible on a standard karyotype, a chromosome deletion or duplication probably involves more than 3 to 5 million bases (Mb) of DNA
- A high proportion of genes are involved in the development and functioning of the brain, thus a child with a cytogenetically visible chromosome abnormality is likely to have developmental delay in association with other malformations, rather than an isolated congenital malformation, e.g. an isolated CHD
- Identifies common chromosomal aneuploidies (e.g. trisomy 13, trisomy 18, trisomy 21, monosomy X), large structural changes (e.g. Cri du chat/5p minus syndrome), structural rearrangements, mosaicism

» Fluorescence in situ hybridisation (FISH)

- This method uses fluorescence-tagged single-stranded DNA targeted probes to hybridise with a specific targeted DNA sequence
- This technique is most commonly applied in the diagnosis of microdeletion syndromes, e.g. Prader–Willi/Angelman syndromes, 22q11.2 deletion syndrome, Miller–Dieker syndrome, and Williams syndrome where the chromosome deletion is generally too small to be seen on a standard karyotype

» Chromosomal microarray analysis (CMA)

- This is a DNA-based method of measuring gains and losses of DNA throughout the human genome and is able to identify chromosomal abnormalities, including submicroscopic abnormalities that are too small (50–100 kilobases) to be detected by conventional karyotyping.
- It is recommended as the first-tier test in the genetic evaluation of infants and children with unexplained intellectual disability, multiple congenital anomalies or autism spectrum disorder and has a diagnostic yield of 15–20%.
- This method cannot detect balanced changes such as inversions, insertions or balanced translocations as there is no net loss or gain in chromosomal material in these rearrangements.
- Variants of uncertain significance (microdeletion/microduplication) can be difficult for clinicians to interpret.

» Practical points

- For standard karyotype and/or FISH studies on peripheral blood, send 3–5 ml of blood in a sodium heparin or lithium heparin tube (green-topped) to the cytogenetics laboratory. For these investigations, the patient's blood should be drawn using sterile technique.
- For CMA, send 3–5 ml of blood in an EDTA tube (purple-topped) to the cytogenetics laboratory.

    - A completed consent form must accompany requests for all chromosome studies.

- Molecular/DNA Studies
  - » Molecular studies are not necessary if the diagnosis is clinically unambiguous, e.g. in Marfan syndrome, the diagnosis is based on clinical criteria (Revised Ghent nosology).
  - » Indications for undertaking molecular studies include:
    - When the diagnosis is not clear clinically
    - When the parents are at risk of a second affected child and would like prenatal diagnosis
  - » Next generation sequencing (NGS) allows massively parallel sequencing of multiple genes to identify single nucleotide variants (SNVs) or small insertions and/or deletions (indels):
    - Single-gene or multiple gene panel (e.g. RASopathy panel, aortopathy panel)
    - Whole exome sequencing (WES): Sequencing of ~1.5% of the genome that codes for proteins (30 Mb, 180000 exons). Non-coding regions are not sequenced.
    - Whole genome sequencing (WGS): Sequencing of the entire genome of 3 billion base pairs
  - » Potential limitations of molecular studies:
    - Genetic heterogeneity of a syndrome, i.e. more than one gene involved; for example, in tuberous sclerosis, where pathogenic variants in at least two genes *TSC1* (chromosome locus 9q34) and *TSC2* (chromosome locus 16p13.3) have been identified
    - Inability to identify all pathogenic variants in a gene, e.g. in Marfan syndrome, in which there are many pathogenic variants possible in the *FBN1* gene, some unique to only a few families
    - Variants of uncertain significance (SNVs/indels) can be difficult for clinicians to interpret
  - » Pre-test genetic counselling is mandatory for all patients who undergo molecular genetic testing. It is also mandatory to offer post-test genetic counselling to these individuals.
  - » Practical points:
    - For molecular/DNA studies, send 3–5 ml of blood in an EDTA tube (purple-topped) to the DNA laboratory.
    - A completed consent form must accompany requests for molecular/DNA studies.
- Biochemical/Metabolic Laboratory Testing
  - » Some genetic disorders presenting with dysmorphic features can be diagnosed with biochemical or metabolic tests. Examples include:

- Storage disorders, e.g. the mucopolysaccharidoses: Urine glycosaminoglycans (GAGs) analysis
- Peroxisomal disorders, e.g. Zellweger syndrome: Plasma very long chain fatty acids (VLCFAs) analysis

After the Diagnosis is Made

When informing parents about the diagnosis, special points to note include:

- Enough time set aside by the clinical staff
- Meeting in a quiet and private place
- Both parents should be present

Often, it is a time of ambivalence for the parents. While they may be relieved that there is finally an explanation for the medical or developmental condition that their child has had, there is also understandably a sense of loss and grief, as they may feel that they have 'lost' a normal child. Referral to a medical social worker or even a psychologist may be necessary.

A multi-disciplinary approach is often required to address the individual medical problems the child may have. Besides the medical aspects, attention must also be paid to the social and psychological problems the child and his family may face. If there are relevant support groups, e.g. Down Syndrome Association of Singapore, contact details should be made available.

What if No Diagnosis is Identifiable?

In such situations, although no underlying cause is identified, the individual medical and developmental problems should receive the appropriate attention and management.

Further diagnostic options available to the clinician are:

- Showing photographs of undiagnosed patients to fellow geneticists. Advances in information technology have made international expertise more readily available.
- Following the patients over time. In some syndromes, the physical features become more apparent with age. Furthermore, new syndromes may be described and new diagnostic tools become available. With the passing of time, a previously undiagnosed syndrome may become clear.
- Reviewing of genetic test results over time, e.g. genome sequencing data.

Conclusion

The approach to a child with suspected genetic syndrome is based on a systematic approach of history-taking and clinical examination, followed by ordering the relevant laboratory investigations. Checking textbooks of syndromes and computerised databases, as well as discussing with fellow geneticists and with our colleagues in the laboratories, is often helpful in coming to an overall diagnosis. Finally, effective communication with the child's parents is very important, during the diagnostic process, when a syndrome diagnosis is made and also when no syndrome can be identified.

Bibliography

1. Jones KL, *et al.* (eds.). (1997) *Smith's Recognizable Patterns of Human Malformation, 5th ed.* Philadelphia, PA: WB Saunders.
2. Carey JC, Cassidy SB, Battaglia A, *et al.* (eds.). (2020) *Cassidy and Allanson's Management of Genetic Syndromes.* John Wiley & Sons.
3. Gorlin RJ, Cohen MM Jr, Hennekam RCM (eds.). (2001) *Syndromes of the Head and Neck, 4th ed.* New York, NY: Oxford University Press.
4. Online Mendelian Inheritance in Man, OMIM®. (2022) An Online Catalog of Human Genes and Genetic Disorders. McKusick-Nathans Institute of Genetic Medicine, Johns Hopkins University. Baltimore, MD. https://omim.org/
5. Hunter AG. (2002) Medical genetics: 2. The diagnostic approach to the child with dysmorphic signs. *CMAJ* **167**(4):367–372.

CHAPTER 58

Common Genetic Conditions

Koh Ai Ling; Lai Hwei Meeng, Angeline

Definitions

- Syndrome
  - » Derived from Greek, meaning 'running together'
  - » Refers to a group of features that occur together consistently and implies a common specific cause, though the cause may not be known at present
- Sequence
  - » Refers to a group of features, resulting from a cascade of events initiated by a single primary factor, e.g. in the Potter Sequence, the cascade of events is renal agenesis, lack of fetal urine, severe oligohydramnios, pulmonary hypoplasia and restricted intrauterine space, compressed facial appearance and limb deformities like talipes
- Association
  - » Refers to a group of features that occur together commonly, but not as consistently as in a syndrome, e.g. the VATER/VACTERL association

Chromosome Disorders

Trisomy 21 (Down Syndrome)

- Incidence
  - » 1 in 650 live births, can vary between 1 in 600 and 1 in 2000 amongst different populations
  - » Overall incidence rises after the maternal age of 35 years
- Features
  - » Diagnostic features in the neonate: Hypotonia, poor Moro reflex, hyperextensibility of joints, excess skin on back of neck, flat facial profile, slanted palpebral fissures, anomalous auricles, dysplasia of pelvis, dysplasia of middle phalanx of fifth finger, single palmar crease. All have at least four features, and 89% have six or more features
  - » Dysmorphic features: Brachycephaly, late closure of fontanelles, third fontanelle, hypertelorism, upslanting palpebral fissures, epicanthic folds, Brushfield spots (rarely seen in Asians), small nose, low nasal bridge, open mouth with protruding tongue, short neck, short broad hands, single palmar

crease, hypoplasia of the middle phalanx of the fifth finger with clinodactyly, wide gap between first and second toes
    - Short stature
    - Developmental delay, intellectual disability. Intelligence Quotient (IQ) is typically between 25 and 50
    - Congenital heart defects (CHD) in about 40% of cases. The common defects are ventricular septal defect (VSD), atrio-ventricular septal defect, atrial septal defect, Tetralogy of Fallot (FT) and patent ductus arteriosus (PDA)
    - Gastrointestinal malformations in about 15% of cases, including tracheooesophageal fistula (TEF), pyloric stenosis, duodenal atresia, annular pancreas, Hirschsprung disease and imperforate anus
    - Haematologic disorders: Neonatal polycythaemia, transient abnormal myelopoiesis (TAM) and acute leukaemia (characteristically AML-M7). The incidence of leukaemia in Down syndrome is about 1%.
    - Thyroid disorders are common, thus annual thyroid function tests are recommended
- Cause
    - 95% have trisomy for chromosome 21, due to non-disjunction
    - 4–5% have an unbalanced translocation, in which a chromosome 21 is attached to another chromosome, most commonly chromosome 14, either arising *de novo* or being transmitted from one of the parents
    - <1% have mosaic trisomy 21
- Diagnosis
    - Karyotype
    - In the case of an unbalanced translocation, parental karyotyping is indicated
- Recurrence risks
    - For trisomy 21, the recurrence risk after one affected child is generally accepted to be 1% for women younger than 37 years and twice the maternal age-related risk for women 37 years and older
    - For Down syndrome due to unbalanced translocations, the recurrence risk is affected by which another chromosome is involved in the translocation, whether the translocation is *de novo* or inherited, and if inherited, whether the origin is paternal or maternal
    - For D-G translocations, i.e. involving one of the group D chromosomes (13, 14 or 15), 50% arise *de novo* and 50% are inherited. If the father is the balanced translocation carrier, the recurrence risk is 2–5%. If the mother is the balanced translocation carrier, the recurrence risk is 10%. These actual recurrence risks are much lower than the theoretical risk, which is 1 in 3 or 33%
    - For G-G translocations, i.e. involving one of the group G chromosomes (21 or 22), 90% arise *de novo* and 10% are inherited. For inherited 21/22 translocations, the recurrence risk is 4%. For inherited 21/21 translocations, all viable zygotes will have translocation Down syndrome, i.e. the recurrence risk is 100%

Trisomy 18 (Edward Syndrome)

- Incidence: About 1 in 8000 live births
- Features
  - » Pre- and postnatal growth restriction
  - » Polyhydramnios and decreased fetal activity
  - » Dysmorphic features: Prominent occiput, micrognathia, low-set malformed ears, overlapping flexed fingers, prominent calcaneus, short sternum, undescended testes
  - » Severe intellectual disability
  - » Neonatal hypotonia, followed by the development of hypertonia
  - » CHD in about 85% of cases, including valvular heart disease, VSD, PDA, etc.
  - » Urogenital and gastrointestinal anomalies
- Shortened life expectancy: 5% survive to 12 months of age. 70% of deaths are due to cardiopulmonary arrest, with central apnoea being a major factor in the neonatal period and infancy.
- Cause: Majority have trisomy for chromosome 18, which is associated with advanced maternal age
- Diagnosis: Karyotype
- Recurrence risk: 0.5% for trisomy 18 after one affected child

Trisomy 13 (Patau Syndrome)

- Incidence: About 1 in 30000 live births
- Features
  - » Mean birthweight is 2600 g. Postnatally, they characteristically have feeding difficulties and failure to thrive.
  - » Dysmorphic features: Microcephaly, scalp defects (commonly at the vertex), sloping forehead, microphthalmia, hypotelorism, cleft lip (lateral or median), micrognathia, malformed ears, short neck, redundant nuchal skin, postaxial polydactyly, flexed fingers, undescended testes
  - » Severe developmental disability
  - » Holoprosencephaly
  - » CHDs and structural renal anomalies are common
  - » An interesting haematologic finding is that of nuclear projections in polymorphonuclear leukocytes, which has been reported in 25–80% of cases
- Shortened life expectancy: 5 to 10% survive to >12 months of age. Cardiopulmonary arrest is the most common cause of death; central apnoea may be an important factor.
- Cause: Majority have trisomy for chromosome 13, which is associated with advanced maternal age
- Diagnosis: Karyotype
- Recurrence risk: Low (~0.5%) for trisomy 13

Turner Syndrome

- Incidence
  - About 1 in 3000 liveborn girls
  - This is one of the most common chromosome disorders at conception, but the majority (about 98–99%) miscarry, usually in the early stages of pregnancy
- Features
  - In neonates, lymphoedema of hands and feet and excess nuchal skin
  - Short stature — Mean untreated adult height is about 145 cm
  - Pubertal failure, infertility due to streak gonads
  - Dysmorphic features: Webbed neck, increased carrying angle of elbows, broad (shield) chest, widely spaced nipples, narrow hyperconvex nails, multiple-pigmented naevi
  - CHDs in 23%, most commonly bicuspid aortic valve, coarctation of the aorta and aortic valve disease
  - Structural renal anomalies
  - Majority have normal intelligence, but may have specific learning difficulties
  - Hypothyroidism, diabetes mellitus and inflammatory bowel disease occur more frequently in girls and women with Turner syndrome, than in the general population
  - Patients with a 45,X/46,XY karyotype have an increased risk of gonadoblastoma
- Cause
  - 50% have 45,X karyotype
  - About 20% have isochromosome X
  - About 30% have mosaicism (45,X/46,XX or 45,X/46,XY)
  - A small proportion have other rarer karyotypes
- Diagnosis: Karyotype
- Management
  - Growth hormone treatment
  - Oestrogen replacement therapy at puberty
  - Surveillance for associated complications

Fragile X Syndrome

- Incidence:
  - 1 in 4000 males
  - This is the most common form of inherited intellectual disability
- Features
  - Intellectual disability of variable severity
  - Dysmorphic features: Macrocephaly, long face, prominent jaw (which develops during adolescence), big ears, post-pubertal macro-orchidism
  - Delayed developmental milestones
  - Shy personality
  - Behavioural problems: Autism spectrum disorder, attention deficit hyperactivity disorder and hyperactivity

- Cause
  - » Most commonly due to a variant in the *FMR1* gene on the long arm of the X chromosome (locus Xq27.3). This locus is designated FRAXA.
  - » The *FMR1* gene consists of a sequence of CGG triplet repeats. Normally, there are 5–55 CGG triplet repeats.
  - » In a full mutation, there are >200 CGG triplet repeats. All males and about 35% of females with a full mutation will have features of the syndrome.
  - » *FMR1* alleles with 55–200 CGG triplet repeats are pre-mutation alleles. When female pre-mutation carriers pass the pre-mutation alleles to their offspring, the allele is unstable and the number of CGG triplet repeats may increase. If the number of CGG triplet repeats increases to >200, their offspring will have the full mutation. When male pre-mutation carriers transmit the pre-mutation allele to their children, the allele remains stable and does not expand.
  - » About 20% of female premutation carriers have premature ovarian failure (cessation of menses below 40 years of age). This information would be helpful for reproductive planning.
  - » Fragile X tremor ataxia syndrome (FXTAS) occurs in individuals who have the *FMR1* premutation and is characterised by late-onset, progressive cerebellar ataxia and intention tremor, cognitive impairment and psychiatric disorders. It is more common in male premutation carriers (40%) than in female premutation carriers (16–20%).
  - » A few other fragile sites on the long arm of the X chromosome have been described, but only FRAXE (chromosome locus Xq28) has been shown to have phenotypic effect.
- Diagnosis
  - » DNA analysis: This is the method of choice for the diagnosis of Fragile X syndrome to detect CGG trinucleotide repeat expansion in *FMR1*. It identifies not only affected males but also differentiates pre-mutation alleles from normal alleles. In a child with intellectual disability, chromosome microarray analysis (CMA) should also be done to exclude other chromosomal abnormalities.
  - » The inheritance of Fragile X syndrome is X-linked. There are implications for the extended family of the affected person, thus carrier testing should be offered to relevant members of the extended family.

Contiguous Gene Deletion Syndromes

22q11.2 Deletion Syndrome/Velocardiofacial Syndrome (VCFS)

- Incidence: 1 in 4000
- Features
  - » Dysmorphic features: Long face, flat malar region, prominent nose with squared nasal root, hypoplastic alae nasi, narrow nasal passages, long philtrum, thin upper lip, slender and tapering fingers

   - Cleft palate, submucous cleft palate, velopharyngeal incoordination or incompetence (resulting in nasal regurgitation, hypernasal voice and recurrent serous otitis media)
   - CHDs, including VSD, right-sided aortic arch, FT, pulmonary atresia with VSD, interrupted aortic arch. Conotruncal defects are the most characteristic CHD.
   - Learning difficulty and mild intellectual disability
   - Structural renal anomalies in about 35% of cases
   - T-lymphocyte dysfunction and hypocalcaemia in infancy may occur, which are features of DiGeorge syndrome.
   - Psychiatric illness in up to 20% of affected adults, including an increased risk of schizophrenia
- Cause
   - Submicroscopic deletion of chromosome 22q11.2
   - Inheritance is autosomal dominant, with variable expressivity
   - Majority of cases represent *de novo* variants; about 15% have inherited the microdeletion.
- Diagnosis
   - CMA or fluorescence *in situ* hybridisation (FISH)
   - Parents of affected children should be offered testing, as clinical features may be very mild. If one parent also has a 22q11.2 deletion, the risk of recurrence for future children is 1 in 2 or 50%.
   - The acronym 'CATCH 22', which was coined for the phenotypic features found in this condition, is regarded as derogatory and should not be used.

Williams Syndrome

- Incidence: 1 in 10000 to 1 in 20000 births
- Features
   - Dysmorphic features: Epicanthic folds, periorbital fullness, stellate iris pattern, flat midface, depressed nasal bridge, anteverted nostrils, long philtrum, thick lips
   - Growth deficiency
   - Infantile hypercalcaemia
   - CHDs, most commonly supravalvular aortic stenosis and pulmonary artery stenosis
   - Intellectual disability
   - Unique personality characteristics: Overfriendliness, empathy, generalised anxiety, specific phobias and attention deficit disorder
- Cause
   - Submicroscopic deletion of chromosome 7q11.23 that includes the elastin (ELN) gene in 95% of patients
   - Inheritance appears to be autosomal dominant, but almost all cases represent new variants and are sporadic. Parent-to-child transmission is rare because affected adults rarely reproduce.
- Diagnosis: CMA or FISH

Other Disorders

Noonan Syndrome

- Incidence: 1 in 2500 live births
- Features
  - » Short stature
  - » Dysmorphic features: Hair may be wispy in infancy and become curly and woolly in childhood. The facial features change with age.
  - » Facial features in the neonate: Tall forehead, hypertelorism, downslanting palpebral fissures, epicanthic folds, depressed nasal root, upturned nasal tip, low-set and posteriorly angulated ears, excessive nuchal skin
  - » Features in infancy and childhood: Relatively large head, hypertelorism, downslanting palpebral fissures, ptosis, hooded eyelids, low-set and posteriorly rotated ears, broad or webbed neck, characteristic chest deformity (pectus carinatum superiorly and pectus excavatum inferiorly), undescended testes
  - » CHDs in about 65%, most commonly dysplastic pulmonary valve and/or pulmonary valve stenosis. Hypertrophic cardiomyopathy, obstructive or non-obstructive, occurs in 20–30%
  - » Feeding difficulties in early infancy are common, occurring in 77% of cases. These range from mild difficulties with poor suck to severe difficulties requiring prolonged tube feeding
  - » Mild intellectual disability in 35%. Mean IQ ranges from 64–127. There may be specific learning problems, especially with speech and articulation.
  - » Structural renal anomalies
  - » Lymphatic abnormalities, including lymphedema
  - » Bleeding abnormalities in 50–65%, including factor XI, XII or VIII deficiency, von Willebrand Disease and platelet dysfunction
- Cause
  - » Heterozygous pathogenic variants in *PTPN11* (ch12q24.1), *SOS1* (ch2p22.1), *KRAS* (ch12p12.1), *BRAF* (ch7q34), *RAF1* (ch3p25.2), *NRAS* (ch1p13.2), *SOS2* (ch14q21.3) and biallelic compound heterozygous pathogenic variants in *LZTR1* have been identified in about 80% of people with Noonan syndrome
  - » Most of the early cases appeared to be sporadic, but recent reports indicate parent-to-child transmission in 30–75%, with mostly autosomal dominant in inheritance and highly variable expressivity.
  - » Most common developmental disorder within the RASopathy family of disorders caused by germline variants in genes encoding components belonging to the Ras and mitogen-activated protein kinase (MAPK) signalling pathway that interacts with extracellular growth factors to regulate cell proliferation, differentiation and senescence
  - » Other RASopathies include Noonan syndrome with multiple lentigines (NSML), Costello syndrome, cardiofaciocutaneous (CFC) syndrome, other Noonan-like syndrome, Legius syndrome and neurofibromatosis type 1
- Diagnosis: DNA analysis (e.g. multigene RASopathy panel)

Neurofibromatosis Type 1 (NF1)

- Incidence: 1 in 3000 live births
- Features
  - » Cardinal features
    - ■ Cutaneous features: multiple *café au lait* spots, intertriginous (axillary, inguinal) freckling, neurofibromata
    - ■ Ocular findings: Lisch nodules, optic glioma
    - ■ Musculoskeletal features: Bony lesions including dysplasia of sphenoid bone, dysplasia or thinning of long bone cortex
  - » Juvenile xanthogranuloma, naevus anaemicus
  - » Learning difficulties/behavioural problems in 50–80% of affected individuals
  - » Scoliosis
  - » Hypertension (can be secondary to renal artery stenosis, coarctation of the aorta, pheochromocytoma)
  - » Risk of other tumours
    - ■ Malignant peripheral nerve sheath tumours in about 10% of affected individuals, especially in adolescence or early adulthood
    - ■ Non-optic gliomas (e.g. brainstem, cerebellum)
    - ■ Haematological malignancies — juvenile chronic myelogenous leukaemia, myelodysplastic syndrome
- Cause
  - » Pathogenic variants in the *NF1* gene on 17q11.2 that encodes neurofibromin
  - » Whole-gene deletions of *NF1* gene occur in 4–5% of individuals with NF1
  - » About half of all affected individuals have the disorder as the result of the *de novo* pathogenic variant and the condition is autosomal dominant in inheritance with highly variable expressivity
- Diagnosis
  - » The diagnosis is primarily based on clinical diagnostic criteria for NF1 that was developed during the National Institutes of Health Consensus Development Conference in 1987 and revised in 2021.
  - » In an individual who does not have a parent with NF1, the diagnosis is established in at least two of the following criteria:
    - ■ Multiple *café au lait* spots (six or more) >5 mm in greater diameter in prepubertal individuals and >15 mm in greatest diameter in postpubertal individuals
    - ■ Neurofibromata of any type (two or more) or plexiform neurofibromata (one or more)
    - ■ Freckling in the axillary or inguinal regions
    - ■ Optic glioma
    - ■ Lisch nodules (two or more) or two or more choroidal abnormalities
    - ■ Distinctive bony lesion — dysplasia of the sphenoid bone, anterolateral bowing of the tibia or pseudoarthrosis of a long bone

    - A heterozygous pathogenic *NF1* variant with a variant allele fraction of 50% in apparently normal tissue (e.g. white blood cells)
  - A child of a parent with NF1 can be diagnosed if one or more of these criteria are met
  - As each of the diagnostic manifestations has different ages of presentation, patients who do not fulfil the diagnostic criteria during the infantile period should be followed up to look for other major clinical manifestations with a later age of onset. For example, *café au lait* spots are mostly present at birth and increase in number thereafter but skin-fold freckling and Lisch nodules usually develop later in childhood
  - Genetic testing using DNA analysis of the *NF1* gene is indicated in:
    - Individuals in whom the possibility of NF1 remains high but do not fulfil the diagnostic criteria
    - A young child with a tumour (e.g. optic glioma) in the absence of other diagnostic features of NF1, in whom establishing a diagnosis of NF1 would be important to guide the management
    - An adult with NF1 if prenatal testing in a current pregnancy or preimplantation genetic testing for future pregnancy is anticipated

Marfan Syndrome

- Incidence: 1 in 5000 to 1 in 10000
- Features
  - Tall stature and disproportionately long limbs, resulting in a decreased upper-to-lower-segment ratio and an increased arm span-to-height ratio
  - Other musculoskeletal features: Arachnodactyly, reduced elbow extension, pectus excavatum or carinatum, flat feet, scoliosis
  - Facial features: Dolichocephaly, downslanting palpebral fissures, enophthalmos, malar hypoplasia, retrognathia
  - Cardiovascular abnormalities: Mitral valve prolapse is common. Progressive aortic root dilatation is the most severe abnormality and may result in increasing aortic regurgitation and heart failure or aortic dissection and rupture. These are the leading causes of death in people with Marfan syndrome
  - Ocular abnormalities: Lens dislocation in 50–80% of cases (usually upward), flat cornea, increased axial length of the globe, hypoplastic iris or ciliary muscle
  - Pulmonary apical bullae, spontaneous pneumothorax (frequency is low: 4.4%)
- Cause
  - Autosomal dominant inheritance, with very high penetrance. About 25% of patients represent *de novo* variants.
  - Pathogenic variants in the fibrillin 1 (FBN1) gene (chromosome locus 15q21.1). Multiple pathogenic variants of all sorts have been found, and the majority identified in not more than one unrelated individual. Pathogenic variants in *FBN1* gene are also found in other conditions, e.g. familial aortic aneurysm and familial ectopia lentis. Thus, finding a pathogenic variant in *FBN1* does not necessarily confirm the presence of Marfan syndrome. DNA

analysis is usually embarked on, if there are considerations about prenatal diagnosis or preimplantation genetic diagnosis

- Diagnosis
  - » The diagnosis is primarily based on clinical criteria using the 2010 Revised Ghent Nosology for Marfan syndrome (See Table 14.1).

Table 14.1 2010 Revised Ghent Nosology for Marfan Syndrome

Diagnosis of Marfan syndrome is made if	
In the absence of family history:	• Aortic root dilatation Z score ≥2 AND Ectopia lentis • Aortic root dilatation Z score ≥2 AND *FBN1* pathogenic variant • Aortic root dilatation Z score ≥2 AND Systemic score ≥7 points* • Ectopia lentis AND *FBN1* pathogenic variant associated with aortic root dilatation
In the presence of family history:	• Ectopia lentis AND family history of Marfan syndrome • A systemic score ≥7 points AND family history of Marfan syndrome • Aortic root dilatation z score ≥2 above 20 yr old, ≥3 below 20 yr old and also family history of Marfan syndrome
Systemic score (score ≥7 indicates systemic involvement)	
Features	**Score (points)**
• Wrist AND thumb sign	3
• Wrist OR thumb sign	1
• Pectus carinatum deformity	2
• Pectus excavatum or chest asymmetry	1
• Hindfoot deformity	2
• Plain pes planus	1
• Reduced upper/lower segment ratio# AND increased arm span/height ratio (>1.05)	1
• Scoliosis > 20° OR thoracolumbar kyphosis	1
• Protrusio acetabuli	2
• Reduced elbow extension (<170°)	1
• Facial features (3 of 5 present) • Dolichocephaly • Downward-slanting palpebral fissures • Enophthalmos • Retrognathia • Malar hypoplasia	1
• Skin striae	1
• Spontaneous pneumothorax	2
• Dural ectasia	2
• Myopia > 3 diopters	1
• Mitral valve prolapse	1

*After exclusion of Loeys–Dietz, Shprintzen–Goldberg, and vascular Ehlers–Danlos syndromes
#Upper segment/lower segment <1 (age 0–5 years); <0.95 (age 6–7 years); <0.9 (age 8–9 years); <0.85 (age above 10 years)

» In general, besides clinical examination, at least two specific studies are necessary for diagnosis: cardiac evaluation, including echocardiography, and slit-lamp eye examination.
» Genetic testing using DNA analysis of the *FBN1* gene is indicated in patients with suspected Marfan syndrome who do not fulfil clinical diagnostic criteria

Bibliography

1. Gorlin RJ, Cohen MM Jr, Hennekam RCM (eds.). (2001) *Syndromes of the Head and Neck, 4th ed.* New York, NY: Oxford University Press.
2. Jones KL, *et al.* (eds). (1997) *Smith's Recognizable Patterns of Human Malformation, 5th ed.* Philadelphia, PA: WB Saunders.
3. Carey JC, Cassidy SB, Battaglia A (eds.). (2020) *Cassidy and Allanson's Management of Genetic Syndromes.* Hoboken, NJ: John Wiley & Sons.
4. Hall B. (1964) Mongolism in newborns: A clinical and cytogenetic study. *Acta Paediatr Scand* **154**(Suppl):1–95.
5. Firth HV, Hurst JA. (2017) *Oxford Desk Reference: Clinical Genetics and Genomics*. Oxford: Oxford University Press.
6. Friedman JM. (1993–2021) Neurofibromatosis 1. In: Adam MP, Ardinger HH, Pagon RA, *et al.* (eds.) *GeneReviews*® [Internet]. Seattle: University of Washington. https://www.ncbi.nlm.nih.gov/books/NBK1109/
7. Legius E, Messiaen L, Wolkenstein P, *et al.* (2021) Revised diagnostic criteria for neurofibromatosis type 1 and Legius syndrome: An international consensus recommendation. *Genet Med* **23**(8):1506–1513.
8. Loeys BL, Dietz HC, Braverman AC, *et al.* (2010) The revised Ghent nosology for the Marfan syndrome. *J Med Genet* **47**(7):476–485.

CHAPTER 59

Inborn Errors of Metabolism

Koh Ai Ling; Ting Teck Wah; Tan Ee Shien; Teo Siak Hong

Introduction

Although individually rare, Inborn Errors of Metabolism (IEMs) collectively have an incidence of about 1:3000–3500 in Singapore. The National Expanded Newborn Screening (NENS) laboratory in our institution has been screening samples of Singaporean children since 2006.

The most opportune time to diagnose an IEM is soon after birth when the baby is asymptomatic. Often, metabolic decompensation can occur within the first week of life resulting in critical illness. Severe morbidity and mortality can result from the first presentation alone.

Newborn Screening

Which Conditions do we Screen for?

Expanded newborn screening allows us to screen for several IEMs, including amino acid disorders, organic acidurias and fatty acid oxidation defects (FAODs), and non-IEM conditions, including congenital adrenal hyperplasia (CAH), cystic fibrosis (CF) and severe combined immunodeficiency (SCID) (see Table 14.2).

Normal screening results indicate that the individual has a very low risk of having one of the listed disorders but do not completely rule out the possibility. Where there is clinical concern for an IEM, a metabolic physician should be consulted, even in the face of normal screening result. Please also note that there are many IEMs that cannot be detected by this extended newborn screen. Where there is clinical concern, a metabolic physician should be consulted.

Practical Aspects

When to do the Test?

The ideal window for testing is between 24 and 72 hours of life, although samples are still acceptable up to 7 days of life. Since some of these conditions present in the first few days of life, early sampling is preferred. The levels of these metabolites vary in the first few weeks of life and so samples taken after 7 days of life give difficulties in reliable interpretation. In particular, FAODs metabolites may have normalised.

Preterm babies should also have their samples taken at 24–72 hours of age with further samples as required based on the preterm baby protocol.

What is Needed?

One drop of blood obtained via heel prick should be allowed to saturate each circle on the newborn screening card. The cards should be allowed to fully air dry (for 3–4 hours) and sent to the newborn screening lab within 24 hours of collection.

Table 14.2 National Expanded Newborn Screening Programme

Primary Targets	Secondary Conditions	Other Conditions
Conditions that the programme aims to detect	Conditions that may be identified while investigating abnormal results for the primary targets	
Amino acid disorders - Phenylketonuria including biopterin defects - Maple syrup urine disease - Citrullinaemia type 1 - Argininosuccinic aciduria - Tyrosinaemia type 1 - Homocystinuria (pyridoxine unresponsive)	Amino acid disorders - Hyperphenylalaninaemia - Arginase deficiency - Citrin deficiency - Hypermethioninaemia - Tyrosinaemia Types 2 and 3	IEM - Galactosaemia - Biotinidase deficiency
Organic acid disorders - Propionic acidaemia - Methylmalonic acidaemia (MUT) - Cobalamin A/B defect - Isovaleric acidaemia - β-ketothiolase deficiency - Glutaric aciduria type 1 - Malonic aciduria - 3-hydroxy-3-methylglutaryl-CoA lyase deficiency - Multiple carboxylase deficiency	Organic acid disorders - 3-methylcrotonyl-CoA carboxylase deficiency - 2-methyl-3-hydroxybutyric aciduria - 3-methylglutaconyl-CoA dehydratase deficiency - Isobutyryl-CoA dehydrogenase deficiency - 2-methylbutyryl-CoA dehydrogenase deficiency/short branch chain acyl-CoA - Ethylmalonic encephalopathy - Cobalamin C/D defect	Non-IEM - Congenital adrenal hyperplasia - Cystic fibrosis - Severe combined immunodeficiency
Fatty acid oxidation disorders - Primary carnitine deficiency/carnitine uptake deficiency - Medium chain acyl-CoA dehydrogenase deficiency - Very long chain acyl-CoA dehydrogenase deficiency - Long chain hydroxy acyl-CoA dehydrogenase deficiency - Trifunctional protein deficiency	Fatty acid oxidation disorders - Carnitine palmitoyltransferase deficiency type 1 - Carnitine palmitoyltransferase deficiency type 2 - Carnitine-acylcarnitine translocase deficiency - Multiple acyl-CoA dehydrogenase deficiency/glutaric aciduria type 2 - Short chain acyl-CoA dehydrogenase deficiency - Medium/short chain hydroxy acyl-CoA dehydrogenase deficiency - Medium chain ketoacyl-CoA thiolase deficiency	

Clinical Manifestations in the Neonatal and Early Infancy Period

- Acute metabolic encephalopathy
- Seizures or neurological deficit
- Hypotonia
- Jaundice and liver dysfunction
- Cardiac disease (e.g. cardiomyopathy)

Approach

History

- Typical clinical presentation
  - » Usually non-specific and subtle
  - » Lethargy or irritability
  - » Poor feeding
  - » Vomiting
  - » Floppy, seizures
  - » Failure to regain birth weight during neonatal period
- Pattern of presentation — well initially with development of symptoms (e.g. poor feeding, lethargy) later on or overwhelming neurological symptoms (e.g. seizures) during early neonatal period
- Birth history is usually unremarkable
- Consanguinity
- Family history of IEM, early neonatal death

Clinical Examination

- Few with dysmorphic features
- Hypotonia/hypertonia
- Jaundice, hepatomegaly
- Respiratory distress
- Cardiomegaly, heart failure

First-Line Metabolic Investigations

- Blood gas pH and bicarbonate
- Blood glucose
- Plasma lactate
- Plasma ammonia
- Plasma amino acid profile
- Plasma acylcarnitine
- Urine organic acid
- Urine (or blood) ketones

Biochemical Abnormalities that may Suggest IEMs

- Severe persistent high anion gap metabolic acidosis

- Severe lactic acidosis
- Respiratory alkalosis (may suggest urea cycle defect [UCD])
- Persistent hypoglycaemia, ketotic or non-ketotic
- Severe ketonuria (abnormal during neonatal period)
- Hyperammonaemia

High Anion Gap Metabolic Acidosis

- Anion gap is defined as the difference between the serum Na^+ and the sum of serum Cl^- plus HCO_3^- (Normal anion gap = 7–16 mmol/L)
- Metabolic acidosis with raised anion gap reflects an increase in an unmeasured anion that may be suggestive of an IEM causing acidosis
  - » Organic acids — organic acidaemias (methylmalonic acidaemia (MMA), propionic acidaemia (PA), isovaleric acidaemia (IVA), glutaric aciduria [GA] type I)
  - » Lactic acidosis — primary lactic acidosis, mitochondrial disorders, organic acidaemias, FAODs, gluconeogenesis defects
  - » Ketosis (especially in neonates) — ketolytic defects (marked unanticipated ketosis without fasting), most IEMs except FAODs
- Hypoglycaemia, and/or hyperammonaemia in the presence of significant acidosis are highly suggestive of IEM

Lactic Acidosis

- Lactic acidosis >2 mmol/L
- Hyperlactataemia is due to the elevation of pyruvate, the NADH/NAD ratio, acidosis or both
- Based on Cohen–Woods classification, lactic acidosis can be due to:
  - » Tissue hypoxia or hypoperfusion (Type A) secondary to asphyxia/hypoxia, decreased cardiac output/left ventricular failure, severe anaemia, carbon monoxide poisoning
  - » Underlying disease process (Type B1) — sepsis, renal failure, hepatic failure, seizures
  - » Toxin or drug mediated (Type B2) — ethanol, methanol, ethylene glycol, salicylates
  - » Inborn or acquired error of metabolism (Type B3) — primary lactic acidosis, mitochondrial disorders, organic acidaemias, aminoacidopathies, glycogen storage disorders (GSDs)
- Majority of the cases are caused by hypoxia, hypoperfusion due to sepsis, myocardial dysfunction.
- Lactic acidosis with ketosis is a nearly constant finding in most IEMs (except in pyruvate dehydrogenase, [PDH], deficiency and FAOD), whereas ketosis is absent in most hyperlactataemias secondary to tissue hypoxia.
- Sampling and handling errors can give spurious results. The blood sample should be a free-flowing venous or arterial sample to avoid spurious elevations. The blood sample tube should be placed in a biohazard specimen bag and then immersed into another bag with crushed ice and sent down to the lab immediately.

Hyperammonaemia

- Hyperammonaemia
  - » >100 µmol/L in neonates
  - » >50 µmol/L in children
  - » >35 µmol/L in adults
- Acute hyperammonaemia is a **medical emergency** for which immediate action must be taken to minimise permanent brain damage. If in doubt, a metabolic physician should be consulted.
- The work up of an encephalopathic child of unknown cause should always include the measurement of ammonia. Persistent hyperammonaemia will lead to cerebral oedema and brain herniation if left untreated.
- Severe hyperammonaemia (>500 µmol/L) is either caused by a UCD (especially with respiratory alkalosis, no ketosis) or by an organic acidaemia (PA, MMA, IVA with metabolic acidosis, ketosis).
- Sampling and handling errors can give spurious results. The blood sample should be a free-flowing venous or arterial sample to avoid spurious elevations. The blood sample tube should be placed in a biohazard specimen bag and immersed into another bag with crushed ice and sent down to the lab immediately.
- To consider high caloric nutrition with no protein and sodium benzoate in severe hyperammonaemia in acute decompensation of UCD.

Basic Principles in Acute Management

- The main aim in the acute management of IEMs is to stop further build-up of potential toxic metabolites by promoting anabolism and preventing catabolism.
- Stop the offending substance during acute decompensation.
- Supportive care
  - » Cardiorespiratory support
  - » Neurological
    - ▪ Neuroprotection in acute encephalopathy
    - ▪ Seizure management
  - » Fluid and electrolyte/acid-base correction and maintenance
    - ▪ To consider sodium bicarbonate/acetate correction in persistent severe metabolic acidosis due to IEMs
    - ▪ Correction of hypoglycaemia
  - » Treat underlying infection
- High calorie hydration/nutrition
  - » Dextrose
    - ▪ 1 g dextrose provides 3.4 kcal
    - ▪ To provide intravenous (IV) dextrose 10%/sodium chloride 0.9% with electrolyte supplementation as first line of hydration/nutrition during acute decompensation

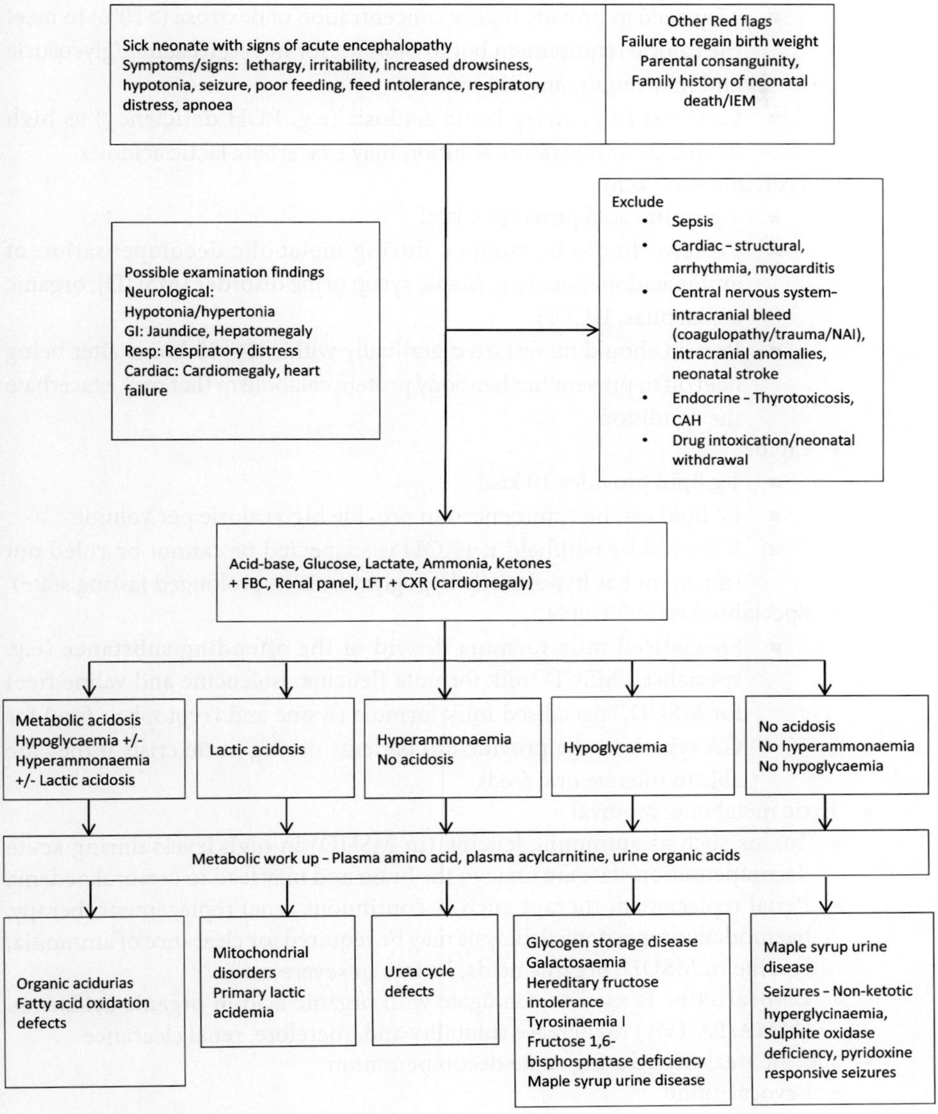

Figure 14.1 Approach to a neonate with suspected IEM.

        - May need to provide higher concentration of dextrose (>10%) to meet the calorie requirement but to monitor for hyperglycaemia/glycosuria and may require insulin infusion
        - Cautious in primary lactic acidosis (e.g. PDH deficiency) as high dextrose concentration solution may exacerbate lactic acidosis
    - Protein/amino acid
        - 1 g amino acid provides 4 kcal
        - Protein should be stopped during metabolic decompensation of aminoacidopathies (e.g. Maple syrup urine disorder [MSUD], organic acidaemias, UCDs)
        - Protein should be restarted gradually within 24–48 hours after being held off to prevent further body protein catabolism that may exacerbate the condition
    - Lipid
        - 1 g lipid provides 10 kcal
        - IV lipid can be commenced to provide high calorie per volume
        - It should be withheld if FAOD is suspected or cannot be ruled out (if patient has hypoketotic hypoglycaemia in prolonged fasting state)
    - Specialised milk formula
        - Specialised milk formula devoid of the offending substance (e.g. specialised MSUD milk formula (leucine, isoleucine and valine free) for MSUD, specialised milk formula (lysine and tryptophan free) for GA type I can be provided to patients during acute crisis if they are able to tolerate oral feeds
- Toxic metabolite removal
    - Toxins such as ammonia, leucine (in MSUD) in high levels during acute decompensation state are toxic to the brain and may lead to cerebral oedema
    - Renal replacement therapy such as continuous renal replacement therapy, haemodialysis, peritoneal dialysis may be required for clearance of ammonia, leucine in MSUD, organic acids, lactate in severe cases
    - Levocarnitine is used to conjugate with organic acid in organic acidaemia (MMA/PA/IVA) to increase solubility and, therefore, renal clearance
- Specific treatment during acute decompensation
    - Levocarnitine
        - Conditions: Primary carnitine deficiency, GA type I, organic acidaemia (MMA/PA/IVA), Mitochondrial Encephalopathy, Lactic acidosis, and Stroke-like episodes (MELAS)
    - L-arginine
        - Conditions: UCDs, MELAS

- » Sodium benzoate
    - Ammonia scavenger by conjugating with glycine for renal excretion
    - Conditions: Hyperammonaemia in UCDs, organic acidaemia (MMA/PA/IVA)
- » Sodium dichloroacetate
    - Conditions: Primary lactic acidosis

Bibliography

1. Saudubray JM, Baumgartner MR, Walter J (eds.). (2016) *Inborn Metabolic Diseases, 6th ed.* Berlin: Springer International Publishing.
2. Ellaway CJ, Wilcken B, Christodoulou J. (2002) Clinical approach to inborn errors of metabolism presenting in the newborn period. *J Paediatr Child Health* **38**(5):511–517.
3. Champion MP. (2010) An approach to the diagnosis of inherited metabolic disease. *Arch Dis Child Educ Pract Ed* **95**(2):40–46.

SECTION 15

HAEMATOLOGY

CHAPTER 60

Anaemia

Lee Ming Wei; Rajat Bhattacharyya; Lam Ching Mei, Joyce

General Approach to Anaemia Definition

True anaemia occurs when there is a decrease in the circulating red cell mass, leading to impaired ability to meet the body's demand for oxygen. Spurious anaemia occurs when there is a dilutional effect of an increase in plasma volume, e.g. in fluid overload and cardiac failure.

Clinical Symptoms

Symptoms include fatigue, breathlessness, dizziness, headaches and blackouts.

Severity of clinical symptoms depends on:

- Severity of anaemia
- Speed of onset — Gradual onset better tolerated
- Age and cardiovascular status of patient — Better tolerated in young

History

- Previous blood tests and transfusion history — For comparison
- Duration of symptoms — Recent or longstanding
- Family history — Consanguinity, congenital anaemias, gallstones
- Dietary history — Goat's milk ingestion, meat intake, vegans
- Drugs and exposure to toxic chemicals
- Blood loss — Including menstrual history
- Abnormal bruising
- History of other illnesses — Diarrhoea, signs of hypothyroidism, autoimmune disorders
- Medical history — Neonatal hyperbilirubinaemia in G6PD deficiency

Clinical Examination

- Stature — Short in Fanconi anaemia
- Skin and sclera — Pallor, jaundice, purpura, bruises, petechiae
- Signs of nutritional deficiencies — Iron, ascorbic acid
- Signs of chronic illness — Thyroid, renal
- Cardiovascular — Heart failure

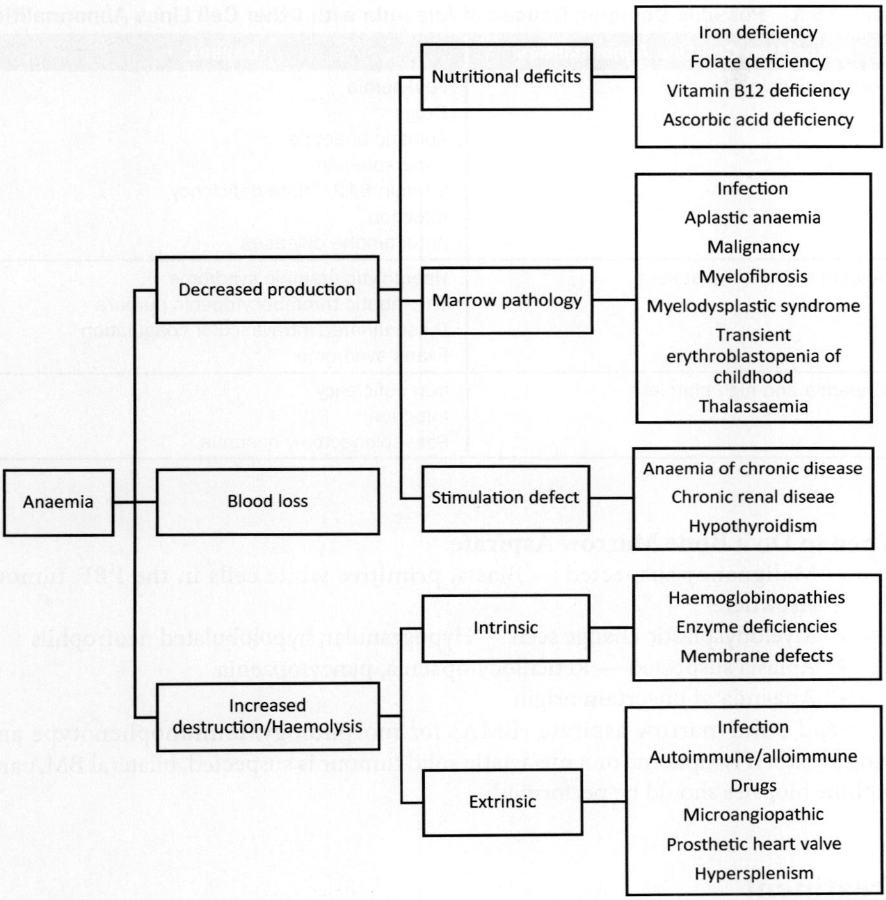

Figure 15.1 Causes of true anaemia.

- Organomegaly — Lymph nodes, liver, spleen
- Rectal examination (if necessary) — Melaena

Investigations

Full blood count (FBC), **peripheral blood film (PBF)** and **reticulocyte count** can give a lot of information and help in deciding what further investigations need to be done.

Blood investigations like liver function test (LFT), renal panel, thyroid function test (TFT), iron studies, haemoglobin (Hb) electrophoresis, alpha thalassaemia mutation, direct Coombs test (DCT), autoimmune markers, Vitamin B12 and folate are ordered on the basis of the suspected diagnosis.

Table 15.1 Possible Common Causes of Anaemia with Other Cell Lines Abnormalities

Associated Cell Line Abnormalities	Causes
Pancytopaenia	Leukaemia Drugs Aplastic anaemia Hypersplenism Vitamin B12/folate deficiency Infection Autoimmune diseases
Anaemia and low platelets	Haemolytic uraemic syndrome Thrombotic thrombocytopenic purpura Disseminated intravascular coagulation Evans syndrome
Anaemia and high platelets	Iron deficiency Infection Post-splenectomy anaemia

When to Do a Bone Marrow Aspirate

- Malignancy suspected — Blasts, primitive white cells in the PBF, tumour elsewhere
- Myelodysplastic change seen — Hypogranular, hypolobulated neutrophils
- Aplasia suspected — Reticulocytopaenia, pancytopaenia
- Anaemia of uncertain origin

Send bone marrow aspirate (BMA) for morphology, immunophenotype and cytogenetics. If lymphoma or a metastatic solid tumour is suspected, bilateral BMA and trephine biopsies should be performed.

Treatment

- Treat underlying condition. In iron deficiency, remember to continue treating for at least 3 months after Hb normalises and a minimum of 6 months to replenish body iron stores.
- Treat symptoms of anaemia, e.g. heart failure.
- Transfuse when there is ongoing blood loss/haemolysis or if there is symptomatic anaemia. In longstanding anaemia, there is no need to transfuse if Hb is stable and patient is not symptomatic.
- If Hb is very low, correct anaemia slowly in stages, e.g. if Hb is 3 g/dL, correct to Hb of 5 g/dL on first day, then to Hb of 7 g/dL the next day.

Useful Formulae in Anaemia

Volume of packed cell transfusion (ml) = (Desired Hb minus Current Hb in g/dL) × (Body weight in kg) × 3.5

Mentzer Index = Mean corpuscular volume (MCV)/Red blood cell (RBC) (<13 more likely thalassaemia trait, >13 more likely iron deficiency)

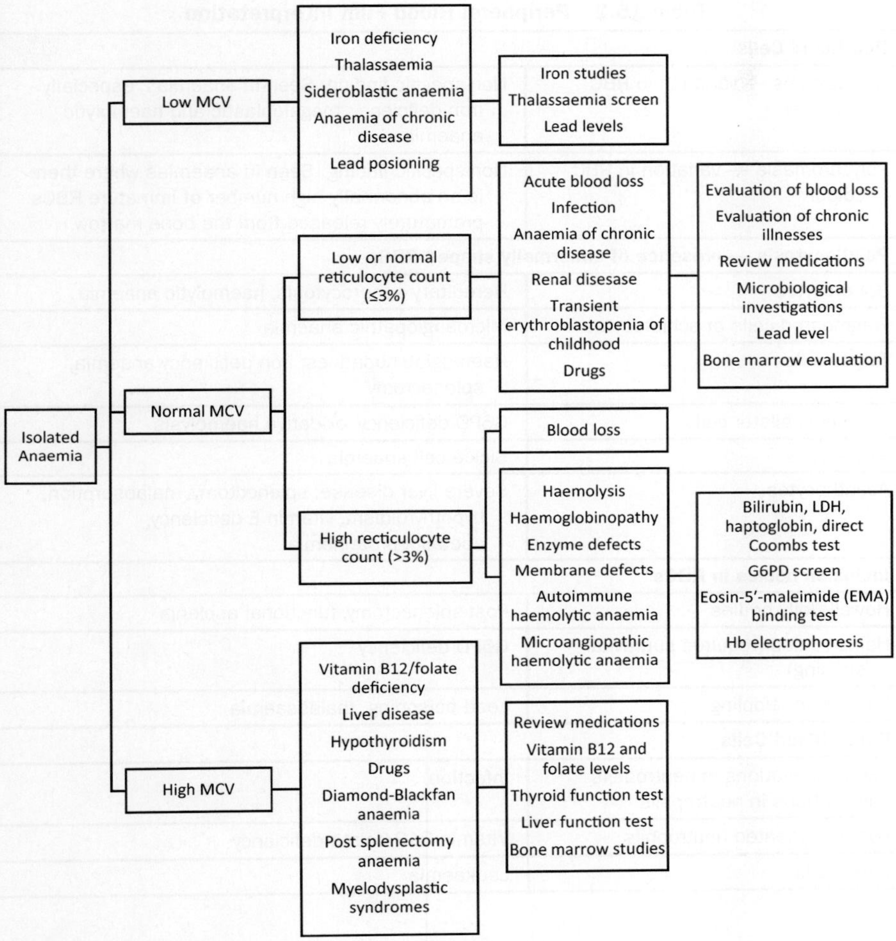

Figure 15.2 Practical approach to isolated anaemia.

Iron Deficiency Anemia

Iron deficiency is an important cause of anaemia in children, and often presents as a mild to moderate microcytic, hypochromic anaemia. Chronic iron deficiency can result in other non-haematological consequences, including effects on neurocognition and immunity. Causes of iron deficiency anaemia (IDA) include nutritional insufficiency, gastrointestinal blood loss, malabsorption syndromes, menstrual losses, infants on an exclusive fresh cow's milk diet.

Diagnostic Workup

Conditions that can produce a hypochromic, microcytic anaemia and be confused with IDA include hereditary anaemias (commonly thalassaemia in Singapore) and anaemia

Table 15.2 Peripheral Blood Film Interpretation

Red Blood Cells	
Anisocytosis — variation in RBC diameter	Non-specific finding. Seen in anaemias, especially iron deficiency, megaloblastic and haemolytic anaemia
Polychromasia — variation in RBC colour	Non-specific finding. Seen in anaemias where there is an abnormally high number of immature RBCs prematurely released from the bone marrow
Poikilocytosis — presence of abnormally shaped RBCs	
Spherocytes	Hereditary spherocytosis, haemolytic anaemia
Fragmented cells or schistocytes	Microangiopathic anaemia
Target cells	Haemoglobinopathies, iron deficiency anaemia, splenectomy
Bite cells, blister cells	G6PD deficiency, oxidative haemolysis
Sickle cells	Sickle cell anaemia
Acanthocytes	Severe liver disease, splenectomy, malabsorption, hypothyroidism, vitamin E deficiency, abetalipoproteinemia
Inclusion bodies in RBCs	
Howell–Jolly bodies	Post-splenectomy, functional asplenia
Heinz bodies (requires supravital staining)	G6PD deficiency
Basophilic stippling	Lead poisoning, thalassaemia
White Blood Cells	
Toxic granulations in neutrophils Vacuolations in neutrophils	Infection
Hypersegmented neutrophils	Vitamin B12/folate deficiency
Blast cells	Leukaemia

of chronic disease. The initial workup should always include a thalassaemia screen to exclude the concomitant thalassaemia trait. However, it should be noted that co-existing iron deficiency can artifactually result in a low HbA_2 level, masking the diagnosis of the beta-thalassaemia trait. A repeat thalassaemia screen should be performed if microcytosis persists despite correction of iron deficiency.

Common laboratory tests used to diagnose iron deficiency include:

- **Serum iron** — There is diurnal variation with higher serum values late in the day. Levels also fluctuate with dietary iron intake. Serum iron cannot be used on its own to diagnose iron deficiency.
- **Serum transferrin/total iron binding capacity (TIBC)** — Transferrin is the carrier protein of iron in the blood and is assayed directly as serum transferrin or indirectly as the TIBC of the patient. This has limited utility on its own, but has some value when used to derive the **transferrin saturation.**
    - » Transferrin saturation = Serum iron/TIBC

- » Iron deficiency is more likely to be present when the transferrin saturation is <15%
- **Serum ferritin** is a sensitive parameter for the assessment of iron stores in healthy subjects. However, ferritin is an acute phase reactant and may be elevated in the presence of chronic inflammation, infection, malignancy or liver disease. Values of <30 mcg/L are suggestive of iron deficiency in children. A serum ferritin level of >100 mcg/L suggests that iron deficiency is unlikely to be present.
- **Soluble transferrin receptor** is upregulated when the iron supply is inadequate and is a useful measure of iron status as it is not affected by inflammation or infection. Serum levels are directly proportional to the degree of iron deficiency. This test is available only in some specialised laboratories in Singapore.
- **Bone marrow iron staining** is considered the gold standard for the diagnosis of iron deficiency, but is not routinely performed due to the invasive nature of the test.

Management

Successful treatment of IDA in infants and children lies in appropriate dosing and scheduling of oral iron therapy, dietary modifications and follow-up assessment for response.

- **Oral iron therapy** with 3–6 mg/kg/day of elemental iron. The supplement should be given between meals and with juice (not milk, as iron is chelated by calcium in milk). See Table 15.3 for a summary of the elemental iron content of common iron supplements.
- **Dietary modifications** — Iron-containing complementary foods should be introduced at 4–6 months of age. Exclusive feeding with fresh cow's milk for infants younger than 12 months is not advised as it is a poor source of iron. High iron-content food products include red meats, cereals fortified with iron and dark green leafy vegetables.
- **Parenteral iron therapy** should be reserved for patients with severe, persistent anaemia who have proven intolerance to oral supplements, malabsorption or poor compliance to oral therapy. Parenteral iron should be used with caution because of the risk of anaphylaxis. Oral iron preparation should not be administered at the same time as intravenous (IV) iron infusion as absorption of iron is reduced. Oral iron therapy should only be commenced at least 5–7 days after iron infusion. See Table 15.3 for a summary of the elemental iron content of common iron therapy preparation.
  - » A patient's total iron deficit can be calculated using the Ganzoni formula. However, it is not commonly used in clinical practice as parenteral iron preparations usually state specific dosing requirements. See Table 15.4 for a summary of the dosing recommended for parenteral iron preparations.
  - » Ganzoni formula:
  - » Iron deficit (mg) = Body weight (kg) × (Target Hb [g/dL] – Actual Hb [g/dL]) × 2.4 + iron stores (mg)*

Table 15.3 Iron Therapy and their Elemental Iron Content

Iron Therapy	Elemental Iron Content
Oral Iron Therapy	
Iron polymaltose drops	50 mg per ml 2.5 mg/drop
Iron polymaltose tablet	100 mg per 100 mg tablet
Iron polymaltose (Floron)	30 mg per capsule
Ferrous gluconate (Sangobion®)	30 mg per capsule
Intravenous Iron Therapy	
Iron sucrose (Venofer®)	100 mg per 5 ml
Ferric carboxymaltose (Ferinject®)	500 mg in 10 ml

Table 15.4 Parenteral Iron Therapy Dosing

Parenteral Iron Therapy	Dosing
Iron sucrose (Venofer®)	3 mg/kg Max. 7 mg/kg/dose or 300 mg/dose, whichever is lower Do not give more than 3 doses per week.
Ferric carboxymaltose (Ferinject®) For ≥14 yr old and ≥35 kg	15–20 mg/kg Max. 20 mg/kg/dose or 1000 mg/dose, whichever is lower Do not administer a single dose more frequently than once a wk.

*Iron stores: Can use 500 mg for ≥35 kg patient or 15 mg/kg for <35 kg patients

- **Red cell transfusions** should only be reserved for patients with severe, symptomatic anaemia compromising end-organ function. Administer with caution to avoid precipitating cardiac failure.

Assessment of Response to Therapy

Response to iron replacement therapy can be monitored with serial reticulocyte counts and Hb assessments. After therapeutic doses of oral iron, a reticulocytosis should be seen within 72 hours. Hb should rise by at least 1 g/dL within 4 weeks and should be monitored subsequently every 2–3 months until it reaches the age-adjusted normal range. Iron supplements should then be continued for a minimum of 3 more months to replace storage iron pools. Early discontinuation of iron therapy will frequently lead to a recurrence of iron deficiency.

The most common causes for non-responders to iron supplements are compliance failures and intolerance to medication as iron formulations do result in gastric irritation. Ongoing gastrointestinal blood loss or other causes of anaemia also have to be evaluated in non-responders.

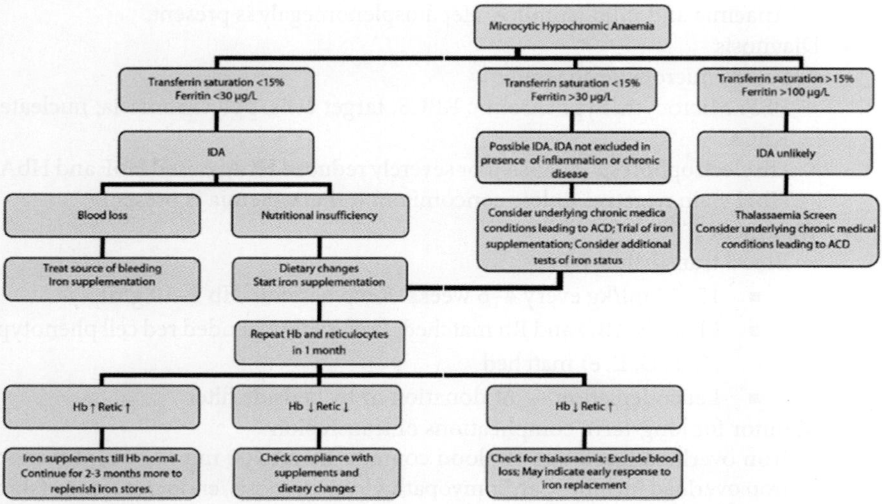

Figure 15.3. Approach to diagnosis, management and assessment of treatment response in iron deficiency anaemia.

ACD — anaemia of chronic disease; Hb — haemoglobin; IDA — iron deficiency anaemia; Retic — reticulocytes; Transferrin saturation — serum iron/total iron binding capacity

Thalassaemia

Thalassaemia is the most common genetic disease in the world. About 4% of the population of Singapore carries the alpha or beta thalassaemia gene. Adult Hb comprises 2 alpha (α) and 2 beta (β) globin chains in a tetramer (α2β2). Defect in any of the globin chains will cause thalassaemia — α globin chain defect causing α thalassaemia and β globin chain defect causing β thalassaemia.

Beta (β) Thalassaemia

Two β-globin genes are present — one on each chromosome 11. More than 300 mutations have been described in this gene with a resultant reduction in the production of normal β-globin chains.

β Thalassaemia Minor or Trait

Clinically asymptomatic. Presents with microcytic anaemia (Hb 9–11 g/dL). PBF shows microcytosis, hypochromia, target cells. Hb electrophoresis shows raised HbA_2, which in conjunction with microcytic anaemia is diagnostic of β thalassaemia trait. No treatment or routine follow-up is necessary. However, family screening, genetic counselling and referral to the National Thalassaemia Registry (NTR) are important.

β Thalassaemia Major

- Clinical Presentation
  - » Presents at <1 year of age, usually at 3–6 months of age.

  - Anaemia and mild jaundice. Hepatosplenomegaly is present.
- Diagnosis
  - Severe microcytic anaemia.
  - PBF: Microcytic hypochromic RBCS, target cells, polychromasia, nucleated RBCs.
  - Hb electrophoresis — Absent or severely reduced HbA, raised HbF and HbA_2. HbH stain negative unless concomitant α thalassaemia is present.
- Treatment
  - Blood transfusion
    - 15–20 ml/kg every 4–6 weeks. Keep baseline Hb 9–10 g/dL.
    - Blood is ABO and Rh matched. Preferably extended red cell phenotype (C, c, D, E, e) matched
    - Leucodepletion — At donation or by bedside filter
- Monitor for long-term complications of transfusion
  - Iron overload (each bag of blood contains about 200 mg of iron). Effects of iron overload include: Cardiomyopathy, liver cirrhosis, endocrinopathy (short stature, delayed puberty, hypothyroidism, hypoparathyroidism, diabetes mellitus), skin pigmentation
  - Risk of blood-borne infections — Hepatitis B, Hepatitis C, HIV, Syphilis, Malaria, Cytomegalovirus.
- Iron Chelation
  - Desferrioxamine (DFO)
    - Start when serum ferritin >1000 mcg/L. Usually after 10–20 transfusions and 18–24 months of age.
    - Dose 20–50 mg/kg/day, 5–7 days/week. Start at a lower dose and increase slowly.
    - Infuse subcutaneously over 8–12 hours each night.
    - Side effects: Painful swelling at injection sites, visual and auditory neurotoxicity, osteoporosis.
    - Increases risk of *Yersinia enterocolitica* infection; Stop during diarrhoea and abdominal pain.
    - Concomitant Vitamin C 50–100 mg 1 hour after start of injection daily helps iron excretion.
  - Deferiprone (Ferriprox/L1)
    - First oral iron chelator licensed for use
    - Particularly effective for myocardial iron removal
    - Dose 75–100 mg/kg/day TDS given with meals
    - Risks: Agranulocytosis (<1%)—regular FBC monitoring is recommended, arthralgia of large joints, transaminitis.
  - Deferasirox (ExJade)
    - Oral iron chelator
    - Dose 20–30 mg/kg/dose once daily before meals. To be dissolved in water or apple juice.

        - Side effects — Skin rash, gastrointestinal disturbances, renal toxicity (glomerulopathy/tubulopathy)
        - Licensed for use in children older than 2 years
    - » Oral chelators can be combined with DFO in severe iron overload conditions.
- Splenectomy for Hypersplenism
    - » Can be considered when older than 5 years. Reduces requirement for transfusion.
    - » Mostly by laparoscopic approach with minimal morbidity.
    - » Indications: Transfusion requirement >220 ml/kg/year, hypersplenism, mechanical discomfort.
    - » Pneumococcal, meningococcal and *Haemophilus Influenzae B* vaccinations before splenectomy.
    - » Penicillin prophylaxis after splenectomy: 250 mg BD long term.
    - » Risks of thrombosis, pulmonary hypertension, infections by encapsulated organisms to be considered before performing splenectomy.
- Haematopoietic Stem Cell Transplantation (HSCT)
    - » Only curative option in thalassaemia. However, treatment-related morbidity and mortality is around 10%.
    - » HLA-matched sibling HSCT is the best option with >80% thalassaemia-free survival rate.
    - » Alternate donor transplant, including matched unrelated donor, cord, haploidentical transplants are also possible options.
- Supplements
    - » Folic acid 1–5 mg once a day
    - » Vitamin C 50–100 mg once a day if on DFO therapy
    - » Calcium supplements

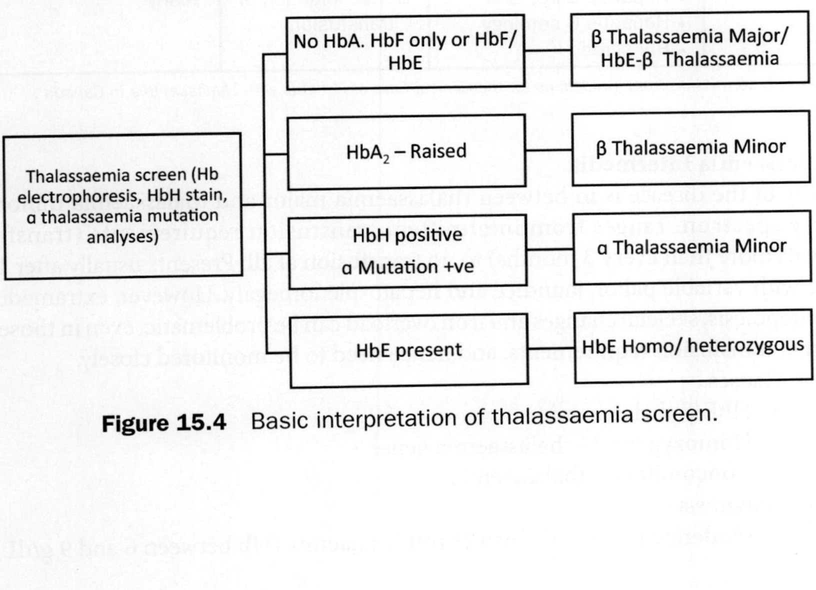

Figure 15.4 Basic interpretation of thalassaemia screen.

Table 15.5 Recommended Investigations for Beta (β) Thalassaemia Major Patients

System	Investigation	Age to Start	Frequency of Monitoring
Iron Load	• Serum ferritin • Liver iron content » Liver MR » Liver biopsy • Cardiac iron load (MR)	• Before initiation of transfusion • After 10–20 transfusions • 10 yr	• Every 3 to 6 mth • Yearly (Biopsy not routine) • Every 1–2 yr
Chelation-associated	• Audiometry • Eye review • Chelation-specific lab tests	• After commencing chelation	• Yearly • Yearly • Yearly
Liver Function	Liver function test	Before initiation of transfusion	Every 3 mth
Cardiac Function	• Physical examination • Echocardiogram, MUGA scan, or cardiac MRI T2*	• At diagnosis • 10 yr	• Every 6 mth • Every 1–2 yr
Endocrine Function	• Height (standing and sitting) • Puberty staging • Serum TSH • Serum calcium and phosphate • Random blood glucose	• At diagnosis • 10 yr • 12 yr • 12 yr • Pre-transfusion	• Every 6 mth • Yearly till completion of puberty • Yearly • Yearly • Every 6 mth
Bone	DEXA bone densitometry scan	10 yr	Every 1–2 yr
Infections	• Hepatitis BsAg, sAb • Hepatitis C serology • HIV screen	Before initiation of transfusion	Yearly

Adapted with permission from 'Guidelines for the Clinical Care of Patients with Thalassaemia in Canada'.

β Thalassaemia Intermedia

Severity of the disease is in between thalassaemia major and thalassaemia minor. The disease spectrum ranges from intermittent transfusion requirements (transfusion intervals more than every 3 months) to no transfusion at all. Presents usually after 1 year of age with variable pallor, jaundice and hepatosplenomegaly. However, extramedullary haematopoiesis, skeletal changes and iron overload can be problematic, even in those with minimal transfusion requirements, and hence need to be monitored closely.

- Causes
  - » HbE/β thalassaemia
  - » Homozygous β+ thalassaemia genes
  - » Concomitant α thalassaemia
- Diagnosis
  - » Moderate microcytic hypochromic anaemia (Hb between 6 and 9 g/dL)

- » PBF shows hypochromic microcytic RBCs, target cells, polychromasia, nucleated RBCs
- » Hb electrophoresis: No or severely reduced HbA, raised HbF and presence of HbE (in HbE/β thalassaemia)

- Treatment
  - » Folic acid — 1–5 mg once a day
  - » Transfusion as necessary, during intercurrent infections, growth failure, skeletal changes
  - » Splenectomy may be considered in case of significant enlargement of spleen
  - » Hydroxyurea (hydroxycarbamide) may reduce transfusion requirement and extramedullary haematopoiesis

Alpha (α) Thalassaemia

α Thalassaemia Minor

(1 or 2 gene deletion or non-deletional mutation)

- Clinically asymptomatic
- Diagnosis
  - » FBC parameters may show microcytosis and hypochromia in 2-gene deletion.
  - » However, single gene deletion can present with a completely normal FBC and are called silent carriers.
  - » Diagnosis can be done only by genetic testing as Hb electrophoresis and HbH stains are normal.
  - » HbH stain may be positive for HbH inclusion bodies in two-gene deletion carriers.
  - » DNA analysis shows either one or two alpha gene deletions or rarely non-deletional changes like Hb Constant Spring (-α/αα, -α/-α, --/αα, -α/αcs).
- Treatment
  - » No treatment or follow-up is necessary. Lifespan is normal. However, family screening, genetic counselling and referral to the NTR is important.

Haemoglobin H (HBH) Disease

- Clinical Presentation
  - » Clinical presentation is that of thalassaemia intermedia, unless concomitant non-deletional α thalassaemia is present (e.g. Hb Constant Spring), resulting in a more severe phenotype
  - » Usually presents with pallor, mild jaundice and hepatosplenomegaly
  - » However, early presentation in infants is also possible
- Diagnosis
  - » PBF shows microcytosis, hypochromia and striking poikilocytosis
  - » HbH stain shows typical golf ball appearance (HbH Inclusion bodies)
  - » DNA analysis commonly shows --/-α or --/αcs
- Treatment
  - » Folic acid supplementation 1–5 mg/d
  - » Blood transfusion as necessary (infections, growth failure, skeletal changes, etc.)
  - » Splenectomy if significant splenomegaly causing mechanical discomfort and hypersplenism

Fetal Hydrops Syndrome/Bart's Hydrops Fetalis

- Clinical Presentation
  - » Maternal toxaemia during pregnancy
  - » Hydrops fetalis
  - » Stillbirth or early postnatal death
- Diagnosis
  - » Should be suspected antenatally in case of fetal hydrops and investigated appropriately
  - » FBC shows very severe anaemia. HbH band in Hb electrophoresis may be seen
  - » DNA analysis shows –/– (no α chains)
- Treatment
  - » Prevention is the best therapeutic strategy because of the severity of the disease.
  - » It may be possible to do fetal transfusions at regular intervals and early delivery followed by transfusions after birth and early transplant. There are some reported survivors in literature.

Co-Inheritance of α & β Thalassaemia

Since the prevalence of both α and β gene defects are common in Southeast Asia, co-inheritance of α and β thalassaemia in various combinations are not uncommon. This actually reduces the severity of the clinical presentation as the globin chain imbalance is less, causing less haemolysis. DNA analysis for both α and β thalassaemia genes is important to make the exact diagnosis. Family screening, appropriate genetic counselling are important, along with referral to the NTR.

Genetic Counselling and Prenatal Diagnosis

In Singapore, all citizens and permanent residents with confirmed thalassaemia should be referred to the NTR. The NTR collates national data on thalassaemia, provides free counselling on thalassaemia and offers thalassaemia screening to family members at subsidised rates.

Couples who are both heterozygous for the same type of thalassaemia carry a 25% risk of having a child with thalassaemia major phenotype. Through counselling and screening, these couples can be prospectively identified and offered the option of prenatal diagnosis. The preferred method for prenatal diagnosis is by chorionic villus sampling, and this is done at around 12 weeks of gestation and the sample is then subjected to DNA analysis. Providing a confirmed genetic diagnosis will enable the couple to make an informed decision about the pregnancy, especially in cases of homozygous β thalassaemia and 4-gene deletion α thalassaemia, where the clinical phenotype is predicted to be thalassaemia major and fetal hydrops, respectively.

Pre-implantation genetic diagnosis (PGD) is now possible by selecting embryos that are not affected by thalassaemia. Theoretically, if there is an older sibling with thalassaemia major, PGD for thalassaemia can be combined with tissue matching with the affected sibling, with a view to providing tissue-matched stem cells for transplantation in the affected sibling. However, this practice carries ethical concerns and may not be widely acceptable.

Bibliography

1. Chew ECS, Lam JCM. (2012) Diagnosis and management of iron deficiency anaemia in children — a clinical update. *Proc Sing Health* **21**(4):278–285.
2. World Health Organization. (2001) Iron deficiency anaemia: assessment, prevention, and control — a guide for program managers. Geneva: World Health Organization. WHO/NHD/01.3.
3. Weatherall DJ, Clegg JB. (2001) *The Thalassaemia Syndromes, 4th ed.* Blackwell Science.
4. Cao A, Rosatelli MC, Monni G, Galanello R. (2002) Screening for thalassaemia: A model of success. *Obstet Gynecol Clin North Am* **29**(2):305–328, vi-vii.
5. Olivieri NF. (1999) The beta-thalassemias. *N Eng J Med* **341**(2):99–109.
6. Thalassemia International Federation. (2007) Guidelines for the clinical management of thalassaemia. No:9 ISBN:978-9963-623-59-4. Available form: www. thalassaemia.org.cy.
7. Thalassaemia International Federation. (2009) Guidelines for the clinical care of patients with thalassemia in Canada. http://www.thalassemia.ca/wp-content/uploads/Thalassemia-Guidelines_LR.pdf
8. Thalassaemia International Federation. (2013) Guidelines for the management of Non Transfusion Dependent Thalassaemia (NTDT). https://issuu.com/internationalthalassaemiafederation/docs/ntdt-final-combined No 19 ISBN 978-9963-717-03-3

CHAPTER 61

Bleeding Disorders

Lee Ming Wei; Rajat Bhattacharyya; Lam Ching Mei, Joyce

Physiology of Haemostasis

Haemostasis refers to the maintenance of vascular integrity when there is injury, at the same time limiting the clot to the site of injury without systemic propagation. It involves an interplay between platelets, the vascular endothelium and the coagulation factors. It consists of a primary phase, which results in the production of a platelet plug and a secondary phase with activation of procoagulant proteins resulting in the formation of a cross-linked fibrin clot.

When uncontrolled, the haemostatic response can lead to thrombosis and tissue damage. The patency of vessels in normal, uninjured tissues is maintained by natural inhibitors of coagulation, consisting of:

- Tissue factor pathway inhibitor
- Antithrombins
- Protein C/Protein S pathway
- The fibrinolytic system, which degrades fibrin and is necessary to allow for complete wound healing

Workup of a Child with Suspected Bleeding Disorder

History

- Nature of the bleed:
  - » Location and type — Bleeding from skin, mucosal surfaces, petechiae and purpura are typically seen in thrombocytopaenia, whereas joint, muscle, soft tissue bleeds and palpable ecchymoses are more likely to be seen in a coagulation defect.
  - » Duration — Bleeding that stops and then recurs quickly is suggestive of a true underlying bleeding disorder.
  - » Time of onset — Acute bleeds that have occurred recently over a period of days to weeks without prior history is suggestive of an acquired disorder; bleeding shortly after birth (e.g. oozing when cord separates, post-circumcision) suggests a congenital condition.
  - » Menorrhagia in pubertal females — Up to 20% girls with menorrhagia at menarche have now been recognised to have a bleeding disorder.

  - Any precipitating factors, e.g. trauma, dental extractions and surgery — Bleeds precipitated by relatively minor injuries or surgery are more likely to be due to a significant underlying bleeding disorder.
- Family history and pedigree:
  - Ask about bleeding history from all members of the family, especially in male relatives to exclude X-linked disorders.
  - Haemophilia can result in abnormal bleeding in a female carrier.
  - Menstrual history and obstetric history of female relatives.
- Drug history:
  - Aspirin, non-steroidal anti-inflammatory drugs (NSAIDs)
  - Anticonvulsants and antibiotics (e.g. penicillins) causing drug-induced thrombocytopaenia
  - Warfarin, low molecular weight heparins

Clinical Examination

- Skin for petechiae/purpura/telangiectasia
- Bleeding from nasal and oral mucosae
- Pallor and other signs of anaemia
- Joints — Swelling or chronic changes (e.g. contractures) secondary to repeated bleeding episodes
- Deep tissue bleeds and intramuscular (IM) swelling
- Systemic illness, e.g. liver or collagen vascular disease
- Evidence of non-accidental injuries

Investigations

- Full blood count (FBC) with a peripheral blood smear — look at all three cell lines:
  - Haemoglobin (Hb) may be decreased if there is significant blood loss.
  - Bicytopaenia or pancytopaenia may indicate bone marrow failure syndromes or infiltrating marrow lesions like leukaemia/lymphoma.
  - Platelet counts to determine severity of thrombocytopaenia. Platelet morphology to look at the size of the platelets. A decreased count may be the result of platelet clumping from EDTA-dependent antibodies (spurious thrombocytopenia). Large platelets are seen in Bernard–Soulier Syndrome and May–Hegglin anomaly. Decreased platelet size may indicate Wiskott–Aldrich Syndrome. Platelet morphology is important, as a mean platelet volume from an automated count may not accurately reflect the platelet size.
- Prothrombin time (PT) and activated partial thromboplastin time (aPTT):
  - Surveys the secondary phase of haemostasis.
  - Normal ranges are age-dependent. In newborns, PT and aPTT may be mildly raised due to immaturity of the coagulation system. Most revert to adult levels by 6 months of age.
  - The PT evaluates the extrinsic and common pathway.

    - » The INR is commonly reported with the PT. However, this should be used only to guide warfarin therapy and not as a laboratory test of coagulation.
    - » The aPTT evaluates the intrinsic system and common pathway.
    - » See Table 15.6 for interpretation of an abnormal platelet, PT and/or aPTT results.
- Mixing studies of PT and aPTT:
    - » Abnormal PT and aPTT results without a history of bleeding should be followed by a mixing study unless obvious clinical signs of bleeding are present, indicating a likely bleeding disorder.
    - » This is performed by mixing equal volumes of a patient's plasma with pooled normal plasma containing normal levels of clotting factors.
    - » If the PT or aPTT normalises, a factor deficiency may be present.
    - » If the PT or aPTT is persistently prolonged beyond the upper limit of the normal range, an inhibitor may present (e.g. specific factor inhibitor, lupus anticoagulant)
    - » Note that the presence of a lupus anticoagulant only causes an *in-vitro* prolongation of the PT or aPTT and does not result in any clinical bleeding symptoms.
- Factor assays:
    - » When the aPTT mixing study indicates a likely factor deficiency, quantitate factors VIII, IX, XI and the von Willebrand factor, as these deficiencies are associated with clinical bleeding.
    - » Deficiencies in factor XII, prekallikrein and high molecular weight kininogen can cause an increase in the aPTT but are not associated with clinical bleeding.
    - » When the PT mixing study indicates a factor deficiency, factor VII should be quantitated.
- Thrombin time (TT):
    - » Laboratory test looking at the time required for a clot to form when thrombin is added to plasma. Increased TT can be due to:
        - ■ Low fibrinogen activity
        - ■ Dysfunctional fibrinogen
        - ■ Presence of fibrin split products
        - ■ Heparin contamination
    - » The reptilase clotting time can be used to exclude heparin contamination as the action of reptilase is not affected by heparin. It will be normal if the TT is prolonged due to heparin contamination.
- Fibrinogen measurement:
    - » Fibrinogen can be measured quantitatively and functionally to detect hypofibrinogenaemia and dysfibrinogenaemia
- Platelet aggregation studies:
    - » These measure the degree and pattern of platelet aggregation after the addition of platelet agonists (adenosine diphosphate [ADP], adrenaline, collagen, thrombin, arachidonic acid, and ristocetin)
    - » Allows for the diagnosis of storage pool defects, Bernard–Soulier Syndrome and Glanzmann thrombasthaenia

Table 15.6 Interpretation of Laboratory Studies used to Diagnose Bleeding Disorders

Platelets	PT	aPTT	Differential Diagnosis	Follow-up Studies
N	N	N	• Mild vWD • Platelet dysfunction • Factor XIII deficiency • Defects of fibrinolysis	• vWD studies • Platelet aggregation tests • 5M urea clot lysis test • Factor XIII assay • $\alpha 2$ antiplasmin assay
N	N	↑	• Congenital factor deficiency, e.g. Haemophilia A/B • Specific factor inhibitor/ lupus anticoagulant • vWD • Heparin contamination	• aPTT mixing study • Factor VIII, IX, XI, XII assays • vWD studies • Lupus anticoagulant • TT/Reptilase time
N	↑	N	• Factor VII deficiency • Specific factor inhibitor • Vitamin K deficiency • Liver disease • Warfarin effect	• PT mixing study • Factor VII assay • LFT
N	↑	↑	• Factor inhibitors/lupus anticoagulant • Combined factor deficiencies/isolated Factor II/V/X deficiency • Vitamin K deficiency • Hypofibrinogenaemia/ dysfibrinogenaemia • High dose warfarin/heparin	• PT/aPTT mixing studies • Factor assays • Lupus anticoagulant • LFT • Fibrinogen assays • TT/Reptilase time
↓	↑	↑	• Disseminated intravascular coagulopathy • Liver dysfunction • Kasabach • Merritt Syndrome	• Factor assays, D-dimer • Fibrinogen assays • LFT
↓	N	N	• Acute/chronic immune thrombocytopaenia • Autoimmune thrombocytopaenia • Platelet production defect/ marrow failure syndromes • Malignancy • Platelet consumption • Platelet sequestration	• ANA/dsDNA • Complement • Bone marrow studies

ANA: antinuclear antibody; aPTT: activated partial thromboplastin time; dsDNA: double-stranded DNA; LFT: liver function test; PT: prothrombin time; TT: thrombin time; vWD: von Willebrand disease.

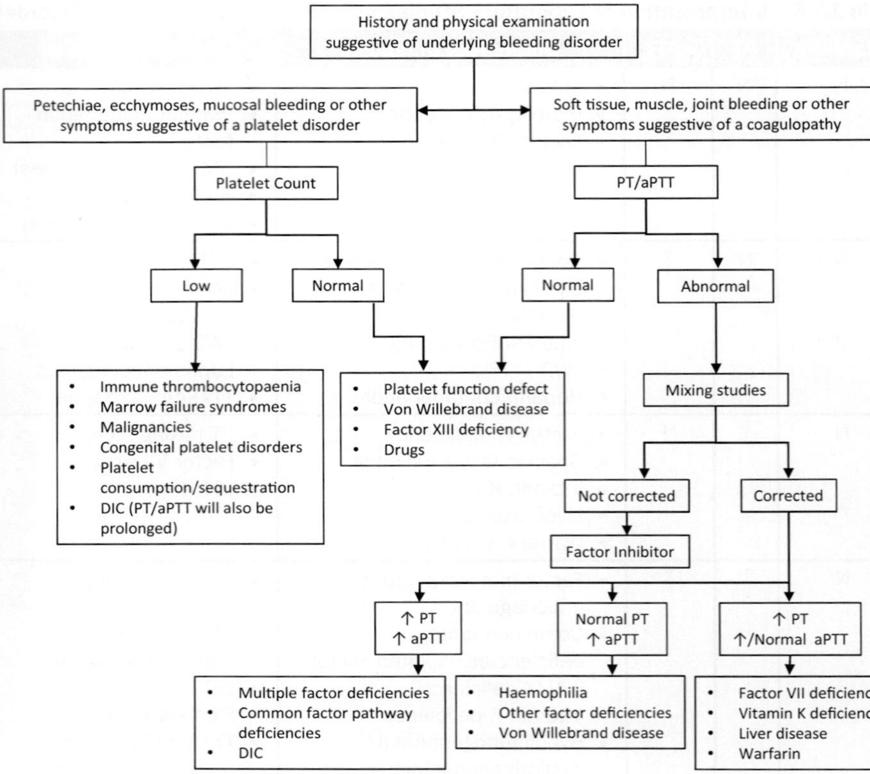

Figure 15.5 Algorithm for investigation of a bleeding child.

aPTT: activated partial thromboplastin time; DIC: disseminated intravascular coagulopathy; PT: prothrombin time

Flow cytometry assays allow for the direct detection of the platelet-surface glycoprotein expression, which is absent in Bernard–Soulier Syndrome and Glanzmann thrombasthaenia

Thrombocytopaenia

This is defined as a platelet count of <100 × 10^9/L. A low platelet count needs to be confirmed by a review of the peripheral smear, especially in an asymptomatic child. False values (pseudothrombocytopaenia) can arise from aggregation of platelets in the syringe caused by agglutination by EDTA antibodies or from a clotted sample.

Causes of Thrombocytopaenia

- Platelet destruction/consumption
  - » Immune-mediated

        - Immune thrombocytopaenia (ITP)
        - Autoimmune thrombocytopaenia
        - Drug-induced
        - Post-transfusion purpura
    - Non-immune mediated
        - Haemolytic uraemic syndrome (HUS)
        - Thrombotic thrombocytopaenic purpura (TTP)
        - Disseminated intravascular coagulopathy (DIC)
        - Giant haemangioma (Kasabach–Merritt Syndrome)
        - Mechanical heart valves
- Impaired platelet production
    - Congenital disorders
    - Fanconi anaemia
    - Bernard–Soulier Syndrome
    - Wiskott–Aldrich Syndrome
    - Amegakaryocytic thrombocytopaenia
- Chromosomal disorders
    - Trisomy 13, 18
- Acquired
    - Aplastic anaemia
    - Malignant marrow infiltration
    - Myelofibrosis
    - Drug-induced
- Platelet sequestration
    - Hypersplenism

Immune Thrombocytopaenia

ITP is an acute self-limiting condition with a peak incidence between 1 and 6 years of age and usually lasting <12 months in duration. Children younger than 1 year or older than 10 years tend to have a more chronic course. ITP is a diagnosis of exclusion based on a suggestive history and absence of findings indicating an alternative cause of thrombocytopaenia.

The onset is acute, usually after an antecedent viral illness 2–3 weeks earlier. Symptoms include the sudden onset of petechiae, purpura, epistaxis, oral mucosal bleeding and, less commonly, haematuria and gastrointestinal tract bleeding.

Physical examination usually reveals a healthy child with no evidence of pallor, weight loss or chronic illness. There should be no hepatosplenomegaly, lymphadenopathy or skeletal defects.

Investigations

- FBC and peripheral blood film (PBF)
    - Thrombocytopaenia should be the only finding, without evidence of involvement of other cell lines. The PBF should be examined to exclude spurious thrombocytopaenia or abnormal platelet morphology.

- Autoimmune markers (anti-nuclear antibody, double-stranded DNA antibodies, complement)
  - » This is not mandatory but can be screened if there is any suggestive history or signs of an underlying autoimmune disorder, especially in older children.
- Viral serologies/polymerase chain reaction
  - » This is not mandatory, but can be useful to find out if an underlying viral aetiology can be identified, especially in very young infants.
- Bone marrow studies
  - » This is only indicated if there is any evidence of bone marrow pathology, e.g. involvement of other cell lines, abnormal blasts, organomegaly. A bone marrow aspirate (BMA) is **not routinely required** for the diagnosis of ITP. It may be performed prior to the commencement of corticosteroid therapy in some institutions to exclude an underlying leukaemia, as steroids can mask an early presentation of haematological malignancies, but this is also not mandatory.

Management

The decision to offer conservative or medical treatment remains controversial as there is no universally accepted 'safe' platelet level. However, observational studies have shown a lower rate of major spontaneous haemorrhages if the platelet count is $\geq 20 \times 10^9$/L. A careful discussion should be held with the family regarding risks and benefits of treatment options.

- Conservative
  - » Most children will recover spontaneously without any medical treatment within 12 months
  - » However, care must be taken to avoid contact sports, rough play and IM injections
  - » Drugs that interfere with platelet function, e.g. aspirin, NSAIDS, should be avoided
- Intravenous immunoglobulin (IVIG)
  - » Blocks Fc receptors on reticuloendothelial organs, e.g. spleen, responsible for the destruction of antibody-coated platelets
  - » Dose is between 1 and 2 g/kg
  - » Response in platelet count is expected within 72 hours
  - » Adverse effects include fever, nausea, headache, anaphylaxis and serum sickness
  - » Slowing the rate of IVIG infusion may alleviate side effects
- Corticosteroids
  - » Interferes with the production of anti-platelet antibodies by B-lymphocytes
  - » A BMA is not mandatory, but may be performed according to institutional practice before commencing steroid therapy as it can mask an early presentation of leukaemia
  - » Choice of corticosteroids includes prednisolone 2–4 mg/kg/day up to 120 mg daily for 5–7 days or dexamethasone 0.6 mg/kg/day up to 40 mg per day for 4 days
  - » Repeated courses may be necessary for long-term remission

Chronic Immune Thrombocytopaenia

About 10–30% of children with acute ITP develop chronic persistent thrombocytopaenia beyond 12 months of duration. An underlying autoimmune disorder/collagen vascular disease has to be excluded, especially in older children. Patients with chronic ITP may not always need treatment, especially if the platelet counts remain $\geq 20 \times 10^9$/L as the platelet count alone does not predict the risk of haemorrhage.

Spontaneous recovery can still occur a few years after the original diagnosis. In refractory, symptomatic patients, treatment options include thrombopoietin receptor agonists, rituximab, azathioprine, danazol, vinca alkaloids and splenectomy.

Neonatal Thrombocytopaenia

The platelet count in both pre-term and term infants at birth is the same as adult values ($150–400 \times 10^9$/L) as platelet production is established towards the end of the first trimester of pregnancy. The incidence of thrombocytopaenia in the neonatal intensive care setting is ~25%.

Causes

- In a 'sick' infant
  - » Placental insufficiency
  - » Perinatal asphyxia
  - » Congenital viral infection (TORCHES infection)
  - » Necrotising enterocolitis
  - » Neonatal sepsis
  - » Congenital heart disease
- In a 'well-looking' infant
  - » Neonatal alloimmune
  - » Thrombocytopaenia
  - » Maternal autoimmune thrombocytopaenia
  - » Wiskott–Aldrich Syndrome
  - » Amegakaryocytic thrombocytopaenia
  - » Trisomy 13, 18 (there will be characteristic syndromic features)

Management

Management of neonatal thrombocytopaenia is dependent on the clinical condition of the child. There are no widely accepted guidelines for platelet transfusions in neonates. Factors to consider include the gestational age of the infant, the underlying condition of the child, whether any active bleeding is present and if any invasive procedures are being performed. As a general rule, platelets should be given to thrombocytopaenic neonates when the degree of thrombocytopaenia alone or in combination with other complications results in an unacceptable risk of haemorrhage, and they should be given in tandem with aggressive therapy for the underlying conditions precipitating the thrombocytopaenia. Most centres would aim to keep the platelet count above $20–50 \times 10^9$/L.

Neonatal Alloimmune Thrombocytopaenia (NAIT)

This is a condition similar to the rhesus haemolytic disease of the newborn where the mother produces anti-platelet antibodies directed against paternal platelet antigens present in fetal platelets. The incidence has been quoted as 1 in 1000 pregnancies although it is believed to be rarer in Asian populations. Human platelet antigen 1a (HPA-1a) is the most common antigen implicated.

Presentation

- 40% can occur in the first pregnancy with no prior sensitisation.
- The typical presentation is a well-looking newborn with petechiae and purpura.
- However, about 20% of neonates can present with an intracranial bleed.
- The degree of thrombocytopaenia can be very severe with platelet counts frequently $<10 \times 10^9$/L.
- Resolution of the thrombocytopaenia occurs in 3–6 weeks after delivery.

Investigation

- There is no confirmatory test for the diagnosis of NAIT.
- However, the diagnosis is highly suggestive if an anti-platelet antibody can be demonstrated in the mother with the corresponding platelet antigen shown to be present on the father and infant.

Management

- For the affected neonate, cranial imaging should be performed to exclude intracranial haemorrhage.
- If clinically indicated, transfusion with antigen-negative platelets is preferable. However, antigen typing of platelet units is not routinely done in Singapore. Transfusion with maternal or random platelets is the next best option.
- IVIG at a dose of 1–2 g/kg can also be used to increase the platelet count.
- The risk of NAIT and its consequences increases with each subsequent pregnancy.
- Management of future pregnancies needs to be coordinated with a specialist obstetrician, as monitoring of fetal platelet counts, maternal administration of corticosteroids/IVIG or intrauterine platelet transfusions may be necessary.

Congenital Bleeding Disorders

Haemophilia A and B

Most patients with congenital bleeding disorders will be issued a local *Medik Awas* (Medic Alert) card, as well as the World Federation of Haemophilia (WFH) card, stating their diagnosis and treatment plans.

Table 15.7 Clinical Characteristics of Haemophilia A and B

Severity	Clotting Factor Level % Activity	Bleeding Episodes	Usual Age of Diagnosis
Mild	>5–40%	Severe bleeding with major trauma or surgery	Often later in life
Moderate	1–5%	Occasional spontaneous bleeding, severe bleeding with trauma or surgery	Before age 5–6 yr old
Severe	<1%	Spontaneous bleeding, predominantly in joints and muscles	1st year of life

Background

Haemophilia is an X-linked bleeding disorder affecting males. The prevalence of Haemophilia A and Haemophilia B in Singapore is 1 in 10000 male births and 1 in 50000 male births, respectively. Haemophilia A is Factor VIII deficiency.

Haemophilia B is Factor IX deficiency.

The bleeding phenotype of patients with haemophilia is dependent on the baseline Factor VIII or Factor IX activity (Table 15.7).

The standard treatment for severe haemophilia includes regular replacement therapy with clotting factor concentrates (prophylaxis) to prevent bleeds.

A group of children is being treated with non-factor replacement therapy, such as emicizumab, which is a bispecific antibody mimicking the action of Factor VIII. This is given as a subcutaneous injection weekly to once a month. Children **without inhibitors** who are treated with emicizumab should be treated with the usual recommended doses of Factor VIII according to body weight and bleed severity.

Management of Acute Bleeds in Haemophilia

Assessment

- Prompt bleeding or suspected bleeding in the head, neck, chest, gastrointestinal tract and abdominal regions should be treated with clotting factor immediately, even before assessment is complete.
- Clotting factor replacement should not be delayed by diagnostic imaging.
- Assess site and extent of bleeding and the impact on function.

Management

- Most bleeds will require factor replacement except for bruises and minor soft tissue injuries that do not impact function and mobility.
- Invasive procedures such as arterial puncture, lumbar puncture must only be performed after clotting factor replacement.
- Prompt clotting factor replacement reduces pain and long-term consequences of bleeding.

- Avoid IM injections, aspirin or NSAIDs.

General Measures for Bleeds

R.I.C.E.S. for Joint and Muscle Bleeds

For muscle and joint bleeds RICES will limit bleeding and reduce pain.

Initiate on Arrival

- R = Rest (in position)
- I = Ice (cold pack to reduce bleeding and pain)
- C = gentle Compression bandage
- E = Elevation
- S = Splint

Venous Access

- Venous access is often the major fear and stressor for children with haemophilia and their parents. Use distraction and relaxation techniques. Ask parents about their preferred method for distracting/comforting their children.
- Treat veins with care; they are the lifeline for patients with haemophilia. Apply pressure for 3 minutes post-venepuncture.

Analgesia

- Paracetamol/codeine is sufficient in most cases; morphine or tramadol can be used for severe pain.
- Splinting/immobilisation is an effective adjunct for reducing severe pain.
- Avoid using products containing aspirin or NSAIDS (e.g. ibuprofen, diclofenac) as these potentially interfere with platelet function.

Antifibrinolytic therapy (Tranexamic acid)

- Often helpful for mucosal bleeding (most common form of bleeding), e.g. mouth bleeds, epistaxis, menorrhagia.
- Reduces breakdown of blood clots and is effective for treating and preventing recurrence of mouth bleeds and epistaxis.
- May be given alone or as adjunct to desmopressin (DDAVP)/factor concentrate.
- Dose of tranexamic acid (500 mg tablets) is 15–25 mg/kg/dose (max.: 1.5 g/dose) TDS orally for 5–7 days.
- **Contraindicated** in **haematuria**

Table 15.8 Suggested Doses of Tranexamic Acid

Weight (kg)	Tranexamic Acid
<20	250 mg tds
20–30	500 mg tds
30–40	750 mg tds
>40	1000 mg tds

Table 15.9 Doses of Factor VIII for Bleeds

Site of Bleed	Desired Factor VIII level (% of normal)	Factor VIII dose (IU) per kg body weight	Duration (Days)	Comments
Joint	40–60	25	1–3	
Muscle (Minor)	40–60	25	1–3	
Muscle (Major) including ileopsoas bleeds • Initial • Maintenance	 • 80–100 • 30–60	 • 50 • 25	 • 1–2 • 3–5 or longer as prophylaxis during physiotherapy	Calf and forearm bleeds may lead to compartment syndrome and be limb-threatening. Consult haematologist and orthopaedic surgeon. Involvement of ileopsoas muscle may be associated with significant blood loss into the retroperitoneal area.
Gastrointestinal tract	80–100	50	1–6	Tranexamic acid is helpful
Epistaxis	30–50	25	1–2	Use tranexamic acid 25 mg/kg 8 hourly for 5–7 d as an adjunct therapy
Oral mucosa	30–50	25	1–2	
Dental extraction	50–100	25	1–2	
Haematuria	30–100	50	3–5	Tranexamic acid is contraindicated
Central Nervous System • Initial • Maintenance	 • 80–100 • 50	 • 50 • 25	 • 1–7 • 8–21	Factor replacement should not be delayed by imaging; it should be administered prior to imaging if suspicion is high. Urgently consult with Haematology and Neurosurgeon required.
Retropharyngeal • Initial • Maintenance	 • 80–100 • 50	 • 50 • 25	 • 1–7 • 8–14	
Retroperitoneal	80–100	50	3–5	
Surgery (major) • Pre-Op • Post-Op	 • 80–100 • 30–50	 • 50 • 25		Bleeding risk and duration of cover will depend on the type of surgery

Physiotherapy

- Referral to physiotherapy for joint and muscle bleeds is essential.
- Physiotherapy should commence as soon as pain has subsided and bleeding has been controlled.

Specific Clotting Factor Replacement in Haemophilia A

Factor VIII

Dose of Factor VIII (IU) = Body weight (kg) × 0.5 IU/kg × desired increase in plasma Factor VIII (%). Doses should be rounded to the nearest **whole vial size** to avoid wastage.

Dose of Factor VIII for surgical procedures:
Major surgical procedures require Factor VIII levels to be raised to 100% (i.e. 50 IU/kg). Maintain circulating Factor VIII activity of 80–100% for the first 7 post-operative days and 30–50% for up to the 14th post-operative day. The duration of bleeding risk should be discussed with the surgeon and used to guide factor replacement therapy.

Dose of Factor VIII for dental extractions:

- Minor dental extractions
  - » Factor VIII activity of 50% before extraction.
  - » To maintain levels of at least 50% for treatment of persistent oozing.
- Major dental procedures
  - » Loading dose = 50 IU/kg followed by
  - » Maintenance dose = 15 IU/kg every 8–12 hours for the first 1–2 days, then same dose 1–2 times a day for 5 days or until wound is adequately healed.

Tranexamic acid should be given up to the 7th post-operative day for all dental procedures.

Desmopressin (DDAVP)

- Releases stored Factor VIII into the circulation.
- To be used only in patients with mild Haemophilia A where there is documented evidence in the medical record of safe and satisfactory response to a DDAVP challenge
- Not adequate for haemostasis in major bleeding
- Generally not recommended in young children (<3 years) due to documented reports of hyponatraemia and seizures. Relatively contraindicated in children with previous seizure disorders.
- **IV Desmopressin:** 0.3 mcg/kg infusion (to monitor BP and pulse during infusion)
- **Intranasal Desmopressin:** 150 mcg (for patients <50 kg); 300 mcg (for patients >50 kg)

Management Options for patients with Factor VIII Inhibitors

- Some patients may develop inhibitors (antibodies that bind to Factor VIII or IX) in the course of haemophilia treatment, which renders treatment with normal factor replacement therapy ineffective.
- This occurs in approximately 20% to 30% of people with Haemophilia A and 3% of people with Haemophilia B on factor replacement therapy.
- The severity of the inhibitor is determined using the Bethesda assay (BU). A high titre inhibitor is any inhibitor that is >5 BU.
- Treatment options for acute bleeds include:
  - » Swarming with Factor VIII:
    - ▪ Only effective if inhibitor level <5 BU
    - ▪ Initial Dose: 70–140 IU/kg bolus

- Maintenance: 4–14 IU/kg/h of continuous infusion (dose should be adjusted according to target plasma Factor VIII levels)

» Activated prothrombin complex concentrate (APCC/Factor eight inhibitor bypassing activity [FEIBA])

- Initial Dose: 50–100 IU/kg/dose, depending on severity of haemorrhage. Dosing Interval: Up to 4 times a day
- *Avoid concomitant use of tranexamic acid with APCC due to increased risk of thrombosis. **Avoid the use of APCC for patients on emicizumab (Hemlibra).**

» Activated Factor VIIa (Novoseven)

- Initial Dose: 90 mcg/kg/dose to be repeated 2 hourly until bleeding stops.
- Single doses of up to 270 mcg/kg can be administered for severe bleeds.

• Long-term treatment options include:

» Immune Tolerance Induction (ITI), which is an immune system 'desensitisation' technique used to eliminate inhibitory antibodies to clotting factor.

» Prophylaxis with emicizumab (Hemlibra), which is a bispecific antibody mimicking the action of Factor VIII

» **Note that patients with inhibitors who are on prophylaxis with emicizumab should NOT be treated with FEIBA/prothrombin complex concentrate due to the risk of developing microangiopathic haemolytic anaemia. They should be treated with recombinant Factor VIIa for acute bleeds.**

Specific Clotting Factor Replacement in Haemophilia B

Factor IX

Dose of Factor IX (IU) = Body weight (kg) × 1.0 IU/kg × Desired increase in plasma Factor IX (%). Doses should be rounded to the **nearest whole vial** size to avoid wastage.

Dose of Factor IX for surgical procedures:

Major surgical procedures require Factor IX levels to be raised to 100% (i.e. 100 IU/kg). Maintain circulating Factor IX activity of 80–100% for the first 7 post-operative days and 30–50% for up to 14 post-operative days. The duration of bleeding risk should be discussed with the surgeon and used to guide factor replacement therapy.

Dose of Factor IX for dental extractions:

• Minor dental extractions

» Factor IX activity of 50% before extraction.

» To maintain levels of at least 25% for treatment of persistent oozing.

• Major dental procedures

» Loading dose = 100 IU/kg followed by

» Maintenance dose = 30 IU/kg every 8–12 hours for the first 1–2 days, then same dose 1–2 times a day for 5 days or until wound is adequately healed.

Table 15.10 Doses of Factor IX for Bleeds

Site of Bleed	Desired Factor IX Level, % of normal	Factor IX dose per kg Body Weight	Duration (Days)	Comments
Joint	40–60	50	1–3	
Muscle (Minor)	40–60	50	1–3	
Muscle (Major) including ileopsoas bleeds • Initial • Maintenance	 • 80–100 • 30–60	 • 80 • 50	 • 1–2 • 3–5 or longer as prophylaxis for physiotherapy	Calf and forearm bleeds may lead to compartment syndrome and be limb-threatening. Consult haematologist and orthopaedic surgeon. Involvement of ileopsoas muscle may be associated with significant blood loss.
Gastrointestinal tract	60–80	75	1–6	Tranexamic acid is helpful
Epistaxis	30–50	50	1–2	Use tranexamic acid 25 mg/kg 8 hourly for 5–7 d as an adjunct therapy
Oral mucosa	30–50	50	1–2	
Dental extraction	50–100	50	1–2	
Haematuria	30–100	75	3–5	*Tranexamic acid is **contraindicated**
Central Nervous System • Initial • Maintenance	 • 80–100 • 30	 • 100 • 30	 • 1–7 • 8–21	Factor replacement should not be delayed by imaging; it should be administered prior to imaging if suspicion is high. Urgent consult with Haematology and Neurosurgeon required.
Retropharyngeal				
• Initial • Maintenance	• 80–100 • 50	• 100 • 50	• 1–7 • 8–14	
Retroperitoneal	80–100	100	3–5	
Surgery (major) • Pre-op • Post-op	 • 80–100 • 30–50	 • 100 • 50		Bleeding risk and duration of cover will depend on the type of surgery

Tranexamic acid should be given up to the 7th post-operative day for all dental procedures.

Von Willebrand Disease

Background

Von Willebrand disease (vWD) is the most common inherited bleeding disorder affecting up to 1% of the population, with most cases caused by a mild quantitative deficiency of the von Willebrand factor (vWF). Quantitative or qualitative deficiencies of vWF cause inadequate platelet adhesion and secondary deficiency of Factor VIII. It affects males and females equally. It is characterised by easy bruising, bleeding from mucosal membranes (particularly epistaxis, oral mucosa and menorrhagia) and post-operative bleeding (see Table 15.11) in more severe cases.

Table 15.11 Phenotypes of von Willebrand Disease

	vWF Defect	Typical Bleeding Pattern
Type 1 (common)	Mild to moderately reduced levels of vWF	Typically associated with mild bleeding
Type 2 (uncommon)	Abnormal structure and function of vWF, several variants including: 2A — Decreased formation of high molecular weight vWF multimers, interfering with collagen binding 2B — Abnormal affinity of platelets, leading to significant thrombocytopaenia 2M — Decreased affinity of the vWF molecule for platelet glycoproteins 2N — Decreased affinity of the vWF molecule for Factor VIII can present with symptoms similar to haemophilia	Variable bleeding pattern
Type 3 (rare)	Severe quantitative defect of vWF	Patients may behave like those with moderate to severe haemophilia

Management of Acute Bleeds in vWD Patients

Antifibrinolytic Therapy (Tranexamic Acid)

- Bleeds in patients with mild vWD tend to be minor and occur from mucosal surfaces. Treatment with tranexamic acid is usually sufficient to control bleeding.
- May be given alone or as an adjunct therapy to DDAVP/ factor concentrate.
- Dose of tranexamic acid is 25 mg/kg/dose TDS orally for 5–7 days.
- Referral to the ENT surgeon may be required for local control of bleeds from epistaxis.

Desmopressin (DDAVP)

- Patients with mild to moderate Type 1 vWD can be treated with DDAVP when there is documented evidence in the medical record of safe and satisfactory response to a DDAVP challenge.
- Occasionally effective in Type 2 vWD, never effective in Type 3 vWD
- **Contraindicated in Type 2B vWD as it worsens thrombocytopaenia**
- Expect two- to three-fold increase in Factor VIII/vWF level.
- Generally not recommended in young children (younger than 3 years) due to documented reports of hyponatraemia and seizures. Relatively contraindicated in children with previous seizure disorders.
- **IV Desmopressin:** 0.3 mcg/kg infusion (to monitor BP & pulse during infusion)
- **Intranasal Desmopressin:** 150 mcg (for patients <50 kg), 300 mcg (for patients >50 kg)

Table 15.12 Desired Factor VIII Level for Bleeds in von Willebrand Disease

Type of Bleeding	Desired Factor VIII Level (%)
Oral mucosa/epistaxis/menorrhagia	30–50
Gastrointestinal	60–80
Joint/muscle	80–100
CNS bleed	80– 100

Factor VIII/vWF Plasma Concentrate for vWD

- An intermediate purity plasma-derived product containing both Factor VIII and vWF concentrate can be used to treat bleeding episodes in vWD.
- Dose of factor concentrate to be used will depend on clinical severity of disease and bleed and is dosed according to the target **Factor VIII** level.
- *Please **round up** the **dose** to the **nearest whole vial** size. Do not waste any factor.
- The dose of Factor VIII/vWF concentrate to be given should be calculated based on the formula:
  - » Dose of factor = Body weight (kg) x (Desired Factor VIII level [%] – Baseline Factor VIII level [%]) / 2

If patients with vWD need surgery, the paediatric haematologist should be consulted as the dose needs to be adjusted according to the bleeding risk.

Desired Factor VIII level for dental extractions:

- Minor dental extractions
  - » Target Factor VIII activity of 30–50% before extraction
- Major dental extractions
  - » Target Factor VIII activity of 50–100% before major extraction or other invasive procedures

Tranexamic acid should be given up to the 7th post-operative day for all dental procedures.

Other Bleeding Disorders

Haemorrhagic Disease of Newborn

Newborn infants have lower levels of Vitamin-K-dependent clotting factors (Factors II, VII, IX, X) due to poor transplacental passage of Vitamin K and low levels stored in the neonatal liver. Endogenous production of Vitamin K in the infant gut occurs only after a few weeks when the intestinal microflora is established. Infants who have not been given exogenous IM or oral Vitamin K after birth are at risk of developing haemorrhagic disease of newborn (HDN).

Presentation

Most common sites of bleeding are from the umbilicus, mucous membranes, gastrointestinal tract, circumcision and venepuncture sites. Haematomas can occur at sites of trauma, including sites related to instrumental delivery. Intracranial bleeding is a risk.

- Early HDN
  - » Presentation is within first 24 hours.
  - » Associated with maternal medications, e.g. anticonvulsants affecting Vitamin K metabolism.
- Classic HDN
  - » Presents 2–7 days after birth.
  - » Seen in infants who did not receive Vitamin K prophylaxis at birth.
- Late HDN
  - » Presents 2–12 weeks after birth.
  - » Most commonly seen in breastfed infants who did not receive Vitamin K prophylaxis at birth as human milk is low in Vitamin K content.
  - » Can also be seen in infants with chronic diarrhoea, malabsorption syndromes and chronic antibiotic therapy.

Management

- Severe episodes of bleeding can be treated with fresh frozen plasma–prothrombin complex concentrate.
- Vitamin K can be given subcutaneously with local pressure if bleeding is not severe. Avoid IM injections because of the risk of haematoma.
- IV Vitamin K can be given; however, it must be administered as a slow infusion due to the risk of anaphylactic reactions.

Disseminated Intravascular Coagulopathy

DIC is an acquired clinicopathological syndrome characterised by systemic activation of coagulation leading to generation of fibrin clots that cause microvascular thrombosis and organ failure, as well as concomitant consumption of platelets and coagulation factors that can result in bleeding. Causes include sepsis, malignancies (commonly seen in acute promyelocytic leukaemia), haemolytic transfusion reactions, toxins and trauma.

Clinical features include signs of bleeding into skin and mucosa at multiple sites. There is oozing from venepuncture sites, petechiae and purpura. There can be fulminant bleeding from internal organs such as the gastrointestinal tract, brain and lungs, leading to shock and end-organ failure. At the same time, microvascular thrombi in arterial and venous sites also contribute to end-organ failure, especially in the kidneys and brain.

Diagnosis

- The diagnosis of DIC is based on a combination of clinical features supported by relevant laboratory tests.
- Suggestive laboratory findings include:
  - » Thrombocytopaenia
  - » Red cell fragmentation seen on the PBF
  - » Prolonged PT, aPTT

   - Low fibrinogen
   - Raised markers of fibrinolysis — Raised D-dimer, fibrin degradation products

Management

- The underlying cause of DIC must be treated.
- Management is mainly supportive, with correction of any factors that can further precipitate or worsen DIC, including hypotension, hypoxia and hypothermia.
- Maintain platelet counts >50 × 10^9/L.
- Fresh frozen plasma/cryoprecipitate to correct coagulopathy if there is active bleeding.
- Maintain fibrinogen >1 g/L.

Bibliography

1. Srivastava A, Santagostino E, Dougall A, *et al.* (2020) WFH guidelines for the management of hemophilia, 3rd ed. *Haemophilia* **26**(6):1–158.
2. Neunert C, Terrell DR, Arnold DM, *et al.* (2019) American Society of Hematology 2019 guidelines for immune thrombocytopenia. *Blood Adv* **3**(23):3829–3866.

CHAPTER 62

Thrombosis and Thrombophilia

Rajat Bhattacharyya; Lam Ching Mei, Joyce

Introduction

Venous and arterial thrombosis are rare events in children. The incidence of venous thromboembolism (VTE) in children at a general paediatric population level is extremely low, reported as 0.07–0.14 per 10000 children. In hospitalised children, this rate is increased 100–1000 times to 58 per 10000 admissions; hence, neonatal and paediatric thrombosis is mostly seen in tertiary care hospitals. Risk factors for thrombosis in children differ from adults and nearly 95% of VTE in children are provoked events. The most common precipitating factor is the presence of a central venous access device (CVAD), which is responsible for almost 90% of VTE in neonates and 60% in older children. The highest rate of thrombosis in children occurs in two age groups — neonatal period and adolescents older than 13 years. Rudolph Virchow in the 19th century had described reasons for development thrombosis in a very simple way, which is known as Virchow's triad and still holds true. These include blood vessel injury (endothelial damage), stasis (slowing of blood flow) and changes in constituents of blood (hypercoagulability), and these can explain all thrombotic events.

Predisposing Conditions

- Indwelling catheters (most important risk factor)
- Infection/trauma/surgery/vascular malformation/cardiac disease/prosthetic valves
- Inflammatory diseases — Systemic lupus erythematosus, rheumatoid arthritis, inflammatory bowel disease
- Renal diseases — Chronic renal failure, nephrotic syndrome
- Drugs — High-dose steroids, asparaginase
- Inherited thrombophilias

Symptoms and Signs

- VTE
    - » Warmth, tenderness and swelling of a limb
    - » Inability to flush or draw blood from an indwelling catheter

  - Chest pain, haemoptysis, palpitations (pulmonary embolism [PE])
  - Headache, neurological impairment (cerebral venous sinus thrombosis)
- Arterial thrombosis
  - Neurological symptoms, e.g. hemiplegia (paediatric stroke), convulsion
  - Impaired limb perfusion

Radiological Investigations

- Doppler ultrasound to diagnose upper or lower limb deep venous thrombosis/ catheter-related thrombosis.
- Upper limb thrombosis may require computed tomography (CT) venography or magnetic resonance (MR) venography as Doppler ultrasound may be relatively insensitive for the detection of intra-thoracic thrombosis.
- CT pulmonary angiography (CTPA) is recommended as the imaging modality for suspected PE.
- CT or MR imaging of the brain with MR angiography and MR venography for diagnosis of paediatric stroke.

Thrombophilia Testing

Thrombophilia refers to a genetic predisposition to the development of venous and arterial thromboembolic disease. The contribution of inherited thrombophilia in paediatric thrombosis is unknown, as the majority of young children who develop thrombosis have multiple risk factors. Thrombophilia was detected in one case series in 60% of adolescents with unprovoked thrombosis. The utility of thrombophilia testing during an acute event is controversial, as thrombosis itself will result in transient changes in serum levels of antithrombotic proteins. Thrombophilia testing is advisable in adolescents with unprovoked VTE and in children with a positive family history for VTE but has little value in neonates and children with a first episode of provoked thrombosis, e.g. catheter-related VTE. The identification of an inherited thrombophilia does not influence the acute management of thrombosis in a child, but may influence the need for long-term anticoagulation, depending on the clinical situation.

Whom to Test

- Routine testing in unselected children with a first episode of VTE, especially if catheter-related, is **not recommended.**
- Consider testing if there are recurrent episodes of unprovoked VTE.
- Adolescents with spontaneous, unprovoked VTE.
- Testing of asymptomatic children with a positive family history is controversial and should only be made after careful discussion with the family.

What to Test

- Protein C, Protein S, Antithrombin
- Factor V Leiden*, Prothrombin G20210A* gene mutation

- Lupus anticoagulant, anticardiolipin antibody of immunoglobulin M (IgM) and IgG, anti-beta 2 glycoprotein 1 antibody of IgM and IgG
- Fasting homocysteine

(* Prevalence in Asians is <1%)

When to Test

- Testing for thrombophilia in the acute setting may result in an incorrect diagnosis of inherited thrombophilia as levels of Protein C, Protein S and antithrombin may show a transient decrease during acute thrombosis and during therapy with heparin and warfarin.
- Thrombophilia testing should ideally be carried out when the acute event has resolved and anticoagulants have been taken off for at least 6 weeks.
- Genetic tests are not affected during an acute episode and can be performed any time.

Management of Venous Thromboembolism

The aims of anticoagulant therapy (ACT) in children with VTE include:

- Reducing the risk of thrombus extension and embolisation
- Reducing the risk of recurrent thrombosis
- Reducing the incidence of post-thrombotic syndrome

Anticoagulant Therapy

- Low molecular weight heparin (LMWH) — subcutaneous
  - » Usually used as first-line therapy for management of acute VTE.
  - » Monitored using serum Anti-Xa levels, targeting a therapeutic level of 0.5–1 U/ml.
  - » Caution should be exercised in children with renal impairment as LMWHs are renally excreted.
  - » Anticoagulant effect is only partially reversed by protamine and withholding therapy for 24 hours for therapeutic dosing before any surgical intervention is necessary.
- Unfractionated heparin (UFH) — intravenous
  - » Indicated in situations where quick reversal is necessary for bleeding risk as the half-life is shorter (60 minutes) compared to LMWH (4 hours).
  - » Anticoagulant effect can be 100% neutralised by protamine.
  - » Disadvantages include the intravenous route of administration and need for frequent monitoring of activated partial thromboplastin time (aPTT) every 4–6 hours to achieve the therapeutic target of between 60 and 80 seconds. Ideally heparin should be monitored by Anti-Xa levels with a desired level of 0.35–0.7 U/ml, but this is time consuming, and round the clock availability of a testing facility is a challenge.
- Warfarin
  - » Vitamin K antagonist.

  - » Indicated where long-term anticoagulation therapy (ACT) is required beyond 6 to 12 months.
  - » Multiple interactions with other medications and food.
  - » Monitored using international normalised ratio (INR), usually targeted between 2 and 3 for management of VTE.
- Duration
  - » Duration of ACT is guided by reason (provoked or spontaneous), presence of ongoing risk factors and also vascular recanalisation.
  - » Shorter duration is recommended (6 weeks to 3 months) for provoked thrombosis with resolution of risk factors and establishment of venous flow in the area of thrombosis.
  - » For unprovoked thrombosis, longer duration of up to 6 to 12 months is recommended. However, the risk benefit ratio of recurrence of thrombosis and bleeding has to be assessed individually and the duration decided based on these factors.
  - » General principles include:
    - ■ Catheter-related VTEs — ACT for 6 weeks to 3 months
    - ■ Secondary VTE with risk factors — ACT for no more than 3 months, or until resolution of the precipitating factor
    - ■ First unprovoked VTE — ACT for 6 to 12 months
    - ■ Recurrent unprovoked VTEs — Consider long-term ACT

Thrombolytic Therapy

- The use of thrombolytic therapy is usually not indicated in the majority of children with VTE, but may be considered in the presence of extensive life-threatening venous thrombosis or in critical organ ischaemia such as intra-cardiac/PE with haemodynamic instability or impaired limb perfusion.
- Tissue plasminogen activator is the preferred agent for thrombolysis.

Recommendations in Specific Areas of Thrombosis

- PE
  - » Children with symptomatic PE should be anticoagulated. Thrombolysis followed by ACT is indicated only if there is life-threatening haemodynamic compromise.
- CVAD-related thrombosis
  - » ACT for 6 weeks to 3 months is recommended for symptomatic thrombosis. If the line is functioning and required for treatment, then line removal is not necessary.
  - » A non-functioning line should be removed after initiation of ACT for 3–5 days.
  - » Asymptomatic thrombosis can be monitored radiologically and treated if there is progression. ACT for 6 weeks to 3 months is also reasonable.
- Cerebral sinus venous thrombosis (CSVT)

- » ACT is recommended even in the presence of haemorrhage because the bleeding is usually secondary to venous hypertension from the thrombosis and obstruction.
  - » In the presence of significant haemorrhage, close radiological monitoring and starting ACT if there is progression of thrombus is also reasonable.
- Renal vein thrombosis (RVT)
  - » Unilateral RVT — ACT should be considered, especially if there is progression into the inferior vena cava to reduce long-term renal complications.
  - » Bilateral RVT — ACT is necessary. Thrombolysis followed by ACT is recommended for life-threatening bilateral RVT.
- Portal vein thrombosis (PVT)
  - » ACT is recommended in PVT if there is occlusive thrombus, post-liver transplant or idiopathic PVT.
- Neonatal thrombosis
  - » CSVT in neonates — Evidence for benefit of ACT is less established but generally recommended as there is evidence that the risk of progression is reduced without an increased risk of mortality or morbidity with anticoagulation.
  - » Catheter-induced arterial thrombosis, e.g. peripheral or umbilical artery thrombosis — Treat with a short course of anticoagulation for 5–7 days with UFH or LMWH and catheter removal.
  - » Neonatal arterial ischaemic stroke (AIS) — If there is no cardioembolic source, then ACT is not recommended as the recurrence risk is extremely low.
- Arterial thrombosis
  - » AIS in children should be treated with UFH or LMWH until a cardioembolic cause, including dissection, has been excluded and then continued with aspirin (3–5 mg/kg/day) for at least 2 years.
  - » AIS associated with vasculopathy should be treated with heparin for at least 3 months and then further therapy should be guided by repeat vascular imaging.
  - » Recurrent AIS should be treated with ACT continued long term.

Direct Oral Anticoagulants

- Oral administration, short onset of action, predictable pharmacological profile with low risk of food and drug interactions, and no need for routine laboratory assessment of anticoagulant activity are major advantages of direct oral anticoagulants (DOACs), especially in paediatric population.
- The direct thrombin inhibitors, e.g. dabigatran and direct oral factor Xa inhibitors (e.g. rivaroxaban, apixaban and edoxaban) have been approved or are currently under clinical trials in children.
- Dabigatran and rivaroxaban, when compared to standard anticoagulation, showed similarly low recurrence rate of thrombosis and bleeding in paediatric VTE (DIVERSITY and EINSTEIN Jr trials). Similar results were found in its use

in CVAD-associated thrombosis (EINSTEIN-Jr CVC-VTE trial), establishing its safety and efficacy.

- As more safety and efficacy data are available from ongoing trials of DOACs in the paediatric population, they are likely to replace long-term use of warfarin and heparin in the future.

Bibliography

1. Monagle P, Chan AKC, Goldenberg NA, *et al.* (2012) Antithrombotic therapy in neonates and children: Antithrombotic therapy and prevention of thrombosis, 9th ed. American College of Chest Physicians Evidence-Based Clinical Practice Guidelines. *Chest* **141**(2):e737S–e801S.
2. Andrew M, David M, Adams M, *et al.* (1994) Venous thromboembolic complications (VTE) in children: First analyses of the Canadian Registry of VTE. *Blood* **83**(5):1251–1257.
3. Revel-Vilk S, Chan A, Bauman M, Massicotte P. (2003) Prothrombotic conditions in an unselected cohort of children with venous thromboembolic disease. *J Thromb Haemost* **1**(5):915–921.
4. Tarango C, Schulman S, Betensky M, Goldenberg NA. (2018) Duration of anticoagulant therapy in pediatric venous thromboembolism: Current approaches and updates from randomized controlled trials. *Expert Rev Hematol* **11**(1):37–44.
5. Monagle P, Cuello CA, Augustine C, *et al.* (2018) American Society of Hematology 2018 Guidelines for management of venous thromboembolism: Treatment of pediatric venous thromboembolism. *Blood Adv* **2**(22):3292–3316.
6. Rossor T, Arichi T, Bhate S, *et al.* (2018) Anticoagulation in the management of neonatal cerebral sinovenous thrombosis: A systematic review and meta⊠analysis. *Dev Med Child Neurol* **60**(9):884–891.
7. Mikler J, Samoš M, Bolek T, *et al.* (2019) Direct oral anticoagulants: Novel approach for the treatment of thrombosis in pediatric patients? *Pediatr Cardiol* **40**(7):1431–1438.
8. Connor P, Sánchez van Kammen M, Lensing AW, *et al.* (2020) Safety and efficacy of rivaroxaban in pediatric cerebral venous thrombosis (EINSTEIN-Jr CVT). *Blood Adv* **4**(24):6250–6258.
9. Halton J, Brandao LR, Luciani M, *et al.* (2021) Dabigatran etexilate for the treatment of acute venous thromboembolism in children (DIVERSITY): A randomised, controlled, open-label, phase 2b/3, non-inferiority trial. *Lancet Haematol* **8**(1):e22–e33.

CHAPTER 63

Transfusion Therapy

Lam Ching Mei, Joyce

Transfusion of red cells and other blood components in paediatrics may be required in clinical situations such as acute blood loss, bone marrow failure and in preparation for major surgical procedures. However, transfusion of blood products is associated with a definite risk of adverse reactions and should only be carried out when the expected benefits are likely to outweigh the potential hazards.

Safety Issues Related to Transfusion of Blood Products

There must be a clear, documented clinical indication for transfusion. Informed consent should be obtained from parents or guardians prior to transfusion of blood components. The person giving consent should be informed of the benefits, risks and potential complications associated with transfusion of blood components.

Correct patient identification is critical when taking blood samples for group and cross matching and when transfusing blood components to patients. **Errors in mislabelling and patient identification can result in an incompatible blood transfusion, which has potentially fatal consequences for the patient.**

Determining the Choice of ABO Groups for Blood Components

- Persons who are ABO Group A have red cells expressing antigens and have circulating Anti-B antibodies in plasma.
- Persons who are ABO Group B have red cells expressing antigens and have circulating Anti-A antibodies in plasma.
- Persons who are ABO Group AB have red cells expressing both A-antigens and B-antigens and do not have any circulating Anti-A or Anti-B antibodies in plasma.
- Persons who are ABO Group O have red cells that do not express either the A-antigen or B-antigen and have circulating Anti-A and Anti-B antibodies in plasma.
- A pack of red cells of a particular ABO blood group is expected to contain the corresponding red cell antigens.

- Platelets, fresh frozen plasma (FFP) and cryoprecipitate contain large amounts of plasma and are expected to carry antibodies associated with the corresponding ABO blood group.
- The choice of ABO groups for transfusion of different blood components can thus be summarised below:

Table 15.13 Choice of ABO Groups for Blood Components

	ABO Group of Blood Component to be Transfused		
Patient's ABO Group	**Red Cells**	**Platelets**	**FFP**
A First Choice Second Choice	 A O	 A AB	 A AB
B First Choice Second Choice	 B O	 B AB	 B AB
AB First Choice Second Choice	 AB A/B	 AB A/B	 AB —
O First Choice Second Choice	 O —	 O A/B	 O A/B

Red Cell Transfusions

- The aim of red cell transfusions is to increase the oxygen-carrying capacity of the blood by increasing haemoglobin (Hb) concentration in patients with anaemia.
- The decision to transfuse should not be merely based on a 'number' but on a clinical indication.
- There are few large studies looking at the effectiveness of Hb transfusion thresholds in children.
- In general, red cell transfusion may be beneficial, especially in symptomatic patients or in patients with ongoing blood loss when Hb <7 g/dL.
- There is usually very little indication for red cell transfusion when the Hb is >10 g/dL.
- By consensus, see Table 15.14 for the transfusion triggers based on haemoglobin levels used in paediatrics.
- The volume of red cells to be transfused can be calculated using the formula
  - » Volume to be transfused (ml) = (Desired Hb minus Current Hb in g/dL) × (Body weight in kg) × 3.5
- The volume of red cells to be transfused is usually between 10 and 15 ml/kg and should not exceed 20 ml/kg.
- A transfusion of 10 ml/kg of red cells is expected to raise the Hb by 2–2.5 g/dL. However, this is variable and dependent on the underlying clinical condition of the child.

Table 15.14 Common RBC Transfusion Triggers

Clinical Situation	Hb Transfusion Trigger (g/dL)
Neonate in intensive care	10–12
Patients undergoing chemotherapy Stable Unstable/febrile	 7 8
Patients with chronic anaemia on regular transfusion therapy	9

Platelet Transfusions

- The degree of thrombocytopenia does not always correlate with bleeding severity, especially in conditions such as immune thrombocytopenia.
- The decision for platelet transfusion should not be based on platelet counts alone but on the clinical situation and other risk factors for bleeding.
- There are also few large studies looking at the effectiveness of platelet transfusion thresholds in children.
- By consensus, see Table 15.15 for the common transfusion triggers based on platelet counts used in paediatrics.
- The volume of platelets to be transfused is 10 ml/kg or 4 units/m^2 — this is expected to raise the platelet count by 30–50 × 10^9/L.
- In Singapore, platelets for paediatric patients can be ordered either as single units of 'apheresed platelets paediatric' (APP) or 'cell-separated platelets' (CSP).
- 1 unit of CSP is equivalent to 4–6 units of APP.
- In general, children weighing >40 kg should be transfused with a unit of CSP.

Table 15.15 Common Platelet Transfusion Triggers

Clinical Situation	Platelet Transfusion Trigger (x10^9/L)
Neonate	25–50
Bone marrow failure (e.g. aplastic anaemia)	10–20
Patients undergoing chemotherapy Stable Unstable/febrile	 10 20
Prior to lumbar puncture	50
Prior to surgical procedures	50–80
Prior to neurosurgical procedures	100

Fresh Frozen Plasma Transfusions

- FFP contains coagulation factors, fibrinogen, albumin and immunoglobulins.
- FFP should not be transfused merely to correct an 'abnormal' PT or APTT without a prior assessment of the underlying cause of coagulopathy.

- The indications for FFP transfusion include:
  - » Reversal of warfarin overdose, in combination with prothrombin complex concentrate (PCC) and Vitamin K
  - » Acute disseminated coagulopathy
  - » Coagulopathy associated with liver disease
  - » Clotting factor deficiencies for which no alternative clotting factor concentrates are available, e.g. Factor XI deficiency
  - » Massive transfusion
- The recommended dose of FFP is 10–15 ml/kg.

Cryoprecipitate

- Cryoprecipitate contains high amounts of Factor VIII, von Willebrand factor, fibrinogen and Factor XIII.
- It is **not recommended** for clotting factor deficiencies where specific clotting factor concentrates are available (e.g. Haemophilia A and B).
- Because of the higher concentration of fibrinogen in cryoprecipitate compared to FFP, it is useful in clinical situations where potential volume overload is an issue.
- Indications for use of cryoprecipitate include:
  - » Hypofibrinogenaemia
  - » Disseminated intravascular coagulopathy
  - » Advanced liver disease
  - » Massive transfusion
- The recommended dose of cryoprecipitate is 5–10 ml/kg.

Modified Blood Components

Leucodepleted/'CMV-Negative' Blood Products

- White blood cells present in red cells and platelets are associated with various adverse effects such as non-haemolytic febrile transfusion reactions, HLA alloimmunisation and transmission of intracellular organisms, such as cytomegalovirus (CMV).
- In Singapore, due to the high CMV seropositive rate, 'CMV-negative' blood products are not obtained from CMV-seronegative individuals, but are produced from leucoreduction of donated blood.
- From 2012, a change in the production method of platelets resulted in all platelet concentrates in Singapore being leucodepleted. There is thus no need to specially request for 'CMV-negative'/leucodepleted platelets.
- However, universal leucodepletion of red cells is still not practised in Singapore. Hence, special requests for 'CMV-negative'/leucodepleted red cells must be made when indicated.

- Indications for use of leucodepleted blood components include but are not limited to:
  - » Haematopoietic stem-cell transplant recipients
  - » Solid organ transplant recipients
  - » Immunocompromised patients at risk of infection with intracellular organisms
  - » Congenital immunodeficiencies
  - » Premature neonates
  - » Intrauterine transfusions
  - » Patients experiencing frequent non-haemolytic febrile transfusion reactions

Irradiated Blood Products

- Transfusion-associated graft-versus-host disease (TA-GvHD) is a potential complication of transfusion of any blood component containing viable T lymphocytes when there is a disparity in the histocompatibility antigens between the donor and recipient.
- Gamma irradiation of red cells and platelets renders T-lymphocytes non-viable.
- Irradiation of blood products hence prevents TaGVHD mediated by donor T-lymphocytes.
- FFP is an acellular blood product and does not require irradiation
- Indications for use of irradiated blood components include but are not limited to:
  - » Intrauterine transfusions
  - » Congenital immunodeficiency, especially in T-cell immunodeficiency syndromes, e.g. DiGeorge syndrome, severe combined immunodeficiency
  - » Haematopoietic stem cell transplant patients
  - » Patients treated with purine analogues, e.g. fludarabine
  - » Transfusion from first- and second-degree relatives
  - » All granulocyte products

Washed Red Cells

- Washing of red cells removes the majority of plasma and plasma proteins from the unit.
- There is a red cell loss of 10–20% associated with the procedure.
- Units of washed red cells must be used within 24 hours as the procedure is carried out in an open system.
- Indications for use of washed cells include:
  - » Patients with IgA deficiency
  - » Patients with a history of severe anaphylactic transfusion reactions or recurrent allergic transfusion reactions
  - » Patients with haemolytic uraemic syndrome, although this is not necessary if the patient is already planned to receive products containing plasma, e.g. platelets, FFP

Massive Blood Transfusion

- Massive transfusion in children is defined as a transfusion of more than 40 ml/kg.
- In cases of massive bleeding, e.g. in polytrauma, the lethal triad includes coagulopathy, acidosis and hypothermia.
- Massive blood loss may result in coagulopathy due to consumption of coagulation factors, as well as reduced activity of coagulation factors from prolonged shock, hypoxia, hypothermia.
- In addition, there are dilutional effects of blood replacement on coagulation proteins and platelets. This occurs because packed red cell transfusions are essentially devoid of plasma and platelets.
- Hence, with a massive transfusion of blood for haemodynamic resuscitation, there is a concurrent need to correct the coagulopathy with early use of FFP, platelets and cryoprecipitate.
- A ratio of at least 1 FFP:2RBC is recommended in early resuscitation of a major bleed.
- Platelets in 15–20 ml/kg aliquots are to be considered after every 40 ml/kg.
- Ratios should be modified accordingly once laboratory parameters are available.
- A Massive Transfusion Protocol should be in place to ensure rapid provision of blood components for children with massive bleeds (See Figure 15.6).
- Both acidosis and hypothermia interfere with the normal functioning of the coagulation system and should be avoided in massive blood loss situations.
- Other complications of massive blood transfusion include:
  - » Hypocalcaemia due to large amounts of citrate given with blood transfusion, since blood is anticoagulated with citrate.
  - » Hyperkalaemia due to potassium leakage from RBCs after prolonged blood storage or irradiation

Adverse Transfusion Reactions

- An adverse transfusion reaction is defined as an undesirable response in a patient temporally associated with the administration of a blood component.
- Transfusion reactions can be acute (presenting within 24 hours) or delayed.
- It is important to recognise a transfusion reaction as many of the early signs and symptoms can be non-specific, including fever, chills, rigors and urticarial rash.
- Allergic reactions and febrile non-haemolytic transfusion reactions are **common** but **less serious,** whereas acute haemolytic transfusion reactions, bacterial contamination of blood products and transfusion-related acute lung injury (TRALI) are **less common** but **life-threatening.**

What to Do when an Adverse Transfusion Reaction is Suspected

- **All suspected transfusion reactions must be reported to the issuing blood bank.**
- Any ongoing transfusion of the suspected unit must be stopped immediately.
- Monitor the patient's vital signs.
- Do an immediate clerical check at the bedside to detect any misidentification and major ABO mismatch. **This is the most common cause of an acute haemolytic transfusion reaction.**

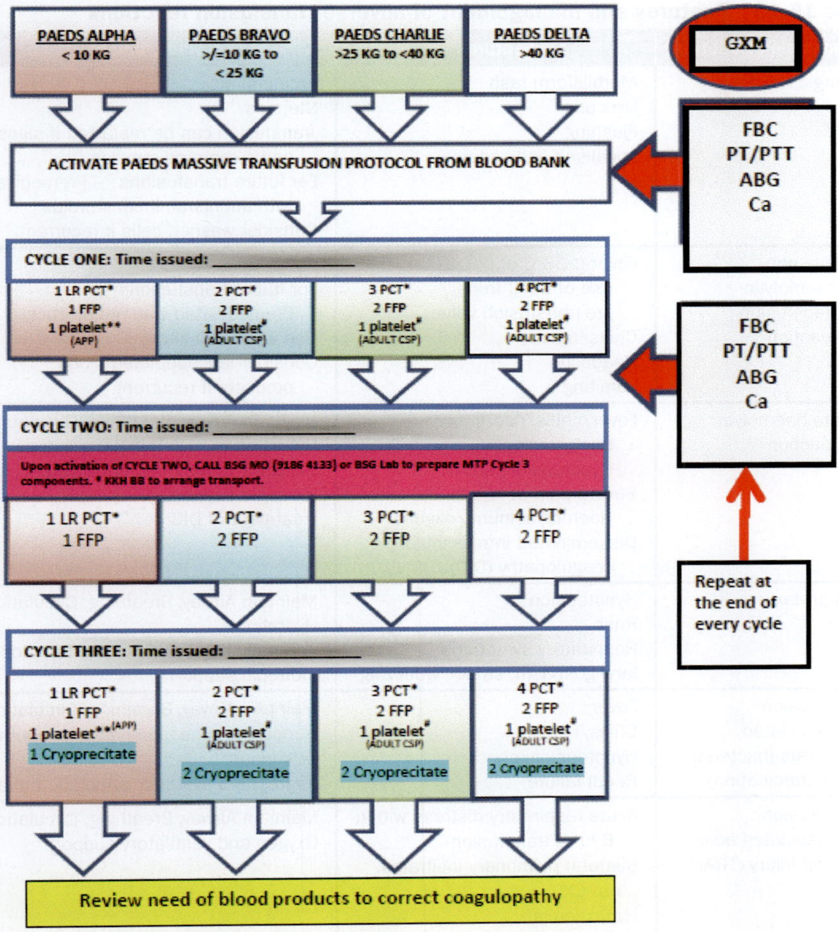

Figure 15.6 Paediatric massive transfusion protocol.

*LR PCT = Leucocyte-reduced packed cells

** APP = Apheresed platelets

- Maintain intravenous access for treatment if necessary.
- Coordinate with the blood bank regarding samples to collect for investigation of the suspected transfusion reaction.
- Do not initiate any further transfusions without consultation with the blood bank/haematologist.
- See Figure 15.7 for the various approaches to diagnosing the likely type of adverse transfusion reaction depending on the presenting symptoms
- See Table 15.16 for the features and management of the various types of adverse transfusion reactions

Table 15.16 Features and management of adverse transfusion reactions

Transfusion Reaction	Features	Management
Allergic reaction	Morbilliform rash Urticaria Flushing Localised angioedema	Antihistamines Steroids Transfusion can be restarted if signs and symptoms subside For future transfusions — Premedicate with antihistamines/steroids Consider washed cells if recurrent
Febrile non-haemolytic transfusion reaction	Fever (≥38°C or a rise of ≥1°C from pre-transfusion value) Chills/rigors Headache Vomiting	Antipyretics For future transfusions — Premedicated with antipyretics Use white cell filter Consider leucodepleted blood products if recurrent
Acute haemolytic reaction	Fever/chills/rigors Back/flank pain Hypotension/shock Severe pain at IV site Haemoglobinuria/oliguria Disseminated intravascular coagulopathy (DIC)	Maintain Airway, Breathing, Circulation Hydration to maintain urine output Diuretics to maintain urine output Inotropic support Treatment of DIC
Anaphylaxis	Hypotension Rash Respiratory symptoms — laryngospasm, stridor, wheezing	Maintain Airway, Breathing, Circulation Hydration Adrenaline, Antihistamines, Steroids Inotropic support
Transfusion-associated sepsis (bacterial contamination)	Fever Chills/rigors Hypotension/shock Renal failure	Maintain Airway, Breathing, Circulation Supportive management, e.g. inotropic support Appropriate systemic antibiotic therapy
Transfusion-associated acute lung injury (TRALI)	Acute respiratory distress within 6 hr of transfusion Bilateral pulmonary infiltrates on CXR Hypoxaemia No evidence of circulatory overload	Maintain Airway, Breathing, Circulation Oxygen and ventilatory support
Transfusion-associated circulatory overload (TACO)	Acute respiratory distress Hypertension/tachycardia Evidence of left heart failure Pulmonary oedema on CXR	Maintain Airway, Breathing, Circulation Oxygen and ventilatory support Diuretics
Transfusion-associated graft- versus-host disease (TaGVHD)	Fever Gastrointestinal symptoms Rash Hepatitis Pancytopenia	Immunosuppression Prevent by transfusing irradiated blood products for patients at risk

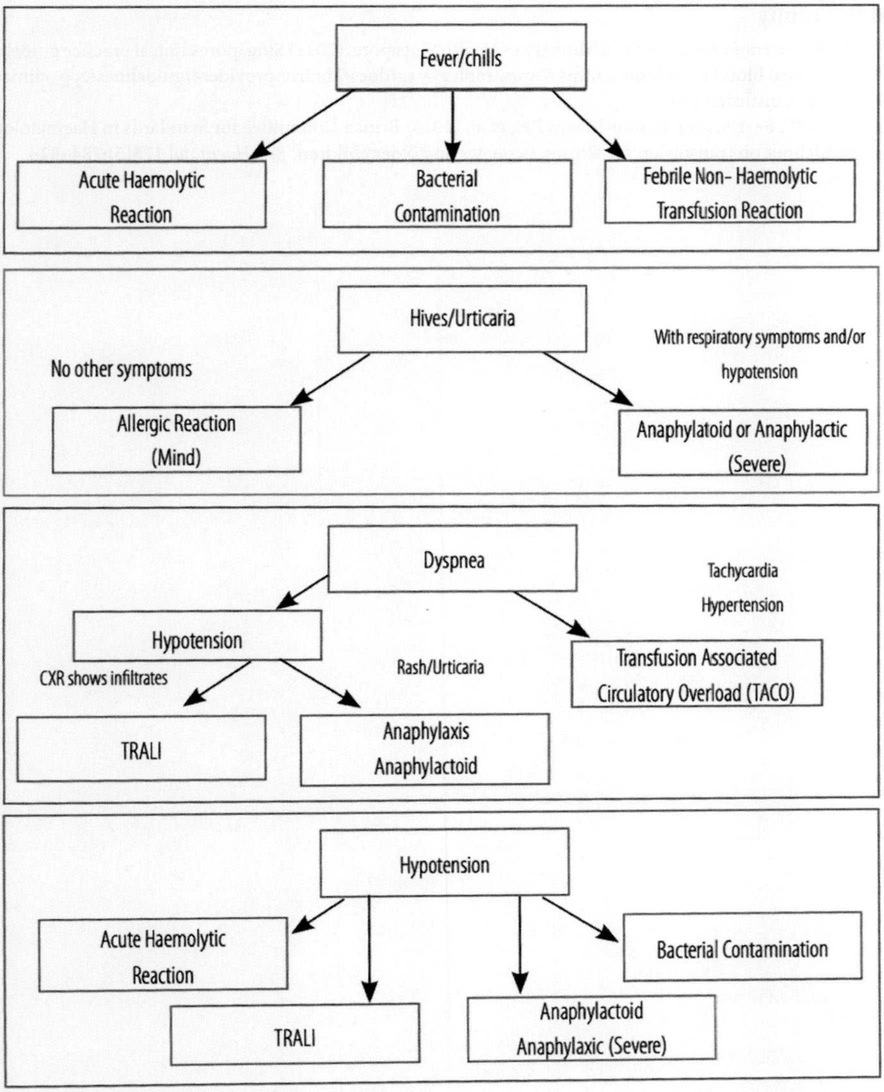

Figure 15.7 Approach to diagnosing the type of transfusion reaction based on presenting symptom.

Source: HSA-MOH Clinical Practice Guideline on Clinical Blood Transfusion 2011, Pages 63–64

Bibliography

1. Health Sciences Authority and Ministry of Health Singapore. (2011) Singapore clinical practice guideline on clinical blood transfusion. https://www.moh.gov.sg/docs/librariesprovider4/guidelines/cpg_clinical-blood-transfusion.pdf
2. New HV, Berryman J, Bolton-Maggs PH, *et al.* (2016) British Committee for Standards in Haematology. Guidelines on transfusion for fetuses, neonates and older children. *Br J Haematol* **175**(5):784–828.

SECTION 16

INFECTIOUS DISEASES

CHAPTER 64

The Febrile Child

Karen Donceras Nadua

Definition and General Principles

Fever is defined as a regulated elevation of the body's core temperature in response to an insult that triggers the body's inflammatory defences. The most commonly cited definition of fever is a body temperature measurement of ≥38°C.

Rectal temperature is the closest approximate of core temperature; however, due to comfort, oral, axillary and tympanic measurement methods are generally preferred. Axillary measurement can be used at any age. Tympanic thermometers are not reliable for infants less than 6 months old. Regardless of the method of measurement used, it is important to be consistent.

While infection is an important and common cause of fever in a child, other causes that trigger the body's inflammatory response should also be considered, such as immune-mediated and autoimmune diseases, neoplastic diseases and drugs.

Fever without Source

- Fever without source (FWS) is defined as fever with no apparent cause.
- The extent and tempo of investigations for FWS depend on the child's age, immune status, height and duration of fever, and clinical status.
  - » For example, neonates have underdeveloped immune systems and are at higher risk for serious bacterial infections (SBIs, such as urinary tract infection [UTI], bacteraemia, meningitis, lobar pneumonia, osteomyelitis). A normal physical examination is insufficient to rule out SBI for this age group; therefore, a thorough workup for SBIs and empiric antibiotics are warranted, regardless of clinical condition.
  - » In older children, viral infections are more common as causes of fever, and antibiotics are often not necessary, especially if the child is clinically well.
- FWS can be a diagnostic dilemma in children aged ≥1 month to 36 months, as occult bacteraemia can occur in young well-appearing infants. This incidence of occult bacteraemia due to *Streptococcus pneumoniae* has greatly declined with increasing vaccine coverage.
  - » Management of this age group is dependent on clinical assessment, sometimes in conjunction with laboratory tests.

Approach

- History

    » To include: Exposure history such as sick contact and travel history, history of immunodeficiency or immunosuppression, history of chronic illness, vaccination history, drug history (including pre-treatment with antibiotics).
- Clinical examination
    » Assess vital signs, perfusion and consciousness, and stabilise as necessary.
    » Thorough physical examination to look for occult infection, such as otitis media, sinusitis, osteomyelitis and septic arthritis, and meningitis and central nervous system infection.
- Red flags that warrant immediate attention and evaluation of a child with FWS
    » Toxic or ill-appearing child or unstable vital signs
    » Age ≤28 days
    » Immunocompromised
    » Underlying chronic illness resulting in reduced physiologic reserves, e.g. congenital cyanotic heart disease
- Initial investigations
    » The laboratory tests (see Table 16.1) below are often used in conjunction with clinical assessment of the child with FWS. Be aware of the limitations of these tests and that they have limited sensitivity in detecting SBIs in the current setting of lower incidence of *S. pneumoniae* occult bacteraemia.
    » UTI is the most common SBI in young children. For febrile children age ≤24 months, urinalysis and urine culture should be done if he/she is ill enough to warrant immediate antimicrobial therapy or if risk factors for UTI are present. These risk factors are: temperature ≥39°C, boys with fever ≥24 hours, girls less than 12 months of age, girls with fever >2 days, and absence of another source of infection.

Table 16.1 Laboratory Tests

	Cut-off	Notes
Full blood count		
- Total white blood cells count	≥15 x 10^9 cells/L	
- Absolute neutrophil count	≥10 x 10^9 cells/L	
- Immature band count	≥1.5 x 10^9 cells/L	
C-reactive protein (CRP)	≥20 mg/L	Rises 6–8 hr after onset of infection; can also rise in other conditions, such as other inflammatory diseases, trauma and burns.
Procalcitonin	≥0.5 ng/ml	Rises earlier than CRP at 3 to 4 hr after onset of infection and is more specific for invasive bacterial infection.

» Chest X-ray (CXR) should only be performed if there is clinical indication as pneumonia in the absence of symptoms and lower respiratory tract signs is highly uncommon.

- Initial management (see Table 16.2)

Table 16.2 Initial Management

	Relevant History Needed	Management
Age ≤ 28 d	Thorough antenatal and birth history, to include: - maternal setup for sepsis: prolonged rupture of membranes (≥18 hr), peripartum fever, per-vaginal discharge - Maternal Group B streptococcus (GBS) colonisation - If colonised, whether she received adequate intrapartum prophylaxis (1 dose of intravenous [IV] Penicillin given at least 4 hr before birth) - Presence of maternal genital ulcers, history of herpes simplex infection in pregnancy	All neonates with fever must be hospitalised for investigation and treatment. <u>Full septic workup</u>: Full blood count C-reactive protein (CRP) or Procalcitonin Blood culture Urinalysis Urine culture Perform lumbar puncture for cerebrospinal fluid studies: microscopy, biochemistry, bacterial culture, PCR for enterovirus, par-echovirus, herpes simplex virus After obtaining microbiological studies, start empiric antibiotics**: - IV Ampicillin meningitic dose - IV Gentamicin If herpes infection is suspected or confirmed, add IV Acyclovir.
Age >1 mth to 3 mth*	As per clinical approach and to include additional history above.	Admit the child for investigation and observation. Assess clinical status. For unwell infants, full septic workup and empiric antibiotics** are recommended as above. For well-appearing young infants, the following can be considered: - Do full blood count, CRP or procalcitonin, blood culture, urinalysis, and urine cultures and closely observe the child. - If urinalysis is suggestive of UTI, then do urine cultures, blood cultures and start empiric antibiotics for UTI. - If urinalysis is normal, but total white blood cells, CRP or procalcitonin are elevated, then consider doing a partial OR full septic workup with blood, urine cultures +/− lumbar puncture and start empiric antibiotics** (IV Ampicillin + IV Gentamicin or IV Ceftriaxone). - If fever is persistent and the urine culture is negative, reassess the child for other sources of infection such as meningitis and consider performing a lumbar puncture.

Table 16.2 (*Continued*)

	Relevant History Needed	Management
Age >3 mth to 36 mth	As per clinical approach	The child can be managed in the outpatient or inpatient setting. Assess clinical status. For well-appearing infants and children, place the child under close observation; no initial blood tests or antibiotics are needed. Do urinalysis for those at risk for UTI (as above). Re-evaluate in 24 to 48 hr if fever persists. Consider full blood count, CRP or procalcitonin, urinalysis, respiratory viral PCR tests, chest X-ray (CXR) if clinically indicated.
Older children	As per clinical approach	The child can be managed in the outpatient or inpatient setting. Assess clinical status. If child is well-appearing, then no investigations or antibiotics are needed. Re-evaluate after 2 to 3 d if fever persists. Consider full blood count, CRP or procalcitonin, respiratory viral PCR tests, CXR if clinically indicated.

*Refer to your Institution's Guideline on Neonatal and Infantile Pyrexia
**Refer to your Institution's Antimicrobial Guidelines for empirical antibiotic choice and dosage

Fever of Unknown Origin in Children

- FWS can evolve into Fever of Unknown Origin (FUO), which is defined as temperature ≥38°C for at least one week with no source identified.
- In FUOs where the cause is eventually identified, the most common conditions are infectious (50%), followed by collagen-vascular (10–20%) and oncologic (10%).
  - » FUO is often an uncommon presentation of a common disease.
  - » Presence of constitutional symptoms may be due to oncologic or autoimmune diseases. In endemic countries including Singapore, tuberculosis (TB) should also be considered.
  - » Parents should be counselled that a child with FUO may have a prolonged stay and may require multiple investigations.

Approach

- A comprehensive history and a detailed physical examination will help direct the evaluation of an FUO with targeted investigations.
- It is useful to identify the clinical syndrome of the FUO (such as fever with rash, fever with cervical lymphadenopathy, pneumonia, meningitis).
- History
  - » Demographics — age, sex, ethnicity
  - » Objective documentation of fever, fever pattern
  - » Onset of symptoms — whether community acquired or nosocomial

        - If nosocomial — recent admissions, surgeries or procedures, presence and duration of catheters and lines, colonisation with multi-drug resistant organisms
    - Presence of constitutional symptoms
    - Sick contacts, including exposure to TB
    - Zoonotic exposure
    - Travel history and geographic exposure
    - Host immune status — Is the patient neutropenic or immunodeficient?
    - Vaccination history
    - Detailed drug history
- Clinical Examination
    - Examination is guided by history. If there is no localising source, a thorough physical examination is needed to look for occult infection, such as otitis media, sinusitis, osteomyelitis and septic arthritis, and meningitis and other central nervous system infection.
- Investigations
    - Investigations will be directed by findings from the history and physical examination.
    - Initial investigations should include full blood count, renal panel, liver function test, urinalysis, and urine and blood cultures.
    - Other investigations to consider:
        - Inflammatory markers such as C-reactive protein, procalcitonin, erythrocyte sedimentation rate.
        - Radiology tests if there is clinical indication.
- Management
    - Empiric antibiotics can be started after relevant cultures are obtained. The choice of antibiotics depends on the clinical syndrome identified.
        - If a child is well-appearing, antibiotics may be held off. Instead, the child will require serial reviews to look for change in clinical status or appearance of new localising signs and symptoms.
    - Non-essential medications should be stopped as drugs can also cause FUO.
    - If the initial investigations' yield is negative and FUO persists, then the child will need to be referred to the paediatric infectious disease specialist and more invasive investigations or detailed imaging may be needed.

Bibliography

1. Adam HM. (2013) Fever: Measuring and managing. *Pediatr Rev* **34**(8):368–370.
2. Antoon JW, Potisek NM, Lohr JA. (2015) Pediatric fever of unknown origin. *Pediatr Rev* **36**(9):380–390.
3. Arora R, Mahajan P. (2013) Evaluation of child with fever without source: Review of literature and update. *Pediatr Clin N Am* **60**(5):1049–1062.
4. Hernandez-Bou S, Trenchs V, Batlle A, *et al.* (2015) Occult bacteraemia is uncommon in febrile infants who appear well, and close clinical follow-up is more appropriate than blood tests. *Acta Paediatr* **104**(2):e76–e81.
5. Long SS. (2016) Diagnosis and management of undifferentiated fever in children. *J Infect* (72 Suppl):S68–S76.

6. Sanders S, Barnett A, Correa-Velez I, *et al.* (2008) Systematic review of the diagnostic accuracy of C-reactive protein to detect bacterial infection in nonhospitalized infants and children with fever. *J Pediatr* **153**(4):570–574.
7. Trippella G, Galli L, De Martino M, *et al.* (2017) Procalcitonin performance in detecting serious and invasive bacterial infections in children with fever without apparent source: A systematic review and meta-analysis. *Expert Rev Anti Infect Ther* **15**(11):1041–1057.

CHAPTER 65

Common Viral Infections

Tan Woon Hui, Natalie; Chong Chia Yin; Thoon Koh Cheng

Chickenpox (Varicella)

Introduction

- **Incubation period**
  - » Eight to 21 days, generally 14 to 16 days.
  - » Can be as long as 28 days in patients given passive immunisation.
- **Infectious period**
  - » Two days before onset of rash until all scabs have dried up (about 1 week, longer in immunocompromised patients).
- **Transmission**
  - » Person-to-person direct contact
  - » Chickenpox and disseminated herpes zoster: Airborne and droplet spread of respiratory secretions and vesicle fluid
  - » For herpes zoster: Direct contact with or droplet spread of vesicle fluid

Clinical Features

- Prodrome of fever, cough, malaise and pruritus
- Generalised maculopapular rash that progresses to clear vesicles, then cloudy vesicles and finally scabs
- Skin lesions start over the face or trunk, appear in crops and spread outward to the limbs
- Oral ulcers can occur
- Fever generally lasts 3 to 5 days
- Suspect secondary bacterial infections if fever lasts >5 days
- Mild, atypical and inapparent infections can occur

Complications

- Secondary bacterial infections: cellulitis, necrotising fasciitis
- Varicella pneumonitis
- Encephalitis, cerebellar ataxia, meningitis, transverse myelitis
- Reye's syndrome
- Thrombocytopenia
- Hepatitis
- Arthritis

- Glomerulonephritis
- Disseminated varicella
- Long term: Herpes zoster

Treatment

- Immunocompetent patients
  - » Oral acyclovir only if:
    - Secondary contact case in a family
    - Older than 12 years
    - Chronic skin or pulmonary conditions
    - On long-term salicylate therapy
    - On short- or long-term, intermittent or aerosolised steroids
  - » Start oral acyclovir within 72 hours (preferably within 24 hours) of rash onset
  - » Intravenous (IV) acyclovir for complicated varicella, e.g. encephalitis, disseminated varicella
- Immunocompromised patients
  - » IV acyclovir until all lesions have crusted, then oral acyclovir for another 3 days
- Acyclovir Dose
  - » Oral 20 mg/kg/dose Q6H
  - » IV younger than 1 month: 10 mg/kg/dose Q8H
  - » IV older than 1 month: 500 mg/m^2/dose Q8H
- Isolation
  - » From 8 days after exposure until all lesions have scabbed
  - » Patient is contagious from about 2 days before onset of illness
  - » If given varicella immunoglobulin (VZIG), isolate until 28 days after exposure
- Immunocompetent patients exposed to chickenpox
  - » If no history of previous chickenpox, assume patient is susceptible to varicella. Varicella vaccine can be offered. It may prevent or modify the illness provided it is given within 72 hours of exposure, i.e. index case is at Day 1 to 2 of illness. May not protect against disease if the patient was exposed at the same time as the index case.
  - » The vaccine is given as two doses subcutaneously 3 months apart in children 12 years or younger, or 6 to 10 weeks apart if older than 12 years.
- Immunocompromised patients exposed to chickenpox
  - » Ask patient for previous history of chickenpox
  - » Check patient's record for varicella antibody result (if previously done)
  - » If varicella immunity is unknown, screen patient's blood for varicella-zoster virus (VZV) IgG antibody (call Virology Lab for urgent testing)
  - » If result shows antibody positive, no action is required
  - » If result shows antibody negative, give VZIG within 10 days of exposure. Please refer to your institution's Varicella Post-Exposure Prophylaxis Protocol.
  - » Dose: 25 IU/kg, or 1 ml/kg (vials of 125 IU/5 ml)
  - » Do NOT overdose, as this may lead to fluid overload and hyperviscosity

  - » Refer to ID/Infection Control team to implement post-exposure prophylaxis protocol
- Discharge if fit, otherwise isolate from other patients for 28 days (from date of exposure).
- If patient is susceptible to chickenpox but has received IV immunoglobulin (IVIG at 400 mg/kg) in the past 3 weeks, VZIG is not required.

Bone Marrow Transplant Patients

- VZIG should be given within 10 days of exposure if significant exposure has occurred to the following group of Bone Marrow Transplant (BMT) patients, regardless of previous varicella antibody result:
  - » Patients who are undergoing conditioning regimen
  - » Allogeneic patients <24 months after BMT
  - » <24 months after BMT and on immunosuppressive therapy
  - » Acute or chronic Graft-versus-host Disease
  - » Varicella antibody negative BMT patient undergoing conditioning treatment, who is exposed to VZV vaccine and having a varicella-like rash

Neonates

- Give VZIG within 96 hours of exposure if:
  - » Mother develops chickenpox within 5 days before delivery till 2 days after delivery
  - » Hospitalised, is premature >28 weeks of gestation and mother has no history of chickenpox and is varicella antibody negative
  - » Hospitalised, is premature <28 weeks of gestation, or <1 kg regardless of maternal history or varicella antibody status

Types of Significant Exposure for Susceptible Persons

- Household: Residing in the same household
- Playmate: Face-to-face indoor play
- Hospital:
  - » Varicella patient in the same 2 to 4 bedroom or adjacent beds in a large ward
  - » Face-to-face contact with an infectious patient or staff member, or a visit by a person deemed contagious
  - » Herpes zoster: Intimate contact (e.g. touching or hugging) with a person deemed contagious

Dengue Fever

Introduction

- **Causative agent**
  - » Dengue virus, serotypes 1 to 4
- **Incubation period**

- » 3 to 14 days, usually 5 to 7 days
- **Infectious period**
  - » 1 day before until 5 days after the onset of illness, during the period of viraemia
- **Transmission**
  - » *Aedes aegypti* and *Aedes albopictus* mosquitoes, which bite during the day

Clinical Features

- An acute febrile illness lasting 2 to 7 days, associated with two or more of the following:
  - » Maculopapular rash, flushing or petechiae, with islands of sparing
  - » Headache
  - » Retro-orbital pain
  - » Myalgia
  - » Arthralgia

Dengue Haemorrhagic Fever (DHF)

- All the following four criteria must be fulfilled:
  - » Fever, or recent history of acute fever
  - » Haemorrhagic manifestations: Bruising and bleeding at venepuncture sites, gums or the gastrointestinal tract. Other examples are epistaxis, a positive tourniquet test or petechiae
  - » Low platelet count ($<100 \times 10^9$/L)
  - » Objective evidence of plasma leakage:
    - ▪ Elevated haematocrit
    - ▪ Low serum protein
    - ▪ Ascites
    - ▪ Pleural or pericardial effusions
- The following suggest impending decompensation:
  - » Severe abdominal pain
  - » Prolonged vomiting
  - » Abrupt change from fever to hypothermia
  - » Change in level of consciousness (irritability or somnolence)

Dengue Shock Syndrome (DSS)

- The four criteria for DHF, and
- Evidence of circulatory failure:
  - » Rapid and weak pulse
  - » Narrow pulse pressure of <20 mmHg
  - » Hypotension
  - » Cold, clammy skin
  - » Altered mental status
- Usually develops 3 to 6 days after onset of symptoms.

Table 16.3 2009 WHO Revised Dengue Case Classification

Dengue without Warning Signs Fever and two of the following: • Nausea, vomiting • Rash • Aches and pains • Leukopenia • Positive tourniquet test
Dengue with Warning Signs** Dengue as defined above with any of the following: • Abdominal pain or tenderness • Persistent vomiting • Clinical fluid accumulation (ascites, pleural effusion) • Mucosal bleeding • Lethargy, restlessness • Liver enlargement >2 cm • Laboratory: increase in haematocrit concurrent with rapid decrease in platelet count ** Requires strict observation and medical intervention
Severe Dengue Dengue with at least one of the following criteria: • Severe Plasma Leakage leading to: » Dengue shock syndrome » Fluid accumulation with respiratory distress • Severe bleeding as evaluated by clinician • Severe organ involvement » Liver: AST or ALT ≥1000 » CNS: impaired consciousness » Failure of heart and other organs

ALT: alanine aminotransferase; AST: aspartate aminotransferase

- Signs of possible decompensation:
  - » Disappearance of fever
  - » Drop in platelets
  - » Increase in haematocrit

Other Complications

- Central nervous system: Encephalopathy, encephalitis, aseptic meningitis, transverse myelitis, Guillain–Barre Syndrome
- Myocarditis
- Transaminitis
- Haemoglobinuria — Intravascular haemolysis
- Vertical transmission to newborn babies

Investigations

- Full blood count: Thrombocytopenia, leukopenia or lymphocytosis with atypical lymphocytes, neutropenia, raised haematocrit
- Dengue serology and non-structural protein 1 (NS1) antigen assay

<u>Not routine, only if child is unwell/has possible features of pre-shock/shock:</u>

- Renal panel: Hyponatraemia
- Liver function test: Elevated transaminases (AST > ALT)
- Coagulation studies: Prolonged prothrombin time and activated partial thromboplastin time
- Group and crossmatch: May need transfusion
- Chest X-ray if chest signs present, or work of breathing increased (pleural effusion)

Management

- Routine
  - » Usually only supportive care is required
  - » Paracetamol for fever (avoid non-steroidal anti-inflammatory drugs)
  - » Complete rest in bed if platelet count $<50 \times 10^9$/L
  - » No intramuscular injections
  - » Intravenous access
  - » Monitor vital signs including blood pressure least every 4 hours
  - » Strict intake/output (I/O) chart. Maintain hydration
  - » Daily platelet count and haematocrit from Day 3 of illness
  - » Dengue is a notifiable disease — Notify Ministry of Health (MOH) via Communicable Diseases Live and Enhanced Surveillance (CDLENS) within 24 hours
- Hypovolaemia
  - » In patients with a rising haematocrit or falling platelet count, administer an IV bolus of normal saline (10 to 20 ml/kg), followed by a maintenance dextrose/saline infusion
  - » Stop IV fluids when the haematocrit <40% and adequate intravascular volume is present; avoid volume overload
- Bleeding
  - » Platelet transfusion only for active bleeding
  - » Fresh frozen plasma is indicated if there is a consumption coagulopathy
  - » Use whole blood or packed cells to replace blood loss
  - » Oxygen can be given for patients with respiratory symptoms
- Further Management
  - » Some indications for admission to Children's Intensive Care Unit are:
    - ■ Requirement for continuous monitoring
    - ■ Requirement for inotropic support
    - ■ Significant bleeding, especially in the setting of severe thrombocytopenia or coagulopathy
    - ■ Evidence of end-organ hypoperfusion, e.g. altered mental status, oliguria despite fluids
    - ■ Respiratory compromise, e.g. secondary to pleural effusions

Hand, Foot and Mouth Disease and Herpangina

Introduction

- Caused by Enteroviruses (EVs)
- About 25 EVs have been shown to cause Hand, Foot and Mouth Disease (HFMD), especially EV71, Coxsackie A16, A6 and echoviruses
- A variant of HFMD is herpangina, which presents with mouth ulcers but no rash, and is due to the same group of EVs
- **Incubation period**
  - » Three to five days (2 days to 2 weeks)
- **Contagious period**
  - » Virus excretion occurs from a few days before, during the acute stage of illness and continues for 3 to 4 weeks from the saliva and 6 to 12 weeks from the faeces
- **Transmission**
  - » Direct contact with saliva, nasal secretions and fluid from vesicles
  - » Oral-faecal transmission via contaminated food, drink and fomites

Clinical Features

- Generally a mild disease affecting young children
- Recovery in about 1 week
- Typically presents with fever for up to 5 days:
  - » Mouth ulcers
  - » Vesiculo-papular rash lasting 7 to 10 days over the palms, soles and buttocks
  - » Sometimes there are papules over the shins
- Herpangina patients have multiple mouth ulcers over the posterior pharynx, buccal mucosa and tongue, but no rash
- Complications are rare: Myocarditis, pulmonary oedema, interstitial pneumonitis, brainstem encephalitis, aseptic meningitis, acute flaccid paralysis and even death

Management

- Isolate the patient in a single room or cohort patients with the same disease condition.
- Symptomatic treatment with close attention to hydration.
- Close monitoring for complications:
  - » Vomiting, change in sensorium, seizures, myoclonic jerks
  - » Hypertension/hypotension, tachycardia out of proportion to fever (normally pulse increases by about 10 bpm above baseline for every 1°C rise in temperature)
  - » Raised total white cell count
- IVIG is a possible therapy for patients with complicated disease.
- Medical certificate for 10 days after onset of illness.
- No swimming for next 3 months in order to decrease transmission to susceptible hosts.
- For complicated patients, in addition to throat swab, send stools and vesicular fluid for EV PCR +/− EV culture.

Bibliography

1. Pickering LK (ed). (2009) *Red Book: Report of the Committee on Infectious Diseases, 28th ed.* Elk Grove Village, IL: American Academy of Pediatrics.
2. Centers for Disease Control and Prevention; Infectious Disease Society of America; American Society of Blood and Marrow Transplantation. (2000) Guidelines for preventing opportunistic infections among hematopoietic stem cell transplant recipients. *Biol Blood Marrow Transpl* **6**(6a):7–83.
3. Istúriz RE, Gubler DJ, Brea del Castillo J. (2000) Dengue and dengue hemorrhagic fever in Latin America and the Caribbean. *Infect Dis Clin N Am* **14**(1):121–140.
4. Radakovic-Fijan S, Graninger W, Muller C, *et al.* (2002) Dengue hemorrhagic fever in a British travel guide. *J Am Acad Dermatol* **46**(3):430–433.
5. Mayers DL. (1999) Exotic virus infections of military significance. Hemorrhagic fever viruses and pox virus infections. *Dermatol Clin* **17**(1):29–40.
6. Dengue fever. In: Goh KT, Paton N, Lam MS, Wong SY (eds.) (1998) *Physician's Guide to Communicable Diseases in Singapore.* Communicable Disease Centre, and Quarantine and Epidemiology Department, Ministry of the Environment, pp. 15–17.
7. Halstead SB. (2000) Dengue fever/dengue haemorrhagic fever. In: Behrman RE, Kliegman RM, Jenson HB (eds.) *Nelson's Textbook of Pediatrics, 16th ed.* Philadelphia, PA: WB Saunders, pp. 1005–1007.
8. World Health Organization. (2009) Dengue: guidelines for diagnosis, treatment, prevention and control, Geneva.
9. American Academy of Pediatrics. (2009) Enterovirus (Nonpolio) infections (Group A and B Coxsackieviruses, Echoviruses, and Enteroviruses). In: Pickering LK (ed.) *Red Book: Report of the Committee on Infectious Diseases, 25th ed.* Elk Grove Village: American Academy of Pediatrics, pp. 287–288.
10. Lee TC, Guo HR, Su HJ, *et al.* (2009) Diseases caused by enterovirus 71 infection. *Pediatr Infect Dis J* **28**(10):904–910.

CHAPTER 66

Common Bacterial Infections

Tan Woon Hui, Natalie; Chong Chia Yin; Thoon Koh Cheng

Bacterial Meningitis

Introduction

The three most common organisms causing haematogenously acquired bacterial meningitis in otherwise healthy children (beyond the neonatal period) are *Streptococcus pneumoniae, Neisseria meningitidis* and *Haemophilus influenzae* Type b (Hib).

Symptoms and Signs

- Fever
- Headache
- Photophobia
- Vomiting
- Neck stiffness
- Back pain
- Myalgia
- Rash
- Confusion and disorientation
- Lethargy
- Seizures
- Kernig's and Brudzinski's signs
- Sixth nerve palsy (suggesting raised intracranial pressure [ICP])
- Papilloedema (uncommon)
- Coma

Symptoms and signs are dependent on the patient's age and the duration of illness. Infants may not have neck stiffness but may be irritable and have inconsolable crying. They may also feed poorly and have vomiting and diarrhoea. A bulging fontanelle may indicate raised ICP but is not a highly sensitive or specific sign for meningitis. Grunting respirations indicate a critically ill infant.

Investigations

- Lumbar puncture (LP) — Cerebrospinal fluid (CSF) for cell count, gram stain and culture:
  - » Cells — Predominantly polymorphs (normal CSF WBC: younger than 1 month <20/uL, 1–2 months old <10/uL, older than 2 months <5/uL; and no polymorphs)

- » Protein — Elevated (normal CSF protein in children: younger than 1 month 0.3–1.2 g/L, 1 to 3 months old 0.2–0.6 g/L, older than 3 months 0.1–0.4 g/L)
- » Glucose — Reduced (normal CSF glucose concentration should be approximately two-third of serum levels; younger than 6 months 2.0–5.6 mmol/L, older than 6 months 2.4–4.3 mmol/L)
- » Pressure — Accepted upper limit during LP with patient in the left lateral decubitus position is 150 mm of water in older children and 85–110 mm of water in younger children. A normal range between 0–60 mm of water has been reported in neonates.
- » Latex agglutination tests for detection of polysaccharide antigen is most reliable for Hib (85–95%), followed by *S. pneumoniae* (50–75%) and *N. meningitidis* (33–50%)
- » Polymerase chain reaction for detection of *N. meningitidis*
- » Contraindications to LP:
  - ■ Signs of raised ICP
  - ■ Cardiorespiratory instability
  - ■ Infection in the area through which the LP needle will pass
  - ■ Evidence of coagulopathy
- » Interpretation of blood-contaminated CSF ('Traumatic Taps'):
  - ■ Traumatic LPs occur in up to 20% of cases. Simple calculations to correct for blood contamination are based on the assumption that the ratio of white to red cells in the CSF attributable to blood contamination is approximately 1:500
  - ■ Another approach would be to determine the Observed: Predicted WBC (O:P) ratio: CSF WBC (Predicted) = CSF RBC x Blood WBC/ Blood RBC.
  - ■ The predicted value is subtracted from the actual or observed CSF WBC.
  - ■ True CSF leucocytosis exists when the observed CSF WBC count is greater than the predicted WBC count (although this method appears to offer better sensitivity and specificity than using the CSF white to red cell ratio alone, it may overcorrect the WBC count)
  - ■ It has been suggested by some authors that contamination of the CSF by less than 10000 red cells × 10^6 does not influence the CSF white cell count and many authorities still believe that it is safer to interpret blood contaminated CSF using the same criteria as a non-contaminated CSF.

- Full blood count
- C-reactive protein (CRP) — Useful in distinguishing bacterial from viral meningitis but has the limitation of low specificity.
- Procalcitonin — Rises earlier than CRP at 3–4 hours after onset of infection and is more specific for invasive bacterial infection.
- Blood culture — Positive in most children with bacterial meningitis, especially that caused by Hib or *S. pneumoniae*

- Serum or blood glucose at the time of LP

Management

- Please refer to your institution's antimicrobial guidelines for meningitis therapy.
- Dexamethasone administered just before or concurrently with the first dose of intravenous (IV) antibiotics significantly diminishes the incidence of neurologic and audiologic deficits due to Hib meningitis. Early administration also improves outcome in pneumococcal meningitis. The recommended dose of IV dexamethasone is 0.2 mg/kg/dose Q8H for 2–4 days.
- Supportive care — Unless the patient is mildly affected, the initial care should be in the children's Intensive Care Unit, as most life-threatening complications occur early and require urgent intervention.

Prognosis and Sequelae

- The mortality rate is <5–10% for the three most common pathogens. Case fatality rate and neurological sequelae are greatest with pneumococcal meningitis.
- Sensorineural hearing loss is the most common sequelae. It occurs in 20–30% of patients after *S. pneumoniae* meningitis and in 5–10% of cases after meningitis due to Hib or *N. meningitidis*. Hearing should be tested within 1 month of discharge to detect hearing loss as early as possible.

Prevention

- Hib conjugate vaccine has had a dramatic impact on reducing the incidence of invasive Hib disease.
- Pneumococcal conjugate vaccine (Prevenar 13) is part of the National Childhood Immunisation Programme (NCIP) in Singapore. Children older than 2 years who are at risk of developing invasive pneumococcal disease should also receive the 23-valent polysaccharide vaccine in addition to the conjugate vaccine.
- Quadrivalent meningococcal conjugate vaccine against A, C, Y and W-135 strains is recommended for high-risk children (e.g. asplenia). Meningococcal serogroup C conjugate vaccine is routinely administered in some countries.
- Chemoprophylaxis:
  - Meningococcal disease (see 'Meningococcal Infections')
  - Hib — Rifampicin prophylaxis is recommended for all household contacts
    - 0–3 months: 10 mg/kg once daily for 4 days
    - 3 months to 12 years: 20 mg/kg once daily for 4 days
    - >12 years and adults: 600 mg once daily for 4 days

Meningococcal Infections

- Caused by *Neisseria meningitidis*
- Can result in bacteraemia, meningitis, septic shock, disseminated intravascular coagulation and focal infections
- Usually serogroups A, B, C, W-135 and Y

- Vaccination available against A, C, W-135 and Y
- Children with terminal complement defects, properdin deficiencies, functional or anatomic asplenia are at high risk for meningococcal infections
- Incubation period 1–10 days, usually <4 days

Treatment

- IV Penicillin G (300000 units/kg/day), *or*
  IV Ampicillin (200–400 mg/kg/day), *or*
  IV Ceftriaxone (100 mg/kg/day) or Cefotaxime 300 mg/kg/day (if IV drip contains calcium)
- Treat for 5 to 7 days if meningitis, 10 to 14 days if septic shock
- Give Rifampicin to eradicate nasopharyngeal carriage, unless the primary treatment was with Ceftriaxone

Transmission and Precautions

- Droplet transmission of respiratory tract secretions
- Respiratory isolation for 24 hours after initiation of effective therapy
- Place the patient in a single room
- When a single room is not available and cohorting is not achievable, maintain spatial separation of at least 3 ft between the infected patient and other patients and visitors
- Wear a mask during examination or when suctioning of patients with suspected meningitis/meningococcal infection within 24 hours of initiation of therapy

High-risk Contacts for which Chemoprophylaxis is Recommended

- Household contact, especially children
- Childcare or nursery school contact during the previous 7 days
- Direct exposure to patient's secretions during the 7 days before the onset of disease, e.g. kissing, sharing toothbrushes or eating utensils
- Frequently sleeps or eats in same dwelling as index patient
- Mouth-to-mouth resuscitation
- Unprotected contact during endotracheal intubation

Prophylaxis Regime for Meningococcal Exposure

- Healthcare workers and adult household contacts
  - » PO Rifampicin 10 mg/kg/dose (max. 600 mg) Q12H × 2 days, *or*
  - » IM Ceftriaxone 250 mg × 1 dose (pregnancy), *or*
  - » PO Ciprofloxacin 500 mg × 1 dose (liver dysfunction)
- Children
  - » PO Rifampicin:
    - Older than 1 month: 10 mg/kg/dose (max. 600 mg) Q12H × 2 days
    - Younger than 1 month: 5 mg/kg/dose (max. 600 mg) Q12H × 2 days,

  or
  - » IM Ceftriaxone 125 mg × 1 dose (younger than 15 years)
- Note: 1 capsule Rifampicin = 150 mg

- Prophylaxis for medical and nursing personnel NOT routinely recommended. Prophylaxis is ONLY recommended for staff who have had unprotected direct droplet exposure (such as mouth-to-mouth resuscitation, intubation or suctioning) within 24 hours of initiation of effective antibiotic therapy

Bibliography

1. Pickering LK (ed.). (2009) *Red Book: Report of the Committee on Infectious Diseases, 28th ed.* Elk Grove Village, IL: American Academy of Pediatrics.
2. Mandell GL, Bennett JE, Dolin R (eds.). (2010) *Mandell, Douglas and Bennett's Principles and Practice of Infectious Diseases, 5th ed.* Philadelphia, PA: Churchill Livingstone.

CHAPTER 67

Tuberculosis

Tan Woon Hui, Natalie; Karen Donceras Nadua;
Chong Chia Yin; Thoon Koh Cheng

Introduction

- Caused by *Mycobacterium tuberculosis*
- Acid-fast bacillus (AFB)
- Transmission usually air-borne

Presentation

- History of contact with an adult with active tuberculosis (TB)
- Risk of disease in exposed children highest in infancy (43% vs. 5–10% in adults)
- Higher risk of extrapulmonary disease in children
- Higher mortality rates if <4 years

Latent TB Infection (LTBI)

- Asymptomatic infection with no abnormal physical findings
- Positive or reactive mantoux test (MTT) or T spot TB
- Chest X-ray (CXR) may be normal or show only granulomas or calcification in the lung, regional lymph nodes or both
- LTBI may evolve into active TB disease

TB Disease

- Pulmonary tuberculosis (PTB):
  - » Most asymptomatic
  - » Early manifestations include fever, weight loss, cough, night sweats and chills
- TB Lymphadenitis:
  - » Most common form of extrapulmonary TB
  - » Usually cervical, supraclavicular and submandibular nodes
  - » Can be unilateral or bilateral
  - » Lymph nodes generally firm and rubbery, non-tender and fixed to underlying tissues
  - » Can progress to affect several nodes
  - » May be associated with active PTB
- Meningitis/miliary TB (rare):

   - Miliary disease is a disseminated form of TB which occurs when massive bacteraemia causes disease in two or more organs
   - Clinical manifestations are protean depending on the site of involvement
- Other extrapulmonary involvement includes pericardium, pleura, abdominal viscera, bone/joint, kidney.

Diagnosis

- CXR findings:
   - Hilar adenitis
   - Segmental lesions
   - Collapse or consolidation
   - Calcification occurs >6 months after infection
   - Multiple lung foci or cavitation
   - Pleural effusions (rare)
   - Miliary disease
- Positive MTT and/or Interferon Gamma Release Assay (IGRA)
   - MTT
      - Site: Clean volar surface of left forearm
      - 0.1 ml of tuberculin injected intradermally
      - 26 G tuberculin needle angled upwards
      - Tense intradermal wheal 6–10 mm should be obtained immediately during injection
      - Do not cover or dress the injection site
      - Read mm of induration 48–72 hours later (transverse diameter only)
      - Incubation period from infection to a positive MTT is 2–12 weeks (median 3–4 weeks)
      - 10% of immunocompetent children with culture-documented disease do not have an initial reactive MTT
      - Children who are immunosuppressed, or who have viral infections (especially measles, varicella and influenza), and miliary TB are often anergic and do not demonstrate a reactive MTT
      - Positive mantoux reaction:
         - **Induration** >10 mm (younger than 12 years)
>15 mm (older than 12 years)
>5 mm (any age) if no previous BCG and exposure to contagious index patient or immunosuppressed patient
         - **Vesiculation or pustular reaction of any size**
   - Interferon Gamma Release Assay (IGRA)
      - Two main tests
         - T-spot TB
         - Quantiferon Gold

- Positive microbiology Investigations
  » Specimens collected according to site of suspected infection should be sent for AFB smear, AFB culture, TB nucleic acid amplification tests (PCR)

Site	Specimen
PTB	3 specimens from gastric lavage (early morning) or sputum or induced sputum ± bronchoalveolar lavage ± pleural fluid
Lymphadenitis	Biopsy and histology of the affected lymph node(s)
Meningitis	Cerebrospinal fluid

  » Isolation of *M. tuberculosis* by culture from the above specimens establishes the diagnosis of TB
  » Organisms are isolated from fewer than 50% of children and 75% of infants with PTB
  » Culture material should be obtained from children with evidence of TB disease, especially when:
    - An isolate from the source case is not available
    - Immunocompromised, e.g. Human immunodeficiency virus (HIV) infection
    - Extrapulmonary disease

Treatment

Site of TB	Drugs and Duration of Treatment
PTB, Lymphadenitis	6 months: 2 months HRZ, followed by 4 months of HR; or 9 months of HR; or 2 months HRE followed by 7 months of HR
Extrapulmonary	9–12 months: 2 months HRZE, followed by 7–10 months of HR

(H: Isoniazid; R: Rifampicin; Z: Pyrazinamide; E: Ethambutol)

- If drug resistance is suspected, initial therapy should include a fourth drug, either ethambutol or streptomycin, until drug susceptibility results are available
- Pyridoxine is recommended if:
  » Diet deficient in milk and meat/nutritional deficiencies
  » Symptomatic HIV-infected children
  » Breastfed infants and their mothers
  » Pregnant adolescents and women
- Complete TB notification form on diagnosis
- Refer to TB Control Unit for Daily Observed Therapy (DOT) if compliance is a problem or multi-drug-resistant (MDR) TB

Persons at Increased Risk for Drug-Resistant TB Infection or Disease

- History of treatment for active TB
- Source case for the contact received treatment

- Contacts of a patient with a drug-resistant contagious TB disease
- Foreign-born persons
- Residents of areas where the prevalence of drug-resistant TB is documented to be high
- Persons whose source case has positive smears for AFB or cultures after 2 months of appropriate anti-TB therapy

Chemoprophylaxis

- Indicated for contacts with:
  - » Reactive MTT or T-spot TB but clear CXR, *or*
  - » MTT/T-spot TB conversion when retested after 8–12 weeks.
- Rifampicin 4 months daily (if Rifampicin-susceptible)

Newborn Infant Whose Mother (or Other Household Contact) has LTBI or TB Disease

Management of the newborn infant whose mother (or other household contact) has LTBI or TB disease (see Table 16.4):

- Based on categorisation of the maternal or household contact infection
- Protection of the infant from infection is of paramount importance
- Separation of the infant from the mother or household contact should be avoided when possible

Infection Control and Prevention

- The following children are considered contagious, and standard and airborne precautions must be observed:
  - » Cavitating or extensive PTB
  - » Positive sputum AFB smears
  - » Laryngeal involvement
  - » Open abscess
- Nurse in a negative-pressure isolation room
- Doors to the room should be kept closed at all times
- All procedures should be carried out within the room
- No cough-inducing procedures, e.g. chest physiotherapy
- High-filtration TB (N95) masks on entry into room. Use a surgical mask on the patient, if movement out of the room is necessary
- Limit visitors
- Do not allow children or immunosuppressed visitors
- All family members who are visitors may require CXR to rule out active PTB as well (consult infectious disease specialist)
- De-isolate if sputum or gastric lavage for AFB smear negative × 3, and no cough

Table 16.4 Management of the Newborn Infant Whose Mother (or other household contact) has LTBI or TB Disease

Circumstances	Recommendations	Remarks
Mother or household contact has a **normal** chest X-ray, asymptomatic	No separation required Give BCG vaccine	The mother usually needs treatment of LTBI, i.e. chemoprophylaxis. The newborn infant needs no special evaluation or therapy. The positive MTT result could be a marker of an unrecognised case of contagious TB within the household, thus other household members should have a MTT and further evaluation.
Mother or household contact has an **abnormal** chest X-ray	Infant should be separated from mother or contact until evaluation is complete If TB disease is found, isolation should continue until the mother or contact is receiving appropriate anti-TB therapy Evaluate infant for TB disease. Test mother or contact for HIV	Other household members should have a MTT and further evaluation
Mother or household contact has clinical or radiographic evidence of possibly contagious TB	• The infant should be evaluated for congenital TB and tested for HIV infection » An MTT, a CXR, a LP and appropriate cultures should be performed promptly » *Placenta should be sent for histology and AFB smears and cultures* » Regardless of the MTT results, treatment of the infant with congenital TB should be initiated promptly with isoniazid, rifampicin, pyrazinamide ± streptomycin • If the infant is receiving treatment, separation is not necessary • If congenital TB is excluded, give BCG vaccine and isoniazid until the infant is 3–4 mth of age, at which time the MTT should be repeated • If the MTT at 3 mth is positive, the infant should be reassessed for TB disease. If disease is not present, isoniazid should be continued for at least 9 mth • If the MTT at 3 mth is negative and the mother and other household contacts with TB have good adherence and response to treatment and are no longer contagious, isoniazid may be discontinued • If the mother (or household contact) has disease due to drug-resistant TB or has poor adherence to treatment and DOT is not possible, the infant should be given BCG vaccine and separated from the ill mother or household members. The infant and mother or contact should be on DOT therapy	TB in the mother or contact should be reported immediately to the Department of Clinical Epidemiology so that investigation of all household members can be performed promptly All contacts should have a MTT, chest X-ray and physical examination The infant should be evaluated at monthly intervals during treatment Note: Patients with multiple drug-resistant TB should be on DOT therapy

Bibliography

1. Pickering LK (ed.). (2009) *Red Book: Report of the Committee on Infectious Diseases, 28th ed.* Elk Grove Village, IL: American Academy of Pediatrics.
2. Jacobs RF, Starke JR. (2003) Mycobacterium tuberculosis. In: Long SS, Pickering LK, Prober CG (eds.) *Principles and Practice of Pediatric Infectious Diseases, 2nd ed.* Philadelphia, PA: Churchill Livingstone, pp. 791–810.
3. Jensen PA, Lambert LA, Lademarco MF, *et al.* (2005) Guidelines for preventing the transmission of Mycobacterium tuberculosis in health-care settings, 2005. *MMWR Recomm Rep* **54**(RR-17):1–141.

CHAPTER 68

Incubation and Isolation Periods for Infectious Diseases

Tan Woon Hui, Natalie; Chong Chia Yin; Thoon Koh Cheng

Disease	Incubation Period	Isolation of Patient
Chickenpox	8–21 d (up to 28 d if VZIG is given)	From school and non-immune friends, until last vesicle has dried (1 wk after appearance of rash)
Diphtheria	3–6 d	Droplet precautions for patients and carriers with pharyngeal diphtheria until two cultures from both the nose and throat are negative Contact precautions for patients with cutaneous diphtheria until two negative cultures of skin lesions Cultures should be taken at least 24 hr apart after stopping antibiotics
Enterovirus infection	3–6 d	Contact precautions for duration of hospitalisation
Rubella	14–23 d	Droplet precautions for 7 d after the onset of rash
Measles	8–12 d	Airborne precautions for 5 d after appearance of rash
Meningococcal infection	1–10 d	Droplet precautions until 24 hr after initiation of effective therapy
Mumps	14–21 d	Droplet precautions until 5 d after onset of parotid swelling
Poliomyelitis	7–21 d	Contact precautions for duration of hospitalisation or until stool cultures are negative
Rabies	Average 4–6 wk	Standard precautions for duration of illness
Typhoid Fever	Usually 1–2 wk	Enteric precautions for duration of illness and until stool cultures are negative (three consecutive specimens obtained at least 48 hr after stopping antibiotics)
Whooping Cough	Usually a week (range 6–20 d)	Droplet precaution for 5 d after starting antibiotics; if unable/unwilling to start antibiotics, precautions for 14 d

Bibliography

1. Pickering LK (ed.). (2009) *Red Book: Report of the Committee on Infectious Diseases, 28th ed.* Elk Grove Village, IL: American Academy of Pediatrics.
2. Mandell GL, Bennett JE, Dolin R (eds.). (2010) *Mandell, Douglas and Bennett's Principles and Practice of Infectious Diseases, 5th ed.* Philadelphia, PA: Churchill Livingstone.

CHAPTER 69

Immunisations

Thoon Koh Cheng; Tan Woon Hui, Natalie; Karen Donceras Nadua

Golden Rules in Vaccination

- All vaccines can be administered at the same visit concurrently with other vaccines.
  - No intervals are required between two or more inactivated vaccines.
  - No intervals are required between live and inactivated vaccines. However, for a live vaccine, do consider the expected side effects of the live vaccine (e.g. for measles, mumps and rubella [MMR] or varicella vaccine, fever or rash can occur 5–14 days after vaccination) when administering an inactivated vaccine at a later date.
  - Two or more different live or intranasal vaccines should be given on the same day, or at an interval of at least 28 days apart (except yellow fever after measles/MMR vaccine, and Bacillus Calmette-Guerin [BCG] before or after oral poliovirus vaccine [OPV]).
- Inactivated vaccines are generally not affected by circulating antibody to the antigen.
  - No intervals are generally required between blood products and inactivated vaccines.
- Live vaccines may be affected by circulating antibody to the antigen.
  - An interval is required between blood products and live vaccines (e.g. 11 months after intravenous immunoglobulins for Kawasaki Disease).
- Vaccine doses should not be given at less than minimum intervals or minimum ages recommended for a particular dose of a specific vaccine.
  - Vaccine doses given up to 4 days before the minimum interval or age can be counted as valid, but should not be abused for scheduling purposes.
- For combination vaccines, the minimum intervals for the individual components must still be met unless otherwise specified by the manufacturer.

- It is not necessary to restart the series or add doses when trying to catch-up for any delayed vaccination series.
- A contraindication is a condition in a recipient that greatly increases the chance of a serious adverse reaction. A precaution is either a condition in a recipient that might increase the chance or severity of an adverse reaction or which might compromise the vaccine's ability to produce immunity.
  - » True contraindications are rare (e.g. true anaphylaxis or allergies to vaccine components, encephalopathy not due to another identifiable cause occurring within 7 days of pertussis vaccination, use of live vaccines in pregnant or immunocompromised persons).
  - » In persons with bleeding disorders (e.g. haemophilia), where the disease severity is mild to moderate, vaccines should be given in the route recommended by the manufacturer due to safety and efficacy concerns (e.g. intramuscular [IM], use a 23-gauge needle and apply direct pressure for ≥2 minutes). Where the disease is severe, then IM vaccination may cause harm, and the route of vaccination must be decided by the primary physician and benefits and risks clearly explained to parents (especially regarding potential loss of efficacy and more severe local reactions to IM vaccines given via subcutaneous/intradermal route); alternatively, when anti-haemophilia or other similar therapy are given, this should be followed by vaccination in the recommended route.
- Healthy household contacts of immunocompromised persons should receive MMR, varicella and influenza vaccines when indicated (risk of wild-type infections outweigh risk of live vaccine-related infections, which are mostly mild). Rotavirus vaccine should also be offered to these healthy household contacts though available data is much less compared with the above.
- Unscientific allegations of connections between vaccines or vaccine components (e.g. MMR or thimerosal with autism) should be vigorously defended.
  - » However, we should still work with patients and parents who refuse the vaccines on these grounds, in the hope that they might change their minds.
- For travel-related vaccines, remember there is no vaccine for lack of common sense, e.g. petting wild monkeys/dogs, having unprotected sex, eating uncooked/unwashed food.

National Childhood Immunisation Schedule

ANNEX A

National Childhood Immunisation Schedule (NCIS)
(from birth to age 17 years, effective from 1 November 2020)

Vaccine	Birth	2 months	4 months	6 months	12 months	15 months	18 months	2-4 years	5-9 years	10-11 years	12-13 years	13-14 years	15-17 years
Bacillus Calmette-Guérin (BCG)	D1												
Hepatitis B (HepB)	D1	D2		D3									
Diphtheria, tetanus and acellular pertussis (paediatric) (DTaP)		D1	D2	D3			B1						
Tetanus, reduced diphtheria and acellular pertussis (Tdap)										B2			
Inactivated poliovirus (IPV)		D1	D2	D3			B1			B2			
Haemophilus influenzae type b (Hib)		D1	D2	D3			B1						
Pneumococcal conjugate (PCV10 or PCV13)			D1	D2	B1								
Pneumococcal polysaccharide (PPSV23)								One or two doses for children and adolescents age **2-17 years with specific medical condition or indication**					
Measles, mumps and rubella (MMR)					D1	D2							
Varicella (VAR)					D1	D2							
Human papillomavirus (HPV2 or HPV4)											D1 (Females)	D2 (Females)	
Influenza (INF)				Annual vaccination or per season for all children age 6 **months to <5 years (6-59 months)**					Annual vaccination or per season for children and adolescents **age 5-17 years with specific medical condition or indication**				

Recommended ages and doses for all children

Recommended for children with specific medical conditions or indications

Footnotes:

- **D1, D2, D3:** Dose 1, dose 2, dose 3
- **B1, B2:** Booster 1, booster 2
- **10-11, 12-13, 13-14 years:** Primary 5, Secondary 1, Secondary 2 (Tdap, IPV, HPV (for females) and MMR (as catch-up) vaccines are provided as part of Health Promotion Board's school-based vaccination programme)
- **HepB:** Doses 2 and 3 are recommended to be given as part of the 6-in-1 vaccine at 2 and 6 months, respectively
- **MMR:** Only the dose 2 is recommended to be given as part of the MMRV vaccine

Reproduced from MOH Circular No. 180/2020

Bibliography

1. National Center for Immunization and Respiratory Diseases. (2011) General recommendations on immunization — recommendations of the Advisory Committee on Immunization Practices (ACIP). *MMWR Recomm Rep* **60**(2):1–64. Erratum in: *MMWR Recomm Rep* (2011) Jul 29; **60**:993.
2. Centers for Disease Control and Prevention. (2020) *CDC Yellow Book 2020: Health Information for International Travel.* Oxford: Oxford University Press.
3. Ministry of Health Singapore. (2020) Changes to the national childhood immunisation schedule. MOH Circular No. 180/2020. https://www.cfps.org.sg/assets/1-Circular-for-GPs/4-MOH-Cir-180-2020-13Jul2020-Updates-to-NCIS-doctors-1.pdf

SECTION 17

NEONATOLOGY

CHAPTER 70

Classification of Newborn Babies

Tan Pih Lin; Khoo Poh Choo

Newborn babies can be classified according to their gestational age, birth weight and other physical attributes.

Gestational Age

Obstetric Methods

- Last menstrual period (LMP): Gestation age (GA) can be calculated from the first day of LMP. The estimated date of delivery (40 weeks' gestation) is calculated by adding 1 year and 7 days to the first day of LMP, then subtracting 3 months from that.
- Ultrasound: Most reliable method, especially if performed within the first trimester. Various measurements may be used such as crown-rump length, biparietal diameter, femur length and abdominal circumference.

Neonatal Methods

- Dubowitz Score (see Figure 17.1): Performed 12–24 hours after birth.
- Ballard Score (see Figure 17.2): A simplified version of the Dubowitz Score. Infant does not need to be alert or vigorous. Accuracy is ± 2 weeks.

The best estimate of neonatal GA is determined from both obstetric and neonatal methods. If the two methods differ from each other by >2 weeks, it is customary to take the neonatal estimate.

- Extreme preterm: <28 weeks
- Very preterm: 28 weeks to <32 weeks
- Moderate preterm: 32 weeks to <34 weeks
- Late preterm: 34 weeks to <37 weeks
- Term: 37 weeks to <42 weeks
- Post-term: GA at birth is >42 weeks

Weight

- Extremely Low Birth Weight (ELBW): <1000 g
- Very Low Birth Weight (VLBW): <1500 g
- Low Birth Weight (LBW): <2500 g

Neurological Criteria

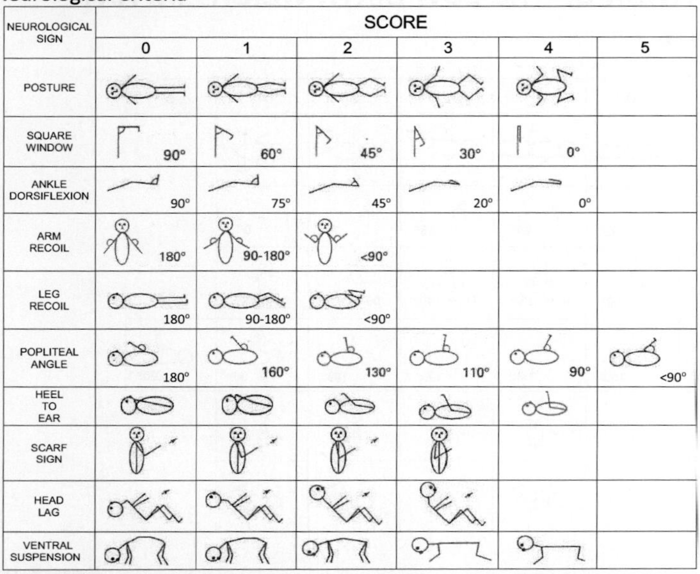

SCORE:

Neurological ________

Superficial ________

Total ________

Score	Gest.
10	27.2
12	27.8
14	28.3
16	28.8
18	29.4
20	29.9
22	30.4
24	30.9
26	31.5
28	32.0
30	32.5
32	33.0
34	33.6
36	34.1
38	34.6
42	35.7
44	36.2
46	36.7
48	37.3
50	37.8
52	38.3
54	38.9
56	39.4
58	39.9
60	40.4
62	41.0
64	41.5
66	42.0
68	42.6

GESTATION AGE BY:

DATES	
ULTRASOUND	
SCORE	

WEIGHT:

LGA >90 centile	
AGA	
SGA <10 centile	

Examiner:

____

DUBOWITZ SCORING SYSTEMS FOR EXTERNAL (superficial) CRITERIA

External Sign \ Score	0	1	2	3	4
Edema	Obvious edema of hands and feet: pitting over tibia	No obvious edema of hands and feet; pitting over tibia	No edema		
Skin texture	Very thin, gelatinous	Thin and smooth	Smooth; medium thickness; rash; superficial peeling	Slight thickening; superficial cracking and peeling, especially of hand and feet	Thick and parchment-like; superficial or deep cracking
Skin colour	Dark red	Uniform pink	Pale pink; variable over body	Pale: only pink over ears. lips, palms, or soles	
Skin opacity	Numerous veins and venules clearly seen. especially over abdomen	Veins and tributaries seen	A few large vessels clearly seen over abdomen	A few large vessels seen indistinctly over abdomen	No blood vessels
Lanugo	No lanugo	Abundant; long and thick over whole back	hair thinning, especially over lower back	Small amount of lanugo and bald areas	At least half of back devoid of lanugo
Plantar creases	No skin creases	Faint red marks over anterior half of sole	Definite red marks over > anterior half; indentations over < anterior third	Indentations over > anterior third	Definite deep indentations over > anterior third
Nipple formation	Nipple barely visible. no areola	Nipple well defined; areola smooth and flat, diameter < 0.75 cm	Areola stippled, edge not raised, diameter < 0.75 cm	Areola stippled, edge raised. diameter > 0.75 cm	
Breast size	No breast tissue palpable	Breast tissue on one or both sides, < 0.5 cm diameter	Breast tissue both sides; one or both 0.5 – 1.0 cm	Breast tissue both sides: one or both > 1 cm	
Ear form	Pinna flat and shapeless, little or no incurving of edge	Incurving of part of edge of pinna	Partial incurving whole of upper pinna	Well-defined incurving whole of upper pinna	
Ear firmness	Pinna soft, easily folded, no recoil	Pinna soft. easily folded, slow recoil	Cartilage to edge of pinna but soft in places, ready recoil	Pinna firm. cartilage to edge, instant recoil	
Genital, male Genital, female (with hips half abducted)	Neither testis in scrotum Labia majora widely separated, labia minora protruding	At least one testis high in scrotum Labia majora almost cover labia minora	At least one testis right down Labia maioia completely cover labia minora		

Figure 17.1 Dubowitz score.

From Dubowitz V, Dubowitz I, Goldberg C. (1970) Clinical assessment of gestational age in the newborn infant. *Journal of Pediatrics* **77**:7.

CLASSIFICATION OF THE LOW-BIRTH-WEIGHT INFANT

Neuromuscular Maturity

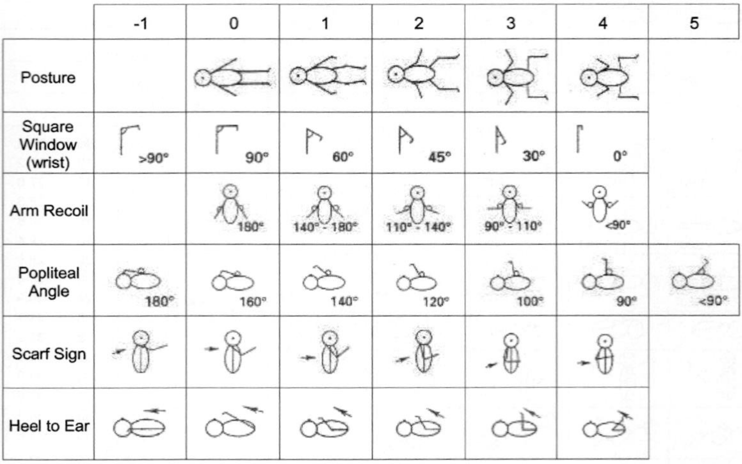

Physical Maturity

	-1	0	1	2	3	4	5
Skin	Sticky friable transparent	Gelatinous red translucent	Smooth pink visible veins	Superficial peeling &/or rash few veins	Cracking pale areas rare veins	Parchment deep cracking no vessels	Leathery cracked wrinkled
Lanugo	none	sparse	abundant	thinning	bald areas	mostly bald	
Plantar Surface	heel–toe 40–50mm: -1 <40mm: -2	>50mm no crease	faint red marks	anterior transverse crease only	creases ant. 2/3	creases over entire sole	
Breast	Imperceptible	barely perceptible	flat areola no bud	stippled areola 1–2mm bud	raised areola 3–4mm bud	full areola 5-10mm bud	
Eye/Ear	lids fused loosely: -1 tightly: -2	lids open pinna flat stays folded	sl. curved pinna; soft ready recoil	well-curved pinna; soft but ready recoil	formed & firm instant recoil	thick cartilage ear stiff	
Genitals Male	scrotum flat smooth	scrotum empty faint rugae	testes in upper canal rare rugae	testes descending few rugae	testes down good rugae	testes pendulous deep rugae	
Genitals Female	clitoris prominent labia flat	prominent clitoris small labia minora	prominent clitoris enlarging minora	majora & minora equally prominent	majora large minora small	majora cover clitoris & minora	

Maturity Rating

Score	Weeks
-10	20
-5	22
0	24
5	26
10	28
15	30
20	32
25	34
30	36
35	38
40	40
45	42
50	44

Figure 17.2 Ballard score.

Maturational assessment of gestational age: Ballard score. (From Ballard JL, Khoury JC, Wedig K, *et al.* (1991) New Ballard Score, expanded to include extremely premature infants. *Journal of Pediatrics* **119**: 417–423. Reprinted with permission.)

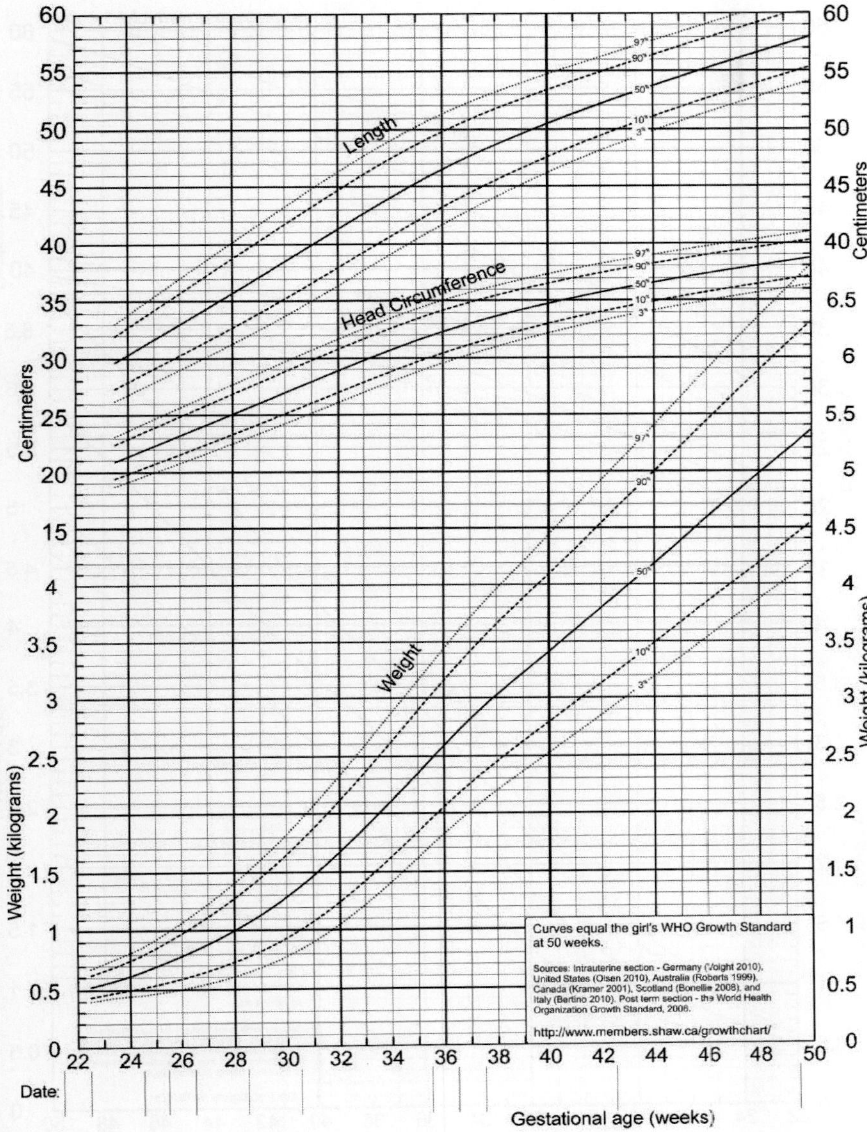

Figure 17.3 Fenton growth chart–girl.

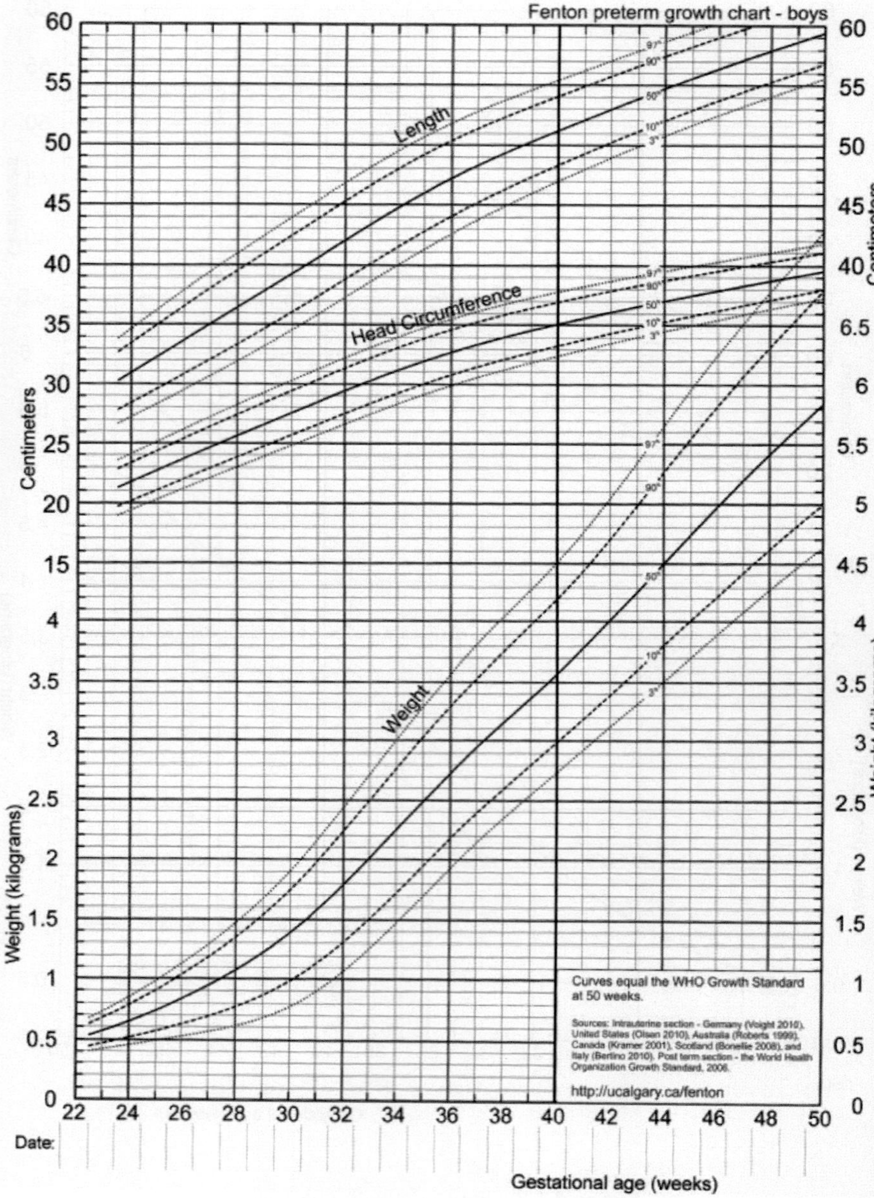

Figure 17.4 Fenton growth chart–boy.

Relative Size

Plot parameters into growth chart (see Figures 17.3 and 17.4).

- Small for gestational age (SGA): Birth weight <10th percentile for estimated GA
- Appropriate for gestational age (AGA): Birth weight between 10th and 90th percentile for estimated GA
- Large for gestational age (LGA): Birth weight >90th percentile for GA

Symmetrical and Asymmetrical Growth Retardation

In symmetrical growth retardation, the baby is small but the growth parameters (head circumference, length and weight) are proportionate to each other. This pattern commonly occurs in early pregnancy and may be related to a genetic syndrome, intra-uterine infection or constitutional.

In asymmetrical growth retardation, head growth is relatively spared as compared to length and weight. Babies are born appearing wasted and malnourished. Typically, this happens in late pregnancy. Common causes include placental insufficiency, pregnancy induced hypertension and multiple pregnancies.

Bibliography

1. Ballard JL, Novak KK, Driver M. (1979) A simplified score for assessment of fetal maturation of newly born infants. *J Pediatr* **95**(5 Pt 1):769–774.
2. Dubowitz LM, Dubowitz V, Goldberg C. (1970) Clinical assessment of gestational age in the newborn infant. *J Pediatr* 77(1):1–10.
3. Fenton, Tanis R, Kim, Jae H. (2013) A systemic review and meta-analysis to revise the Fenton growth chart for preterm infants. *BMC Pediatr* **13**:59.

CHAPTER 71

Newborn Resuscitation

Quek Bin Huey; Abdul Haium Abdul Alim

Introduction

Approximately 1–10% of newborns delivered in hospital require active resuscitation. Majority only requires simple stabilisation. Goal of newborn resuscitation is to deliver healthy, breathing, pink babies OR when not possible, to transfer seriously asphyxiated babies to the Neonatal Intensive Care Unit (NICU) in as good condition as possible!

Changes from in-utero to ex-utero environment:

- Lungs expand with the first cry or few breaths
- Lungs are filled with air whilst fluid is absorbed
- Increase in blood flow to the lungs
- Gas exchange takes place
- Closure of intra and extra cardiac shunts
- Oxygen transported to tissues of other parts of the body

Failure or disruption of these changes results in failure of gas exchange, persistence of foetal circulation, increasing acidosis and hypoxia. If this asphyxia is prolonged, it leads to cell death, and eventually permanent neurological damage and even death.

The phases of asphyxia consist of:

- Primary apnoea — the breathing becomes deeper and more rapid, then regular breathing ceases and consciousness is lost. Heart rate (HR) is still maintained, and at this phase, the baby will respond to stimulation.
- Secondary apnoea — if the insult continues, the baby will start to gasp and go into terminal or secondary apnoea. The HR and blood pressure fall, and there is increasing acidosis. The baby will require active resuscitation with positive pressure ventilation and even chest compression.

The baby in secondary apnoea will die without intervention and may die despite intervention. Primary and secondary apnoea may occur in utero. It is not possible to distinguish at birth. Thus, when faced with an apnoeic baby at birth that does not respond to simple interventions, active resuscitation must be started immediately.

Health professionals who attend to delivery of newborns must thus be proficient in at least the initial steps of stabilisation and resuscitation and be able to work as a team for effective resuscitation. They should be accredited in neonatal resuscitation (such as the Singapore Neonatal Resuscitation Course [SNRC]). The recommendations for newborn stabilisation are constantly being updated based on best available evidence. The most recent guidelines come from the International Liaison Committee on Resuscitation (ILCOR) 2020 Consensus on Science and Treatment Recommendations (CoSTR), updated

Paediatric & Neonatal resuscitation guidelines from the American Heart Association and European Resuscitation Council in 2021, and the Singapore Resuscitation and First Aid Council (SRFAC) Neonatal & Paediatric Resuscitation Guidelines Workgroup 2021.

The guidelines are organised in alignment with the newborn resuscitation algorithm processes:

- Anticipate need and preparation
- Umbilical cord management — Delayed cord clamping
- Initial steps — **A**irway and temperature maintenance
- **B**reathing (Positive pressure ventilation [PPV])
- **C**hest compression
- **D**rugs — Medications
- Post-resuscitation care

Preparation

Preparation involves anticipation of high risk pregnancies, preparation of appropriate equipment, as well as adequate personnel at delivery.

Anticipation

- Quick history:
  - » What is the expected gestational age? This determines the equipment needed.
  - » How many babies are expected?
  - » Is the amniotic fluid clear? If meconium or heavily blood stained — be prepared for full resuscitation.
  - » Are there any additional risk factors?
    - ■ Antepartum, e.g. maternal diabetes, maternal hypertension, maternal haemorrhage, maternal infection, prolonged rupture of membranes.
    - ■ Intrapartum, e.g. prolapsed cord, maternal sedation, abnormal foetal heart tracing, abruptio placenta.
  - » What is the plan for cord management?
- Pre-brief: Identify roles (e.g. team leader, assign some in charge of airway, circulation, documentation, etc.), anticipate problems → Call for help early!

Equipment

- Use a check-list:
  - » Thermoregulation
    - ■ Overhead radiant warmer, warm towels, polyethylene bag for newborns <33 weeks' gestation, woollen cap.
  - » Airway
    - ■ Bulb suction or appropriate size suction catheter, set suction pressure at 80–100 mmHg, meconium aspirator if liquor thickly stained with meconium.
    - ■ Equipment for intubation: Laryngoscope and appropriate size endotracheal tube (ETT) for gestation.

- » Breathing
  - ■ Oxygen source and blender, pulse oximeter
  - ■ Ambu-bag or T-piece (preferred for preterm deliveries)
  - ■ Appropriate size facemasks
- » Circulation
  - ■ ECG leads — if available
  - ■ Drugs: Adrenaline, normal saline
  - ■ Umbilical venous catheter (UVC)

Personnel

- At every birth, there should be one dedicated person who is capable of initial steps & PPV.
- If additional risk factors are present, then a team with advanced skills, including a team leader should be present. The team should do a pre-briefing to go through role assignments during resuscitation and identify the risk factors.

Umbilical Cord Management

Cord clamping may be delayed up to 30–60 seconds for vigorous term or preterm newborns (American Academy of Paediatrics/ILCOR recommendation 2020). However, do follow your hospital guidelines with regard to delayed cord clamping. The vigorous infant can be placed at the level of the introitus or on the mother's abdomen before the cord is clamped.

Airway: Initial Assessment & Stabilisation

Assessment begins immediately after birth and continues throughout the resuscitation process until vital signs have normalised. The neonatal resuscitation algorithm is shown in Figure 17.5.

Assess the newborn immediately after delivery with these four questions:

- Is the infant term?
- Does the baby have a good cry and good breathing effort?
- Is the baby vigorous with good tone?
- Is the liquor clear?

If the answers to the above questions are **Yes**, then the infant may have **routine care** and can stay with the mother. Dry the baby and continue temperature control by putting baby skin to skin with mother. Ensure the baby's airway is open and continue ongoing evaluation of breathing and activity.

Initial Stabilisation

If the answers to the above questions are **No**, then the baby needs to be stabilised, with emphasis on temperature and airway.

- **Dry** → Place baby under the radiant warmer and dry the infant using pre-warmed towels. If it is a premature baby under 33 weeks' gestation, place immediately in a polyethylene bag without drying. Put on a woollen cap as heat loss is maximal from the head. Temperature of baby should be monitored throughout resuscitation.

- **Position** → Open the airway by placing head in a slightly extended position or use a shoulder roll.
- **Stimulate** → If the newborn is not vigorous or does not cry after the above manoeuvers, stimulate by gently flicking the soles of the feet or rubbing the back.
- **Suction** → Only if secretions are present. Suction the mouth followed by the nose if there are secretions. Suction pressure should not exceed 100 mmHg, and depth should not go beyond 5 cm from the level of the lips. Not all babies need suction, and keep in mind that it can cause bradycardia.

If the newborn does not breathe well or cry after initial stabilisation, initiate **bag and mask ventilation** (i.e. breathe for the baby!). PPV **should not be delayed for more than 1 minute** after birth. You should also call for help for more assistance and a pulse oximeter should be placed over the baby's right hand or wrist. An extra person should also be in charge of the documentation of the resuscitation process. Check HR by auscultating the chest. Count number of heart beats in 6 seconds, and times 10 for HR in 1 minute.

Management of Meconium Stained Amniotic Fluid

When meconium is observed in the amniotic fluid, and the newly born infant is depressed, the initial steps should be performed, including suctioning of the oropharynx for meconium. If infant continues to be depressed, start PPV as per guidelines. Intra-tracheal suction should be performed if there is suspected obstruction of airway from meconium, and if personnel capable of intubation are present.

Breathing: Positive Pressure Ventilation

Indications:

- Apnoea or gasping
- HR less than 100/min
- Oxygen saturation below the target range despite free-flow oxygen or continuous positive airway pressure

Rate: Rate of bagging is 40 to 60 breaths per minute.

Oxygen: Start ventilation with room air (21% oxygen) for term and premature babies 33 weeks' gestation and above. For premature babies less than 33 weeks' gestation, start at 21 to 30% oxygen. Refer to the targeted pre-ductal saturation according to age in minutes in Figure 17.5.

Ventilation is the most important and effective step in newborn resuscitation. If done correctly, establishment of adequate ventilation will restore circulation. If you are performing effective ventilation, you should see adequate chest excursion with each inflation and equal air entry. The HR will start to improve (above 100/min), the baby should start to breathe spontaneously, the saturation will improve (look more pink) and tone should also improve.

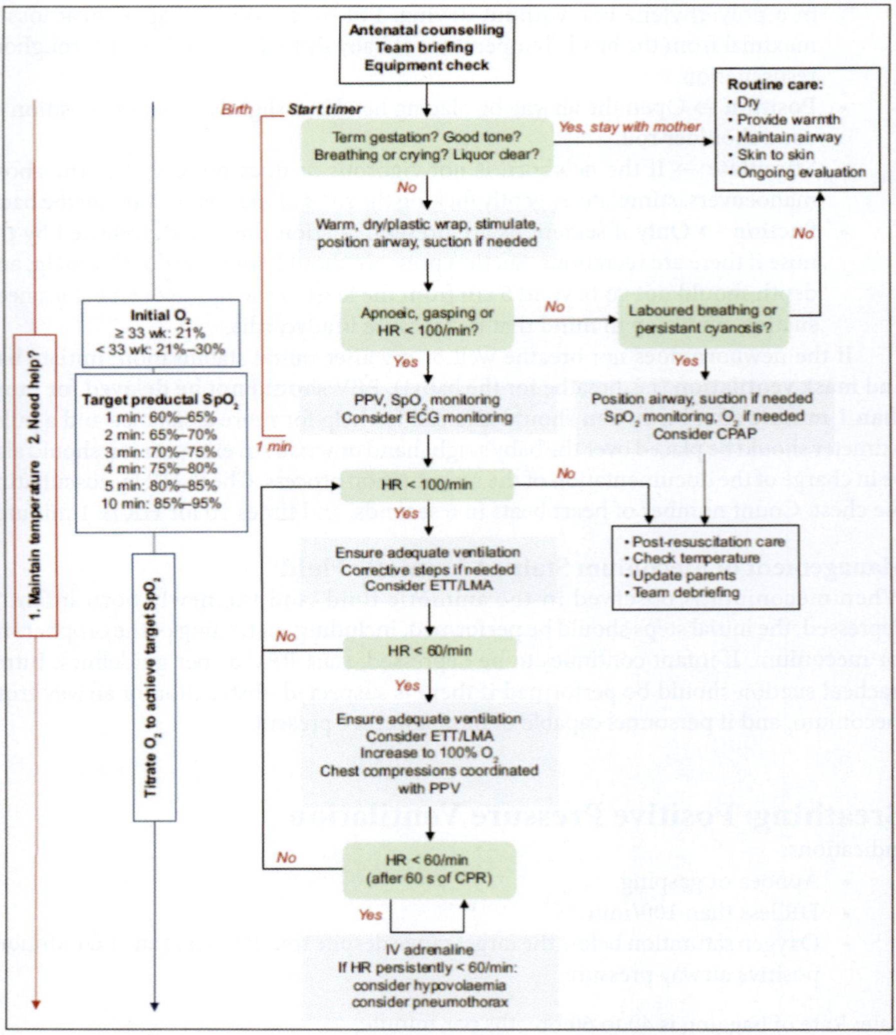

Figure 17.5 Newborn resuscitation algorithm (Chart) — 2021.

CPAP: continuous positive airway pressure; CPR: cardiopulmonary resuscitation; ECG: electrocardiography; ETT: endotracheal tube; HR: heart rate; IV: intravenous; LMA: laryngeal mask airway; O_2: oxygen; PPV: positive pressure ventilation; SpO_2: oxygen saturation

Assessment of response after PPV:

- Check HR after 15 seconds of commencing PPV and assess chest movement (chest rise).
- If chest movement observed, continue PPV for another 15 seconds → total 30 seconds.
- If no chest movement observed → Perform ventilation corrective steps (MR. SOPA – see Table 17.1), then administer PPV for 30 seconds.

Table 17.1 Ventilation Corrective Steps (MR. SOPA)

	Corrective Steps	Actions
M	Mask adjustment	Reapply the mask, consider 2 hand technique
R	Reposition airway	Place head neutral or slightly extended
Try PPV and reassess chest movements		
S	Suction mouth and nose	Use bulb syringe or suction catheter
O	Open mouth	Open the mouth and lift the jaw forward
Try PPV and reassess chest movements		
P	Pressure increase	Increase the pressure in 5–10 cmH_2O increments, maximum 40 cmH_2O
Try PPV and reassess chest movements		
A	Alternative airway	Place an endotracheal tube or laryngeal mask airway
Try PPV and assess chest movement and breath sounds		

Re-assess HR after **30 seconds of PPV with good chest movement**. If HR improves to more than 100/min, check breathing. Stop PPV if continued good HR and sustained good respiratory effort and tone. If still apnoeic, continue PPV until respiratory effort improves. If HR drops to less than 60/min, start chest compression with coordinated PPV.

Chest Compression

Indication: HR less than 60/min after 30 seconds of effective PPV.

The baby should ideally have an advanced airway placed by this time, i.e. ETT or laryngeal mask. If ECG leads are available, it should be placed to allow continuous heart rate monitoring as cardiopulmonary resuscitation is taking place. Always ventilate baby at the same time with oxygen increased to 100%. The frequency should be 3 compressions to 1 ventilation with an aim to deliver 90 to 120 compressions in 1 minute. The 'two thumb' technique (Figure 17.6) is preferred. Both thumbs should meet over the sternum with fingers around the chest wall with the sternum compressed to one-third of the antero-posterior chest dimension.

Assessment of response after chest compression:

- Check HR after 60 seconds of coordinated chest compression with ventilation.
- If HR remains less than 60/min, consider drugs.

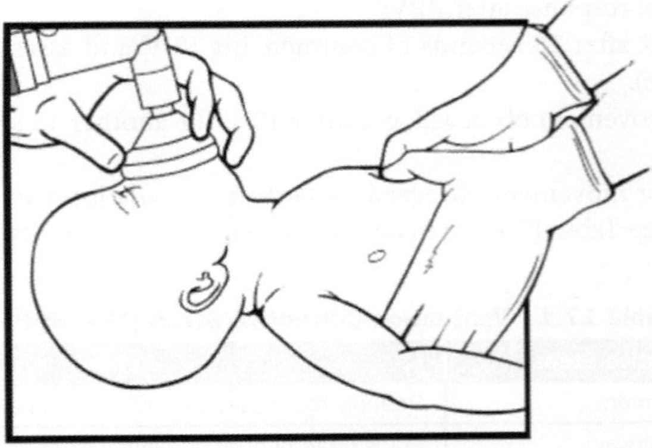

Figure 17.6 'Two-thumb' technique.

Drugs — Medications

- Adrenaline
  - » Indication: HR less than 60/min despite at least 30 seconds of effective PPV followed by 60 seconds of coordination PPV and chest compression
  - » Dose:
    - ▪ Intravenous (preferred route) — 0.1 to 0.3 ml/kg of 1:10000 as rapid bolus. Can be repeated in 3 to 5 minutes.
    - ▪ ETT (less effective) — 0.5 to 1 ml/kg of 1:10000
- Normal saline
  - » Indication: Evidence of volume or blood loss, hypovolaemic shock
  - » Dose: 10 ml/kg over 10 to 20 minutes

Blood can also be considered if evidence of significant blood loss such as maternal abruptio placentae.

UVC should be inserted for intravenous access.

Chest compression can be moved to head of the bed to free up space for UVC insertion

Post Resuscitation Care

- Check temperature
- Secure all tubes — ETT, UVC
- Inform NICU of admission
- Post resuscitation debrief should be done after each resuscitation. It should be a team-centred approach where the team members talk to each other and identify the areas of resuscitation that went well, and what can be improved upon. The team leader's role is to facilitate the discussion, focusing on teamwork and communication.

Conclusion

Effective resuscitation is also dependent on these key behavioural skills:

- Know your environment
- Use available information
- Anticipate and plan
- Clearly identify a team leader
- Communicate effectively
- Delegate workload optimally
- Allocate attention wisely
- Use available resources
- Call for help when needed
- Maintain professional behaviour

Remember:

- Time is life
- Speed is essential
- Be prepared
- Know what you're doing!
- Be cool (Do not panic!!!!!)
- Do not be over-optimistic (Expect the worst and be prepared for it)

Bibliography

1. Biswas A, Ho SKY, Yip WY, *et al.* (2021) Singapore neonatal resuscitation guidelines 2021. *Sing Med J* **62**(8):404–414.
2. Yeo CL, Biswas A, Ee KTT, *et al.* (2017) Singapore neonatal resuscitation guidelines 2016. *Sing Med J* **58**(7):391–403.
3. Wyckoff MH, Wyllie J, Aziz K, *et al.* (2020) Neonatal life support: 2020 international consensus on cardiopulmonary resuscitation and emergency cardiovascular care science with treatment recommendations. *Circulation* **142**(16):S185–S221.
4. Aziz K, Lee CHC, Escobedo MB, *et al.* (2020) Part 5: Neonatal Resuscitation: 2020 American Heart Association Guidelines for Cardiopulmonary Resuscitation and Emergency Cardiovascular Care. *Circulation.* **142**(16 Suppl 2):S524–50.
5. Madar J, Roehr CC, Ainsworth S, *et al.* (2021) European Resuscitation Council Guidelines 2021: Newborn resuscitation and support of transition of infants at birth. *Resuscitation.* **161**:291–326.
6. Perlman JM, Wyllie J, Kattwinkel J, *et al.* (2015) Part 7: Neonatal Resuscitation: 2015 International Consensus on Cardiopulmonary Resuscitation and Emergency Cardiovascular Care Science with Treatment Recommendations. *Circulation.* **132**(16 Suppl 1):S204–41.
7. Wyckoff MH, Aziz K, Escobedo MB, *et al.* (2015) Part 13: Neonatal Resuscitation: 2015 American Heart Association Guidelines Update for Cardiopulmonary Resuscitation and Emergency Cardiovascular Care. *Circulation.* **132**(18 Suppl 2):S543–60.
8. Wyllie J, Perlman JM, Kattwinkel J, *et al.* (2015) Part 7: Neonatal resuscitation: 2015 International Consensus on Cardiopulmonary Resuscitation and Emergency Cardiovascular Care Science with Treatment Recommendations. *Resuscitation.* **95**:e169–201.

CHAPTER 72

Breastfeeding

Chua Mei Chien; Pooja Agarwal Jayagobi; Tong Wing Yee

Benefits

Breast milk is the preferred food for babies. A rich body of scientific evidence supports the advantages of breastfeeding for both mother and baby. Beyond the nutritional benefits and psychological bonding, breastfeeding protects the baby from infections, allergic disorders and reduces the risk of metabolic diseases, such as obesity, type 2 diabetes mellitus and cardiovascular disease. Therefore, it is the professional and moral obligation of healthcare providers to advocate breastfeeding and support the mother and baby in every possible way. Any period of breastfeeding is better than no breastfeeding at all.

The current recommendation is **exclusive breastfeeding** with no supplementary fluids until 6 months of age. Thereafter, appropriate complementary foods are gradually introduced. Baby can be breastfed up to 2 years of age or longer. The following are some of the benefits of breastfeeding:

- Protection against infection
  - » Breast milk contains many anti-infective agents, including secretory IgA, lactoferrin, macrophages and leukocytes, and reduces:
    - ■ Respiratory tract infections
    - ■ Otitis media
    - ■ Viral diseases
    - ■ Diarrhoeal diseases by promoting the growth of healthy and non-pathogenic bacteria in the intestine, preventing *Escherichia coli* from binding with the intestinal mucosa
    - ■ The risk of necrotising enterocolitis (NEC) in premature infants
- Protection against atopy and allergy
  - » Breastfed babies are less likely to develop eczema, asthma and other atopic diseases. Breastfeeding is especially beneficial for babies who are at high risk of developing atopic diseases due to a strong family history of allergy.
  - » Breast milk contains species-specific protein. Complete breastfeeding delays introduction of foreign proteins such as cow's milk protein.
- Nutritional benefits
  - » Breast milk provides adequate nutrition for term babies up to 6 months of age.
  - » The composition of breast milk evolves to reflect the changing nutritional needs as the baby gets older.

- » Breast milk contains many compounds (e.g. omega-3 fatty acids) that are not present in infant formulae.
- » The iron in breast milk is much more easily available to the baby although the quantitative amount is lower compared to the level in cow's milk.
- Other benefits
  - » Breastfeeding does not require special preparation or a clean water supply; it is relatively pathogen-free, economical and comes at a neutral temperature.
  - » Promotes mother — infant bonding.

Characteristics of Human Milk

- Colostrum
  - » Produced in the first few postpartum days.
  - » Yellowish in appearance.
  - » Rich in immunoglobulins, especially secretory IgA and other anti-infective components to boost passive immunity in the baby.
- Transitional milk
  - » Gradually appears several days postpartum.
  - » Increases in volume, caloric content and water-soluble vitamins.
  - » Immunoglobulin components are less than colostrum.
- Mature milk
  - » There is a great biological variation in the characteristics of milk between individuals and even in the same individual at different phases of lactation.
  - » As the baby matures, human milk undergoes considerable variation to keep up with the baby's nutritional needs.
  - » Large part is water, and fat content is most variable.
  - » Caloric density is about 67 calories/100 ml.
  - » Fore milk
    - ▪ Early part of the feeding.
    - ▪ More dilute and contains less fat.
  - » Hind milk
    - ▪ Later part of the feeding.
    - ▪ More concentrated and contains more fat.
    - ▪ As the energy content is higher in the hind milk, it is important to empty the breast completely during feeding.

Stool and Urine Pattern in Breastfed Babies

Breastfed babies have characteristic stool and urine patterns. This helps in the assessment of the adequacy of feeding.

- First 24 hours
  - » Passes meconium 1–2 times
  - » Passes urine once or twice

- 24–48 hours
  - » More meconium, appearance of transitional stool
  - » Passes urine 2–4 times over 24 hours
- 48–72 hours
  - » Transitional stool changing to yellowish breastmilk stool
  - » Urination frequency increases to 3–4 times over 24 hours
- Beyond 72 hours
  - » Frequent loose yellowish stool
  - » Passes urine 6–8 times over 24 hours
  - » Failure to pass adequate amounts of urine and delayed appearance of yellowish mature stools are objective indicators of inadequate feeding

The Baby-Friendly Hospital Initiative (WHO/UNICEF)

The Baby Friendly Hospital Initiative (BFHI) accreditation ensures that exclusive breastfeeding is promoted and protected. An accredited baby-friendly hospital is fully compliant to the 10 steps to successful breastfeeding as well as the international code of marketing of breastmilk substitutes.

Ten Steps to Successful Breastfeeding

- A written breastfeeding policy that is routinely communicated to all healthcare staff.
- Training all healthcare staff in skills necessary to implement this policy.
- Antenatal education to inform all pregnant women about the benefits and management of breastfeeding.
- Achieving skin-to-skin contact between mother and baby within 5 minutes of birth for at least 1 hour for both vaginal births and caesarean births without general anaesthesia (GA). Skin to skin can be performed for births after GA once the mother is alert.
- Showing mothers how to breastfeed with proper latching and positioning and how to maintain lactation, even if they should be separated from their infants.
- Giving newborn infants no food or drink other than breast milk unless medically indicated. Supplemental feeding if indicated for medical reasons should be given by cup or spoon feeding to avoid nipple confusion.
- Practising rooming-in to allow mothers and infants to remain together 24 hours a day. Medical examination and procedures should be done by the bedside whenever possible.
- Encouraging breastfeeding on demand with no restriction on the frequency and duration of feeding. Early and frequent feeding of at least 8 to 12 times a day helps establish mother's milk supply, promotes clearance of meconium, reduces incidence of jaundice and minimises breast engorgement.
- Giving no artificial teats or pacifiers to breastfeeding infants.
- Ensuring mothers have access to community breastfeeding support groups and other breastfeeding resources on discharge from the hospital or clinic.

International Code of Marketing of Breastmilk Substitutes

Full compliance with the International Code of Marketing of Breastmilk Substitutes is also vital in the protection of exclusive breastfeeding. The hospital and healthcare providers are not to solicit or accept sponsorships or gifts from companies producing or marketing breastmilk substitutes.

Monitoring the Adequacy of Feeding

The mother-and-baby dyad should be monitored closely and frequently in the first week to assess adequacy of feeding and to allow the identification and correction of breastfeeding difficulties. An adequately breastfed baby has the following characteristics:

- Good suck and swallow pattern
- Frequent feeding at least 8–12 times a day
- Normal frequency of urine and stools — See 'Stool and Urine Pattern in Breastfed Babies'
- Acceptable weight loss (<7% by Day 3 of life)
- Full-term breastfed babies most often regain birth weight by 10–14 days; a weight loss of >7% of the birth weight during the first week calls for a comprehensive review of the mother-and-baby dyad.

Contraindications to Breastfeeding

A positive hepatitis B serology and Venereal Disease Research Laboratory (VDRL) test are NOT contraindications to breastfeeding.

There are very few contraindications to breastfeeding:

- Galactosaemia in the baby
- Maternal psychosis
- Maternal active tuberculosis
- Maternal human immunodeficiency virus (HIV)
- Maternal herpes with active lesion on the breast
- Maternal chemotherapy or radiotherapy for cancer treatment
- Selected medication: Radioactive iodine, anti-malaria drugs

Some drugs have no data on breastfeeding safety and alternatives should be offered whenever available.

Pasteurised Donor Human Milk

When the mother's own milk is inadequate, contraindicated or not available, pasteurised donor human milk (PDHM) is the recommended alternative. PDHM can be provided to eligible infants who are hospitalised or at home.

Current eligibility criteria for referral to our centre's Human Milk Bank are as below:

- Infants with significant illness:
  - » Preterm infants <35 weeks
  - » Infants <1.8 kg

  - » Ex-prems with co-morbidities (e.g. chronic lung disease, necrotising enterocolitis, retinopathy of prematurity)
  - » Congenital heart disease
  - » Gastrointestinal disease
  - » Other medical conditions (e.g. encephalopathy)
- Infants in whom their own mother's milk is contraindicated due to:
  - » Medical conditions (e.g. HIV)
  - » Medical treatment (e.g. chemotherapy)
  - » Significant mental illness
  - » Drug misuse
- Infants in whom their own mother's milk is unavailable:
  - » Adopted infants
  - » Infants whose mothers are deceased
- Other compassionate reasons

Indications for Referral to Lactation Consultants

Lactation consultants are professionally qualified nurses or healthcare professionals who are invaluable in supporting breastfeeding in both hospital and community settings. In Singapore, most hospitals provide lactation support services. These are some general indications for referral to lactation consultants:

- Decreased or insufficient milk supply
- Difficulty in latching-on
- Difficulty with milk expression
- Breast problems: Engorgement, sore nipple, nipple confusion, short or inverted nipples
- High-risk infants: Premature, very-low-birth-weight babies
- Returning to work
- Maternal anxiety

Bibliography

1. ESPGHAN Committee on Nutrition, Agostoni C, Braegger C, *et al.* (2009) Breast-feeding: A commentary by the ESPGHAN Committee on Nutrition. *J Pediatr Gastroenterol Nutr* **49**(1):112–125.
2. Kramer MS, Kamura R. (2012) Optimal duration of exclusive breastfeeding. *Cochrane Database Syst Rev* **2012**(8):CD003517.
3. Section on Breastfeeding. (2012) Breastfeeding and the use of human milk. *Pediatrics* **129**(3):e824–841.
4. Duijts L, Jaddoe VW, Hofman A, Moll HA. (2010) Prolonged and exclusive breastfeeding reduces the risk of infectious diseases in infancy. *Pediatrics* **126**(1):e18–e25.
5. Quigley MA, Kelly YJ, Sacker A. (2007) Breastfeeding and hospitalization for diarrheal and respiratory infection in the United Kingdom Millennium Cohort Study. *Pediatrics* **119**(4):e837–e842.
6. Maffei D, Schanler RJ. (2017) Human milk is the feeding strategy to prevent necrotising enterocolitis! *Semin Perinatol* **41**(1):36–40.
7. Greer FR, Sicherer SH, Burks AW; Committee on Nutrition; Section on Allergy and Immunology. (2019) The effects of early nutritional interventions on the development of atopic disease in infants and children: The role of maternal dietary restriction, breastfeeding, hydrolysed formulas, and timing of introduction of allergenic complementary food. *Pediatrics* **143**(4):e20190281.

8. Martin CR, Ling PR, Blackburn GL. (2016) Review of infant feeding: Key features of breast milk and infant formula. *Nutrients* **8**(5):279.
9. Andreas NJ, Kampmann B, Mehring Le-Doare K. (2015) Human breast milk: A review on its composition and bioactivity. *Early Hum Dev* **91**(11):629–635.
10. UNICEF. (nd) Baby-friendly hospital initiative. https://www.unicef.org/documents/baby-friendly-hospital-initiative

CHAPTER 73

Neonatal Dermatoses

Odattil Geetha; Koh Jean Aan, Mark

Erythema Toxicum

- Very common
- Appears within the first 48–72 hours of life
- Presents as scattered blotchy erythematous macules and papules, occasionally with small pustules
- Mostly occurs on face, trunk and upper extremities
- Baby is generally well
- No specific treatment is necessary, self resolves in a few days or a week

Milia

- Presents as single or multiple small, white papules
- Most commonly appears on the forehead and face, especially the nose bridge
- Ruptures and disappears after few weeks but may take a few months
- No specific treatment is necessary apart from routine cleanliness

Mottling (Cutis Marmorata)

- Scattered areas of erythema with pale areas in-between
- Common following exposure to cold; becoming less obvious with warming
- If baby is unwell, need to exclude pathological associations, e.g. hypothermia, poor perfusion, shock, sepsis, central nervous system disturbances and hypothyroidism

Transient Neonatal Pustular Melanosis

- More common in dark-skinned babies
- Maybe present at birth and last for 4–5 days
- Heterogeneous with pustules and vesicles and areas of dark macules
- Baby is clinically well
- No specific treatment is necessary
- May be confused with neonatal herpes and bacterial infection

Sucking Blister

- Believed to be due to vigorous sucking of the baby either in-utero or immediately after birth
- Presents in the accessible areas such as hand, forearm and lips but may also occur on foot
- Baby is well
- Should not be confused with neonatal herpes, bullous impetigo and epidermolysis bullosa

Acne Neonatorum

- Appears in the first 2–4 weeks of life
- Appears as skin-coloured to pinkish, monomorphic papules, mostly on forehead and face
- Often appears together with features of seborrheic dermatitis
- Most undergo resolution without treatment
- Advise against heavy application of emollients
- Anti-fungal shampoos (e.g. ketoconazole), mild topical corticosteroids with or without topical anti-fungal (e.g. desonide lotion or miconazole/hydrocortisone combination), and a light moisturiser may be used for treatment

Infantile Haemangioma

- Most common vascular tumour in infants and children
- Most common over the head and neck region, they can also affect other sites
- Not present at birth, they appear in the first few weeks of life and undergo a proliferative growth phase in the first 5–6 months of life, followed by a slow growth phase until about 1 year of age
- Will regress or involute thereafter but the rate will depend on the size of the haemangioma
- Regression may result in telangiectasias, skin atrophy or fibrofatty change
- Some large, segmental haemangiomas may be associated with syndromes and abnormalities in other organs:
  - » Facial segmental haemangiomas (PHACE syndrome — Posterior fossa abnormalities, Haemangiomas, Arterial abnormalities, Cardiac abnormalities and Eye abnormalities)
  - » Perineum segmental haemangiomas (PELVIS syndrome — Perineal haemangioma, External genital malformations, Lipomyelomeningocele, Vesicorenal abnormalities, Imperforate anus and Skin tag)
  - » If there are five or more discreet haemangiomas, there is a risk for visceral haemangioma, especially hepatic haemangioma
- Referral to paediatric dermatologists for treatment must be considered in the following circumstances:

  - 'Beard area' and neck haemangiomas — possible airway involvement
  - Periorbital haemangiomas — possible ocular axis occlusion, amblyopia, astigmatism
  - Lip, peri-oral, ear, anogenital and intertriginous region — risk of ulceration
  - Nasal tip haemangiomas
  - Large, segmental haemangiomas of the face and neck — risk of PHACE
  - Large lumbosacral, anogenital haemangiomas — risk of PELVIS
  - Multiple lesions with possible visceral involvement
- Treatment
  - Small, clinically non-significant haemangiomas may be observed for self-involution
  - Topical timolol may be used for small, superficial haemangiomas
  - Oral propranolol may be considered for larger, complicated haemangiomas
  - Other forms of treatment include pulsed dye laser and systemic corticosteroids

Capillary Malformations

- Malformed dilated capillaries in the skin
- Appear as blotches of red or purple skin discolouration on any part of the body
- Always present at birth, although they may become more obvious with time
- Two common capillary vascular malformations:
  - Naevus flammeus (salmon patch, stork bites)
    - Patchy light-red area
    - Common on forehead, eyebrow and nape of neck
    - Blanches on pressure
    - More intense in colour and noticeable when baby is crying
    - Most lesions on the forehead will spontaneously disappear within the first years of life
    - Nape lesions may be permanent
    - Most do not require treatment
  - Port-wine stain
    - Intensely red to reddish-purplish macule
    - Commonly unilateral in distribution
    - If present on forehead or upper eyelids, it can be associated with the Sturge–Weber syndrome.

Mongolian Blue Spot

- Extremely common (up to 75% in Asian babies)
- Large irregular areas of bluish or purplish-blue discolouration
- Mostly on buttock or on the back
- Many disappear in toddler years; some may persist
- No treatment is necessary

Diaper Dermatitis

- Very common, especially after a few months of life
- May be caused by several factors, including irritation from urine and faeces, tight diaper bands, yeast/candida infection and bacterial infection
- Presents with erythema, scaling, fissuring and erosions if severe
- If satellite papules are present, consider secondary candida infection
- If lesions are oozy with pus discharge, consider secondary bacterial infection
- Treatment is with frequent diaper changes, topical moisturisers (e.g. white soft paraffin) and mild topical corticosteroids (e.g. desonide cream) or a combination of corticosteroid and anti-fungal agent (e.g. hydrocortisone/miconazole cream). A course of oral antibiotics may be necessary if evidence of secondary bacterial infection.

Bibliography

1. Paller A, Mancini A. (2020) Hurwitz Clinical pediatric dermatology: A textbook of skin disorders of childhood and adolescence. In: *Cutaneous Disorders of the Newborn, 6th ed.*, Chap. 2. Elsevier Health, pp. 10–36.
2. Schachner LA, Hansen RC. (2011) Pediatric dermatology. In: *Neonatal Skin and Skin Disorders, 4th ed.*, Vol. 1., Chap. 6. Elsevier Health, pp. 299–373.

CHAPTER 74

Birth Trauma

Tan Pih Lin

Risk Factors for Birth Trauma

- **Maternal factors**
  - » Primiparous
  - » Older multipara
  - » Small malformed pelvis
- **Obstetric factors**
  - » Breech position
  - » Precipitous delivery
  - » Abnormal presentation (transverse, face, brow)
  - » Instrumental delivery (forceps or vacuum extraction)
  - » Shoulder dystocia
- **Foetal factors**
  - » Macrosomia
  - » Prematurity

Caput Succedaneum

This is a diffuse swelling of the scalp, resulting from an impairment of venous return due to prolonged delivery. Underlying collection is tissue fluid. It crosses the suture lines and is more pronounced at the time of delivery; the swelling can be indented. This undergoes natural resolution within 1–2 days and no active management is necessary.

Cephalohaematoma

This results from the rupture of blood vessels from the skull to the periosteum. The swelling does not cross the suture line as the blood collects in the sub-periosteum. It may be less noticeable at birth and progressively becomes enlarged as the blood continues to collect. A linear skull fracture may be present. With time, it becomes calcified and forms a distinct bony swelling.

Sub-Galeal Bleed

This results from the rupture of veins between the scalp and dural sinuses. It occurs more commonly with vacuum-assisted deliveries and is a rare but potentially severe form of bleeding in a newborn. Early recognition and management is crucial as it can lead to massive blood loss. The bleeding is diffuse over the scalp and fluctuant in nature. It tends to move towards the dependent side. Observe and monitor in special care nursery/neonatal intensive care unit.

Both cephalohaematoma and sub-galeal bleed can aggravate neonatal jaundice.

Clavicular Fracture

This is more common in a macrosomic baby with shoulder dystocia. Occasionally a 'snap' is heard during delivery. The features include asymmetric Moro reflex and restricted upper extremity movement on the affected side. The fracture may be detected on palpation.

Erb's Palsy

This results from excessive traction of the neck during delivery. The severity varies from mild praxia with spontaneous recovery to more severe permanent damage. This is due to injury to the brachial plexus involving the cervical fifth and sixth nerves. This results in an inability to abduct the extremity at the shoulder, externally rotate the arm and supination. The infant holds the arm in adduction and internal rotation.

Klumpke's Paralysis

This is a more severe form of brachial plexus injury. The nerves involved are the cervical seventh and eighth and first thoracic nerves. It commonly causes paralysis of the hand and may be associated with an ipsilateral Horner's syndrome.

The treatment of Erb's and Klumpke's paralyses is neuro-rehabilitation with an active and passive range-of-motion exercises.

Facial Nerve Palsy

This is usually a peripheral nerve injury due to the compression of the facial nerve between the facial bone and mother's pelvis or obstetric forceps at the time of delivery. The face is asymmetrical with a deviation of the unaffected side during crying, absence of naso-labial fold on the affected side. The infant may not be able to close the eyelid of the affected side and proper eye care is necessary to prevent drying of conjunctiva.

Bibliography

1. Rosenberg A. (2003) Traumatic birth injury. *Neoreviews* **4**(10):e270–e276.
2. Akangire G, Carter B. (2016) Birth injuries in neonates. *Pediatr Rev* **37**(11):451–462.

CHAPTER 75

Neonatal Jaundice

Abdul Haium Abdul Alim

Introduction

Jaundice is the yellowish discolouration of the skin, sclera, and mucous membranes. It occurs due to elevated levels of bilirubin in the blood (hyperbilirubinaemia). It is one of the most common medical conditions affecting newborn infants.

Approximately 60% of neonates born at term and 85% of preterm neonates will develop neonatal jaundice (NNJ). Most of these neonates will develop 'physiological jaundice', which is usually benign. However, when unconjugated serum bilirubin (SB) level is too high, it could cause irreversible brain injury or hearing impairment. It is important, therefore, to identify those neonates at risk of severe neonatal hyperbilirubinaemia and treat them early to prevent the occurrence of acute bilirubin encephalopathy and kernicterus.

The following guidelines are applicable to inpatient management of NNJ in our institution.

Assessment

- All newborn infants should be examined for jaundice at every opportunity in the first 72 hours of life.
- Visual inspection of baby for jaundice should be done preferably in natural light.
- Visual inspection alone should not be relied upon to estimate the severity of jaundice, and all babies with clinically suspected jaundice in the first two weeks of life should have a transcutaneous or SB measurement to estimate the severity of jaundice.
- Neonates with any of the high-risk factors, who are likely to develop severe hyperbilirubinaemia, should be identified early and monitored more closely for NNJ.

Risk Stratification

All newborn infants in the first two weeks of life, who are at risk of NNJ, should be risk stratified for the purpose of management. The high-risk group is more prone to develop severe hyperbilirubinaemia and is at a higher risk for bilirubin-induced neurologic dysfunction.

Table 17.2 Risk Stratification for Neonatal Jaundice

Normal Risk	High Risk for Severe Hyperbilirubinaemia
Any baby who is not in the 'high-risk' category^	1. Visible jaundice within 24 hr of age 2. G6PD deficiency and other haemolytic conditions 3. ABO incompatibility* *defined as Mother Blood Group O, Baby Blood Group A/B, and DCT positive OR Maternal "Anti-A" or "Anti-B" IgG antibody titres ≥128* 4. Rhesus incompatibility 5. Rapidly rising serum bilirubin (>103 μmol/L per day) 6. Late preterm (35–36 wk gestation) 7. Asphyxia (Apgar ≤5 at 1 and 5 min) 8. Family history of severe NNJ in siblings needing exchange transfusion 9. Inadequate breast feeding plus weight loss ≥10% 10. Infants with birth weight of 2000–2500 g * *NB: If the mother's group and antibody titres unknown, manage the baby as 'high-risk' until the results are available*
^The following group of infants in the second week of life (8–14 days of age) could be considered as normal risk. 1. Mother's group and antibody titres still unknown 2. Exclusive breast feeding who had an initial weight loss of ≥10%, which improved and regained birth weight	

Estimation of Bilirubin Levels

- SB measurement is the gold standard for the diagnosis and monitoring of NNJ.
- Transcutaneous bilirubin (TcB) measurements can be used as a screening tool to measure jaundice levels in babies with gestational age of ≥35 weeks and birth weight ≥2 kg.
- Any TcB measurement that are close to phototherapy thresholds needs to be confirmed by SB measurement.

Transcutaneous Bilirubin Action Levels

TcB action levels refer to the TcB level above which babies with NNJ should be subjected to SB confirmation or the TcB level below, which babies can be safely discharged without immediate risk.

The following table could be used as a guide for action levels above which the SB test should be performed for 'normal risk' and 'high risk' babies, respectively.

Serum Bilirubin Measurements

- SB measurement remains the 'gold standard' for jaundice treatment decisions.
- SB should be tested if:

Table 17.3 Transcutaneous Bilirubin Action Levels to Perform SB Measurement (µmol/L)

Normal Risk Infants		High Risk Infants	
Age	**TcB Value**	**Age**	**TcB Value**
0–12 hr		0–12 hr	80
13–24 hr		13–24 hr	120
25–36 hr	160	25–36 hr	140
37–48 hr	180	37–48 hr	160
49–72 hr	200	49–72 hr	180
73–96 hr	220	73–96 hr	200
97–120 hr	220	97–120 hr	200
121 hr–7 d	240	121 hr–7 d	220
8–14 d	≥250	8–14 d	240

» TcB is not available.
» The result of TcB value exceeds the action level to perform SB level
» If the neonate is:
  - Unwell
  - <35 weeks' gestation at birth
  - Clinically appearing jaundiced in less than 24 hours of age
  - Undergoing phototherapy or has undergone phototherapy in last 24 hours (there is insufficient evidence to recommend the use of TcB during or immediately after phototherapy)
» Both venous and capillary SB results should be considered equivalent measures.
» Total SB should be used to determine appropriate treatment rather than the unconjugated fraction of bilirubin for the purpose of NNJ management.

Investigation

In a neonate with significant hyperbilirubinaemia requiring phototherapy or exchange transfusion, the following investigations may be considered to exclude haemolytic disease of the newborn. Additional investigations such as sepsis work-up, renal function or liver function tests could be carried out depending on the clinical presentation.

- Full blood count, including blood film report and reticulocyte count
- Blood group, rhesus type and direct Coomb's test of the baby ('NNJ profile' for baby)
- Blood group, rhesus type and abnormal antibodies of the mother ('NNJ profile' for mother)
- SB, if > 4 hours have elapsed since the last bilirubin determination

Treatment

Phototherapy is a safe, effective, non-invasive and inexpensive method to remove bilirubin from body. Phototherapy involves the exposure of as much of the baby's skin as possible to blue fluorescent lights, which emit wavelengths in the 430–490 nm range.

- Phototherapy decreases the bilirubin level by enhancing the conversion of bilirubin in the exposed skin to a more easily excreted form.
- Increasing the amount of skin exposure to blue lights can enhance bilirubin excretion.
- Use eye covers to prevent damage to the baby's eyes.

Single Blue Phototherapy

- The exposure of one plane of body surface (e.g. either the baby's front or back) to the phototherapy light. Regularly turning the baby helps to maximise the exposure of all surfaces.
- Once started on single blue phototherapy, it is advisable to continue phototherapy at least for 24 hours to maximise efficacy and prevent rebound jaundice.
- Recheck SB level 12–24 hours after starting phototherapy depending on clinical status.

Double Blue Phototherapy

- The simultaneous exposure of two body surface planes to two separate sets of blue lights, i.e. both front and back.
- Recommended if the SB level is above the double blue phototherapy criteria or if the rate of rise of SB is >5 μmol/L/hr despite *being* on single phototherapy.
- Recheck SB level 6–12 hours after starting double phototherapy depending on clinical status.

Intense Phototherapy

- Involves the use of four lights to achieve higher irradiance/light intensity. This maximises exposure of all body surfaces in four planes (front, back, right and left sides).
- Start intense blue phototherapy when SB levels are close to (e.g. within 25 μmol/L) exchange levels or above the exchange level and while exchange transfusion is being arranged.
- Recheck SB level 4–6 hours after starting intense phototherapy depending on clinical status of neonates.

Criteria for Phototherapy

- There are two sets of phototherapy criteria, each tailored to a specific group of babies:
  - » Babies born at <35 weeks' gestation and/or with birth weight <2 kg
  - » Babies born at ≥35 weeks' gestation and with birth weight ≥2 kg (fall under the National NNJ guidelines)

Infants Born <35 Weeks' Gestation and/or with Birth Weight <2 kg

For babies born at less than 35 weeks' gestation or with birth weight less than 2 kg (who do not fall under the standard criteria), the phototherapy guidelines in the Table 17.4 are used.

For this group, abnormal criteria are applied if:

- Jaundice is observed within 24 hours of age
- Blood group incompatibility with positive direct Coomb's test, or antibody titre ≥128
- G6PD deficiency
- Perinatal asphyxia
- Sepsis
- Significant cephalohaematoma or bruising

Double blue lights are used when the SB is <35 μmol/L below the exchange level or the rate of rise of SB is >5 μmol/L/h.

Phototherapy could be stopped if the SB level is 35 μmol/L below the phototherapy start level.

Table 17.4 Phototherapy Guidelines for Infants Born <35 Weeks' Gestation and/or with Birth Weight <2 kg

Birth Weight (g)	Photo Level (μmol/L)		Exchange Level (μmol/L)	
	Normal	Abnormal	Normal	Abnormal
<1250	150	120	220	190
1250–1499	170	140	250	220
1500–1999	200	170	310	270
2000–2499	220	190	340	300
≥2500	260	230	400	340

Infants Born ≥35 Weeks' Gestation and with Birth Weight ≥2 kg

For babies born at ≥35 weeks' gestation or with birth weight ≥2 kg, the phototherapy guidelines in the Tables 17.5 and 17.6 are used.

Monitoring While on Phototherapy

- Ensure adequate feeding and hydration. Add 10–20 ml/kg/day extra feed volume, if tolerated. Monitor vital signs closely.
- Change position of baby frequently to expose different skin area for phototherapy.
- Ensure eyes are covered to prevent glaring and discomfort.

Discontinuation of Phototherapy

- Once the 'off phototherapy' level has been reached.
- There is no need to routinely test for rebound jaundice, unless there are clinical indications.
- The baby can be discharged immediately after discontinuation of phototherapy if it remains clinically well.

Table 17.5 Phototherapy and Exchange Transfusion Thresholds — Infants Born ≥35 Weeks' Gestation and Birth Weight ≥2 kg — Normal Risk

Age	Stop Phototherapy	Single Blue Phototherapy	Double Blue Phototherapy	Intense Blue Phototherapy	Exchange Transfusion
0–12 hr	Please See — Serum Bilirubin Levels in "High Risk Infants" Criteria				
13–24 hr					
25–36 hr	160	200	250	275	300
37–48 hr	185	225	300	325	350
49–72 hr	210	250	300	325	350
73–96 hr	235	275	325	350	375
97–120 hr	235	275	350	375	400
121 hr–7 d	260	300	350	375	400
8–14 d	285	325	375	400	425

Table 17.6 Phototherapy and Exchange Transfusion Thresholds — Infants Born ≥35 Weeks' Gestation and Birth Weight ≥2 kg — High Risk

Age	Stop Phototherapy	Single Blue Phototherapy	Double Blue Phototherapy	Intense Blue Phototherapy	Exchange Transfusion
0–12 hr		100	150	175	200
13–24 hr		150	200	225	250
25–36 hr	135	175	225	250	275
37–48 hr	160	200	250	275	300
49–72 hr	185	225	275	300	325
73–96 hr	210	250	300	325	350
97–120 hr	210	250	300	325	350
121 hr–7 d	235	275	325	350	375
8–14 d	260	300	325	350	375

Use of Intravenous Immunoglobulin

- Systematic review of the use of high dose intravenous immunoglobulin (IVIG) has shown to significantly reduce the need for exchange transfusions.
- It is recommended to consider IVIG infusion (at a dose of 500 mg/kg, slow infusion) as an adjunct to intense blue phototherapy in babies with iso-immunisation from Rhesus or ABO haemolytic disease, where the SB level continues to rise by more than 8.5 μmol/L/h despite the child on phototherapy and adequate hydration.
- The suggested rate of IVIG infusion is:
  - » 0.5 ml/kg/h × 15 min followed by
  - » 1 ml/kg/h × 15 min followed by
  - » 2 ml/kg/h × 15 min followed by
  - » 3 ml/kg/h × 15 min followed by
  - » 4 ml/kg/h until end of infusion

Exchange Transfusion

- Exchange transfusion should be considered if:
  - » SB level reaches the threshold for an exchange transfusion and is not decreasing after hydration and intensive phototherapy for 4–6 hours.
  - » Associated significant neonatal anaemia from haemolysis.
  - » SB levels above the exchange transfusion threshold and clinical signs of encephalopathy. In such infants, intense phototherapy should be commenced urgently, and exchange transfusion should be initiated immediately.
  - » SB level reaches the threshold for an exchange transfusion and there are factors that disrupt the blood brain barrier, e.g. acidosis, asphyxia, sepsis, hypo-albuminemia, hypothermia or prematurity.
- Exchange transfusion needs to be considered as an urgent treatment:
  - » In babies with high levels of bilirubin and who demonstrate any of the clinical features of acute bilirubin encephalopathy.
  - » If SB level is >85 μmol/L above the exchange transfusion threshold. Meanwhile hydrate and start the baby on intensive phototherapy.

Other Considerations

- Feeding
  - » Feeding can be continued; nil by mouth if the baby needs exchange transfusion.
  - » Increase feeds by at least 10% over the usual expected intake.
  - » Continue breastfeeding.
  - » If not near or at the exchange transfusion level, the baby can be taken off the lights for up to 30 minutes to breastfed.
- Parental and caretaker education
  - » Prior to discharging the baby, emphasise the importance of early follow-up:
    - ▪ Especially important for babies discharged before age 48 hours
    - ▪ Emphasise the risks and manifestations of acute bilirubin encephalopathy and its consequences
  - » Breastfed babies:
    - ▪ Give thorough breastfeeding advice
    - ▪ Teach mothers and caregivers the signs of dehydration
  - » Borderline premature babies (35–36 weeks' gestation):
    - ▪ A vulnerable group
    - ▪ Tend to be discharged from hospital as early as full-term well babies because of their larger physical size and apparent maturity
    - ▪ At higher risk of developing jaundice, requiring phototherapy
    - ▪ Advice to parents of this particular group must be particularly instructive

Bibliography

1. American Academy of Pediatrics Subcommittee on Hyperbilirubinemia. (2004) Management of hyperbilirubinemia in the newborn infant 35 or more weeks of gestation. *Pediatrics* **114**(1):297–316.
2. National Institutes for Health and Care Excellence. (2016) Jaundice in Newborn Babies under 28 days. Clinical Guidance (CG98). https://www.nice.org.uk/guidance/cg98/chapter/Recommendations
3. Academy of Medicine and College of Pediatrics and Child Health, Singapore. (2018) Guidelines on evaluation and management of neonatal jaundice.
4. Liu H, Liu W, Tang X, Wang T. (2015) Association between G6PD deficiency and hyperbilirubinemia in neonates: A meta-analysis. *Pediatr Hematol Oncol* **32**(2):92–98.

CHAPTER 76

Respiratory Distress

Kong Juin Yee

Respiratory distress in babies can manifest as many signs/symptoms, including nasal flaring, grunting, tachypnoea, chest wall retractions, tachycardia, cyanosis/desaturations, stridor, carbon dioxide (CO_2) retention, irritability and apnoea (usually the last sign).

General Management Principles

- Overall care: Keep baby in a thermoneutral environment (nurse in an incubator or under a radiant warmer set to maintain skin temperature at 36.5°C by using servo control). Minimise disturbances and handling by grouping together blood sampling and procedures. Any disturbance of a sick baby may cause apnoea, bradycardia and desaturations. Babies who are intubated or on continuous positive airway pressure (CPAP) might sometimes need sedation (morphine drip or chloral hydrate), though this should be used judiciously in the preterm population due to side effects like hypotension and respiratory depression.
- Ongoing monitoring: Continuous monitoring of heart rate, respiratory rate, oxygen saturation (SpO_2) and temperature (servo probe on baby's skin) would be needed. Blood pressure (BP) can be measured non-invasively with an oscillometric BP cuff (may over-read) or with an intra-arterial line (more reliable and continuous). Blood gas (arterial preferred, via peripheral arterial line or umbilical arterial catheter) should be monitored every 4–6 hours, or even more frequently during the acute stage of respiratory illness. When ventilator parameters are changed, follow-up blood gas should be done 30–60 minutes after change. Calculation of the oxygenation index and alveolar-arterial oxygen gradient ($AaDO_2$) should be done with every blood gas when the infant's respiratory illness is severe.
- Investigations: Investigate for cause of respiratory distress (Chest X-ray [CXR]), infection markers, e.g. full blood count, C-reactive protein, blood cultures, blood glucose, nasopharyngeal aspirate for respiratory viruses and cranial ultrasound). Repeat CXR should be considered if any acute or gradual worsening of respiratory status or escalation of ventilator support. If there is a change in nature of secretions, consider sending endotracheal aspirates for gram stain and culture though this should be interpreted with caution as positive results may indicate colonisation as opposed to true infection.

- Treatment: Different modes of ventilatory support can be used depending on the underlying cause for respiratory distress as well as the degree of support needed. Oxygen should be humidified and blended to keep target saturation ranges (term versus preterm) in order to prevent side effects from hyperoxia or hypoxaemia. Treat the underlying causes, for example: surfactant (respiratory distress syndrome [RDS]), antibiotics (infection), caffeine (apnoea of prematurity) while supporting the baby's respiratory status.

Oxygen Delivery

Oxygen is a drug. It should be given judiciously just enough to maintain targeted SpO_2 (88–95% for preterm, and 93–98% for term) with partial pressure of oxygen (PaO_2) of 40–60 mmHg generally. Targeted SpO_2 and PaO_2 might differ depending on clinical conditions, e.g. babies with persistent pulmonary hypertension of newborn (PPHN) might need higher targets, as opposed to babies with cyanotic heart disease, whom lower targets are acceptable. Hence, oxygen blending should be used at all times if available to avoid hyperoxia-related complications.

Oxygen can be delivered to infants without positive pressure via:

- Hood box: Infant's head is placed in a hood infused with humidified oxygen (titrated to desired concentrations with an oxygen concentration analyser placed near the infant to accurately measure the fraction of inspired oxygen (FiO_2) received by the baby)
- Nasal cannula (NC): Usually used in infants with chronic lung disease when they fail to maintain target SpO_2 after depronging from CPAP. High flow NC (with flow 2–6 L per min [LPM]) and low flow NC (with flow 0.5–2 LPM) can be used depending on the need for support. FiO_2 0.21–1.00 should be titrated to aim for SpO_2 within the target range. Some babies with significant chronic lung disease can be discharged home on NC oxygen under home care arrangement using a home oxygen concentrator and SpO_2 monitoring.

Continuous Positive Airway Pressure

In CPAP, a continuous flow (usually 6 LPM) of heated and humidified air (with or without oxygen) is circulated past the infant's airway at a set pressure (usually 5–6 cmH_2O) while the infant breathes spontaneously. FiO_2 and positive end expiratory pressure (PEEP) can be adjusted to keep target SpO_2 range and to provide support for infant's respiratory distress, respectively. It is usually delivered by nasal prongs either via the ventilator circuit or bubble (under water) CPAP system. An orogastric tube should be placed, as CPAP can cause gastric distension interference with lung inflation by pushing up the diaphragm.

CPAP might be contraindicated in babies with gastrointestinal anomalies (mostly obstruction, congenital diaphragmatic hernia), necrotising enterocolitis or immediate post gastrointestinal-related surgical repair. It sometimes causes agitation/excessive crying, especially near term or term babies, hence mild sedation (e.g. chloral hydrate) can be considered to prevent complications like pneumothorax.

Indications

- Disease with low functional residual capacity or poor compliance: RDS, transient tachypnoea of a newborn, pulmonary oedema due to patent ductus arteriosus (PDA)
- Recurrent apnoea: CPAP may reduce or terminate attacks in preterm babies with apnoea of prematurity
- Upper airway or airway closure disease: Obstructive airway (e.g. Pierre Robin syndrome), obstructive sleep apnoea, bronchopulmonary dysplasia, bronchiolitis, tracheomalacia
- As a weaning mode from the mechanical ventilator

Failure of CPAP and Indications for Mechanical Ventilation

- FiO_2 >0.3–0.4 (depending on gestational age and underlying lung disease) when on PEEP 5–6 cmH_2O
- Partial pressure of CO_2 ($PaCO_2$) >65 mmHg on arterial blood gas
- Marked retractions
- Frequent apnoea and bradycardia
- Intractable metabolic acidosis
- Cardiovascular instability or collapse
- Decreased respiratory effort (neuromuscular disease, deep sedation and paralysis)

Trouble shooting before intubation: Exclude errors in blood gas sampling, machine malfunction, improper CPAP application or pressures not achieved (may try chin strap or proper fit of prongs), and nasal obstruction by secretions or water in the tubing. Nasal intermittent mandatory ventilation (NIMV) mode can be considered prior to intubation; however, this might not be appropriate depending on the baby's status and underlying condition.

Mechanical Ventilation

When non-invasive respiratory support, e.g. CPAP/NIMV modes are not sufficient, babies need to be intubated and supported via invasive mechanical ventilation.

Conventional Mechanical Ventilation Mode

The most commonly used mode of conventional mechanical ventilation (CMV) in the neonatal intensive care unit is pressure limited (± volume targeted), time cycled modes and synchronisation with the baby's inspiratory breaths, if any. In addition, volume targeted or volume guarantee (VG) is the preferred mode as it is associated with less ventilator-induced injury, e.g. pneumothorax, hypocarbia, or even serious complications like intraventricular haemorrhage (IVH) in preterm infants.

Following are some general principles regarding CMV in babies:

- Peak inspiratory pressure (PIP): PIP is adjusted to ensure adequate, but not excessive chest movement. It is generally set between 15 and 20 cmH_2O pressure (higher PIP may be needed if the compliance is low). In VG mode, the set PIP serves as the upper limit of pressure allowed for generating the volume prescribed for the baby. If the baby's lungs compliance improves, the actual measured PIP needed to generate prescribed volume might very well be lower than the set PIP (max. PIP); on the other hand, the set PIP might need to be increased in order to achieve the set tidal volume (Tv) if its lungs are stiff.

- PEEP: Usually set at 5–6 cmH_2O. PEEP, when is set too low, can lead to atelectasis of lungs and impairment of oxygenation and gas exchange. PEEP that is inappropriately high over-distends alveoli, causes pneumothoraces, decreases compliance, impedes venous return and diminishes cardiac output (hypotension).
- Tv: This is set as the desired Tv (whatever PIP needed to achieve volume is used, with the safety margin of the set max. PIP). Usually it is set between 4 and 6 ml/kg in newborn babies. This can be difficult when there is a large leak around the ETT, as the machine sensor would have difficulty in accurately measuring the Tv that the baby was actually getting.
- FiO_2: This is adjusted to maintain PaO_2 between 40 and 60 mmHg (target SpO_2 90–95%) in preterm infants and PaO_2 between 50 and 85 mmHg (target SpO_2 92–98%) in term infants. Avoid hyperoxia, as it is associated with increased risk of retinopathy of prematurity in preterm babies.
- Rate: The ventilator rate greatly depends on the clinical status of the baby. Initial setting is usually 30–40 breaths per minute and is adjusted to maintain $PaCO_2$ of 40–50 mmHg or 50–60 mmHg (permissive hypercarbia) in chronic babies if pH is maintained between 7.25 and 7.35. Hypocarbia ($PaCO_2$ <35 mmHg) should be avoided as it will cause reduced cerebral blood flow and is especially harmful in a premature brain as well as babies suffering from hypoxic ischaemic brain injury. Severe hypercarbia >60 mmHg has also been associated with higher risk of IVH, especially in the very preterm infants during the first days of life.
- Inspiratory Time (iT) and Expiratory Time (eT): These two parameters affect the ventilator rate. iT is generally kept between 0.35 and 0.4 s, the longer the better for oxygenation. eT should be longer than iT in order to effectively clear CO_2 from the lungs. Although strategies for ventilation are recommended according to the working diagnosis of the newborn, the response of the individual infant is variable and changes should be made quickly if there is no clinical improvement or deterioration while on mechanical ventilation.
- Ventilator flow rate: This should be adequate to generate required PIP, iT, and allow the wash-out of exhaled CO_2 and compensate for leaks around the endotracheal tube (ETT) and tubing. Generally, it is set at 6–8 LPM.

High Frequency Oscillatory Ventilation Mode

In specific lung pathologies (e.g. PPHN, meconium aspiration syndrome, pulmonary hypoplasia and pulmonary interstitial emphysema) or failure of CMV mode, a different strategy of ventilation like the high frequency oscillatory ventilation (HFOV) mode can be used. HFOV uses a constant distending pressure (mean airway pressure [MAP]) with pressure variations oscillating around the MAP at very high rates. It has been proposed to reduce ventilator-associated lung injury by creating very small tidal volumes for gas exchange.

Recommended settings when transitioning from CMV mode to HFOV mode:

- MAP: 2–3 cmH_2O above the MAP measured on the previous conventional mode. The MAP should be adjusted (titrated up or down by 1–2 cmH_2O) based on the lung expansion seen on CXR performed within 1 hour after being on HFOV mode. Optimal inflation is when the top margin of the right doom of diaphragm is at the 8th to 9th rib with good lung aeration bilaterally. Hypotension is one of the common complications of overdistension of lungs from high MAP, as this impairs venous return (hence filling of the heart) and reduces cardiac output.
- Amplitude (ΔP): The normal starting range for amplitude is generally between 20 and 30. The optimal level is attained when chest wiggle is seen over the chest and transmitted to the umbilical/lower abdominal region.
- Frequency (Hertz): For term infants, 10–12 Hertz (Hz); preterm infants, 12–14 Hz. Frequency should be adjusted only when $PaCO_2$ levels remain out of range despite optimisation of amplitude.
- Inspiratory: Expiratory (I:E) ratio: Commonly set at a 1:2 ratio and not to be adjusted usually.

Clinical assessment of chest expansion/wiggle, air entry, colour and peripheral perfusion is important. Blood gas should preferably be checked 30 minutes after any change in ventilator setting, and also to be repeated after a severely out of range $PaCO_2$ level is detected (both hypocarbia and hypercarbia).

PaO_2 and $PaCO_2$ can be altered independently of one another:

Issues	Conventional Mode	High Frequency Oscillatory Mode
PaO_2 low	Increase FiO_2, increase PIP (in steps of 1–2 cmH_2O), increase I:E ratio, and increase PEEP (in steps of 1 cmH_2O)	Increase MAP (not to overdistend as could impair venous return and cause hypotension)
$PaCO_2$ high	Increase rate (in steps of 5–10 breaths per minute), increase PIP (in steps of 1–2 cmH_2O), increase or decrease PEEP (in order to increase ΔP, defined by PIP-PEEP)	Increase amplitude (by 2 at a time) Decrease frequency (by 1 Hz at a time)

Senior doctors should be consulted to explore possible use of different modes of ventilation (e.g. high frequencies), administration of surfactant, inotropes (dopamine, dobutamine), sedatives and analgesics (choral hydrate, phenobarbitone, morphine sulfate), volume expanders (normal saline, plasma), pulmonary vasodilators (e.g. inhaled nitric oxide [iNO], sildenafil or magnesium sulphate) as well as dexamethasone. In the setting of severe respiratory failure and not responding to maximum ventilatory support and adjuncts, extracorporeal membrane oxygenation can be considered as part of a collaborative decision between paediatric cardiothoracic surgeon, cardiologist, paediatric and neonatal intensivists, with input and consent from parents.

Deterioration During Ventilation

Sudden Clinical Deterioration

- Usually manifests in the form of hypoxia (a fall in SpO_2 or clinically cyanosed), bradycardia or sudden hypercapnia in blood gas.
- Observe for air entry and chest expansion; consider ETT suction and direct laryngoscopy to ensure the tube is in the right position. A disposable endotracheal tube CO_2 ($ETCO_2$) detector can be a great tool to reconfirm that ETT is still in place, as a colour change will indicate correct placement (expired CO_2 changes colour from purple to yellow). An obstructed tube by secretions or pulmonary haemorrhage (especially considered when a baby has a large PDA) can be the reason for this. Consider re-intubation in cases of suspected blocked or dislodged tube, which resolve with good suctioning. T-piece resuscitator (Neopuff™) should be readily available to provide manual positive pressure ventilation or CPAP in between extubation and reintubation episodes.
- Exclude pneumothorax by auscultation or by transillumination. In an emergency situation, a tension pneumothorax can be drained by needle aspiration of the air in pleural space. Otherwise, confirmation with CXR is preferred, especially in extremely low birth weight infants, as a false positive transillumination test can be seen, given their thin chest walls.

Gradual Deterioration

- This is usually accompanied by increased desaturation episodes or lability and/or an increase in $PaCO_2$. As this may be due to a displaced or blocked ETT or air leak as well, these should be excluded first.
- Other possible causes include:
  - » Inappropriate and inadequate ventilator settings: Due to progressive deterioration of underlying disease state (pneumonia, pulmonary oedema from PDA, lobar collapse) that leads to poor compliance and concurrent atelectasis. Consider an increase in PIP, PEEP, iT, rate and/or FiO_2.
  - » Baby fighting against ventilator: Blocked or mal-positioned ETT and inadequate ventilation should be excluded first. Sedation should be given after exclusion of other causes. Synchronisation of ventilation usually avoids this problem.
  - » Worsening RDS: Babies with severe RDS may need a repeated dose of surfactant (can be done 6–12 hours after the last dose, depending on the type of surfactant used) if their FiO_2 requirement gradually increases beyond 0.30 to 0.40, with findings confirmed on CXR.
  - » Infection: Nosocomial infections are common. Maintain vigilance and test appropriately. Consider changing the antibiotic therapy if the baby is already covered with empiric therapy and not improving

» IVH: Pallor, bulging fontanelle, seizures, fall in haemoglobin, sudden desaturation, hypotension and acidosis may indicate IVH. This can be confirmed by bedside cranial ultrasound.
» Hypotension: Check BP. Review fluid volume given to the patient. Consider administration of normal saline/plasma/vasopressors such as dopamine.
» Anaemia: Frequently due to iatrogenic causes such as blood sampling (in the tiny preterm baby) and other causes of blood loss (IVH, haemolytic anaemia).
» Metabolic imbalance: Check blood gases for acidosis, consider laboratory tests for electrolytes, urea, creatinine.
» Poor environmental support: Avoid excessive handling, group and plan procedures, and ensure a thermo-neutral environment.

Refractory Hypoxia

- If the SpO_2 and PaO_2 remains below target despite apparent adequate ventilation and FiO_2 ≥50%, consider the following:
  » The baby is fighting or breathing out of synchrony with the ventilator
  » Increased intra-pulmonary shunting caused by progressive atelectasis or lobar lung collapse
  » Pulmonary hypertension with shunting through the foramen ovale and/or PDA
  » Fixed cyanotic heart disease

Weaning Off the Ventilator

When the baby's condition has improved, ventilator settings should be weaned, whenever possible to prevent lung injury. If the baby is on HFOV mode, amplitude can be weaned by 2 each time to the lower range of 20, while MAP can be reduced in 1–2 cmH_2O steps to 8–10 cmH_2O as long as oxygenation is maintained, before switching to conventional ventilation or extubation. When on CMV mode, PIP can be reduced by 1–2 cmH_2O to 16–18 cmH_2O; set Tv (if on VG mode) to 4–4.5 ml/kg — monitoring inspiratory pressure needed to achieve volume set, the rate can be reduced (to be lower than baby's spontaneous breath but not lower than 25). When weaning is achieved to minimal settings as above, extubation should be considered. To maximise the success of weaning and extubation, sedation and muscle relaxant, if used, should be discontinued or at least reduced to the minimal dose. Administration of a loading dose of caffeine citrate should be considered in preterm infants of ≤34 weeks' gestation to prevent failure of extubation due to apnoea of prematurity. Adjunctive therapy like iNO as well as cardiac inotropes is generally weaned off before planning for extubation. Consider NIMV (especially for the very premature infants with expected low respiratory effort), CPAP or high/normal flow NC after extubation if anticipating baby to not tolerate room air (based on the severity of lung disease and pre-intubation need of support). After extubation, monitor the baby closely for worsening respiratory distress. Blood gas should be followed (30–60 minutes after extubation) if infants is extubated to non-invasive respiratory support and consider performing CXR to evaluate for any atelectasis if clinical worsening post extubation is observed (optional).

Failure to Wean

- Immaturity: Maturation of control of breathing may be delayed in premature baby
- Laryngeal oedema, subglottic stenosis, lower tract obstruction. Nebulised adrenaline can be used, or pre-extubation dexamethasone can be considered.
- Chronic lung disease
- Pulmonary oedema: PDA, fluid overload
- Central nervous system: Severe brain injury from severe IVH and hypoxic ischaemic encephalopathy, or congenital malformations, heavy sedation from medications
- Infection, aspiration of milk, atelectasis
- Metabolic and electrolyte imbalance
- Inadequate nutritional status, anaemia

Bibliography

1. Hermansen CL, Lorah KN. (2007) Respiratory distress in the newborn. *Am Fam Physician* **76**(7):987–994.
2. Goldsmith JP, Karotkin E, Gautham S, Keszler M. (2017) *Assisted Ventilation of the Neonate, 6th ed.* Elsevier.
3. Sweet DG, Carnielli V, Greisen G, *et al.* (2019) European consensus guidelines on the management of respiratory distress syndrome — 2019 Update. *Neonatology* **115**(4):432–450.
4. Keszler M. (2017) Mechanical ventilation strategies. *Semin Fetal Neonatal Med* **22**(4):267–274.
5. Wheeler CR, Smallwood CD. (2020) 2019 Year in review: Neonatal respiratory support. *Respir Care* **65**(5):693–704.
6. Vento G, Tirone C, Paladini A, et al. (2021) Weaning from the Ventilator in Bronchopulmonary Dysplasia. *Clin Perinatol* **48**(4):895–906.
7. Chowdhury O, Wedderburn CJ, Duffy D, Greenough A. (2012) CPAP review. *Eur J Pediatr* **171**(10):1441–1448.
8. Stenson BJ. (2016) Oxygen saturation targets for extremely preterm infants after the NeOProM trials. *Neonatology* **109**(4):352–358.
9. Kinsella JP, Abman SH. (1998) Inhaled nitric oxide and high frequency oscillatory ventilation in persistent pulmonary hypertension of the newborn. *Eur J Pediatr* **157**(Suppl 1):S28–S30.

CHAPTER 77

Neonatal Sepsis

Yeo Kee Thai

Definitions

Neonatal sepsis describes a clinical syndrome related to the systemic infection, typically characterised by the isolation of microbial pathogens from the blood, with or without clinical signs of infection within the first 28 days of life. Early onset sepsis (EOS) is typically defined as infections that occur within the first 72 hours of life and late onset sepsis (LOS) occurs >72 hours of life.

Risk Factors

Early onset infections are typically acquired through *vertical* transmission — ascending infection or acquisition of microorganisms during delivery. The associated risk factor for EOS originates in the antepartum/intrapartum period and includes factors such as maternal intrapartum fever and chorioamnionitis, prolonged rupture of membranes and perinatal microbial colonisation.

Late onset infections occur through *horizontal* transmission of microorganisms, which are acquired from the environment or carers. Risk factors for LOS includes the presence of intravascular devices, exposure to medications such as H_2 blockers and inappropriate antibiotic usage.

Maternal Risk Factors

- Preterm delivery
- *Group B Streptococcus* (GBS) colonisation
- Prolonged rupture of membranes >18 hours
- Clinical chorioamnionitis (maternal fever, uterine tenderness, purulent or foul smelling liquor, maternal tachycardia, foetal tachycardia)
- Maternal urinary tract infection

Infant Risk Factors

Infant risk factors for sepsis are variable but would typically include:

- Prematurity
- Low birth weight
- Male gender

- Presence of intravascular devices
- Skin or mucosal breakdown
- Exposure to H_2 blockers
- Prolonged & inappropriate usage of antibiotics

Causative Organisms

Common organisms responsible for EOS include GBS and gram-negative organisms such as *Escherichia coli*. Other bacterial causes include *Listeria monocytogenes, Streptococcus viridans, Enterococcus* and other gram-negative bacteria.

The epidemiology and distribution of causative organisms for LOS differ across different settings. The commonly reported organisms include gram-negative bacteria (e.g. *E. coli, Klebsiella, Pseudomonas*), *Coagulase negative staphylococcus, Staphylococcus aureus, Enterococcus,* GBS and *Candida*.

Other non-bacterial causes of neonatal sepsis include viral pathogens such as respiratory viral infections (e.g. respiratory syncytial virus, parainfluenza virus, rhinovirus), herpes simplex virus and enteroviruses.

Clinical Presentation

Initial clinical presentation of sepsis can be subtle and non-specific.

Signs include:

- Temperature instability: Hypothermia or hyperthermia
- Cardiovascular: Tachycardia, hypotension
- Respiratory: Apnoea, tachypnoea, nasal flaring, retractions, grunting
- Gastrointestinal: Poor feeding, vomiting, feeding intolerance, jaundice
- Neurological: Lethargy, irritability, seizures

Investigations

- Full blood count: Specifically high or low white cell count, increased immature-to-total neutrophil ratio (>0.20)
- C-reactive protein, procalcitonin
- Blood culture
- Cerebrospinal fluid culture
- Urine microscopy and culture
- Chest X-ray

Prevention

Intrapartum antibiotics prophylaxis is a strategy for the prevention of early onset GBS infection, and studies have documented decreases in the incidence of GBS sepsis.

Indications for intrapartum antibiotics include:

- Positive antenatal cultures for GBS

- Unknown maternal colonisation status with gestation <37 weeks
- GBS bacteriuria during the current pregnancy
- Previous newborn with invasive GBS disease

Appropriate prophylaxis for GBS is penicillin or cefazolin given 4 hours or more before delivery. Antibiotic susceptibility information may be required for women who have an anaphylactic reaction to penicillin. Clindamycin and vancomycin may be considered in these situations.

Antibiotic Regimen

Selection of antibiotic regimen for the treatment of neonatal sepsis is based on local epidemiology and susceptibilities of infecting bacteria. Typical antibiotic regiment in early onset infection include penicillin G/ampicillin and gentamicin. The selection of ampicillin could be considered for the empiric coverage of *L. monocytogenes.* In late onset infection, the choice of antibiotics typically include cloxacillin and an aminoglycoside (gentamicin/amikacin).

In all situations, escalation of antibiotic coverage to agents such as third-generation cephalosporin and carbapenems would depend on the clinical condition and response to initial empiric antibiotics. Considerations should also be made to ensure coverage and treatment for the possibility of meningitis. Antibiotic coverage should be adjusted once the results of the culture and susceptibilities are made available.

Bibliography

1. Shane AL, Sanchez PJ, Stoll BJ. (2017) Neonatal sepsis. *Lancet* **390**(10104):1770–1780.
2. Polin RA; Committee on Fetus and Newborn. (2012) Management of neonates with suspected or proven early-onset bacterial sepsis. *Pediatrics* **129**(5):1006–1015.
3. Goh GL, Lim CSE, Sultana R, *et al.* (2022) Risk factors for mortality from late onset sepsis among preterm very-low-birthweight infants: A single-center cohort study from Singapore. *Front Pediatr* **9**:801955.
4. Yeo KT, de la Puerta R, Tee NWS, et al. (2018) Burden, etiology, and risk factors of respiratory virus infections among symptomatic preterm infants in the Tropics: A retrospective single-center cohort study. *Clin Infect Dis* **67**(10):1603–1609.

CHAPTER 78

Necrotising Enterocolitis

Amudha Jayanthi Anand

Necrotising enterocolitis (NEC) is a condition characterised by varying degrees of mucosal necrosis and is predominantly seen in premature infants. Age of onset depends on gestation:

- Preterm infants: 2 weeks to 3 months of life
- Term infants: First week of life

Incidence of NEC in the very low-birth-weight infants is about 5–7%.

Risk Factors

- Prematurity
- Feeding — formula feeding and rapid advancement of feeds
- Hypotension requiring inotropes
- Perinatal asphyxia
- Polycythaemia
- Severe chorioamnionitis
- Use of H_2 blockers
- Prolonged antibiotic use
- Umbilical catheters
- Maternal cocaine abuse
- Infections: Both bacterial and viral
- Congenital gastrointestinal abnormalities
- Patent Ductus Arteriosus
- Congenital heart disease

Measures to Reduce Risk

- Oral care with colostrum.
- Start trophic feeds early within the first 24 hours if possible.
    - » Avoid nil by mouth and keep on minimal enteral nutrition or non-nutritive feeds of 20 ml/kg/day whenever possible.
- Encourage an exclusive breast milk diet (expressed breast milk or pasteurised donor human milk).
- Strictly adhering to the department/institution's standardised feeding protocol.
- High index of suspicion in at-risk neonates.

- Use probiotics.
- To continue with feeds during blood transfusion and to suspend additives for 48 hours.
- Limit the use of broad spectrum antibiotics. In all cases of presumed sepsis, empirical antibiotics must be stopped if final blood culture is negative.
- Use of high calorie formulas is to be considered after maximising feeding volume to 180 ml/kg/day with human milk and should be prescribed in conjunction with dietician consultation.
- Avoid the use of additives with high osmolality.
  » All oral medications must be diluted with an appropriate dilution guide.
  » It is recommended that only one oral medication should be administered per milk feed.
  » The osmolality of oral feeds should be kept below 450 mOsm/L.

Clinical Features

Non-Specific Signs and Symptoms

- Lethargy
- Tachycardia (Heart rate >160/min)
- Temperature instability
- Apnoea and bradycardia with desaturations
- Systemic hypotension

Abdominal Signs and Symptoms

- Feeding intolerance
- Vomiting
- Increased pre-feed residuals >30%
- Abdominal distension with tenderness and discoloration
- Bloody or bilious gastric aspirates
- Ileus
- Bloody stool

Investigations

- Full blood count (8–24 hourly until stabilisation of neutrophils and platelets), C-reactive protein, blood culture, renal panel, arterial blood gas, blood sugar monitoring, coagulation profile (12–24 hourly until normal), group and crossmatch
  » Non-specific laboratory findings: Neutropaenia, leucocytosis, hyponatraemia, metabolic acidosis, hyperglycaemia, disseminated intravascular coagulopathy (in severe NEC).

- Serial abdominal X-ray (anteroposterior and decubitus view) 6–8 hourly
  - Radiological findings: Fixed dilated bowel loops or 'sentinel loop sign', pneumoperitoneum, portal venous gas, pneumatosis intestinalis (latter two pathognomonic for NEC).
- Stool for rotavirus, enterovirus and bacterial culture (if no stool, send rectal swab)

Table 17.7 Modified Bell Staging Criteria for Necrotising Enterocolitis

Stage	Systemic Signs	Abdominal Signs	Radiographic Signs	Treatment
IA: Suspected NEC	Temperature instability, apnoea, bradycardia, lethargy	Gastric retention, abdominal distension, emesis, occult blood in stools	Normal or mild ileus	Nil orally, antibiotics for 3 d
IB: Suspected NEC	Same as IA	Same as IA and grossly bloody stool	Same as IA	Same as IA
IIA: Confirmed NEC (mild disease)	Same as IA	Same as IA plus absent bowel sounds with or without abdominal tenderness	Intestinal dilatation, ileus, pneumatosis intestinalis	Nil orally, antibiotics for 7–10 d
IIB: Confirmed NEC (moderate disease)	Same as IA, plus mild metabolic acidosis, mild thrombocytopenia	Same IA plus abdominal tenderness, abdominal wall cellulitis and palpable abdominal mass	Same as IIA with portal vein gas	Nil orally, antibiotics for 14 d
IIIA: Advanced NEC (severe disease, bowel intact)	Same as IIB, plus hypotension, bradycardia, respiratory acidosis, metabolic acidosis, disseminated intravascular coagulation, neutropaenia	Same as I and II, plus signs of generalised peritonitis, marked tenderness and distension of abdomen	Same as IIB, plus definite ascites	Nil orally, antibiotics for 14 d, fluid resuscitation, inotropic support, ventilator therapy, paracentesis
IIIB: Advanced NEC (severe disease, bowel perforated)	Same as IIIA	Same as IIIA	Same as IIB, plus pneumoperitoneum	Same as IIIA plus surgery

Management

- Manage Airway, Breathing and Circulation (consider ventilator support in Stage 2 NEC and above)
- Continuous blood pressure monitoring (via intra-arterial insertion)
- Nil by mouth and initiate total parenteral nutrition
- Nasogastric decompression
- Fluid resuscitation: Normal saline bolus 10–20 ml/kg (as required)
  - » Consider fresh frozen plasma for volume expansion if there is associated coagulopathy
- Lumbar puncture (only if stable and clinically indicated)
- Intravenous antibiotics for 7–14 days for definite NEC
  - » Cloxacillin, gentamicin/amikacin and metronidazole
  - » Escalate to cefotaxime/meropenem if there is worsening clinical status
- Fluconazole prophylaxis in Stage 2 NEC and above
- Early referral to paediatric surgeon
  - » Absolute indication for urgent laparotomy is presence of pneumoperitoneum

Prognosis

- Mortality rate between 20 and 40%
- Late complications include cholestasis, stenosis, strictures, short bowel syndrome and malabsorption
- Affected infants have about 25% risk of developing neurodevelopmental delay

Bibliography

1. Bertino E, Giuliani F, Prandi G, *et al.* (2009) Necrotizing enterocolitis: Risk factor analysis and role of gastric residuals in very low birth weight infants. *J Pediatr Gastroenterol Nutr* **48**(4):437–442.
2. Mohammad A, Shah PS. (2012) Transfusion associated necrotizing enterocolitis: A meta-analysis of observational data. *Pediatrics* **129**(3):529–540.
3. Kasivajjula H, Maheshwari A. (2014) Pathophysiology and current management of necrotizing enterocolitis. *Indian J Pediatr* **81**(5):489–497.
4. Srinivasan L, Bokiniec R, King C, *et al.* (2004) Increased osmolality of breast milk with therapeutic additives. *Arch Dis Child Fetal Neonatal Ed* **89**(6):F514–F517.
5. Quigley M, Embleton ND, McGuire W. (2019) Formula versus donor breast milk for feeding preterm or low birth weight infants. *Cochrane Database Syst Rev* **7**(7):CD002971.
6. Sullivan S, Schanler RJ, Kim JH, *et al.* (2010) An exclusively human milk-based diet is associated with a lower rate of necrotizing enterocolitis than a diet of human milk and bovine milk-based products. *J Pediatr* **156**(4):562–567.e1.
7. Gephart SM, Spitzer AR, Effken JA, *et al.* (2014) Discrimination of GutCheck(NEC): A clinical risk index for necrotizing enterocolitis. *J Perinatol* **34**(6):468–475.
8. Autmizguine J, Hornik CP, Benjamin DK Jr, *et al.* (2015) Anaerobic antimicrobial therapy after necrotizing enterocolitis in VLBW infants. *Pediatrics* **135**(1):e117–e125.
9. Bell MJ, Ternberg JL, Feigin RD, *et al.* (1978) Neonatal necrotizing enterocolitis. Therapeutic decisions based upon clinical staging. *Ann Surg* **187**(1):1–7.
10. Walsh MC, Kliegman RM. (1986) Necrotizing enterocolitis: Treatment based on staging criteria. *Pediatr Clin N Am* **33**(1):179–201.

CHAPTER 79

Polycythaemia

Shrenik Vora

Definition

A haematocrit value >65% when obtained from a large, freely flowing peripheral vein.

Pathophysiology

Incidence: 1.5–4% of all live births.

Haematocrit value peaks at 2–4 hours of life due to transudation of fluid out of the intravascular space.

The relationship between haematocrit and viscosity is almost linear till 65% and exponential after that. As the viscosity increases, there is an impairment of tissue oxygenation and perfusion and a tendency to form microthrombi, which may cause severe damage to gut, cerebral cortex, kidneys and adrenal glands.

Aetiology

Causes of polycythaemia in neonates include:

- Intrauterine hypoxia (Due to increased red blood cells [RBC] production as compensation; as suggested by the increased number of nucleated RBCs)
  - » Intra uterine growth retardation
  - » Maternal pregnancy-induced hypertension
  - » Maternal gestational diabetes mellitus
  - » Maternal smoking
  - » Maternal cyanotic heart disease
  - » Post term
- Transfusions:
  - » Delayed cord clamping (>3 minutes)
  - » Holding baby below the level of introitus
  - » Twin-to-twin transfusion
  - » Maternal-foetal transfusion
  - » Perinatal asphyxia
  - » Iatrogenic–blood transfusion
- Other causes:
  - » Dehydration
  - » Trisomy 13, 18, 21
  - » Hypothyroidism, thyrotoxicosis

 » Congenital adrenal hyperplasia
 » Beckwith–Wiedemann syndrome

Clinical Features

Most of the symptoms are non-specific and related to the underlying cause.

- Neurological: Hypotonia, irritability, jitteriness, seizures
- Cardiovascular: Tachycardia, cyanosis

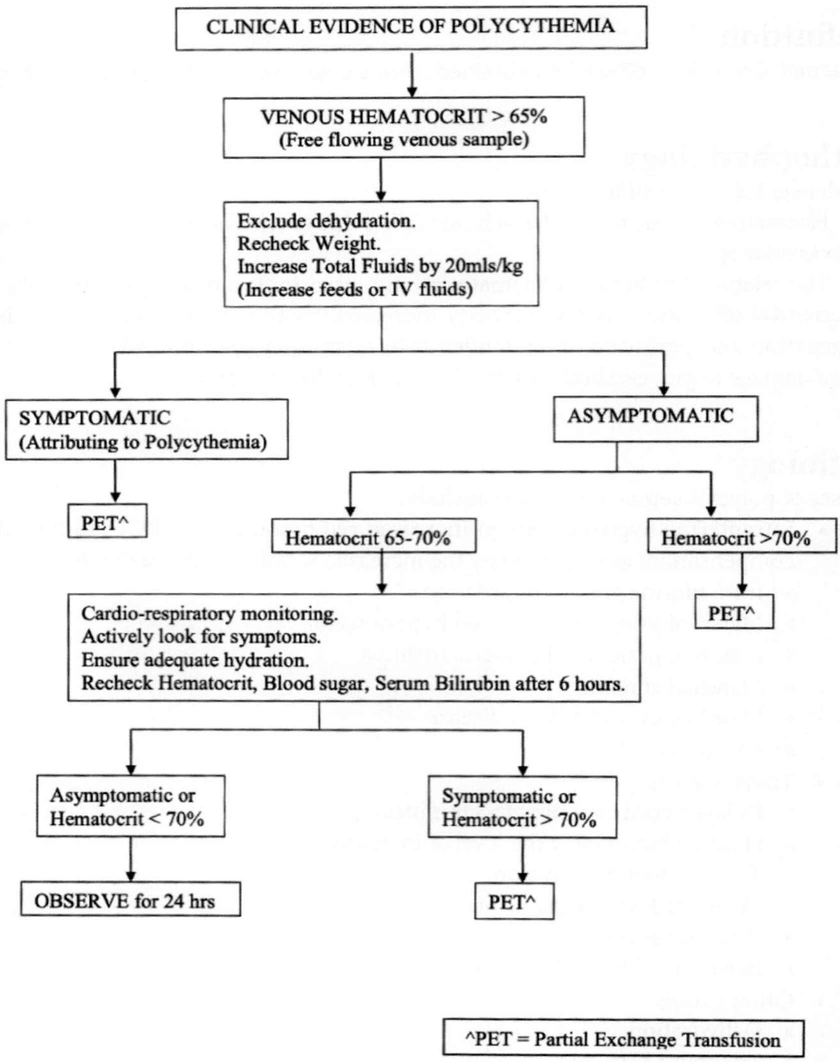

Figure 17.7 Algorithm for management of polycythaemia.

- Respiratory: Respiratory distress
- Gastrointestinal: Poor suck, vomiting, feeding difficulties
- Metabolic: Hypoglycaemia, pathological jaundice
- Haematological: Thrombocytopenia

Management

- Ensure adequate hydration.
- Correct underlying cause and treat complications.
- Definite treatment is partial exchange transfusion (PET) where blood is taken out slowly and replaced with normal saline (preferred) or plasma.
- PET
  - Indications:
    - Symptomatic polycythaemia
    - Haematocrit >70% in asymptomatic infant
  - Target: To attain haematocrit of 55%
  - Route of PET: Intra-arterial line and intravenous line or umbilical venous cannulation
  - Volume of blood exchanged:

$$\text{Volume to be exchanged} = \frac{\text{Blood volume x (Observed haematocrit — desired haematocrit)}}{\text{Observed haematocrit}}$$

[Blood volume = 80 ml/kg in term babies and 90 ml/kg in preterm babies]

Complications

- Neurological: Seizures, strokes, motor deficits, intellectual impairment
- Cardiovascular: Cardiomegaly, increased pulmonary resistance, decreased cardiac output, congestive cardiac failure
- Gastrointestinal: Necrotising enterocolitis, ileus
- Renal: Renal vein thrombosis, renal failure, oliguria
- Others: Priapism, testicular infarct, peripheral gangrene

Bibliography

1. Vora S, Sriram B. (2016) Protocol for management of polycythaemia in neonates. Department of Neonatology, KK Women's and Children's Hospital, Singapore.

CHAPTER 80

Hyperinsulinaemic Hypoglycaemia

Suresh Chandran; Yap Kok Peng, Fabian; Victor Samuel Rajadurai

Hypoglycaemia in newborn infants is defined as plasma glucose levels <3.0 mmol/L in the first 48 hours of life and <3.5 mmol/L beyond that. Hyperinsulinism is suspected when an infant needs >10 mg/kg/min to maintain normoglycaemia (3.5–7 mmol/L) beyond 48 hours of life. While increasing the glucose infusion rate (GIR) in increments of 2 mg/kg/min to maintain glucose levels, critical blood samples, including plasma glucose, insulin, C peptide, ketone bodies, free fatty acids, cortisol and growth hormone, are collected during an episode of hypoglycaemia. Detectable insulin level when hypoglycaemic, along with hypoketonaemia, hypofattyacidaemia and a positive response to glucagon intravenous (IV)/intramuscular (rise in glucose concentration of >1.5 mmol/L within 30 minutes) with normal cortisol and growth hormone levels, is consistent with a diagnosis of hyperinsulinaemic hypoglycaemia (HH). Other causes for hypoglycaemia, including sepsis and inborn errors of metabolism (IEM), should be ruled out.

The attempt to raise the GIR in these infants is achieved by raising the fluid volume or dextrose concentration (up to 30% dextrose concentration) as required. A central line should be secured for a dextrose concentration of more than 12.5%. Target to maintain plasma glucose levels >3.5 mmol/L in order to prevent hypoglycaemic brain injury. Discuss the case with HH Specialist from Neonatology/Endocrinology. Retrieve IEM result. Serum ammonia levels are elevated in infants with Hyperammonaemia/Hyperinsulinism (HI/HA) syndrome, the second-most common cause of congenital hyperinsulinism.

HH can be transient or persistent (genetic or congenital). Transient forms are often seen in infants of diabetic and obese mothers, small for gestational age (SGA) infants, following perinatal asphyxia and in Beckwith–Wiedemann syndrome. Most of them resolve spontaneously with increasing feeds or with short periods of high GIR. A prolonged form of HH is seen in some SGA infants, lasting for 6 weeks to 6 months, who respond well to oral diazoxide (DZX). Recessive mutations in the K_{ATP} channel of the β-cells of pancreas, encoded by the genes ABCC8 and KCNJ11, are the most common cause of congenital hyperinsulinism.

Oral DZX is the drug choice (3–20 mg/kg/day in 2 divided doses) in the treatment of HH. It is a K_{ATP} channel agonist and is effective in most forms of HH, except in diffuse disease due to AR-inherited ABCC8/KCNJ11 mutations. Oral hydrochlorothiazide (1 mg/kg/day in 2 divided doses) should be combined with DZX to combat the fluid retention side effect of DZX. DZX, being 90% protein bound, toxicity could be severe in infants with hypoalbuminaemia. In DZX-responsive infants, on successful weaning of IV dextrose, a safety fast study (SFS) (6 hours fast) can be done to confirm the infant's

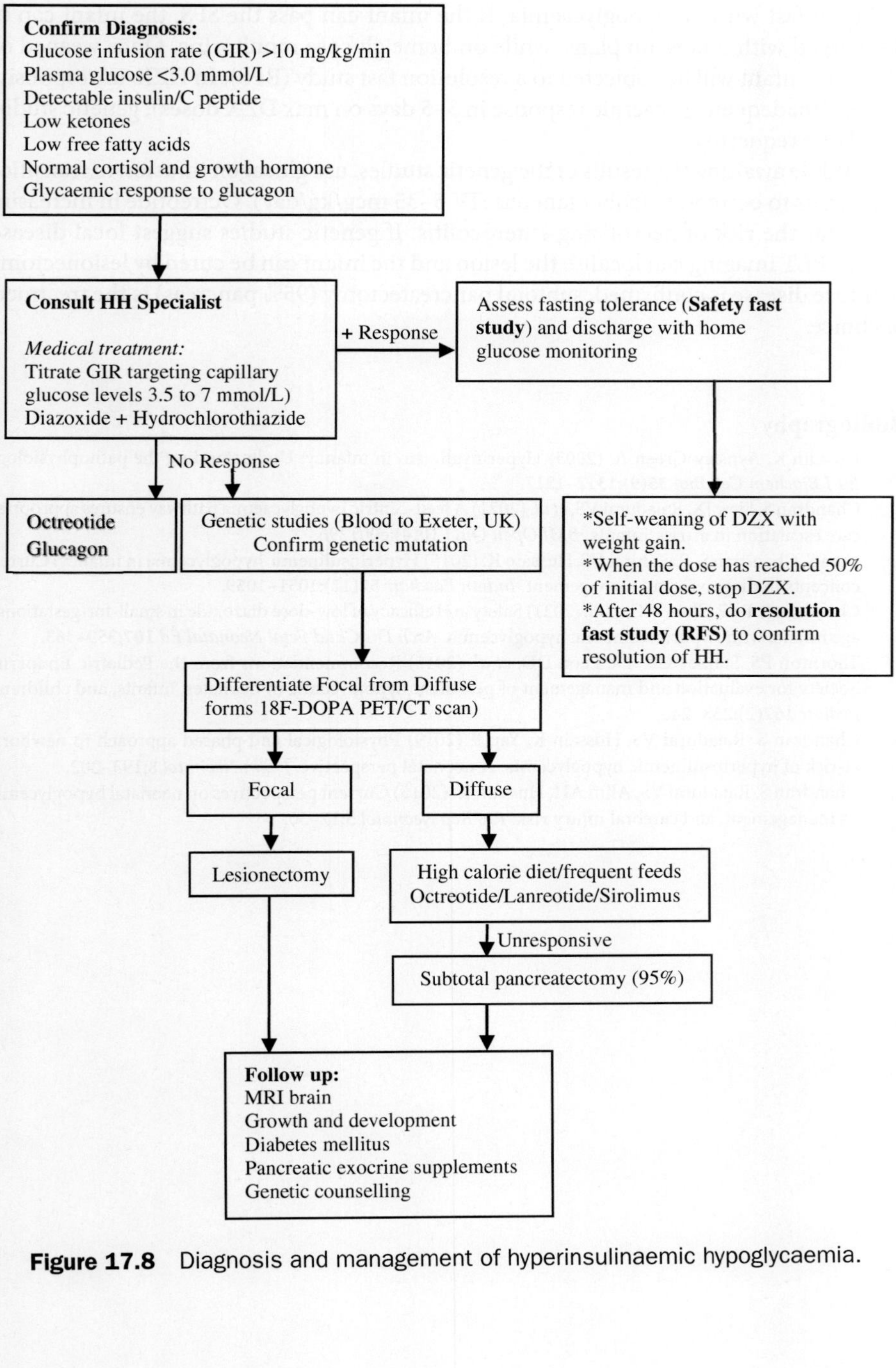

Figure 17.8 Diagnosis and management of hyperinsulinaemic hypoglycaemia.

ability to fast without hypoglycaemia. If the infant can pass the SFS, the infant can be discharged with follow-up plans, while on home glucose monitoring. Once weaned off DZX, the infant will be subjected to a resolution fast study (RFS). In DZX-unresponsive infants (inadequate glycaemic response in 3–5 days on max DZX doses), genetic studies should be requested.

While awaiting the results of the genetic studies, use glucagon infusion to transition the infants to octreotide (subcutaneous /IV 5–35 mcg/kg/day). Octreotide in increasing doses has the risk of necrotising enterocolitis. If genetic studies suggest focal disease, DOPA-PET imaging can localise the lesion and the infant can be cured by lesionectomy. If diffuse disease is confirmed, subtotal pancreatectomy (95% pancreas) is the treatment of choice.

Bibliography

1. Hussain K, Aynsley-Green A. (2003) Hyperinsulinism in infancy: Understanding the pathophysiology. *Int J Biochem Cell Biol* **35**(9):1312–1317.
2. Chandran S, Siew JX, Rajadurai VS, *et al.* (2021) A feed-centric hypoglycaemia pathway ensures appropriate care escalation in at-risk infants. *BMJ Open Qual* **10**(4):e001296.
3. Vora S, Chandran S, Rajadurai VS, Hussain K. (2015) Hyperinsulinemic hypoglycemia in infancy: Current concepts in diagnosis and management. *Indian Paediatr* **52**(12):1051–1059.
4. Chandran S, Rr P, Chua MC, *et al.* (2021) Safety and efficacy of low-dose diazoxide in small-for-gestational-age infants with hyperinsulinemic hypoglycemia. *Arch Dis Child Fetal Neonatal Ed* **107**:359–363.
5. Thornton PS, Stanley CA, De Leon DD, *et al.* (2015) Recommendations from the Pediatric Endocrine Society for evaluation and management of persistent hypoglycemia in neonates, infants, and children. *J Pediatr* **167**(2):238–245.
6. Chandran S, Rajadurai VS, Hussain K, Yap F. (2019) Physiological and phased approach to newborns at-risk of hyperinsulinemic hypoglycemia: A neonatal perspective. *J Clin Neonatol* 8:193–202.
7. Chandran S, Rajadurai VS, Alim AH, Hussain K. (2015) Current perspectives on neonatal hypoglycemia, its management, and cerebral injury risk. *Res Rep Neonatol* **5**:17–30.

CHAPTER 81

Neonatal Seizures

Nirmal Kavalloor Visruthan

Seizure Pattern

Subtle seizures constitute 50% of the seizures in the newborns. They may be in the form of tonic horizontal deviation and jerking of the eyes, repetitive blinking or fluttering of the eyelids, oral and buccal movements (drooling, sucking, yawning), tonic limb posturing, complex purposeless movement ('swimming', 'bicycling'), apnoeas and rhythmic fluctuations of vital signs. Seizures may also present as focal or multifocal clonic seizures, tonic seizures and myoclonic seizures.

Jitteriness Versus Seizure

A number of 'seizure-like' behavioural states may be confused with seizures. These include jitteriness, movement during rapid eye movement (REM) sleep, decorticate and decerebrate posturing, and autonomic dysfunction.

Clinical Features	Jitteriness	Seizures
Abnormality of gaze or eye movements	Absent	Present
Autonomic changes	Absent	Present
Response to stimulation	Yes	No
Movement ease with passive flexion	Yes	No
Predominant movement	Tremor	Jerking

Common Causes

- Hypoxic ischaemic encephalopathy: Seizures usually occur at 12–24 hours of life
- Metabolic (hypoglycaemia, hypocalcaemia, hypo/hypernatraemia)
- Neonatal stroke
- Infections: Meningitis, viral encephalitis, TORCH (Toxoplasmosis, Rubella, Cytomegalovirus and Herpes Simplex) infections
- Intracranial bleeds
- Inborn errors of metabolism
- Neonatal abstinence syndrome
- Congenital malformations: Schizencephaly, lissencephaly, holoprosencephaly

- Epilepsy syndromes
  - » Benign idiopathic neonatal seizures: 'Fifth day fits', benign examination and clinical course
  - » Benign familial neonatal convulsions: Family history of neonatal seizures and spontaneously resolves in a few days to weeks
  - » Early myoclonic encephalopathy: Inherited metabolic disorder including non-ketotic hyperglycinemia
  - » Early infantile epileptic encephalopathy: Ohtahara syndrome
  - » Genetic epilepsy syndromes, e.g. KCNQ2 mutations

Workup

- Perinatal history including family history, risks for sepsis, drug usage, gestational diabetes mellitus and perinatal hypoxia
- Physical examination
- Basic laboratory tests:
  - » Full blood count, C-reactive protein
  - » Renal panel
  - » Calcium, magnesium and phosphate
  - » Blood glucose
- Additional tests:
  - » Lumbar puncture
  - » Plasma ammonia and lactate
  - » Plasma and Cerebrospinal Fluid (CSF) amino acids, urine organic acids
  - » Toxicological screen
- Electroencephalogram (EEG) or amplitude-integrated EEG (aEEG)
- Neuroimaging: Ultrasound, Computed Tomography or Magnetic Resonance Imaging of the brain
- Genetic testing for epilepsy syndromes

Acute Management

See Figure 17.9 for the algorithm for acute management of neonatal seizures.

Hypoxic Ischaemic Encephalopathy

Hypoxic ischaemic encephalopathy (HIE) is a neurological dysfunction affecting newborn infants. Its prevalence ranges from 1–3/1000, and it affects mainly term infants. The major pathological mechanism is decreased cerebral blood flow and oxygen delivery. This results in primary (immediate hypoxic neuronal death) and secondary (cells 'commit' to die over 6 to 72 hours) energy failure. During this 'window of opportunity', hypothermia may have a beneficial effect. The most common causes for HIE are due to intrauterine asphyxia such as placental abruption, cord prolapse and uterine rupture. However, it is

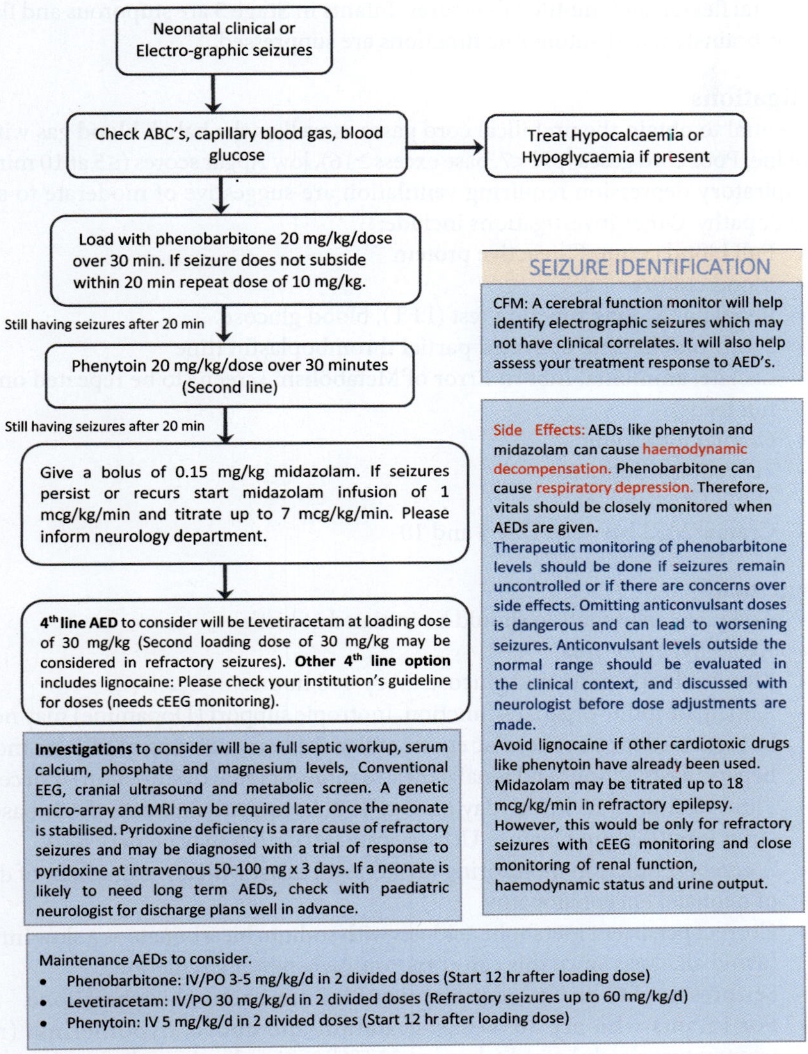

Figure 17.9 Algorithm for acute management of neonatal seizures.

important to rule out reversible causes of neonatal encephalopathy such as metabolic disorders, infections, neonatal stroke and central nervous system malformations.

Stages of Encephalopathy

Sarnat recognised 3 stages of neonatal encephalopathy. **Stage 1** lasts less than 24 hours and is characterised by hyperalertness, uninhibited Moro and stretch reflexes, sympathetic effects and a normal electroencephalogram. **Stage 2** is marked by obtundation, hypotonia, strong distal flexion and multifocal seizures. Infants in **Stage 3** are stuporous and flaccid, and their brainstem and autonomic functions are suppressed.

Investigations

It is essential to obtain the umbilical cord gases as well as the baby's blood gas within 1 hour of life. Poor cord gases (pH <7, base excess ≥16), low Apgar scores (≤5 at 10 minutes) and respiratory depression requiring ventilation are suggestive of moderate to severe encephalopathy. Other investigations include:

- Full blood count, C-reactive protein
- Blood culture
- Renal panel, liver function test (LFT), blood glucose
- Prothrombin time/activated partial thromboplastin time
- Lactate, ammonia, Inborn Error of Metabolism screen (to be repeated once on full feeds)
- Cranial ultrasound
- 2D echocardiogram
- aEEG (if available)
- Cranial MRI between Day 5 and 10

Management

- Adequate resuscitation should be initiated at birth.
- Avoid hyperthermia.
- Monitor blood gases and glucose every 4–6 hours.
- Anticipate multi-organ dysfunction. Inotropic support (Dopamine) may need to be instituted for poor cardiac contractility. Daily monitoring of LFT (to monitor hepatic dysfunction) and renal panel (to monitor renal dysfunction) is necessary.
- Fluid restrict to 50 ml/kg/day on Day 1. Subsequently increase fluids based on strict input/output balance. Urinary catheterisation may be necessary.
- A cerebral function monitoring (aEEG) will assist with an assessment of degree of neonatal encephalopathy.
- Correct persistent metabolic acidosis with sodium bicarbonate as a slow infusion (avoid alkalosis since this can compromise cerebral circulation).
- Seizures need to be treated promptly with intravenous phenobarbitone.
- For infants who are 36 weeks' gestation and above, hypothermia (rectal temperature slowly brought down to 33.5°C) initiated at the earliest and continued for 72 hours has become the standard of care. See Figure 17.10 for the algorithm to decide which babies may qualify for cooling.

Follow-up

- All infants need a full neurological assessment (Dubowitz–Hammersmith) before discharge.
- Neurology follow-up.
- High-risk hearing screen at 3 months of age.
- Developmental examination during neonatal follow-up.

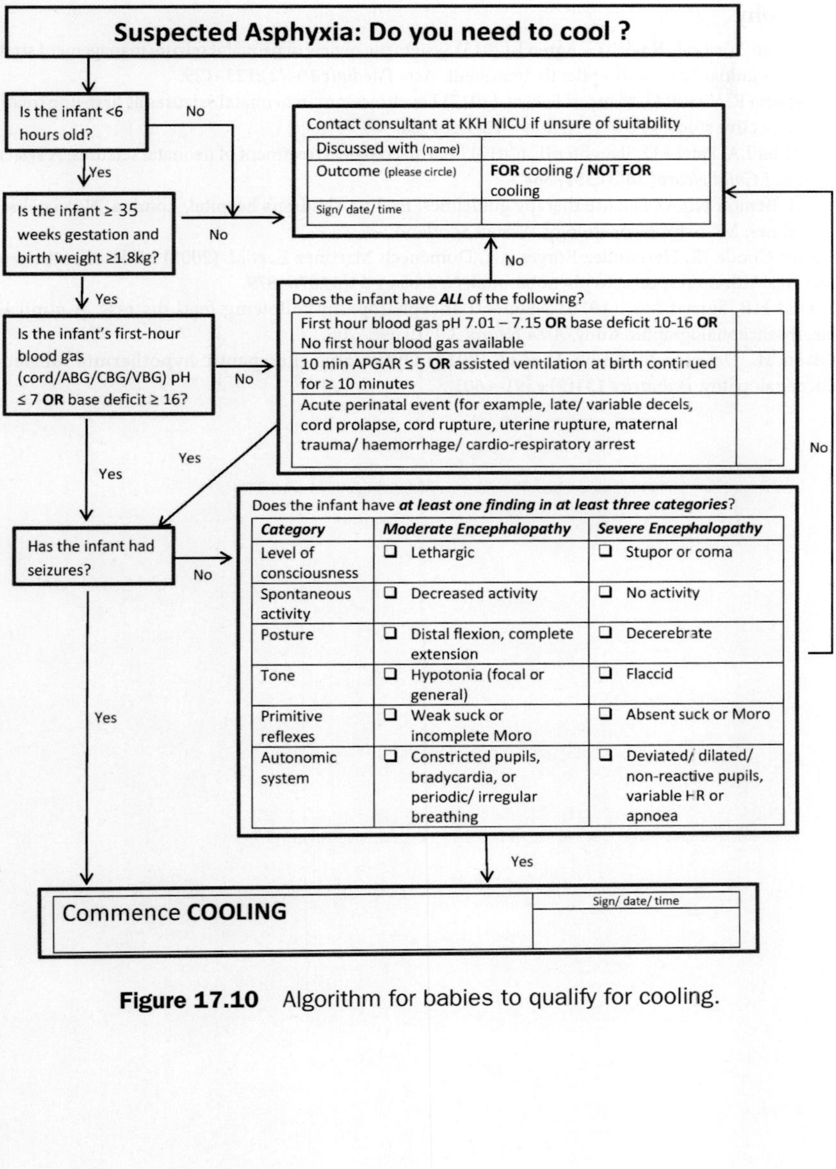

Figure 17.10 Algorithm for babies to qualify for cooling.

Bibliography

1. Hellström-Westas L, Boylan G, Ågren J. (2015) Systematic review of neonatal seizure management strategies provides guidance on anti-epileptic treatment. *Acta Paediatr* **104**(2):123–129.
2. Falsaperla R, Vitaliti G, Mauceri L, *et al.* (2017) Levetiracetam in neonatal seizures as first-line treatment: A prospective study. *J Pediatr Neurosci* **12**(1):24–28.
3. Slaughter LA, Patel AD, Slaughter JL. (2013) Pharmacological treatment of neonatal seizures: A systematic review. *J Child Neurol* **28**(3):351–364.
4. UCSF Benioff NICU, Seizure therapy guidelines; Evelina children's hospital, London, Neonatal seizure guidelines; MCN for Neonatology, West of Scotland.
5. Castro Conde JR, Hernández Borges AA, Doménech Martínez E, *et al.* (2005) Midazolam in neonatal seizures with no response to phenobarbital. *Neurology* **64**(5):876–879.
6. Sarnat HB, Sarnat MS. (1976) Neonatal encephalopathy following fetal distress. A clinical and electroencephalographic study. *Arch Neurol 33*(10):696–705.
7. Olsen SL, Dejonge M, Kline A, *et al.* (2013) Optimizing therapeutic hypothermia for neonatal encephalopathy. *Pediatrics* **131**(2):e591–e603.

SECTION 18

NEPHROLOGY

CHAPTER 82

Haematuria

Leow Hui Min, Esther; Ng Yong Hong

Definition

Microscopic haematuria is defined by the presence of ≥5 red blood cells (RBC)/μL in an uncentrifuged urine sample. The diagnosis of gross haematuria is made when blood is present in the urine that is visible to the naked eye.

A positive urine dipstick is not good enough for diagnosis. A false-positive result may be caused by haemoglobinuria, myoglobinuria or improper use of strips. Urine may be discoloured by drugs, such as rifampicin, or food, such as beetroot. Urate crystals in the urine of infants may cause a pink discolouration to the nappy. Microscopic examination is essential to confirm haematuria.

Localising the Origin of Haematuria (Glomerular versus Non-Glomerular)

- Glomerular bleeding is suggested by the presence of RBC casts or granular casts.
- Urine phase contrast microscopy is performed on a fresh urine specimen. Glomerular haematuria yields RBCs with distortion and variation in shape and size (dysmorphic). Lower tract bleeding gives RBCs, which are uniform in shape and size (isomorphic). Sensitivity and specificity is over 90% in detecting glomerular haematuria. The microscopic haematuria is more likely glomerular in origin if >20–30% red blood cells are dysmorphic.
- Presence of white blood cells (WBC) casts suggests renal inflammation.

Table 18.1 Causes of Discolouration of Urine

Colour of Urine	Causes
Pink/red	Fresh blood (haematuria) Haemoglobinuria, myoglobinuria, porphyrins, urate Foods (e.g. beetroot, rhubarb, blackberries, red dyes, red dragon fruit) Drugs (e.g. chloroquine, chlorpromazine, desferrioxamine)
Brown	Oxidised haem pigment (blood from upper urinary tract or urine left standing for a long time) Bile pigments, methaemoglobinaemia, alkaptonuria Drugs (e.g. metronidazole, chloroquine, primaquine, nitrofurantoin)
Dark yellow or orange	Normal concentrated urine Foods containing carotene (e.g. papaya, carrots, pumpkin, etc.) Drugs (e.g. rifampicin, warfarin)

Table 18.2 Categories of Haematuria

	Symptomatic	Asymptomatic
Gross Haematuria	Symptomatic gross haematuria	Asymptomatic gross haematuria
Microscopic Haematuria	Symptomatic microscopic haematuria	Asymptomatic microscopic haematuria • Intermittent • Persistent • With proteinuria

Causes

Table 18.3 Causes of Haematuria in Children

Glomerular	Familial	• Thin basement membrane • Alport's syndrome • Hereditary angiopathy, nephropathy, aneurysms, muscle cramps syndrome • MYH9 syndromes (associated thrombocytopathies) • CFHR5 nephropathy (Greek Cypriot)
	Primary	• Post-infectious glomerulonephritis (GN) • Glomerulopathy • Membranous nephropathy • Rapidly progressive GN • IgA nephropathy
	Systemic/ secondary	• Systemic lupus erythematosus • Henoch Schönlein purpura • ANCA-associated vasculitis • Anti-glomerular basement GN • Haemolytic Uraemic Syndrome
Non-glomerular	• Infection: » Bacterial: ▪ Upper tract: Pyelonephritis (usually microscopic haematuria) ▪ Lower tract: Cystitis, urethritis, vulvitis, balanitis (gross haematuria is usually seen in cystitis) » Viruses: Adenovirus, cytomegalovirus, BK virus » Rare: Tuberculosis, schistosomiasis • Hypercalciuria with/without stones • Renal calculi • Malignancy » Renal: Nephroblastoma Bladder: Rhabdomyosarcoma • Trauma • Interstitial nephritis • Cystic renal disease • Renal vein involvement: Renal vein thrombosis, nutcracker syndrome • Chemical cystitis (e.g. cyclophosphamide) • Vascular malformations	
Extra-renal	• Strenuous exercise • Bleeding disorders: Haemophilia, thrombocytopaenia, sickle cell haemoglobinopathy • Factitious (e.g. menarche)	

History

- Associated symptoms
  - » Infection: Fever, dysuria, frequency, loin pain
  - » Stone disease: Pain, passage of 'sand'/stones
  - » Acute glomerulonephritis (AGN): Preceding upper respiratory tract infection or skin infection, oedema
  - » Secondary cause: Fever, rashes, arthralgia/arthritis
- Nature of haematuria: Terminal haematuria often suggests local causes such as urethritis/vulvitis
- Previous episodes of gross haematuria
- History of trauma
- Family history: Haematuria, proteinuria, hypertension, renal stones, renal failure, deafness, coagulopathy, polycystic kidney disease
- Drug history, e.g. medications, health supplements or herbal compounds

Clinical Examination

- Local examination
- Evidence of GN: Hypertension, oedema

Gross Haematuria

Investigations (Symptom-directed)

- Urine culture
- Urine calcium/creatinine ratio
- Full blood count
- Renal panel
- Clotting study where appropriate
- Complement level
- KUB (Kidney-Ureter-Bladder) X-Ray for radio-opaque calculi
- Renal ultrasound
- Other imaging studies/biochemical tests where appropriate

Treatment

- Treat underlying cause
- Follow-up till resolution

When to Refer to Paediatric Nephrologists (Inpatient/Outpatient)

- Persistent haematuria following treatment for urinary tract infection, e.g. cystitis
- Recurrent and/or painless gross haematuria
- Hypertension, abnormal renal function, presence of proteinuria or structural anomaly on renal ultrasound

Microscopic Haematuria

Asymptomatic microscopic haematuria is common. It is found in up to 4% of school-going children on urine screening. With repeated testing on three consecutive samples, <0.5% is positive.

What Do I Do in a Child with Microscopic Haematuria?

In the absence of proteinuria and symptoms, repeat urine microscopy. If persistent in at least three samples over one month, then proceed to investigate.

Investigations (Symptom-directed)

- Urinalysis (UFEME)
- Urine culture
- Urine protein/creatinine ratio (uPCR)
- Urine calcium/creatinine ratio
- Urine phase contrast microscopy
- Renal ultrasound
- Others as indicated

How Often Do I Follow Up if the Above Investigations are Normal?

3–6 monthly for a year and at each review, blood pressure, UFEME and uPCR should be performed together with an assessment for the development of new renal or systemic symptoms or family history of renal disease.

What if Protein is Detected?

Proteinuria is defined as uPCR >0.2 mg/mg or 20 mg/mmol creatinine. If proteinuria is detected with a random specimen, proceed to quantitate protein by doing timed urine collection. If >4 mg/m^2/hour, refer to a nephrologist. If <4 mg/m^2/hour, follow-up closely for development of proteinuria at subsequent reviews.

Indications for Renal Biopsy

- Associated significant proteinuria (40 mg/m^2/hour on timed urine collection)
- Azotaemia
- Hypertension
- Recurrent gross haematuria
- Family history of GN
- Systemic diseases (e.g. Systemic lupus erythematosus, ANCA-positive vasculitis)

Bibliography

1. Avner ED, Harmon WE, Niaudet P, *et al.* (2016) *Pediatric Nephrology, 7th ed.* Springer.
2. Milford DV, Robson AM. (2003) The child with abnormal urinalysis, haematuria and/or proteinuria. *Clinical Paediatric Nephrology, 3rd ed.* Oxford: Oxford University Press.
3. Diven SC, Travis LB. (2000) A practical primary care approach to haematuria in children. *Pediatr Nephrol* **14**(1):65–72.

4. Ahmad G, Segasothy M, Morad Z. (1993) Urinary erythrocyte morphology as a diagnostic aid in haematuria. *Sing Med J* **34**(6):486–488.
5. Dalrymple RA, Ramage IJ. (2017) Fifteen-minute consultation: The management of microscopic haematuria. *Arch Dis Child Educ Pract Ed* **102**(5):230–234.
6. Geary DF, Schaefer F. (2016) *Pediatric Kidney Disease, 2nd ed.* Berlin: Springer-Verlag.

CHAPTER 83

Acute Nephritic Syndrome

Leow Hui Min, Esther; Ng Yong Hong

Definition

Sudden onset of symptoms of glomerular injury (haematuria, hypertension, oedema) and varying degrees of renal insufficiency.

Differential Diagnoses

- Post-infectious:
  - Bacterial:
    - Group A ß-haemolytic *Streptococcus* (most common)
    - *Pneumococcus* sp.
    - *Staphylococcus* sp.
    - *Klebsiella* sp.
    - *Meningococcus* sp.
    - *Salmonella typhi*
    - *Mycoplasma pneumoniae*
  - Viral:
    - Human immunodeficiency virus
    - Coxsackie
    - Epstein–Barr
    - Hepatitis B
    - Influenza
    - Mumps
- Primarily renal disease
  - IgA nephropathy
  - C3 glomerulopathy
  - Hereditary nephritis (Alport's Syndrome)
- Systemic involvement
  - Henoch–Schönlein purpura with nephritis
  - Systemic lupus erythematosus (SLE)
  - ANCA-associated vasculitis
  - Anti-glomerular basement membrane disease
  - Infective Endocarditis related
  - Shunt nephritis

History

- Symptoms in relation to underlying cause
  - » History of upper respiratory tract infection 1 to 2 weeks prior to onset of acute glomerulonephritis (AGN)
  - » History of skin infection prior to onset of AGN. Latent period between pyoderma and onset of AGN is variable.
  - » Systemic symptoms: Fever, malaise, anorexia, arthritis, rash (systemic and extra renal symptoms are often seen in SLE nephritis)
- Urinary tract symptoms
  - » Oliguria
  - » Painless gross haematuria (typically described as 'coke', 'tea' or 'smoky')
- Symptoms in relation to fluid overload
  - » Facial swelling and/or generalised oedema
  - » Dyspnoea, exercise intolerance (pulmonary oedema)
- Cerebral complications of hypertension, including headaches, seizures, mental status changes and visual changes
- Family history of autoimmune disorders, renal failure (dialysis/kidney transplantation), haematuria, early onset hearing loss

Physical Examination

- Hypertension
- Oedema, e.g. ascites, pedal and/or periorbital oedema
- Circulatory congestion: Tachypnoea, tachycardia, cardiomegaly, hepatomegaly, raised jugular venous pressure, crepitations in the lungs

Table 18.4 Investigations

Investigation	
Urinalysis (UFEME)	Dysmorphic red blood cell (RBC), RBC casts White blood cell (WBC), WBC casts Proteinuria (proportional to RBC)
Renal panel	Elevated blood urea and creatinine
Full blood count	Anaemia (as in SLE) ± leucocytosis Leucopenia, especially lymphopenia is seen in SLE Thrombocytopenia in SLE
Bacteriological and serological studies	Throat swab (may be negative if treated) Elevated Anti-Streptolysin O titer (ASOT)
Immunological markers	Hypocomplementemia (CH50, C3, C4) Autoimmune markers: Elevated double-stranded DNA, Anti-Nuclear Antibody titers in SLE
Radiology	Chest X-ray: Cardiomegaly, pulmonary congestion/oedema Renal ultrasound: Non-specific echogenic kidneys

Management

- Monitoring: Strict intake and output charting, daily weight, blood pressure monitoring at least 4 hourly or closer interval as determined by clinical severity
- Supportive/symptomatic
  - » Bed rest
  - » Supplemental oxygen and loop diuretics (frusemide) if hypoxia from pulmonary oedema
- Salt and water restriction to insensible water loss (400 ml/m^2/day) plus half urine output
  - » Frequent re-evaluation of fluid status and fluid balance to determine fluid requirement/restriction
- Treatment of hypertension
  - » Drugs that can be used include loop diuretics (frusemide), calcium channel blocker or hydralazine (hydralazine is contraindicated in patients with SLE)
  - » If severe, refer to chapter on Hypertension
- Antibiotics indicated in patients with positive cultures. Penicillin is the drug of choice (erythromycin in allergic individuals) for streptococcal infections

Natural History

Resolution of:

Gross haematuria	2 weeks
Oliguria	2 weeks
Azotaemia	2 weeks
Hypertension	4 weeks
Decreased C3	6 weeks
Proteinuria	6 months
Microscopic haematuria	12 months

Indications for Renal Biopsy

- Severe renal failure of unknown/uncertain aetiology
- Atypical features such as co-existing Nephrotic Syndrome
- Delayed resolution

Prognosis

- Excellent in post-streptococcal AGN, with restoration of renal function in more than 90%
- Rapidly progressing glomerulonephritis (RPGN) in 1%

Bibliography

1. Smith JM, Faizan MK, Eddy AA. (2003) The child with acute nephritic syndrome. *Clinical Paediatric Nephrology, 3rd ed.* Oxford: Oxford University Press.
2. Barratt M, Avner E, Harmon B (eds.). (1999) *Pediatric Nephrology, 4th ed.* Lippincott Williams & Wilkins.
3. Eison TM, Ault BH, Jones DP, *et al.* (2011) Post-streptococcal acute glomerulonephritis in children: clinical features and pathogenesis. *Pediatr Nephrol* **26**(2):165–180.
4. Welch TR. (2012) An approach to the child with acute glomerulonephritis. *Int J Pediatr* 2012:426192.

CHAPTER 84

Nephrotic Syndrome

Chao Sing Ming; Yap Jia Ying, Celeste

Introduction

Nephrotic Syndrome (NS) is a syndrome defined clinically by Kidney Disease: Improving Global Outcomes (KDIGO) 2021 guideline as:

- Heavy proteinuria (nephrotic range) with urine protein/creatinine ratio (uPCR) ≥2 (mg/mg) or urine total protein (UTP) ≥3 g/L (random sample) or ≥40 mg/m^2/h (timed sample) and the presence of either
- Low serum albumin <30 g/L <u>or</u>
- Oedema when serum albumin level is not available

Hyperlipidaemia is not required for the diagnosis of NS.

Over 80% of childhood NS are Idiopathic NS (INS) with no clear cause. It is presumably an immune mediated disorder that leads to glomerular podocyte dysfunction, resulting in increased protein permeability and massive urinary protein loss. The vast majority of INS will show minimal glomerular changes on histology except for podocyte effacement. Other histological diagnoses include Diffuse Mesangial Proliferation, Focal Segmental Glomerulosclerosis (FSGS), rarely membranous and membranoproliferative glomerulonephritis.

INS by itself is not common (incidence of 1.15–16.9 per 100000 children). However, it is an important and prevalent cause of generalised oedema in children and a major presenting symptom of childhood glomerulonephritis.

Non-INS with known causes include genetic causes, secondary to systemic disease like systemic lupus erythematosus (SLE), Haemolytic Uraemic Syndrome (HUS) and IgA nephropathy, and rarer causes include infections, drugs or neoplasia.

Clinical Classifications and Defintions

- Steroid responsiveness is of greater clinical and prognostic value than histology in INS. Renal biopsy is therefore not needed in the management of most children with INS.
- **Clinical response to steroid** therapy and the **clinical course** guide the management and prognosis of INS. Thus, the broad clinical classification into Steroid Sensitive Nephrotic Syndrome (**SSNS**), found in over 80% of patients, and Steroid Resistant Nephrotic Syndrome (**SRNS**), found in 10–20% of patients.

Table 18.5 Definitions (KDIGO 2021)

Complete Remission	Urine total protein (UTP) <0.2 g/L or urine protein/creatinine ratio (uPCR) <0.2 (mg/mg) or dipstick protein nil/trace for 3 or more consecutive days.
Partial Remission	Decrease in proteinuria of ≥50% over presenting value or uPCR between 0.2 and 2 (mg/mg) or dipstick protein 1+ to 2+ or serum albumin 30 g/L or more.
Steroid response/ sensitive	Remission achieved within 4 wk of steroid therapy.
Relapse	UTP ≥ 3 g/L or uPCR ≥2 (mg/mg) or dipstick protein ≥3+ for 3 consecutive days with or without oedema. Oedema is a clear sign of relapse.
Frequent relapses	2 or more relapses within 6 mth of initial response, or 4 or more relapses within any 12-mth period.
Steroid dependence	2 consecutive relapses during steroid treatment or 1 relapse within 2 wk of its cessation.
Steroid resistance	Failure to achieve remission after 4 wk of daily steroid therapy at 60 mg/m^2/d.
Late steroid resistance	Steroid resistance develops after being steroid sensitive previously.

Management of SRNS, being a heterogeneous syndrome, is complex and will not be covered in this chapter.

- The **clinical course** further divides SSNS into no relapse or infrequent relapsing NS, which is seen in about half of SSNS patients and frequent relapsing NS (**FRNS**) or steroid-dependent NS (**SDNS**) in the remaining half. While infrequent relapsing NS responds well to steroid treatment with prolonged remissions, FRNS and especially SDNS require prolonged steroid and steroid sparing immunosuppression therapy to maintain remission, resulting in more side effects of treatment that require regular monitoring.
- The clinical response and clinical course should be clearly defined and firmly established to form the basis of treatment (Table 18.5).

There are several distinct histological types of INS:

1. Minimal Change Disease (MCNS) seen in 80% cases typically presents as SSNS. Variants, including IgM, mesangial proliferation and C1q glomerulonephritis, often present with FRNS and SDNS, which are more difficult to treat.
2. FSGS often presents as SRNS or late steroid resistance.
3. Membranous and membranoproliferative nephropathy are rarer and often present as SRNS.

Investigations

- Confirm diagnosis: Urinalysis, UTP or uPCR, serum albumin. Diagnosis of heavy proteinuria is usually straightforward and does not require timed measurement.

- Full blood count: Haemoconcentration, if present, is due to intravascular contraction and may increase the risk of thrombosis.
- Renal panel: Dilutional hyponatremia due to over-hydration; azotaemia due to pre-renal dehydration.
- Other investigations, e.g. chest X-ray, urine/blood culture are guided by clinical indications.
- Screening tests for systemic disease (e.g. SLE) to be done only if there are clinical suspicion (e.g. systemic symptoms, haematological abnormalities, nephritic symptoms and signs).

Principles of Treatment and Management

1. **To induce remission and treat complications**
   - Prednisolone is the mainstay of treatment (see Tables 18.6 and 18.7).
   - Important to monitor steroid side effects. Explain to parents the side effects and action plans.
   - Complications of NS include:
     » Infections: Cellulitis, spontaneous peritonitis, pneumonia (prone to *Streptococcus pneumoniae* infections and thus empirical use of high dose ampicillin or ceftriaxone), varicella infection, pulmonary tuberculosis.
     » Shock/pre-shock: NS patients are more prone to intravascular contraction from fluid loss. Triggers include diarrhoea, vomiting and sepsis. Look for symptoms of hypovolaemia, oliguria, pre-renal acute kidney injury with low urinary sodium (FeNa <1%) and raised haematocrit.
     » Treat with intravenous (IV) normal saline 20 ml/kg over 1 to 2 hours if urgent or IV 20% albumin 1 g/kg over 2 to 4 hours with continuous blood pressure (BP) and vital signs monitoring.
     » Venous thromboembolism (renal vein, cerebral sinus venous, pulmonary embolism): rare but can be serious and may require anticoagulation.
     » Hyponatraemia with seizures (often due to rapid IV over-hydration). Needs IV albumin and frusemide.
2. **Symptomatic treatment**
   - Most patients do not require albumin and frusemide for the relief of oedema while awaiting response to steroid.
   - Indications for quick relief of oedema include severe ascites, scrotal oedema, labial oedema and hyponatraemia with central nervous system symptoms. As this therapy may not be sustained and effective, repeated infusions may be needed.
   - Note that indiscriminate use of albumin in some patients who do not have signs and symptoms of hypovolaemia can result in rapid intravascular expansion and precipitate pulmonary oedema.
   - IV albumin is given as 20% albumin at 1–1.5 g/kg (preparation as 10 g per 50 ml bottle, avoid wastage) over 4 to 6 hours. IV frusemide 1–3 mg/kg/dose is given at midway and at the end of infusion.
   - Fluid restriction is needed only in severe oedema in an otherwise stable patient (restrict up to two-third normal).

Table 18.6 Prednisolone Regime for Initial Presentation of NS

Duration	Dosage (as a Single Dose)
4 wk	60 mg/m²/d (max. 60 mg)
4 wk	40 mg/m²/alternate days (max. 40 mg)
4 weeks of tapering	30 mg/m²/alternate days (max. 30 mg) for 8 d, 20 mg/m²/alternate days (max. 20 mg) for 8 d, 10 mg/m²/alternate days (max. 10 mg) for 12 d
Total duration should be at least 12 wk	

Table 18.7 Prednisolone Regime for Relapse of NS

Prednisolone as 60 mg/m²/day (max. 60 mg) until complete remission for 5 consecutive days. Maintenance therapy varies according to clinical course.		
Maintenance regimes:		
Relapse	**Duration (maintenance)**	**Dosage (single dose)**
Infrequent	At least 4 wk	Prednisolone at EOD doses starting at 60 mg/m², reducing by 10 mg/m² every 8 d till 10 mg/m²
FRNS and SDNS	EOD prednisolone for 3–6 mth	Use lowest dose to maintain remission without major side effects (usually at the dose when last relapse occurred). Consider steroid-sparing drugs.

$$\text{Surface area } (\text{m}^2) = \sqrt{\frac{\text{Weight (kg)} \times \text{Height (cm)}}{3600}}$$

- No additional salt intake. Strict salt restriction is unnecessary, unlike treatment for acute glomerulonephritis, which can cause significant fluid overload.

3. **Early detection and treatment of relapse**
    - Home monitoring and caretaker education is essential. Refer to patient information pamphlet and nephrotic diary.
4. **Monitor untoward steroid side effects**
    - Monitor growth, BP and refer ophthalmologist to screen for posterior subcapsular cataract or glaucoma if steroid treatment is prolonged beyond 6 months.
    - Refer patients with FRNS and SDNS to nephrology for further management and steroid sparing therapy.

Points to Remember

1. Indications of hospitalisation include:
    - Severe oedema that may require IV albumin/frusemide.
    - Presence or suspect complications (see above).
    - NS with systemic symptoms that require further workup and specific treatment.

2. First clinical response to steroid treatment will be an increase in urine output and weight loss (often before resolution of proteinuria), occurring after 7–10 days of prednisolone treatment.
3. Patient can be safely discharged if clinically stable and caregiver understands clearly home monitoring and action plans (Refer to your institution's clinical pathway for uncomplicated INS). Complete remission occurs after 2–4 weeks of treatment (80% by end of 2 weeks, 90% by end of 3 weeks).
4. Relapses are expected in most patients and parents need to be forewarned and to monitor for possible relapse.
5. Home dipstick protein monitoring to detect early relapse can avoid unnecessary admissions. Intercurrent infection, especially upper respiratory tract infection (URTI), may induce unsustained proteinuria. If there is no oedema and improving trend in urine protein to <3+ after 5 days, treatment for relapse is unnecessary. However, it is important to continue outpatient monitoring.
6. Parent or caregiver education is important for long-term management. Exclude noncompliance in treatment failure (as in most chronic illnesses) and address this issue before considering steroid resistance.
7. Complete resolution of NS can be considered if patient remains well with no proteinuria after 4 consecutive years. A small proportion of patients may continue to relapse into adulthood with a less favourable outcome.

Clinical features for non-MCNS that require referral to nephrologist for renal biopsy and management include:

- Steroid resistance
- Gross haematuria
- Family history of NS
- Hypertension
- Non pre-renal azotaemia
- Evidence of systemic disease
- Relative indication for age of onset <1 year or >12 years (onset <3 months: congenital NS, 3–12 months: possible genetic NS, congenital infections, >12 years: higher risk of non-MCNS).

Treatment Regimes

General Considerations

- Recommended treatment for initial presentation is quite well established with randomised controlled trials and good quality evidence (grade B), while suggested treatment for relapses is less well established (grade C–D).
- Documenting hypoalbuminaemia is not necessary for the diagnosis of relapse.
- Eighty per cent of childhood INS are MCNS with 93% being SSNS. MCNS has an excellent prognosis with no long-term renal morbidity.
- Morbidity is mainly seen in FRNS, especially SDNS due to complications of the nephrotic state and steroid side effects (especially retarded growth, infections,

eye complications, hypertension), which necessitates the use of steroid-sparing drugs (cyclophosphamide, cyclosporine, mycophenolate mofetil, rituximab).
- All immunosuppressive drugs have significant side effects and their use requires documenting clear indications, parental consent, explanation of side effects and regular monitoring.

Treatment of Relapse NS as Outpatient

1. **Non-oedematous patient**
   - Treat after ascertaining sustained proteinuria, i.e. UTP ≥3 g/L or dipstick protein ≥3+ for >3 consecutive days.
   - Unsustained proteinuria may occur with intercurrent infection or URTI, but proteinuria should improve after 3 to 5 days. Up to 25% of the relapses remit spontaneously and therapy is unnecessary.

2. **Oedematous patient** (swelling, sudden weight gain in the presence of significant proteinuria of >2+) should be treated as relapse irrespective of the duration of proteinuria.

Immunisations

- Immunisations with inactivated vaccines (Diphtheria, pertussis and tetanus, pneumococcal, Haemophilus influenzae type B, hepatitis B, influenza, Salk polio, meningococcal), in general, will not be harmful but more likely to be effective when given to a patient who is in remission or on low dose alternate day prednisolone.
- Live attenuated vaccination (Mumps, measles and rubella, oral polio, varicella, Bacillus Calmette-Guerin) may be harmful to patients with ongoing steroid or other immunosuppressive treatment and should be deferred until patient is off treatment for 3 to 6 months.
- Timely pneumococcal vaccination is advisable as patients with NS are particularly prone to pneumococcal infection.
- Consult paediatric infectious disease specialist if in doubt.

Prognosis

Prognosis is excellent in SSNS (<5% progress to chronic renal failure in 10 years) but significant side effects of therapy may incur in FRNS, especially SDNS, and it is crucial to balance efficacy with the side effects of treatment. SRNS, being heterogeneous, has varying prognosis but its prognosis is generally much worse, with 50% patients with FSGS progressing to end-stage renal failure in 5 years.

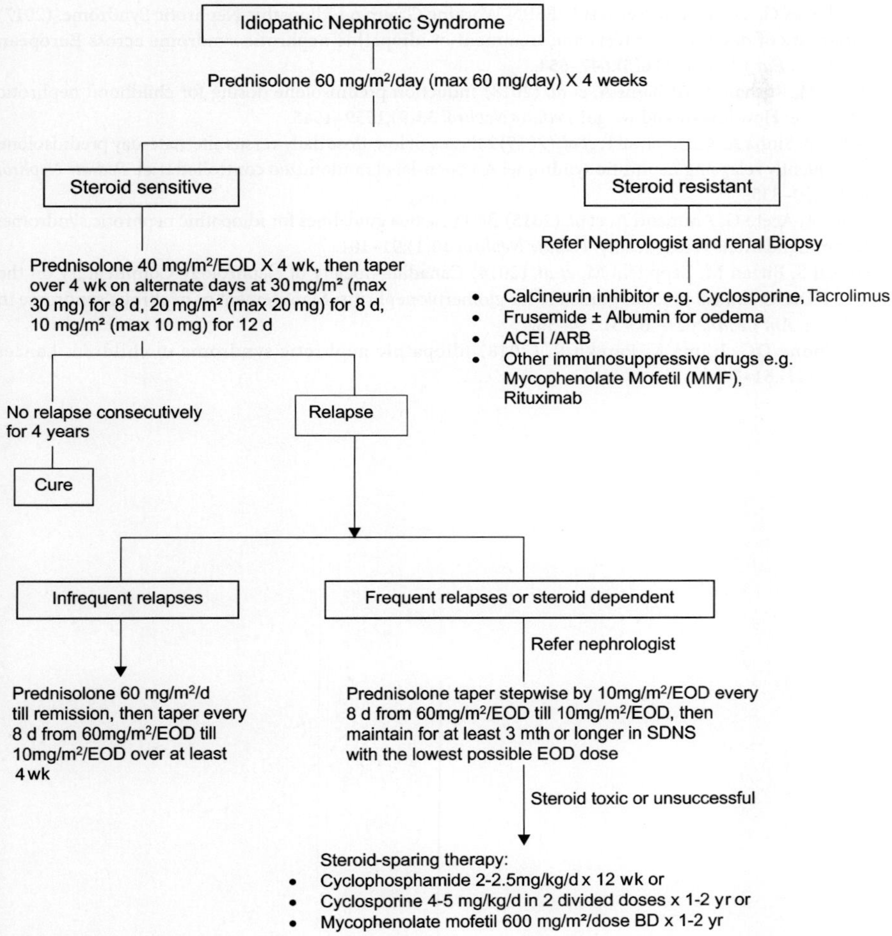

Figure 18.1 Algorithm for the management of childhood idiopathic nephrotic syndrome.

Bibliography

1. Kidney Disease: Improving Global Outcomes (KDIGO) Glomerular Disease Work Group. (2021) KDIGO 2021 Clinical Practice Guideline for the management of glomerular diseases. *Kidney Int* **100**(4S):S1–S276.
2. Hodson EM, Knight JF, Willis NS, Craig JC. (2000) Corticosteroid therapy in nephrotic syndrome: A meta-analysis of randomised controlled trials. *Arch Dis Child* **83**(1):45–51.
3. Esfahani ST, Madani A, Asgharian F, *et al.* (2011) Clinical course and outcome of children with steroid-sensitive nephrotic syndrome. *Pediatr Nephrol* **26**(7):1089–1093.
4. Webb NJA, Woolley RL, Lambe T, *et al.* (2019) Long term tapering versus standard prednisolone treatment for first episode of childhood nephrotic syndrome: Phase III randomised controlled trial and economic evaluation. *BMJ* **365**:l1800.

5. Deschenes G, Vivarelli M, Peruzzi L; ESPN Working Group on Idiopathic Nephrotic Syndrome. (2017) Variability of diagnostic criteria and treatment of idiopathic nephrotic syndrome across European countries. *Eur J Pediatr* **176**(5):647–654.
6. Sibley M, Roshan A, Alshami A, *et al.* (2018) Induction prednisolone dosing for childhood nephrotic syndrome: How low should we go? *Pediatr Nephrol* **33**(9):1539–1545.
7. Yadav M, Sinha A, Khandelwal P, *et al.* (2019) Efficacy of low-dose daily versus alternate-day prednisolone in frequently relapsing nephrotic syndrome: An open-label randomized controlled trial. *Pediatr Nephrol* **34**(5):829–835.
8. Pasini A, Aceto G, Ammenti A, *et al.* (2015) Best practice guidelines for idiopathic nephrotic syndrome: Recommendations versus reality. *Pediatr Nephrol* **30**(1):91–101.
9. Samuel S, Bitzan M, Zappitelli M, *et al.* (2014) Canadian Society of Nephrology Commentary on the 2012 KDIGO clinical practice guideline for glomerulonephritis: Management of nephrotic syndrome in children. *Am J Kidney Dis* **63**(3):354–362.
10. 10. Noone DG, Iijima K, Parekh R. (2018) Idiopathic nephrotic syndrome in children. Lancet 392(10141):61–74.

CHAPTER 85

Hypertension

Leow Hui Min, Esther; Ng Yong Hong

Definition

Defined as average systolic blood pressure (SBP) and/or diastolic blood pressure (DBP) that is ≥95th percentile for gender, age and height on ≥3 occasions.* Refer to blood pressure (BP) level charts below for both genders based on age and height centiles.
**except children with stage 2 hypertension or a child with symptomatic hypertension*

When should Blood Pressure be Measured?

- Children above the age of 3 who are seen in medical care settings should have their BP measured at least once during every clinic visit.
- Children less than 3 years old should have their BP measured in special circumstances:
  - » History of prematurity, very low birth weight or other neonatal complication requiring intensive care
  - » Congenital heart disease (repaired or un-repaired)
  - » Recurrent urinary tract infections, haematuria or proteinuria
  - » Known renal disease or urologic malformations
  - » Family history of congenital renal disease
  - » Solid-organ transplant

Table 18.8 Definitions of Blood Pressure Categories and Stages

	1–13 Years Old	≥13 Years Old
Normal blood pressure	<90th percentile	<120/<80 mmHg
Elevated blood pressure	≥90th percentile to <95th percentile or 120/80 mmHg to <95th percentile (whichever is lower)	120/<80 to 129/<80 mmHg
Stage 1 hypertension	≥95th percentile to <95th percentile + 12 mmHg, or 130/80 to 139/89 mmHg (whichever is lower)	130/80 to 139/89 mmHg
Stage 2 hypertension	≥95th percentile + 12 mmHg, or ≥140/90 mmHg (whichever is lower)	≥140/90 mmHg

Table 18.9 Blood Pressure Levels for Boys by Age and Height

Age	BP Centile		Height Percentile or Measured Height						
		Height Percentile	5%	10%	25%	50%	75%	90%	95%
1		Height in cm	77.2	78.3	80.2	82.4	84.6	86.7	87.9
	50th	SBP/DBP	85/40	85/40	86/40	86/41	87/41	88/42	88/42
	90th	SBP/DBP	98/52	99/52	99/53	100/53	100/54	101/54	101/54
	95th	SBP/DBP	102/54	102/54	103/55	103/55	104/56	105/57	105/57
	95th + 12 mmHg	SBP/DBP	114/66	114/66	115/67	115/67	116/68	117/69	117/69
2		Height in cm	86.1	87.4	89.6	92.1	94.7	97.1	98.5
	50th	SBP / DBP	87 / 43	87 / 43	88 / 44	89 / 44	89 / 45	90 / 46	91/46
	90th	SBP / DBP	100 / 55	100 / 55	101 / 56	102 / 56	103 / 57	103 / 58	104/58
	95th	SBP / DBP	104 / 57	105 / 58	105 / 58	106 / 59	107 / 60	107 / 61	108/61
	95th + 12 mmHg	SBP / DBP	116 / 69	117 / 70	117 / 70	118 / 71	119 / 72	119 / 73	120/73
3		Height in cm	92.5	93.9	96.3	99	101.8	104.3	105.8
	50th	SBP / DBP	88 / 45	89 / 46	89 / 46	90 / 47	91 / 48	92 / 49	92/49
	90th	SBP / DBP	101 / 58	102 / 58	102 / 59	103 / 59	104 / 60	105 / 61	105/61
	95th	SBP / DBP	106 / 60	106 / 61	107 / 61	107 / 62	108 / 63	109 / 64	109/64
	95th + 12 mmHg	SBP / DBP	118 / 72	118 / 73	119 / 73	119 / 74	120 / 75	121 / 76	121/76
4		Height in cm	98.5	100.2	102.9	105.9	108.9	111.5	113.2
	50th	SBP / DBP	90 / 48	90 / 49	91 / 49	92 / 50	93 / 51	94 / 52	94/52
	90th	SBP / DBP	102 / 60	103 / 61	104 / 62	105 / 62	105 / 63	106 / 64	107/64
	95th	SBP / DBP	107 / 63	107 / 64	108 / 65	108 / 66	109 / 67	110 / 67	110/68
	95th + 12 mmHg	SBP / DBP	119 / 75	119 / 76	120 / 77	120 / 78	121 / 79	122 / 79	122/80

5		Height in cm	104.4	106.2	109.1	112.4	115.7	118.6	120.3
	50th	SBP / DBP	91 / 51	92 / 51	93 / 52	94 / 53	95 / 54	96 / 55	96/55
	90th	SBP / DBP	103 / 63	104 / 64	105 / 65	106 / 65	107 / 66	108 / 67	108/67
	95th	SBP / DBP	107 / 66	108 / 67	109 / 68	109 / 69	110 / 70	111 / 70	112/71
	95th + 12 mmHg	SBP / DBP	119 / 78	120 / 79	121 / 80	121 / 81	122 / 82	123 / 82	124/83
6		Height in cm	110.3	112.2	115.3	118.9	122.4	125.6	127.5
	50th	SBP / DBP	93 / 54	93 / 54	94 / 55	95 / 56	96 / 57	97 / 57	98/58
	90th	SBP / DBP	105 / 66	105 / 66	106 / 67	107 / 68	109 / 68	110 / 69	110/69
	95th	SBP / DBP	108 / 69	109 / 70	110 / 70	111 / 71	112 / 72	113 / 72	114/73
	95th + 12 mmHg	SBP / DBP	120 / 81	121 / 82	122 / 82	123 / 83	124 / 84	125 / 84	126/85
7		Height in cm	116.1	118	121.4	125.1	128.9	132.4	134.5
	50th	SBP / DBP	94 / 56	94 / 56	95 / 57	97 / 58	98 / 58	98 / 59	99/59
	90th	SBP / DBP	106 / 68	107 / 68	108 / 69	109 / 70	110 / 70	111 / 71	111/71
	95th	SBP / DBP	110 / 71	110 / 71	111 / 72	112 / 73	114 / 73	115 / 74	116/74
	95th + 12 mmHg	SBP / DBP	122 / 83	122 / 83	123 / 84	124 / 85	126 / 85	127 / 86	128/86
8		Height in cm	121.4	123.5	127	131	135.1	138.8	141
	50th	SBP / DBP	95 / 57	96 / 57	97 / 58	98 / 59	99 / 59	99 / 60	100/60
	90th	SBP / DBP	107 / 69	108 / 70	109 / 70	110 / 71	111 / 72	112 / 72	112/73
	95th	SBP / DBP	111 / 72	112 / 73	112 / 73	114 / 74	115 / 75	116 / 75	117/75
	95th + 12 mmHg	SBP / DBP	123 / 84	124 / 85	124 / 85	126 / 86	127 / 87	128 / 87	129/87
9		Height in cm	126	128.3	132.1	136.3	140.7	144.7	147.1
	50th	SBP / DBP	96 / 57	97 / 58	98 / 59	99 / 60	100 / 61	101 / 62	101/62
	90th	SBP / DBP	107 / 70	108 / 71	109 / 72	110 / 73	112 / 74	113 / 74	114/74
	95th	SBP / DBP	112 / 74	112 / 74	113 / 75	115 / 76	116 / 76	118 / 77	119/77

(Continued)

Table 18.9 (*Continued*)

Age	BP Centile		Height Percentile or Measured Height						
		Height Percentile	5%	10%	25%	50%	75%	90%	95%
	95th + 12 mmHg	SBP / DBP	124 / 86	124 / 86	125 / 87	127 / 88	128 / 88	130 / 89	131/89
10		Height in cm	130.2	132.7	136.7	141.3	145.9	150.1	152.7
	50th	SBP / DBP	97 / 59	98 / 60	99 / 61	100 / 62	101 / 63	102 / 63	103/64
	90th	SBP / DBP	108 / 72	109 / 73	111 / 74	112 / 74	113 / 75	115 / 75	116/76
	95th	SBP / DBP	112 / 76	113 / 76	114 / 77	116 / 77	118 / 78	120 / 78	121/78
	95th + 12 mmHg	SBP / DBP	124 / 88	125 / 88	126 / 89	128 / 89	130 / 90	132 / 90	133/90
11		Height in cm	134.7	137.3	141.5	146.4	151.3	155.8	158.6
	50th	SBP / DBP	99 / 61	99 / 61	101 / 62	102 / 63	103 / 63	104 / 63	106/63
	90th	SBP / DBP	110 / 74	111 / 74	112 / 75	114 / 75	116 / 75	117 / 76	118/76
	95th	SBP / DBP	114 / 77	114 / 78	116 / 78	118 / 78	120 / 78	123 / 78	124/78
	95th + 12 mmHg	SBP / DBP	126 / 89	126 / 90	128 / 90	130 / 90	132 / 90	135 / 90	136/90
12		Height in cm	140.3	143	147.5	152.7	157.9	162.6	165.5
	50th	SBP / DBP	101 / 61	101 / 62	102 / 62	104 / 62	106 / 62	108 / 63	109/63
	90th	SBP / DBP	113 / 75	114 / 75	115 / 75	117 / 75	119 / 75	121 / 76	122/76
	95th	SBP / DBP	116 / 78	117 / 78	118 / 78	121 / 78	124 / 78	126 / 79	128/79
	95th + 12 mmHg	SBP / DBP	128 / 90	129 / 90	130 / 90	133 / 90	136 / 90	138 / 91	140/91
13		Height in cm	147	150	154.9	160.3	165.7	170.5	173.4
	50th	SBP / DBP	103 / 61	104 / 60	105 / 61	108 / 62	110 / 63	111 / 64	112 / 65
	90th	SBP / DBP	115 / 74	116 / 74	118 / 74	121 / 75	124 / 76	126 / 77	126 / 77
	95th	SBP / DBP	119 / 78	120 / 78	122 / 78	125 / 78	128 / 80	130 / 81	131 / 81
	95th + 12 mmHg	SBP / DBP	131 / 90	132 / 90	134 / 90	137 / 90	140 / 92	142 / 93	143 / 93

14		Height in cm	153.8	156.9	162	167.5	172.7	177.4	180.1
	50th	SBP / DBP	105 / 60	106 / 60	109 / 62	111 / 64	112 / 65	113 / 66	113 / 67
	90th	SBP / DBP	119 / 74	120 / 74	123 / 75	126 / 77	127 / 78	128 / 79	129 / 80
	95th	SBP / DBP	123 / 77	125 / 78	127 / 79	130 / 81	132 / 82	133 / 83	134 / 84
	95th + 12 mmHg	SBP / DBP	135 / 89	137 / 90	139 / 91	142 / 93	144 / 94	145 / 95	146 / 96
15		Height in cm	159	162	166.9	172.2	177.2	181.6	184.2
	50th	SBP / DBP	108 / 61	110 / 62	112 / 64	113 / 65	114 / 66	114 / 67	114 / 68
	90th	SBP / DBP	123 / 75	124 / 76	126 / 78	128 / 79	129 / 80	130 / 81	130 / 81
	95th	SBP / DBP	127 / 78	129 / 79	131 / 81	132 / 83	134 / 84	135 / 85	135 / 85
	95th + 12 mmHg	SBP / DBP	139 / 90	141 / 91	143 / 93	144 / 95	146 / 96	147 / 97	147 / 97
16		Height in cm	162.1	165	169.6	174.6	179.5	183.8	186.4
	50th	SBP / DBP	111 / 63	112 / 64	114 / 66	115 / 67	115 / 68	116 / 69	116 / 69
	90th	SBP / DBP	126 / 77	127 / 78	128 / 79	129 / 80	131 / 81	131 / 82	132 / 82
	95th	SBP / DBP	130 / 80	131 / 81	133 / 83	134 / 84	135 / 85	136 / 86	137 / 86
	95th + 12 mmHg	SBP / DBP	142 / 92	143 / 93	145 / 95	146 / 96	147 / 97	149 / 98	149 / 98
17		Height in cm	163.8	166.5	170.9	175.8	180.7	184.9	187.5
	50th	SBP / DBP	114 / 65	115 / 66	116 / 67	117 / 68	117 / 69	118 / 70	118 / 70
	90th	SBP / DBP	128 / 78	129 / 79	130 / 80	131 / 81	132 / 82	133 / 82	134 / 83
	95th	SBP / DBP	132 / 81	133 / 82	134 / 84	135 / 85	137 / 86	138 / 86	138 / 87
	95th + 12 mmHg	SBP / DBP	144 / 93	145 / 94	146 / 96	147 / 97	149 / 98	150 / 98	150 / 99

Adapted from Flynn JT, et al. (2017) Clinical practice guideline for screening and management of high blood pressure in children and adolescents. Pediatrics ***140****(3).*

Table 18.10 Blood Pressure Levels for Girls by Age and Height

Age	BP Centile		Height Percentile or Measured Height						
		Height Percentile	5%	10%	25%	50%	75%	90%	95%
1		Height in cm	75.4	76.6	78.6	80.8	83	84.9	86.1
	50th	SBP / DBP	84 / 41	85 / 42	86 / 42	86 / 43	87 / 44	88 / 45	88 / 46
	90th	SBP / DBP	98 / 54	99 / 55	99 / 56	100 / 56	101 / 57	102 / 58	102 / 58
	95th	SBP / DBP	101 / 59	102 / 59	102 / 60	103 / 60	104 / 61	105 / 62	105 / 62
	95th + 12 mmHg	SBP / DBP	113 / 71	114 / 71	115 / 72	115 / 72	116 / 73	117 / 74	117 / 74
2		Height in cm	86.1	87.4	89.6	92.1	94.7	97.1	98.5
	50th	SBP / DBP	87 / 45	87 / 46	88 / 47	89 / 48	90 / 49	91 / 50	91 / 51
	90th	SBP / DBP	101 / 58	101 / 58	102 / 59	103 / 60	104 / 61	105 / 62	106 / 62
	95th	SBP / DBP	104 / 62	105 / 63	106 / 63	106 / 64	107 / 65	108 / 66	109 / 66
	95th + 12 mmHg	SBP / DBP	116 / 74	117 / 75	118 / 75	118 / 76	119 / 77	120 / 78	121 / 78
3		Height in cm	91	92.4	94.9	97.6	100.5	103.1	104.6
	50th	SBP / DBP	88 / 48	89 / 48	89 / 49	90 / 50	91 / 51	92 / 53	93 / 53
	90th	SBP / DBP	102 / 60	103 / 61	104 / 61	104 / 62	105 / 63	106 / 64	107 / 65
	95th	SBP / DBP	106 / 64	106 / 65	107 / 65	108 / 66	109 / 67	110 / 68	110 / 69
	95th + 12 mmHg	SBP / DBP	118 / 76	118 / 77	119 / 77	120 / 78	121 / 79	122 / 80	122 / 81
4		Height in cm	97.2	98.8	101.4	104.5	107.6	110.5	112.2
	50th	SBP / DBP	89 / 50	90 / 51	91 / 51	92 / 53	93 / 54	94 / 55	94 / 55
	90th	SBP / DBP	103 / 62	104 / 63	105 / 64	106 / 65	107 / 66	108 / 67	108 / 67
	95th	SBP / DBP	107 / 66	108 / 67	109 / 68	109 / 69	110 / 70	111 / 70	112 / 71
	95th + 12 mmHg	SBP / DBP	119 / 78	120 / 79	121 / 80	121 / 81	122 / 82	123 / 82	124 / 83

5		Height in cm	103.6	105.3	108.2	111.5	114.9	118.1	120
	50th	SBP / DBP	90 / 52	91 / 52	92 / 53	93 / 55	94 / 56	95 / 57	96 / 57
	90th	SBP / DBP	104 / 64	105 / 65	106 / 66	107 / 67	108 / 68	109 / 69	110 / 70
	95th	SBP / DBP	108 / 68	109 / 69	109 / 70	110 / 71	111 / 72	112 / 73	113 / 73
	95th + 12 mmHg	SBP / DBP	120 / 80	121 / 81	121 / 82	122 / 83	123 / 84	124 / 85	125 / 85
6		Height in cm	110	111.8	114.9	118.4	122.1	125.6	127.7
	50th	SBP / DBP	92 / 54	92 / 54	93 / 55	94 / 56	96 / 57	97 / 58	97 / 59
	90th	SBP / DBP	105 / 67	106 / 67	107 / 68	108 / 69	109 / 70	110 / 71	111 / 71
	95th	SBP / DBP	109 / 70	109 / 71	110 / 72	111 / 72	112 / 73	113 / 74	114 / 74
	95th + 12 mmHg	SBP / DBP	121 / 82	121 / 83	122 / 84	123 / 84	124 / 85	125 / 86	126 / 86
7		Height in cm	115.9	117.8	121.1	124.9	128.8	132.5	134.7
	50th	SBP / DBP	92 / 55	93 / 55	94 / 56	95 / 57	97 / 58	98 / 59	99 / 60
	90th	SBP / DBP	106 / 68	106 / 68	107 / 69	109 / 70	110 / 71	111 / 72	112 / 72
	95th	SBP / DBP	109 / 72	110 / 72	111 / 73	112 / 73	113 / 74	114 / 74	115 / 75
	95th + 12 mmHg	SBP / DBP	121 / 84	122 / 84	123 / 85	124 / 85	125 / 86	126 / 86	127 / 87
8		Height in cm	121	123	126.5	130.6	134.7	138.5	140.9
	50th	SBP / DBP	93 / 56	94 / 56	95 / 57	97 / 59	98 / 60	99 / 61	100 / 61
	90th	SBP / DBP	107 / 69	107 / 70	108 / 71	110 / 72	111 / 72	112 / 73	113 / 73
	95th	SBP / DBP	110 / 72	111 / 73	112 / 74	113 / 74	115 / 75	116 / 75	117 / 75
	95th + 12 mmHg	SBP / DBP	122 / 84	123 / 85	124 / 86	125 / 86	127 / 87	128 / 87	129 / 87
9		Height in cm	125.3	127.6	131.3	135.6	140.1	144.1	146.6
	50th	SBP / DBP	95 / 57	95 / 58	97 / 59	98 / 60	99 / 60	100 / 61	101 / 61
	90th	SBP / DBP	108 / 71	108 / 71	109 / 72	111 / 73	112 / 73	113 / 73	114 / 73
	95th	SBP / DBP	112 / 74	112 / 74	113 / 75	114 / 75	116 / 75	117 / 75	118 / 75

(Continued)

Table 18.10 (*Continued*)

Age	BP Centile		Height Percentile or Measured Height						
		Height Percentile	5%	10%	25%	50%	75%	90%	95%
	95th + 12 mmHg	SBP / DBP	124 / 86	124 / 86	125 / 87	126 / 87	128 / 87	129 / 87	130 / 87
10		Height in cm	129.7	132.2	136.3	141	145.8	150.2	152.8
	50th	SBP / DBP	96 / 58	97 / 59	98 / 59	99 / 60	101 / 61	102 / 61	103 / 62
	90th	SBP / DBP	109 / 72	110 / 73	111 / 73	112 / 73	113 / 73	115 / 73	116 / 73
	95th	SBP / DBP	113 / 75	114 / 75	114 / 76	116 / 76	117 / 76	119 / 76	120 / 76
	95th + 12 mmHg	SBP / DBP	125 / 87	126 / 87	126 / 88	128 / 88	129 / 88	131 / 88	132 / 88
11		Height in cm	135.6	138.3	142.8	147.8	152.8	157.3	160
	50th	SBP / DBP	98 / 60	99 / 60	101 / 60	102 / 61	104 / 62	105 / 63	106 / 64
	90th	SBP / DBP	111 / 74	112 / 74	113 / 74	114 / 74	116 / 74	118 / 75	120 / 75
	95th	SBP / DBP	115 / 76	116 / 77	117 / 77	118 / 77	120 / 77	123 / 77	124 / 77
	95th + 12 mmHg	SBP / DBP	127 / 88	128 / 89	129 / 89	130 / 89	132 / 89	135 / 89	136 / 89
12		Height in cm	142.8	145.5	149.9	154.8	159.6	163.8	166.4
	50th	SBP / DBP	102 / 61	102 / 61	104 / 61	105 / 62	107 / 64	108 / 65	108 / 65
	90th	SBP / DBP	114 / 75	115 / 75	116 / 75	118 / 75	120 / 76	122 / 76	122 / 76
	95th	SBP / DBP	118 / 78	119 / 78	120 / 78	122 / 78	124 / 79	125 / 79	126 / 79
	95th + 12 mmHg	SBP / DBP	130 / 90	131 / 90	132 / 90	134 / 90	136 / 91	137 / 91	138 / 91
13		Height in cm	148.1	150.6	154.7	159.2	163.7	167.8	170.2
	50th	SBP / DBP	104 / 62	105 / 62	106 / 63	107 / 64	108 / 65	108 / 65	109 / 66
	90th	SBP / DBP	116 / 75	117 / 75	119 / 75	121 / 76	122 / 76	123 / 76	123 / 76
	95th	SBP / DBP	121 / 79	122 / 79	123 / 79	124 / 79	126 / 80	126 / 80	127 / 81
	95th + 12 mmHg	SBP / DBP	133 / 91	134 / 91	135 / 91	136 / 91	138 / 92	138 / 92	139 / 93

14		Height in cm	150.6	153	156.9	161.3	165.7	169.7	172.1
	50th	SBP / DBP	105 / 63	106 / 63	107 / 64	108 / 65	109 / 66	109 / 66	109 / 66
	90th	SBP / DBP	118 / 76	118 / 76	120 / 76	122 / 76	123 / 77	123 / 77	123 / 77
	95th	SBP / DBP	123 / 80	123 / 80	124 / 80	125 / 80	126 / 81	127 / 81	127 / 82
	95th + 12 mmHg	SBP / DBP	135 / 92	135 / 92	136 / 92	137 / 92	138 / 93	139 / 93	139 / 94
15		Height in cm	151.7	154	157.9	162.3	166.7	170.6	173
	50th	SBP / DBP	105 / 64	106 / 64	107 / 64	108 / 65	109 / 66	109 / 67	109 / 67
	90th	SBP / DBP	118 / 76	119 / 76	121 / 76	122 / 77	123 / 77	123 / 78	124 / 78
	95th	SBP / DBP	124 / 80	124 / 80	125 / 80	126 / 81	127 / 82	127 / 82	128 / 82
	95th + 12 mmHg	SBP / DBP	136 / 92	136 / 92	137 / 92	138 / 93	139 / 94	139 / 94	140 / 94
16		Height in cm	152.1	154.5	158.4	162.8	167.1	171.1	173.4
	50th	SBP / DBP	106 / 64	107 / 64	108 / 65	109 / 66	109 / 66	110 / 67	110 / 67
	90th	SBP / DBP	119 / 76	120 / 76	122 / 76	123 / 77	124 / 78	124 / 78	124 / 78
	95th	SBP / DBP	124 / 80	125 / 80	125 / 80	127 / 81	127 / 82	128 / 82	128 / 82
	95th + 12 mmHg	SBP / DBP	136 / 92	137 / 92	137 / 92	139 / 93	139 / 94	140 / 94	140 / 94
17		Height in cm	152.4	154.7	158.7	163.0	167.4	171.3	173.7
	50th	SBP / DBP	107 / 64	108 / 64	109 / 65	110 / 66	110 / 66	110 / 66	111 / 67
	90th	SBP / DBP	120 / 76	121 / 76	123 / 77	124 / 77	124 / 78	125 / 78	125 / 78
	95th	SBP / DBP	125 / 80	125 / 80	126 / 80	127 / 81	128 / 82	128 / 82	128 / 82
	95th + 12 mmHg	SBP / DBP	137 / 92	137 / 92	138 / 92	139 / 93	140 / 94	140 / 94	140 / 94

Adapted from Flynn JT et al. (2017) Clinical Practice guideline for screening and management of high blood pressure in children and adolescents. Pediatrics ***140****(3).*

Table 18.11 Blood Pressure Levels Values for Neonates and Infant (0–1 year of age)

Gestation (weeks)	50th Percentile SBP/DBP (MAP)	95th Percentile SBP/DBP (MAP)	99th Percentile SBP/DBP (MAP)
26	55 / 30 (38)	72 / 50 (57)	77 / 56 (63)
28	60 / 38 (45)	75 / 50 (58)	80 / 54 (63)
30	65 / 40 (48)	80 / 55 (65)	85 / 60 (68)
32	68 / 40 (48)	83 / 55 (62)	88 / 60 (69)
34	70 / 40 (50)	85 / 55 (62)	90 / 60 (70)
36	72 / 50 (57)	87 / 65 (72)	92 / 70 (71)
38	77 / 50 (59)	92 / 65 (74)	97 / 70 (79)
40	80 / 50 (60)	95 / 65 (75)	100 / 70 (80)
42	85 / 50 (62)	98 / 65 (76)	102 / 70 (81)
44	88 / 50 (63)	105 / 68 (80)	110 / 73 (85)

Adapted from Dionne et al. (2012) Hypertension in infancy: Diagnosis, management and outcome. Pediatr Nephrol ***27****(1):17–32.*

- » Malignancy or bone marrow transplant
- » Treatment with drugs known to raise BP
- » Other systemic illnesses associated with hypertension (neurofibromatosis, tuberous sclerosis)
- » Evidence of elevated intracranial pressure

Evaluation of Persistent Asymptomatic Hypertension

<table>
<tr><td>1st consultation</td><td>Elevated blood pressure (90th–95th centile)</td><td>Stage 1 hypertension (95th centile–95th centile + 12 mmHg or 130–139/80–89 mmHg)</td><td>Stage 2 hypertension (>95th centile + 12 mmHg or ≥140/90 mmHg)</td></tr>
<tr><td rowspan="2">Management at 1st consultation</td><td colspan="3">Lifestyle interventions: healthy diet, sleep and physical activity
Nutrition and/or weight management referral</td></tr>
<tr><td colspan="2"></td><td>Upper and lower extremity BP should be checked (right arm, left arm, and 1 leg)</td></tr>
<tr><td>2nd consultation</td><td>6 months later</td><td>1–2 weeks later</td><td>Within 1 week</td></tr>
<tr><td>Management at 2nd consultation</td><td colspan="2">Upper and lower extremity BP should be checked (right arm, left arm and 1 leg)</td><td>ABPM*
Diagnostic evaluation
Subspecialty referral (cardiology or nephrology)</td></tr>
</table>

3rd consultation	6 mth later	3 mth later	
Management at 3rd consultation	Ambulatory Blood Pressure Monitoring (ABPM) Diagnostic evaluation Subspecialty referral (cardiology or nephrology)		

Initial Diagnostic Evaluation

Blood	Full blood count, renal panel, calcium, magnesium, phosphate, uric acid, fasting lipid panel, fasting glucose with HbA1c and insulin level, liver function test, thyroid function test
Urine	Urinalysis (UFEME), urine albumin/creatinine ratio
Imaging	Renal ultrasound with Doppler Study of renal arteries
Others (As Required)	Referral to Sleep Clinic for sleep study if history is suggestive of obstructive sleep apnoea Referral to Cardiology for echocardiogram to look for left ventricular hypertrophy or coarctation of aorta Referral to Ophthalmology to look for hypertensive retinopathy

Further investigations may be required, as indicated by history and physical examination.

Severe Hypertension

- Not rigorously defined, thus leading to confusion at times.
- Useful definition:
  - » BP elevation that fulfils (and usually exceeds) the definition of Stage 2 hypertension and that is accompanied by severe symptoms; physical exam and/or laboratory findings of accelerated hypertension are frequently also present.
  - » 20 mmHg above the 95th percentile.
- Adult definition:
  - » Blood pressures that are 50% above normal BP or >180/120 mmHg.
- Children presenting with severe symptoms need to be treated more rapidly:
  - » It is risky to lower the BP too rapidly, especially in those whose hypertension has been longstanding.
  - » In such patients, a shift in cerebral autoregulation occurs, which in the hypertensive state, protects the brain from excessive perfusion.
  - » Too rapid lowering of the BP in patients with such alterations of cerebral flow might lead to an ischemic stroke from under perfusion of the brain.
- Can be subdivided into hypertensive emergency or hypertensive urgency.

Hypertensive Emergency

- Presence of severe hypertension (as defined above), and
- The presence of end-organ injury, such as cardiac failure (left ventricular hypertrophy, pulmonary oedema), hypertensive retinopathy (papilloedema, exudates and fundal haemorrhages), hypertensive encephalopathy (altered mental state, convulsions), cerebral haemorrhage, cerebral infarction.

Treatment

- All cases of hypertensive emergency should be admitted to the Children's Intensive Care Unit for continuous BP monitoring.
- Aim of treatment is to lower the BP to the desired range gradually so as to minimise hypertensive sequelae, but yet not compromise perfusion to vital organs due to a sudden decrease in BP.
- The ultimate short-term BP goal in such patients should generally be around in the 95th percentile.
- BP should be reduced by no more than 25% of the planned reduction over the first 8 hours, with the remainder of the planned reduction over the next 12 to 24 hours.
- Pay attention to pupillary reactions, consciousness level and neurological examination.
- Saline for volume expansion should be available on standby in case of sudden hypotension.
- Choice of antihypertensive agent:
  - » Depends on aetiology of hypertension.
  - » Antihypertensive with rapid onset of action, short half-life, safe and efficacious is preferred.
  - » Intravenous (IV) route of administration preferred in hypertensive emergency.
  - » See Table 18.12 for the drugs that can be used in hypertensive emergency.
  - » Long-acting oral medications can be introduced after reasonable BP control within 24 to 48 hours of initiation of IV antihypertensive infusion.

Hypertensive Urgency

- Presence of severe hypertension with no evidence of acute end organ damage/ compromise.
- Patients may have symptoms of nausea, headache or blurred vision.

Treatment

- Goal of therapy is reduction of BP over a 24-hour period.
- Choice of either IV or oral antihypertensive. Oral agents can be used to gradually lower BP in patients who are asymptomatic and do not have evidence of immediate end-organ injury.
- The oral drugs that can be used in hypertensive urgency are listed in Table 18.13.

Table 18.12 Drugs used for Hypertensive Emergency

Drug/Route	Class	Dose	Onset of Action	Duration	Precautions
IV labetalol (25 mg/5 ml vial)	α- and β-adrenergic blocker	IV bolus 0.2 to 1 mg/kg/dose (max. 20 mg/dose) over 2 min then IV continuous 0.25 to 3 mg/kg/hr (max. 120 mg/hr) [neonates: 0.25 to 4 mg/kg/hr]	5 to 10 min	3 to 6 hr	Heart block, bradycardia, orthostatic hypotension, avoid in heart failure and asthma
IV sodium nitroprusside (50 mg/2 ml vial)	Direct vasodilator	Initial IV 0.3 to 0.5 µg/kg/min; titrate up every 5 min (max. 10 µg/kg/min)	Instantaneous	1 to 2 min	Nausea and vomiting, cyanide accumulation with prolonged use. Protect from light and monitor blood cyanide level when infusing for >72 hr or in patients with renal failure.
IV hydralazine (20 mg/ml ampoule)	Direct vasodilator	IV bolus 0.1 to 0.5 mg/kg/dose 4 to 6 hourly (max. 20 mg/dose, 3.6 mg/kg/d) IV continuous 12.5 to 50 µg/kg/hr (up to 18 mg/hr); max. 3 mg/kg/d	5 to 15 min	3 to 8 hr	Not preferred in SLE. Tachycardia. Caution in use in coronary artery disease.
IV frusemide (20 mg/2 ml ampoule)	Loop diuretic	IV bolus 1 to 6 mg/kg/dose 6 to 12 hourly (adult initial bolus 80 to 200 mg, subsequently adult 20 to 60 mg 6 to 12 hourly; max. 1500 mg/d) IV continuous 0.05 to 1 mg/kg/hr (adult 10 to 40 mg/hr)	5 min	2 hr	Hypokalaemia. Rapid infusion increases risk of ototoxicity. May exacerbate hypocalcaemia or hyperuricemia
IV esmolol (100 mg/10 ml vial)	β-adrenergic blocker	IV bolus 0.5 mg/kg/dose over 1 min then IV continuous infusion 0.05 to 0.5 mg/kg/min Max. 0.5 mg/kg/min	1 to 2 min	10 to 20 min	Hypotension, avoid in heart failure and asthma, very short acting, profound bradycardia
IV bumetanide (2 mg/4 ml ampoule)	Loop diuretic	IV bolus 0.01 to 0.1 mg/kg/dose 6 to 24 hourly (max. 10 mg/d) IV continuous 0.001 to 0.2 mg/kg/hr (adult 0.5 to 2 mg/hr)	2 to 3 min	4 to 6 hr	More costly than frusemide. Rapid infusion increases risk of ototoxicity. May exacerbate hypocalcaemia or hyperuricemia

Table 18.13 Drugs used for Hypertensive Urgency

Drug/ Route	Initial Dose	Maximum Dose	Precautions
PO nifedipine (immediate release 5 mg/liquid capsule, 10 mg/liquid capsule)	0.2 to 0.5 mg/kg/dose 4 to 6 hourly (10 mg/dose)	3 mg/kg/d, 120 mg/d	Rapid onset hypotension, tachycardia, headache
PO hydralazine (10 mg/tablet)	0.25 to 0.5 mg/kg/dose 8 to 12 hourly (Max. 25 mg/dose)	Max. 7.5 mg/kg/d, 200 mg/d	Not preferred in SLE. Tachycardia. Caution in use in coronary artery disease.
PO propranolol (10 mg/tablet, 40 mg/tablet, 1 mg/ml suspension)	0.25 to 1 mg/kg/dose 8 to 12 hourly (80 mg/dose)	Max. 5 mg/kg/d, 320 mg/d	Avoid in asthma and cardiac failure. Monitor heart rate
PO captopril (12.5 mg/tablet, 1 mg/ml suspension)	0.1 to 0.5 mg/kg/dose 8 to 12 hourly (6.25 mg/dose) Very young neonates and infants: 0.01 to 0.05 mg/kg/dose (Max. 2 mg/kg/d)	6 mg/kg/d, 150 mg/d	Hypotension in high renin states, renal failure and hyperkalaemia. Very young neonates are dosed differently
PO clonidine (25 µg/tablet)	0.5 to 5 µg/kg/dose (Max. 10 µg/kg/dose) 6 to 8 hourly	Max. 25 µg/kg/d, 1200 µg/d	Sedation, bradycardia and xerostomia

Bibliography

1. Dionne JM, Abitbol CL, Flynn JT. (2012) Hypertension in infancy: Diagnosis, management and outcome. *Pediatr Nephrol* **27**(1):17–32.
2. Flynn JT, Kaelber DC, Baker-Smith CM, *et al.* (2017) Clinical Practice Guideline for screening and management of high blood pressure in children and adolescents. *Pediatrics* **140**(3):e20171904.
3. Flynn JT, Tullus K. (2009) Severe hypertension in children and adolescents: Pathophysiology and treatment. *Pediatr Nephrol* **24**(6):1101–1112.
4. Gilmore RM, Miller SJ, Stead LG. (2005) Severe hypertension in the emergency department patient. *Emerg Med Clin N Am* **23**(4):1141–1158.
5. Lande MB, Flynn JT. (2009) Treatment of hypertension in children and adolescents. *Pediatr Nephrol* **24**(10):1939–1949.
6. LexiComp. (nd) Pediatric and neonatal Lexi-drugs online. Hudson, Ohio: Up-to-date. Inc.
7. LexiComp. (nd) LexiComp online. Hudson, Ohio: Up-to-date. Inc.
8. Chandar J, Zilleruelo G. (2012) Hypertensive crisis in children. *Pediatr Nephrol* **27**(5):741–751.
9. Joint Formulary Committee. (2017) British National Formulary 73. London: BMJ Publishing and the Royal Pharmaceutical Society.
10. Paediatric Formulary Committee. (2021) British National Formulary for Children 2020–2021. London: BMJ Publishing and the Royal Pharmaceutical Society.

CHAPTER 86

Urinary Tract Infections and Vesicoureteric Reflux

Chong Siew Le; Chao Sing Ming

Introduction

Urinary tract infection (UTI) is one of the most common bacterial infections seen in children and a leading cause of acute sepsis in infants requiring hospitalisation. Incidence of renal involvement or acute pyelonephritis is high, especially during infancy (up to 80%).

Although the majority of children with UTI have an excellent prognosis, there is a definite risk of renal damage or scarring following pyelonephritis, especially in those with vesicoureteric reflux (VUR) or obstructive uropathy.

Clinical Classification

The epidemiology, pathophysiology and prognosis of UTI are interrelated and differ according to age, sex and, in particular, the site of infection. A useful classification is according to the site of infection (Table 18.14). While more than 80% of patients with

Table 18.14 Clinical Classification of Childhood UTI

Clinical Features	Upper Tract Infection	Lower Tract Infection
Age	Generally <2 yr	Generally >2 yr
Renal involvement	Neonates and young infants are at high risk	No risk
Sex	Female = Male in infancy Female > Male past infancy	Female > Male
Fever	+ (All febrile UTI have presumed pyelonephritis)	–
Voiding problem	–	+
Dysuria	–	+
Frequency	–	+
Suprapubic pain	–	+
Loin pain (older children)	+	–

Table 18.15 Clinical Features of Atypical (complicated) UTI

• Past history of UTI/renal or renal tract abnormality/bladder dysfunction
• Septicaemia/seriously ill
• Poor urine output, raised serum creatinine
• Palpable abdominal mass/bladder
• Persistent fever after 48 hr of appropriate antibiotic treatment
• Uncommon uropathogen, e.g. *Pseudomonas*

upper UTI have typical clinical features of unexplained fever with or without urinary symptoms, it is important to look at clinical features of atypical or complicated UTI (Table 18.15), which may suggest underlying renal/renal tract abnormalities that warrant attention and further investigations, including micturating cystourethrogram (MCU).

Diagnosis and Management

Upper Urinary Tract Infection

- The cardinal symptom of pyelonephritis is unexplained high fever, often with chills and rigors. UTI should be suspected in such instances, especially in infants. Cloudy urine is a more specific symptom than smelly urine.
- A pre-treatment, properly collected mid-steam urine culture, is mandatory to establish a firm diagnosis of UTI.
- Up to 9% patients with pyelonephritis may have equivocal or negative urine culture. If urine culture is equivocal and suspicion of pyelonephritis is high, a DMSA scan can help to establish diagnosis.
- When early initiation of antibiotic treatment is necessary, an invasive method of urine collection (suprapubic tap, catheterisation) is justified. Beware and be ready to collect midstream urine as baby may spontaneously void while being cleaned for the procedure.
- *E. coli* is the commonest uropathogen (>80%). Gentamicin is the recommended first-line antibiotic (93% sensitivity) and ceftriaxone (almost 100%) as an alternative.
- Although ceftriaxone has almost 100% sensitivity, it is used as second-line treatment for fear of the emergence of resistant bacterial strains. However, in patients with compromised renal function, ceftriaxone is the antibiotic of choice.

<u>Urine culture — points to remember</u>:

- Bagged urine specimen is often contaminated and should not be used for the urine culture.
- Label clearly the method used for urine collection as diagnostic criteria vary (see below).

Table 18.16 Urine Culture and Sensitivity Results and Interpretations

Method of Collection	Colony Forming Units/ ml (Pure Growth)	Probability of Infection (%)
Suprapubic tap	Gram-negative bacilli: any count	>99%
	Gram-positive cocci >1000	>99%
Transurethral catheterisation	>100000	95%
	10000–100000	Infection likely
	=1000	Doubtful, repeat if indicated
	<1000	Infection unlikely
Clean catch mid-stream	2 specimens >100000	90%
	1 specimen >100000	80%
	=50000 –100000	Doubtful; repeat if indicated
	<50000	Infection unlikely
Mixed growth		Contamination

- Always obtain fresh urine. Direct plating of urine onto dipslides can be done outside office hours.
- Always interpret culture results with clinical correlations.

Antibiotic Treatment for Uncomplicated Febrile UTI

Choice of Antibiotics	Duration of Treatment
<u>Intravenous (IV) Antibiotics</u>: **First line** • Gentamicin 5–6 mg/kg/d Q24H • Infants <1 mth, add Ampicillin 100 mg/kg/d Q6H (to cover possible enterococci infection). *Precautions for gentamicin therapy*: If serum creatinine elevated for age, ensure adequate hydration and consider second-line antibiotics for fear of gentamicin nephrotoxicity. If continued >48 hr, check gentamicin trough levels. **Second line** • Ceftriaxone 50 mg/kg/DOSE Q24H • Cefotaxime 200–300 mg/kg/d Q6–8H Cefotaxime is preferred in neonates. **<u>Oral antibiotics</u>:** • First-generation cephalosporins, e.g. Cephalexin (50 mg/kg/d Q8H) • Co-amoxiclav (Amoxicillin 80–90 mg/kg/d Q12H)	Total duration: 14 d IV therapy until no fever for 24 hr, then switch to oral therapy according to antibiogram For those with bacteraemia, IV therapy should be continued for 7–10 d

Refer to your institution's antimicrobial guidelines for latest antimicrobial selection and dosing recommendations.

Lower Urinary Tract Infection

- Common in young girls.
- Presents with voiding symptoms — dysuria, frequency, urgency and suprapubic pain. Some may present with urge incontinence or secondary nocturnal enuresis.
- Commonly afebrile.
- Though troublesome and often recurrent, avoid over investigations unless there is suspicion of febrile or upper UTI.
- Essential to perform perineum examination to rule out local inflammation/ infection.
- Presence of phimosis in boys could increase risk of infection.

Antibiotic Treatment of Lower Urinary Tract Infection

Choice of Antibiotics
1. Co-trimoxazole (TMP/SMZ)* TMP 8 mg/kg/d Q12H 2. Nitrofurantoin*: 5–7 mg/kg/d Q6H 3. Cephalexin: 50 mg/kg/d Q8H 4. Trimethoprim: 8 mg/kg/d Q12H (Useful for G6PD deficient patients) (*Screen for G6PD deficiency)

Duration of Treatment
7 d of antibiotics >12 yr old: 3 d TMP/SMZ can be considered instead of the standard 7 d treatment

Approach and Indications for Investigations Following UTI

Principle

- Most of the experimental and clinical evidence strongly supports that both VUR and UTI are responsible for acquired renal scarring and that this damage takes up to 4–6 months to establish, becoming evident on the DMSA scan.
- Once formed, scarring is irreversible and when extensive, it can significantly reduce the function of the affected kidney (<45% differential function on DMSA scan).
- Acute pyelonephritis may heal completely but some may subsequently form scars.
- Dilating VUR (Grade III–V) remains an important risk factor for acute pyelonephritis (APN) and renal scarring and requires further management.

Risk of scarring correlates to:

- Severity of VUR: Dilating VUR (Grade III–V) being at higher risk
- Recurrence of UTI

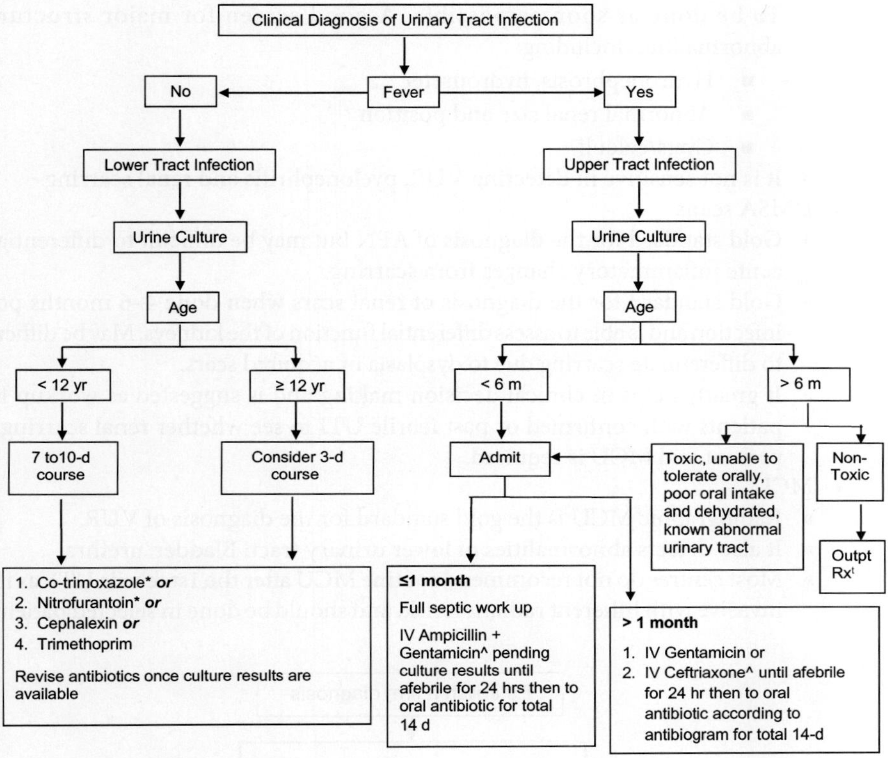

*Contraindicated in children with G6PD deficiency

^ Consider cephalosporin if abnormal kidney function or at risk of kidney injury (e.g. suspected hypoplastic dysplastic kidney)

† Consider outpatient treatment with the following:

- Send properly collected urine for culture
- Treat with oral cephalexin or co-amoxiclav for 14 days
- Revise treatment accordingly to culture and sensitivity result.
- For patient with 1st uncomplicated febrile UTI, to obtain renal US appointment with review at outpatient clinic in 2-4 weeks.

Figure 18.2 Algorithm for the management of uncomplicated febrile UTI in children.

While somewhat controversial, investigations following uncomplicated febrile UTI are basically aimed at discovering any underlying renal and renal tract abnormality that may predispose patient to repeat infections. Parents need to be informed that recurrent UTI is likely to occur in the initial 6–12 months and that they should be advised to be vigilant for possible recurrent UTI when their child has fever of unknown source and the necessary action plan.

Imaging Studies

Investigations include renal ultrasound (US KUB), DMSA scans and MCU, each with its own purpose and merits.

- US KUB

- » To be done as soon as possible. A good screen for major structural abnormalities, including:
  - ■ Hydronephrosis, hydroureter
  - ■ Abnormal renal size and position
  - ■ Cysts/calculi
- » It is not sensitive in detecting VUR, pyelonephritis and renal scarring.

• DMSA scans
- » Gold standard for the diagnosis of APN but may be difficult to differentiate acute inflammatory changes from scarring.
- » Gold standard for the diagnosis of renal scars when done 4–6 months post infection and is able to assess differential function of the kidneys. May be difficult to differentiate scarring due to dysplasia or acquired scars.
- » It greatly helps in clinical decision making and is suggested as workup for patients with confirmed or past febrile UTI to see whether renal scarring is present and MCU is required.

• MCU
- » Radiographic MCU is the gold standard for the diagnosis of VUR.
- » It also detects abnormalities of lower urinary tract: Bladder, urethra.
- » Most centres do not recommend routine MCU after the 1st febrile UTI, as it is invasive with inherent radiation risk, and should be done in selected patients.

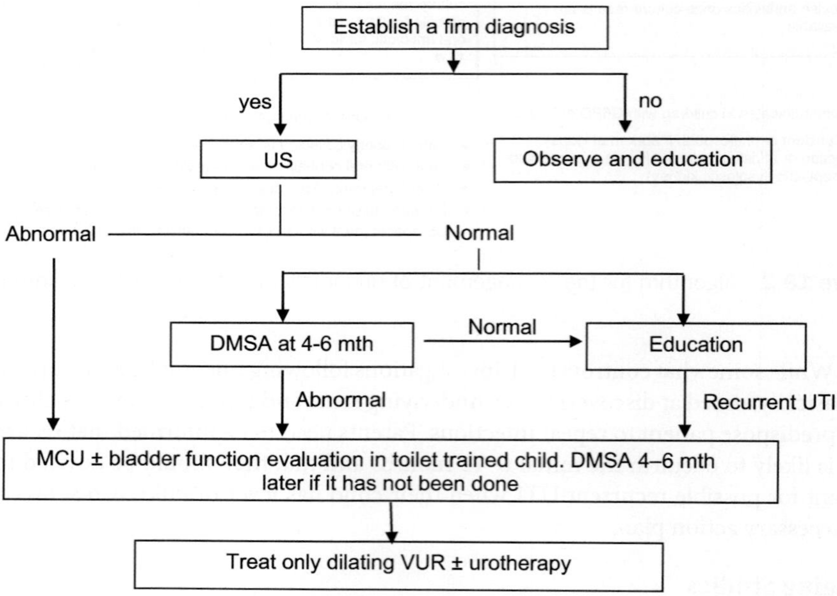

Figure 18.3 Approach to investigations following UTI.

- » Indications generally include:
  - ▪ Atypical/complicated UTI
  - ▪ Abnormal US KUB or DMSA scans
  - ▪ Recurrent UTI

Guidelines for Micturating Cystourethrography

Why MCU

- Gold standard for the diagnosis of VUR.
- Definitive diagnosis of posterior urethral valves (PUV) in boys, especially if bilateral dilated upper tract is present on ultrasound.
- Diagnosis of neuropathic bladder where bladder hypertrophy and trabeculation can be seen on MCU.

Points to Remember

- MCU should only be done when the UTI is adequately treated, usually 2 to 4 weeks after an infection.
- Antibiotic prophylaxis (usually co-trimoxazole 2–3 mg/kg/dose ON) should be started if MCU is indicated.
- Antibiotic cover for the procedure (co-trimoxazole or trimethoprim 8 mg/kg/day in BD dose) for 3 days starting the day before MCU.
- In borderline cases of renal pelvic calyceal dilatation, follow-up US KUB is reasonable before considering MCU.
- In patients with significant hydronephrosis (peripheral calyceal dilatation with or without cortical thinning), especially without hydroureter, MAG-3 scan can be considered to rule out pelvic-ureteric junction obstruction.

Precautions

- Indication must be present. If doubtful, consult senior doctor or renal physician.
- Adequate explanations must be given to parents regarding indications, procedure and possible complications. Risks of procedure are acceptable if indications are present.
- Complications of MCU include:
  - » Infection
    - ▪ Minimise risk by:
      - Proper aseptic technique
      - Co-trimoxazole cover (Trimethoprim if G6PD deficiency)
  - » Trauma
    - ▪ Minimise risk by:
      - Adequate lubrication/local anaesthesia with sterile 1% lignocaine gel
      - Correct-sized catheter depending on patient size

- Advance catheter until urine flows out freely, then advance by about 2 cm before securing with tapes. Catheter length *introduced* should not exceed 4 to 5 cm in neonates and 7 to 10 cm in older children
- Avoid using force when resistance is met and consult senior doctor

- Aftercare
  - » Ensure antibiotic cover and prophylaxis.
  - » To seek medical attention if unable to pee or if symptoms suggestive of UTI develop.

Indications for doing MCU must be clear and the disadvantages include:

- Invasive procedure requiring bladder catheterisation.
- Radiation risk to gonads, especially in females.

Vesicoureteric Reflux

VUR is a heterogeneous group of disorders. It is either a primary developmental disorder with or without renal dysplasia or is secondary to obstruction at the bladder or urethra. In its uncomplicated primary form, only dilating VUR (Grade III–V) needs treatment. The first line of treatment is medical. Indications for surgical treatment are:

- Failed medical treatment
- Associated urological abnormalities, e.g. urethrocele, duplex systems, obstructive uropathy

Medical Treatment

- Prophylactic antibiotics at night to prevent urosepsis. Check G6PD status.
  - » Choice of antibiotic:
    - ■ Co-trimoxazole [if G6PD deficiency or <6 weeks old, to use trimethoprim alone] (2–3 mg/kg/dose trimethoprim ON)
    - ■ Cephalexin (15–20 mg/kg/dose ON)
    - ■ Nitrofurantoin (2 mg/kg/dose ON) for infants >1 month (Avoid in G6PD deficiency)
- All toilet-trained children diagnosed with VUR or persistent VUR should be screened for bowel and bladder dysfunction.
- Regular follow-up
  - » Consider to repeat MCU if recurrent UTI and refer surgeon.
  - » Beyond 5–6 years old and if there is no recurrent UTI, focus should be on renal involvement with long-term follow-up for hypertension and proteinuria if there is significant renal scarring.
  - » If VUR still causes UTI past 5–6 years old, treatment is surgical as there is little chance of spontaneous resolution beyond this age.

When to Refer to the Paediatric Nephrologist

- If VUR is high grade/dilating.

- If VUR is secondary to obstructive uropathy.
- If significant renal scarring is present, especially if differential function <45% (unilateral kidney scarring) or if bilateral kidney scarring with or without impaired kidney function.
- If there are complicated pathologies, e.g. duplex kidney, urethrocele, trabeculated bladder.

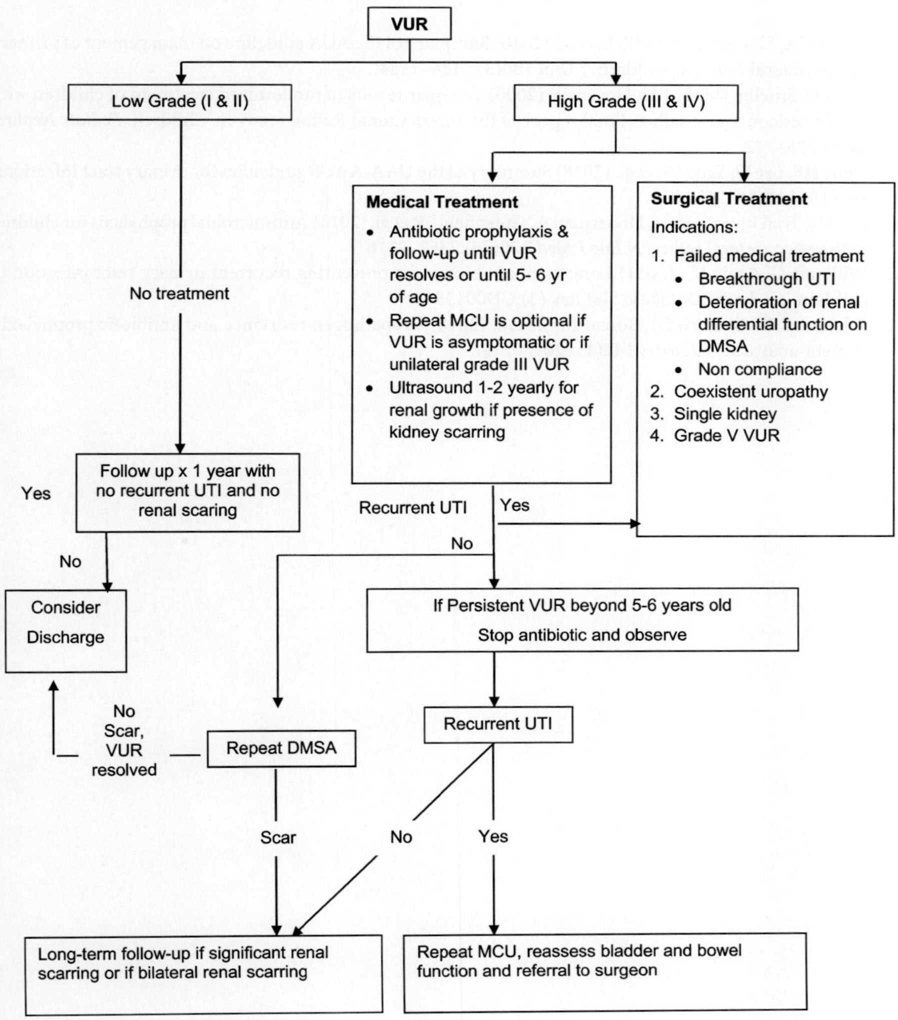

Figure 18.4 Clinical Approach to VUR.

Bibliography

1. Brandström P, Esbjörner E, Herthelius M, *et al.* (2010) The Swedish reflux trial in children. *J Urol* **184**(1):274–297.
2. Subcommittee on Urinary Tract Infection, Steering Committee on Quality Improvement and Management, Roberts KB. (2011) Urinary tract infection: Clinical practice guideline for the diagnosis and management of the initial UTI in febrile infants and children 2 to 24 months. *Pediatrics* **128**(3):595–610.
3. Shaikh N, Ewing AL, Bhatnagar S, Hoberman A. (2010) Risk of renal scarring in children with a first urinary tract infection: A systematic review. *Pediatrics* **126**(6):1084–1091.
4. Müller LSO. (2011) Imaging in urinary tract infection: Top-down or down-up? *Pediatr Radiol* **41**(1):S96–S98.
5. Peters CA, Skoog SJ, Arant BS Jr, *et al.* (2010) Summary of the AUA guideline on management of primary vesicoureteral reflux in children. *J Urol* **184**(3):1134–1144.
6. Jodal U, Smellie JM, Lax H, Hoyer PF. (2006) Ten-year results of randomized treatment of children with severe vesicoureteric reflux. Final report of the International Reflux Study in Children. *Pediatr Nephrol* **21**(6):785–792.
7. Choe HS, Lee SJ, Yang SS, *et al.* (2018) Summary of the UAA-AAUS guidelines for urinary tract infections. *Int J Urol* **25**(3):175–185.
8. RIVUR Trial Investigators, Hoberman A, Greenfield SP, *et al.* (2014) Antimicrobial prophylaxis for children with vesicoureteral reflux. *N Eng J Med* **370**(25):2367–2376.
9. Williams G, Craig JC. (2011) Long-term antibiotics for preventing recurrent urinary tract infection in children. *Cochrane Database Syst Rev* (3):CD001534.
10. Selekman RE, Shapiro DJ, Boscardin J, *et al.* (2018) Uropathogen resistance and antibiotic prophylaxis: A meta-analysis. *Pediatrics* **142**(1):e20180119.

CHAPTER 87

Acute Kidney Injury

Indra Ganesan

Definition

Acute kidney injury (AKI) is an abrupt decrease in glomerular filtration rate (GFR), resulting in the inability of the kidneys to maintain water and electrolyte homeostasis and acid–base balance, resulting in a rise in the serum creatinine.

Classified into:

Oliguric AKI — urine output is <400 ml/m^2/day or <1 ml/kg/h
Non-oliguric AKI — urine output is maintained

Approach

Table 18.17 Causes of Acute Kidney Injury

Pre-renal	Volume depletion	Gastrointestinal losses: Vomiting, diarrhoea Haemorrhage Renal losses: Tubulopathies
	Third space loss	Hypoalbuminaemic states: Nephrotic syndrome, liver disease Burns, crush injury Capillary leak syndrome, septicaemia
	Circulatory failure	Cardiac tamponade, congestive cardiac failure, pericarditis
Renal	<u>Glomerular</u> Glomerulonephritis	Acute nephritic syndrome Post-infectious glomerulonephritis Ig A vasculitis nephritis (previously known as HSP Nephritis)/Ig A nephropathy Lupus nephritis Rapidly progressive glomerulonephritis
	<u>Vascular</u>	Haemolytic-uraemic syndrome Renal artery and vein thrombosis
	<u>Tubulointerstitium</u> Interstitial nephritis	Allergic Post-infectious
	Tubular necrosis	Progress from pre-renal conditions Nephrotoxins — drugs (aminoglycosides, amphotericin, ifosphamide, cisplatin) Radiocontrast dye
	Intratubular obstruction	Pigment injury — haemoglobinuria, myoglobinuria Uric acid nephropathy (tumour lysis syndrome) Crystalluria — acyclovir
Post-renal	Obstructive uropathy	Posterior urethral valve Obstruction of single kidney or bladder Bilateral ureteric obstruction

Distinguishing between Acute Kidney Injury and Chronic Renal Failure

- Features of chronicity include:
  - » Growth failure
  - » Chronic hypertensive retinopathy
  - » Renal osteodystrophy or rickets
  - » Small kidneys on renal ultrasound
- Features such as anaemia, hyperphosphataemia and hypocalcaemia are not distinguishing features as they may occur in AKI.

Differentiation Between Pre-renal, Renal and Post-renal Causes

- **Urine Microscopy**

Cells	Dysmorphic red cells White cells Eosinophils	Glomerulonephritis Pyelonephritis Acute interstitial nephritis
Casts	Red cell Tubular cells/epithelial cells	Glomerulonephritis
Crystals	Uric acid	Tumour lysis

- **Urinary Indices**

Children

	Urine osmolality (mOsm/kg)	Urine sodium (mmol/L)	FENa (%)
Pre-renal	>500	<20	<1
Renal	<350	>40	>1

Neonates

	Urine osmolality (mOsm/kg)	Urine sodium (mmol/L)	FENa (%)
Pre-renal	>400	<20	<2.5
Renal	<400	>50	>2.5

$$\text{Fractional excretion of sodium (FENa)} = \frac{\text{Urine/plasma Na}}{\text{Urine/plasma Cr}} \times 100(\%)$$

- **Renal Ultrasound**

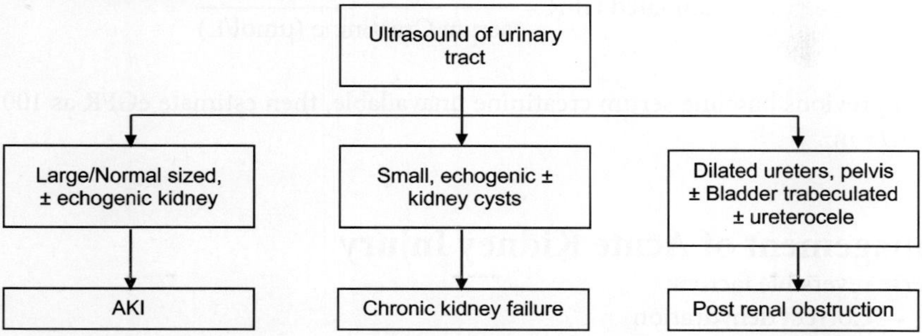

- **Fluid challenge**

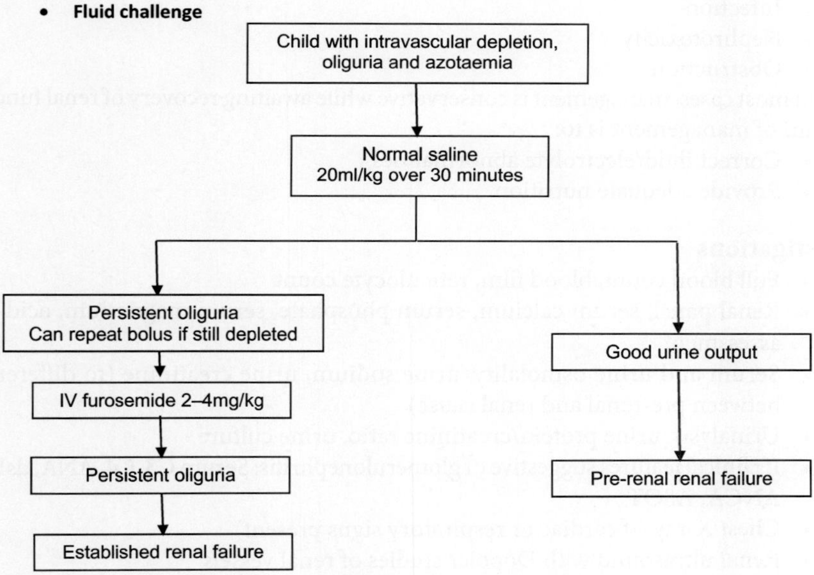

Table 18.18 Staging of Acute Kidney Injury using KDIGO Classification

Stage	Serum Creatinine	Urine Volume
1	Increase to 1.5–1.9 X baseline OR Increase by ≥26.5 μmol/L	<0.5 ml/kg/hr for 6–12 hr
2	Increase to 2.0–2.9 X baseline	<0.5 ml/kg/hr for ≥12 hr
3	Increase to 3.0 X baseline OR Increase of serum creatinine to ≥353.6 μmol/L OR initiation of renal replacement therapy OR Decrease in eGFR to <35 ml/min/1.73 m^2 in patients <18 yr	<0.3 ml/kg/hr for ≥24 hr OR Anuria ≥12 hr

$$\text{Estimated GFR} = \frac{\text{Height (cm)} \times 36.5}{\text{serum Creatinine } (\mu\text{mol/L})}$$

If previous baseline serum creatinine unavailable, then estimate eGFR as 100 ml/min/1.73 m^2.

Management of Acute Kidney Injury

Reverse reversible factors:

- Correct dehydration
- Hypotension
- Infection
- Nephrotoxicity
- Obstruction

In most cases, management is conservative while awaiting recovery of renal function. The aim of management is to:

- Correct fluid/electrolyte abnormalities
- Provide adequate nutrition

Investigations

- Full blood count, blood film, reticulocyte count
- Renal panel, serum calcium, serum phosphate, serum magnesium, acid–base assessment
- Serum and urine osmolality, urine sodium, urine creatinine (to differentiate between pre-renal and renal cause)
- Urinalysis, urine protein/creatinine ratio, urine culture
- If clinical features suggestive of glomerulonephritis: Serum C3, C4, ANA, dsDNA, ANCA, ASOT
- Chest X-ray (if cardiac or respiratory signs present)
- Renal ultrasound with Doppler studies of renal vessels
- Renal biopsy if indicated

Fluid Management

Principle:

- If euvolemic, replace Insensible Water Loss (IWL = 400 ml/m^2/day) plus urine output.
- If fluid overloaded, aim to decrease body weight by 0.5–1% per day.
- Weight gain or hyponatraemia during this phase indicative of fluid overload.
- Intravenous (IV) frusemide (1 mg/kg/DOSE) promotes renal blood flow during the early stage.
- Larger doses of IV frusemide 2 to 4 mg/kg/DOSE over 15 minutes may be required.
- If there is persistent oliguria despite optimisation of medical therapy, renal replacement therapy should be considered.

Electrolyte Management

Hyperkalaemia

- Prompt treatment if T wave changes on ECG or serum potassium >6.0 mmol/L
- Monitor ECG
- Drugs: Refer to chapter on 'Potassium Disorders'.

Hyponatraemia

- Results from fluid overload, need to fluid restrict and IV frusemide.
- If renal salt wasting, then for sodium supplementation.
- Na^+ deficit = 0.6 × Body Weight (kg) × [(Desired Na^+) – (Actual Na^+)]
- Correct slowly, raising serum Na^+ by not more than a maximum rate of 12 mmol/L per day.

Metabolic Acidosis

- Judicious use of sodium bicarbonate.
- Aim for half correction. Formula for calculating bicarbonate replacement = 1/3 × body weight (kg) × base excess.
- Be mindful that bicarbonate replacement will increase CO_2 tension, and an intact respiratory system is needed to eliminate the CO_2 produced.
- Be aware of Ca^{2+} levels as the correction of acidosis will cause shift from ionised to non-ionised form.

Hyperphosphataemia and Hypocalcaemia

- Hyperphosphataemia is managed by dietary phosphate restriction and phosphate binders (calcium carbonate or calcium acetate).
- Calcium-based phosphate binder doses:

Age group	Frequency	Calcium acetate 667 mg/Tab equivalent	Calcium carbonate 625 mg/Tab equivalent
<1 yr	3 to 4 times a day with meals	¼ Tab	
1 to 6 yr		½ Tab	
6 to 12 yr		1 Tab	
12 to 18 yr		2 Tab	

- Doses are titrated based on meal frequency and serum phosphate levels.
- Calcium acetate is preferred where there is hypochlorhydria due to either gut immaturity or the use of medications such as proton-pump inhibitors and H_2 receptor antagonists.

Nutritional Management

- Minimum of 25% of the daily caloric requirement is necessary to reduce ongoing catabolism.
- May require up to 25% dextrose, infused via a central line.
- Protein is restricted to 1 g/kg/day.

Hypertension

Refer to chapter on 'Hypertension'.

Drugs

- Minimise or discontinue nephrotoxic drugs. If necessary, monitor drug levels and side-effects.
- Doses may have to be adjusted in renal impairment.

Dialysis

Aim

Maintain fluid, electrolyte and acid–base balance; remove endogenous and exogenous toxins until renal function recovers.

Indications

The indications are not specific and should be individualised. In children, the dialysis is usually initiated for the indication of fluid overload.

Indications for initiating dialysis include:

- Oliguria/anuria
- Serum urea >35 mmol/L
- Hyperkalaemia >6.5 mmol/L unresponsive to conservative treatment
- Intractable metabolic acidosis (serum bicarbonate <10 mmol/L)
- Pulmonary oedema unresponsive to diuretic therapy
- Symptomatic uraemia — encephalopathy, pericarditis (generally when urea >50 mmol/L)
- Toxins

Modes of Dialysis in AKI

- Peritoneal dialysis
- Haemodialysis
- Continuous venovenous haemodialysis

Outcome

Three phases:

- Oliguric phase: Lasts few days to 6 weeks
- Diuretic phase
- Recovery phase: May last for months

Mortality

Dependent on cause. Overall, about 30%, and usually if coincident with multi-organ failure.

Bibliography

1. Rees L, Webb N, Brogan P (eds.). (2007*) Paediatric Nephrology*. Oxford: Oxford Handbooks in Paediatrics.
2. Avner ED, Harmon WE, Niaudet P, *et al.* (2016) *Pediatric Nephrology, 7th ed.* Springer.
3. Chan JC, Williams DM, Roth KS. (2002) Kidney failure in infants and children. *Pediatr Rev* **23**(2):47–60.
4. Kidney Disease: Improving Global Outcome (KDIGO). (2012) Acute kidney injury work group. KDIGO clinical practice guideline for acute kidney injury. *Kidney Int* **2**:S1–S138.

CHAPTER 88

Nocturnal Enuresis

Chao Sing Ming

Nocturnal Enuresis (NE) is a common, distressing and socially disruptive health problem affecting 5 to 10% of children aged 7 to 10 years old. Prevalence of NE reduces with increasing age by about 15% per annum. However, those ≥5 years who still wet their beds on an average of ≥2 times/week should be given the benefit of treatment without unnecessarily prolonging the distress and consequences of enuresis.

While the cause of NE is largely unknown, it has a strong genetic predisposition and is characterised by two important features that form the basis of its treatment: (1) Failure to awake from sleep in response to signalling of a full bladder, and (2) Urine production in excess of the bladder capacity (a mismatch due to either nocturnal polyuria (NP) or a reduced bladder capacity, or both).

There are two major clinical categories of NE according to the International Children's Continence Society (ICCS): monosymptomatic NE (MNE) and non-monosymptomatic NE (NMNE). It is important to differentiate these two categories as they differ in pathogenesis, clinical features and treatment strategy.

Treatment of MNE is more straightforward when compared to NMNE, by using desmopressin or enuresis alarm as monotherapy with a satisfactory treatment outcome. Treatment outcome may be further improved by better patient selection and expanded therapeutic considerations.

Definitions (ICCS)

Incontinence

Involuntary leakage of urine. It can be subdivided into continuous, intermittent, daytime incontinence and enuresis. Total loss of control and awareness of voiding is seen in neuropathic bladder. Continuous or constant wetting is seen in rare anatomical abnormalities (e.g. ectopic ureter in girls, epispadias). Daytime incontinence is intermittent incontinence with a small amount of urine while awake, and is due to underlying bladder dysfunction.

Nocturnal Enuresis/bedwetting
Intermittent incontinence while asleep, beyond 5 years of age.

Primary Nocturnal Enuresis:
Never been dry for more than 6 months.

Secondary Nocturnal Enuresis:
Been consistently dry for at least 6 months and then bedwetting recurs. Secondary causes (Urinary tract infection [UTI], polyuria) should be excluded.

Monosymptomatic Nocturnal Enuresis:
NE as an isolated problem without symptoms of bladder or bowel dysfunction or other co-morbidities.

Non-monosymptomatic Nocturnal Enuresis:
Usually refers to NE with additional daytime symptoms of an overactive bladder (OAB).

Overactive Bladder:
Frequent micturition, urgency and sometimes urge incontinence. Holding manoeuvres like squatting, crossing legs to stop the urge. Twenty to thirty per cent of patients with NE have daytime symptoms related to an OAB.

Clinical Assessment

A good focused history and careful examination, followed by a simple urinalysis to screen for urinary abnormalities are all that is required. Imaging studies and urodynamic studies should be reserved for those with a complicated history, e.g. febrile UTI or abnormal clinical findings such as cutaneous stigmata of occult spinal dysraphism.

History taking involves assessing the severity of bedwetting, onset, screening for features of NMNE and suggestion of NP, which will help towards determining the choice and success of treatment (See Figure 18.5 for the algorithm on clinical assessment and a checklist).

Evidence of NP in enuresis includes the wetting (> 2 nights) covering large areas or using a diaper weight that exceeds 100% of the expected bladder capacity for age, as documented by a 4- to 7-day bedwetting diary. Co-morbidities in NMNE include bladder dysfunction, bowel dysfunction, behavioural and developmental disorders, sleep apnoea, which may need specialist referral and be separately addressed. It is also important to ask for the history of febrile UTI, which may signify underlying urinary tract abnormalities.

History is usually straightforward and a physical examination is unremarkable. However, it is important not to miss an unusual case of neuropathic bladder, anatomical abnormalities and polyuria from diabetes mellitus or insipidus.

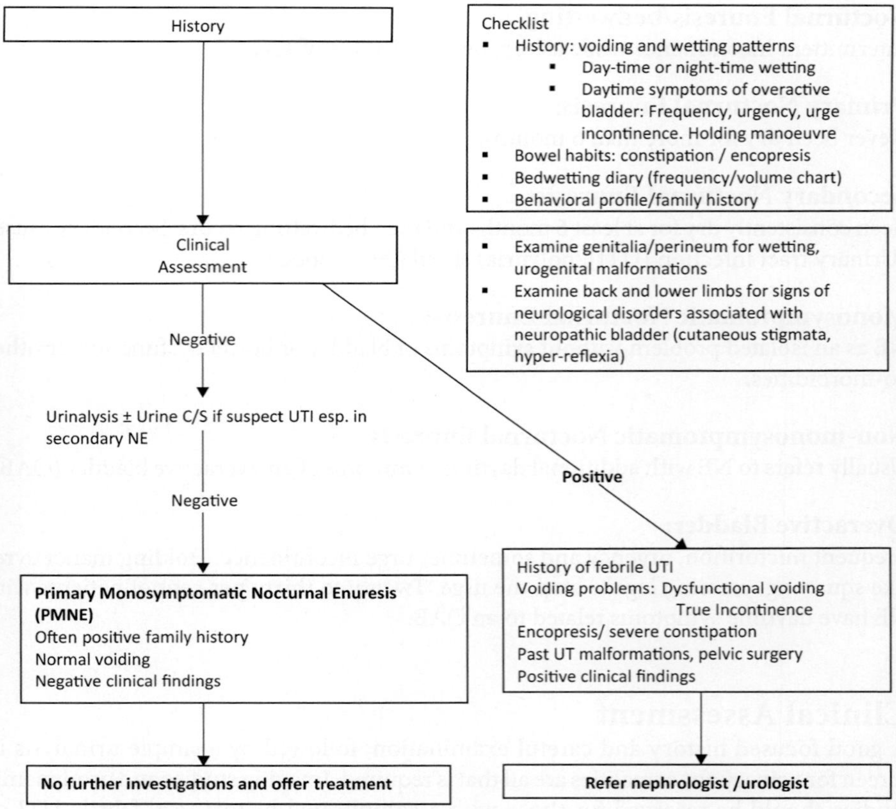

Figure 18.5 Initial clinical assessment of nocturnal enuresis.

Treatment Modalities (See Figure 18.6 for algorithm on treatment guideline for PMNE)

- Desmopressin (DDAVP) and the use of enuresis alarm are two established treatment options that had been found to be effective in clinical trials. Treatment options should be adequately explained (using NE information pamphlets) to parent and patient, guided by individual wetting pattern and choice.
- Daytime problem in NMNE needs to be treated first before enuresis can be successfully treated.
- Anticholinergic like oxybutynin can be useful when NE is associated with OAB.
- Tricyclic antidepressants (imipramine) is not superior to alarm or DDAVP and is not recommended because of its potential fatal side effects when overdosed.

Desmopressin (DDAVP)

- It is widely accepted that NP, as seen in one-third to two-third MNE, is mainly due to a lack of the normal circadian rhythm of nocturnal increase in anti-diuretic hormone or vasopressin (AVP) production, which helps to concentrate and reduce urine volume during sleep.
- DDAVP, a potent synthetic anti-diuretic analogue of AVP, is used to boost the effect of endogenous AVP and invariably improves NP. However, it does not improve the sleep arousal in response to a full bladder and its reported success rate in the treatment of NE is a moderate 50–70%. Relapse rate varies from 30 to 50%.

Considerations to Improve Outcome when using DDAVP

- Best result in patients with NP.
- To be taken 1 hour before sleep with minimal amount of water (alternatively, use lyophilisate DDAVP, if available), in order for DDAVP to reach maximum urine concentrating capacity.
- Restrict fluid 1–2 hours before and 8 hours (average duration of action) after administration.
- Use of bedwetting diary to monitor treatment and to reinforce compliance.
- Tapered withdrawal may help to avoid relapse.
- Combine DDAVP with alarm training when monotherapy fails. Combination with anticholinergic, which has a separate side effect profile for treating daytime symptoms, should only be considered in specialist clinic.

The most serious reported complication of DDAVP treatment is water intoxication due to excessive water intake, as DDAVP reduces water excretion and urine production. This may cause sudden dilutional hyponatraemia and seizures. Patients and caretakers should be forewarned of this serious adverse effect and omit its use whenever water intake becomes necessary, e.g. in acute gastroenteritis. Minor side effects reported include headache, abdominal pain and aggressiveness. Information pamphlets on the safety and precautions of DDAVP treatment is available and should be given to patients for their reference.

Enuresis Alarm

- Enuresis alarm training is effective with a good reported success rate of around 60–80% as it addresses the main problem in NE, which is a lack of arousal from sleep in response to signalling from a full bladder.
- It has a reported relapse rate of 15% but retreatment is often effective. However, its use can be cumbersome and can be trying in the initial period of training.
- Enuresis alarm training has been found to be particularly effective and showed early results in cases of severe bedwetting due to the intensive training involved from frequent bedwetting.

- Proper method of using the alarm also helps to ensure good results. Referral to an occupational therapist has been found to be useful for adherence to the proper method by the patient and caretaker.
- When compared with DDAVP, enuresis alarm training has a more sustained effect when off treatment.

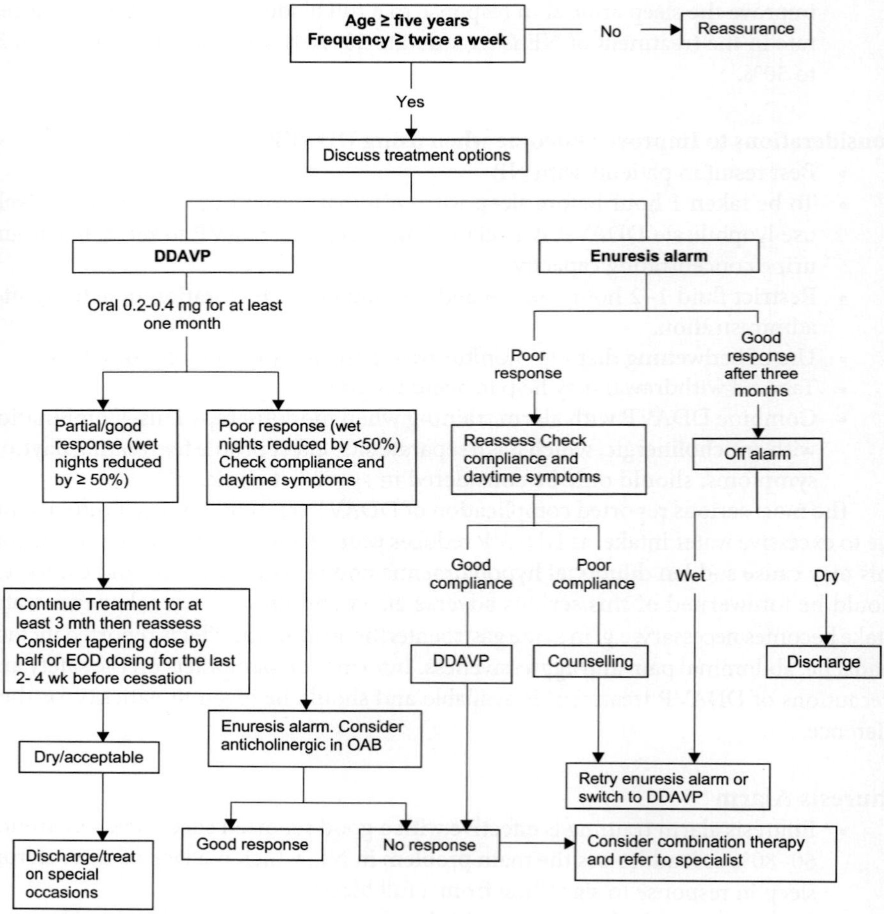

Figure 18.6 Treatment guidelines for Primary MNE.

Bibliography

1. Kuwertz-Broking E, von Gontard A. (2018) Clinical management of nocturnal enuresis. *Pediatr Nephrol* 33(7):1145–1154.

2. Kamperis K, Van Herzeele C, Rittig S, *et al.* (2017) Optimizing response to desmopressin in patients with monosymptomatic nocturnal enuresis. *Pediatr Nephrol* **32**(2):217–226.
3. Baird DC, Seehusen DA, Bode DV. (2014) Enuresis in children: A case-based approach. *Am Fam Physician* **90**(8):560–568.
4. Austin PF, Bauer SB, Bower W, *et al.* (2014) The standardization of terminology of lower urinary tract function in children and adolescents: Update report from the Standardization Committee of the International Children's Continence Society. *J Urol* **191**(6):1863–1865.
5. Chao SM. (2005) Enuresis and voiding disorders. In: Chiu MC, Yap HK (eds.) *Practical Paediatric Nephrology*, pp. 171–178.

CHAPTER 89

Renal Reference Limits

Chong Siew Le

Urine Excretion Indices for Calcium, Urate and Oxalate

Notes

1. Measurement of urine calcium, urate and oxalate is part of the metabolic work up of patients with renal calculi and nephrocalcinosis.
2. High urinary excretion of urine calcium and uric acid have also been found in children with microscopic or gross haematuria.
3. Urinary calcium, uric acid and oxalate excretion are affected by various factors, including age, dietary intake and fluid intake.
4. 24 hours' urine sample has been widely regarded as gold standard for the diagnosis of metabolic abnormalities. However, it is challenging to obtain a proper 24-hour urine specimen in young children, particularly amongst those who are not toilet trained. Hence, spot (random) urine sample for calcium, urate and oxalate to creatinine ratio can be used as a screening test.
5. Spot urine sample for calcium, urate and oxalate to creatinine ratio (consider urine calcium/osmolality for patient with decreased muscle mass), together with other metabolic work up (serum creatinine, sodium, potassium, chloride, bicarbonate, calcium, albumin, uric acid, phosphate, magnesium and urine amino acids), should be routinely performed for patients with renal calculi and nephrocalcinosis. Abnormal spot urine screening tests or metabolic tests should be further evaluated by a timed urine collection where feasible.
6. The urinary reference limits (95th percentile [upper limit]) for calcium/creatinine, calcium/osmolality, urate/creatinine, urate/creatinine, and 24-hour urine calcium, urate and oxalate is detailed in the table below.

Table 18.19 Urinary Reference Limits for Calcium/Creatinine, Calcium/Osmolality, Urate/Creatinine, Oxalate/Creatinine, and 24-Hour Urine Calcium, Urate and Oxalate

Age (year)	Urinary Calcium/ Creatinine (mmol/mmol)	Urine Calcium/ Osmolality	24-hour Urine Calcium	Urinary Urate/ Creatinine (mmol/mmol)	24-hour Urine Urate	Urinary Oxalate/ Creatinine (mmol/mmol)	24-hour Urine Oxalate
$^{1}/_{12}$–$^{6}/_{12}$	2.2	Normal muscle mass: 0.0035 mmol/mmol/kg Decreased muscle mass: >0.00625 mmol/mmol/kg	0.1 mmol/kg/d	1.6	0.11 mmol/kg/d	0.22	<0.5 mmol/1.73 m^2
$^{6}/_{12}$–1	2.2			1.5		0.17	
1–2	1.5			1.4		0.13	
2–3	1.4			1.3		0.10	
3–5	1.1			1.1		0.08	
5–7	0.8			0.8		0.07	
7–10	0.7			0.56		0.06	
10–14	0.7			0.44		0.06	
14–17	0.7			0.40		0.06	

Bibliography

1. Matos V, Van Melle G, Boulat O, *et al.* (1997) Urinary phosphate/creatinine, calcium/creatinine, and magnesium/creatinine ratios in a healthy pediatric population. *J Pediatr* **131**(2):252–257.
2. Matos V, Van Melle G, Werner D, *et al.* (1999) Urinary oxalate and urate to creatinine ratios in a healthy pediatric population. *Am J Kidney Dis* **34**(2):e1.
3. Mir S, Serdaroglu E. (2005) Quantification of hypercalciuria with the urine calcium osmolality ratio in children. *Pediatr Nephrol* **20**(11):1562–1565.
4. Richmond W, Colgan G, Simon S, *et al.* (2005) Random urine calcium/osmolality in the assessment of calciuria in children with decreased muscle mass. *Clin Nephrol* **64**(4):264–270.
5. Geary DF, Schaefer F. (2008) *Pediatric Kidney Disease, 2nd ed.* Springer.

SECTION 19

NEUROLOGY

CHAPTER 90

Headaches and Migraines

Lim Yi Xiu, Jocelyn; Yeo Tong Hong

Introduction

Headaches are common in children and adolescents, with a worldwide prevalence of 60% under 20 years. Females are 1.5 times more likely to get headaches than males. Migraines occur in approximately 8% of these children and adolescents, with a higher incidence in those above 14 years. They are a significant cause of recurrent hospital visits and school absences.

While prevalence is high, most are due to benign causes, most commonly caused by upper respiratory tract infections and primary headaches. Acute headaches with progressive symptoms raise the suspicion of intracranial pathology.

Primary Headache

Primary headaches disorders in children can be broadly categorised into:

- Migraines (with or without aura)
- Complicated migraines (hemiplegic, brainstem, retinal)
- Episodic migraine variants (cyclical vomiting, paroxysmal vertigo, paroxysmal torticollis, abdominal)
- Tension type headaches (episodic or chronic)

Most are typically tension-type headaches and migraines without aura; the two can frequently co-occur.

Secondary Headache

Secondary headaches are most commonly caused by head and neck or systemic conditions (see Table 19.3).

Approach to Headache Evaluation

A comprehensive history and directed clinical neurologic examination are the most sensitive in determining underlying aetiology.

Table 19.1 Diagnostic Criteria of the International Headache Society (IHS) for Tension-Type Headache (TTH)

A.	Infrequent TTH: ≥10 episodes on <1 d per mth on average (<12 d/yr) and fulfilling B to D Frequent TTH: ≥10 episodes on 1–14 d per mth on average for >3 mth (≥12 d and <180 d/yr) and fulfilling B to D Chronic TTH: Headache on ≥15 d per mth on average for >3 mth (≥180 d/yr) and fulfilling B to D
B.	Lasting from 30 min to 7 d
C.	At least two of the following four features: 1. Bilateral location 2. Pressing or tightening (non-pulsating) quality 3. Mild or moderate intensity 4. Not aggravated by routine physical activity (e.g. walking or climbing stairs)
D.	Both of the following: 1. No nausea or vomiting 2. No more than either photophobia or phonophobia
E.	Not better accounted for by another ICHD-3 diagnosis

Table 19.2 Diagnostic Criteria of the International Headache Society (IHS) for Paediatric Migraine Without Aura

A.	≥5 attacks fulfilling criteria B to D
B.	Lasting 4–72 hr (when untreated or unsuccessfully treated)
C.	At least two of the following four features: 1. Unilateral location 2. Pulsating quality 3. Moderate or severe pain intensity 4. Aggravated by or causes avoidance of routine physical activity (e.g. walking or climbing stairs)
D.	At least one of the following accompanying headache: 1. Nausea and/or vomiting 2. Photophobia and phonophobia
E.	Not better accounted for by another ICHD-3 diagnosis

History

Document onset, frequency, time of day, nature of pain, site, duration and severity (impairment of activities more sensitive than pain score). Ask about triggers, relieving factors, prodrome and associated symptoms.

Clinical Examination

- Note: Glasgow Coma Scale (GCS), vital signs, cognition, head circumference
- Complete neurological evaluation, in particular:

Table 19.3 Common Causes of Secondary Headache in Children

Head and Neck Conditions	Systemic Disorders
• Upper respiratory tract infections, sinusitis, allergic rhinitis • Otitis media • Temporomandibular joint pain • Dental disorders • Head injury • Meningitis • Epileptic seizure or following a seizure • Intracranial bleeding • Brain tumour • Idiopathic intracranial hypertension	• Fever • Viral infections • Dehydration • Medication side effect • Hypoglycaemia • Hypercapnia • Hypertension

  - » Signs of meningism
  - » Fundoscopy for papilloedema, abnormal ocular movements
  - » Focal neurological deficits
  - » Gait abnormalities, ataxia, incoordination
  - » Speech abnormalities (quality and quantity)
  - » Abnormal movements — dyskinesia, catatonia
- Directed systemic examination depending on presenting symptoms

Warning Signs

Neuroimaging may be indicated if there is/are:

- signs and symptoms of raised intracranial pressure, including papilloedema
- change in cognition/behaviour or deteriorating school performance
- acute onset, severe or progressive headaches
- early morning vomiting
- headache waking patient up from sleep
- abnormal neurological findings

Management Goals for Primary Headaches

- Eliminate secondary contributory causes — treat allergic rhinitis, sinusitis (imaging only indicated if symptomatic), myopia, dental disorders.
- Manage expectations: Response takes time, triggers are often multi-factorial, including psychological stressors.
- Focus on coping mechanisms and optimising function and daily activities rather than a direct reduction in pain score.

Table 19.4 Key History in the Evaluation of Headache

Characteristics	Primary Headaches		Secondary Headaches	
	Tension Type	Migraine	Benign	Potentially Life-Threatening
Onset *When did headaches begin?*	Chronic		Acute	Acute, worsening
How did it begin? *Precipitants*	Psychosocial stressors, poor sleep		With fever and/or infective symptoms	Trauma/often no precipitant
Location	Diffuse	Usually bifrontal		
Temporal pattern	Non-progressive, episodic	Episodic with well intervals	Resolves with symptomatic treatment	Progressively more severe
Duration *How long does each episode last?*	Can last ‘all day’	Often brief, usually 30–120 min		Persistent, does not go away completely with analgesia
Frequency	Daily or several times weekly	Weekly or less		Persistent, may be nightly, if secondary to raised intracranial pressure (ICP)
Any particular time or circumstance?	e.g. school, bus ride, hunger, heat			Night and/or early morning awakening.
Aura/prodrome		Aura, lethargy, mood change, thirst or food cravings		
Quality and intensity of pain	Traditional terms like band-like or throbbing does not accurately distinguish between the two		Mild to moderate	Severe, non-remitting

(*Continued*)

Table 19.4 (*Continued*)

Characteristics	Primary Headaches		Secondary Headaches	
	Tension Type	Migraine	Benign	Potentially Life-Threatening
Associated symptoms	Concomitant anxiety, low mood or depression, poor social circumstances (parental conflict, bullying)	Nausea, vomiting, anorexia, photophobia, phonophobia, osmophobia	Fever, upper respiratory tract infections, sinusitis	Symptoms can persist between and beyond headache Focal symptoms, e.g. aphasia, weakness, numbness. Lethargy, poor appetite, vomiting, behavioural change.
Impairment of activities *What do you do during the headache?*	Usually continue watching TV or play games. Looks well.	Seek refuge in dark, quiet room. Appears ill.	Usually no impairment.	Activity can be severely impaired.
Triggers, aggravating factors	After school, increased workload, tiredness.	Light, noise, smells, activity	Intercurrent illness	Increased ICP: worse lying down Low ICP: worse sitting/standing
Family history	Often	Often		Not common
Efficacy of medication use	Helpful to identify those at risk of rebound analgesic headaches		Responsive to medications	Exposure to medications that increase risk of idiopathic intracranial hypertension

Non-Pharmacological Interventions

- Lifestyle measures: Good sleep hygiene (keeping bedtime constant even during weekends and holidays), attention to routine, adequate hydration, regular meals and physical activity.
- Empower coping: A headache diary helps to identify triggers and aggravating factors for interventions (e.g. short nap, quick shower, dark/quiet room), helps assess need for prophylactic therapy and its efficacy.
- Education: Understanding natural course, specific headache characteristics, aggravating and relieving factors, medication use/effect.
- Psychological/psychiatric/medical social worker referral if concomitant anxiety, depression, challenging family or school circumstances.
- Cognitive behavioural therapy, relaxation and/or distraction techniques.

Pharmacological Treatments

Acute Symptom Relief

- Use when severe or persistent with restriction of daily activities, despite non-pharmacological measures.
- Consider paracetamol, ibuprofen or naproxen, sumatriptan (age >12 years)
    i. Treatment is more likely to be effective when used earlier within the first hour.
    ii. Treatment is more effective in pain relief than associated symptoms like nausea/vomiting; antiemetics can be prescribed in addition.
    iii. Treatment can be repeated once within a 24-hour period if it is effective but pain recurs.
- Avoid medication overuse: limit pain relievers to ≤2–3 times a week (<15 days/month of paracetamol/NSAIDS, <10 days/month of triptans)

Prophylactic Medication

Migraine prophylaxis aims to reduce the frequency and intensity of attacks and should be considered when there are more than four attacks per month, when there is poor response to symptomatic treatment and daily activities are significantly affected.

Many different classes of drugs have been used including anti-epileptics, antihistamines, anti-depressants, calcium channel blockers, beta blockers and alpha-agonists. However, there is a lack of definitive evidence for efficacy. The placebo effect is also significant in children (~60% of patients).

The decision to start prophylaxis should be made together with the neurologist, parent and child, taking into consideration psychosocial factors, medication side effects and non-pharmacological interventions. It is inappropriate to continue prophylaxis long term once attacks subside.

Bibliography

1. Abu-Arafeh I, Razak S, Sivaraman B, Graham C. (2010) Prevalence of headache and migraine in children and adolescents: A systemic review of population-based studies. *Dev Med Child Neurol* **52:**1088–1097.
2. Antilla P. (2006) Tension-type headache in childhood and adolescence. *Lancet Neurol* **5**:268–274.
3. Roser T, Bonfert M, Heinen F, *et al.* (2013) Primary versus secondary headache in children: A frequent diagnostic challenge in clinical routine. *Neuropediatrics* **44**:34–39.
4. IHS. (2018) The international classification of headache disorders, 3rd edition. *Cephalalgia* **38**(1):1–211.
5. Powers SW, Coffey CS, Chamberlin LA, *et al.* (2016) Trial of amitriptyline, topiramate, and placebo for pediatric migraine. *N Eng J Med* **376**(2):115–124.
6. Oskoui M, Pringsheim T, Holler-Managan Y, *et al.* (2019) Practice guideline update summary: Acute treatment of migraine in children and adolescents. *Neurology* **93**:487–499.
7. Maryam O, Pringsheim T, Billinghurst L, *et al.* (2019) Practice guideline update summary: Pharmacologic treatment for pediatric migraine prevention. *Neurology* **93**:500–509.
8. Papetti L, Ursitti F, Valeriani M, *et al.* (2019) Prophylactic treatment of pediatric migraine: Is there anything new in the last decade? *Front Neurol* **10**:771.

CHAPTER 91

Seizures and Epilepsy

Ngoh Seow Fen, Adeline; Lim Yi Xiu, Jocelyn; Chan Wei Shih, Derrick

Seizures

Definition

A seizure is a transient occurrence of signs and/or symptoms due to abnormal excessive or synchronous neuronal activity in the brain. A seizure is a symptom, not a diagnosis.

Acute Symptomatic Seizures

Seizures that have an obvious and immediate preceding cause. Common causes include:

- Head trauma
- Electrolyte abnormalities (hypoglycaemia, hyponatraemia, hypocalcaemia)
- Central nervous system (CNS) infections (meningoencephalitis, abscesses)
- Structural lesions (tumours, bleeds)
- Ischaemic stroke

These are often isolated events and do not recur when the cause is removed.

Febrile Seizures

Seizures occurring in:

- Children aged 6 months to 6 years old with
- Temperature >38°C (child may only be febrile after the seizure) and
- Absence of CNS infection

Febrile seizures:

- Can be simple: Lasting <15 minutes long, single episode in 24 hours and generalised
- OR complicated (complex): Lasting >15 minutes long, multiple episodes in 24 hours and focal

Management is mostly symptomatic and supportive:

- Identify source of infection and treat accordingly.
- Antipyretics for comfort care. This does not prevent/reduce febrile seizure recurrence.
- Provide Febrile Seizure patient information leaflet.
- Discharge when well with advice for management of acute seizure.
- Consider standby rectal diazepam if febrile seizures are recurrent and/or prolonged in children >1 year old and >10 kg.

Provoked Seizures

Seizures in the context of intercurrent illness (usually gastroenteritis or upper respiratory tract infections) and absence of fever in the preceding 24 hours. Majority do not require treatment. Acute treatment with benzodiazepines and/or phenytoin/phenobarbitone is occasionally required if seizures are recurrent within 24 hours or are prolonged.

Status epilepticus (SE): >30 minutes of continuous seizure activity or multiple seizures without intervening recovery of consciousness. A functional definition of status epilepticus is a seizure persisting beyond 5 to 10 minutes. See Figure 19.1 for the clinical pathway of status epilepticus management.

Epilepsy

In children with no acute cause or triggering factor, a first unprovoked seizure is said to have occurred. Two or more unprovoked seizures at least 24 hours apart constitutes a working diagnosis of epilepsy. In children with significant risk factors such as an abnormal electroencephalogram (EEG) or neuroimaging, epilepsy can also be diagnosed after one unprovoked seizure.

Epilepsy is a disorder of the brain characterised by an enduring predisposition to generate epileptic seizures and by the neurobiological, cognitive, psychological and social consequences of this condition.

Classification of Seizures

The International League Against Epilepsy (ILAE) Seizure Classification was first presented in 1981, dividing seizure types into generalised and partial, with consciousness as a sub-divider. Since then, it has undergone several revisions, with the latest modification in 2017. This revised framework seeks to be more operational and has three non-hierarchal levels of diagnosis:

- Seizure type
- Epilepsy type (focal, generalised, combined generalised and focal, unknown)
- Epilepsy syndrome

Focal seizures — originate within networks in one hemisphere of the brain

- Awareness refers to perception or knowledge of self and environment during a seizure, may be left unspecified if unclear from history.
- Motor onset is subdivided into:
  - » Automatisms — repetitive motor activity, e.g. lip smacking or chewing, finger tapping or fumbling
  - » Atonic — loss of tone
  - » Clonic — rhythmic regular jerking of the limbs, body
  - » Epileptic spasms — sudden flexion/extension/mixed movements of predominantly proximal and truncal muscles. More sustained than myoclonus but shorter than tonic movements

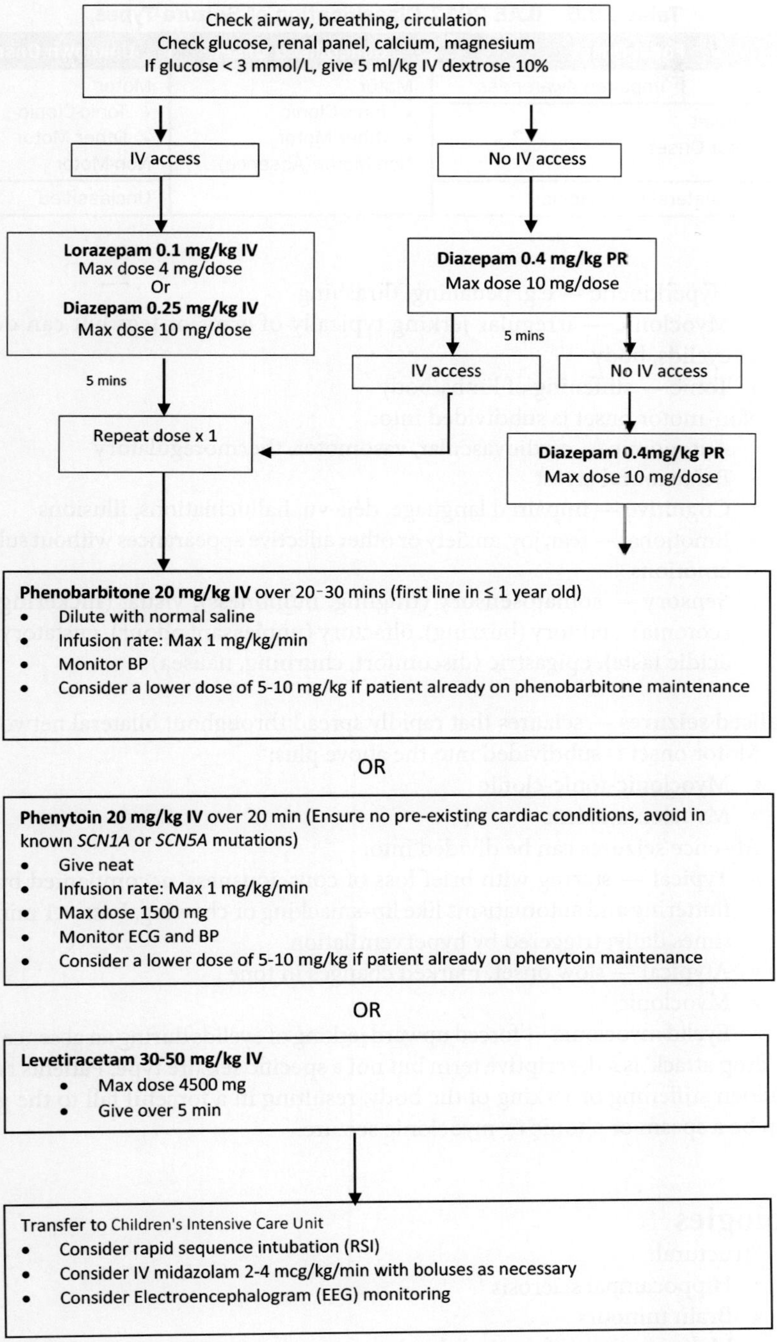

Figure 19.1 Clinical pathway for the management of status epilepticus.

Table 19.5 ILAE 2017 Classification of Seizure Types

Focal Onset		Generalised Onset	Unknown Onset
Aware	Impaired Awareness	Motor • Tonic-Clonic • Other Motor Non-Motor (Absence)	Motor • Tonic-Clonic • Other Motor Non-Motor
Motor Onset Non-Motor Onset			
Focal to bilateral tonic-clonic			Unclassified

  - » Hyperkinetic — e.g. pedalling, thrashing
  - » Myoclonic — irregular jerking typically of arms or legs but can occur in eyelids, body
  - » Tonic — stiffening of limbs/body
- Non-motor onset is subdivided into:
  - » Autonomic — cardiovascular, vasomotor, thermoregulatory
  - » Behavioural arrest
  - » Cognitive — impaired language, déjà vu, hallucinations, illusions
  - » Emotional — fear, joy, anxiety or other affective appearances without subjective emotions
  - » Sensory — somatosensory (tingling, numbness), visual (flickering lights, scotoma), auditory (buzzing), olfactory (unpleasant odour), gustatory (bitter, acidic taste), epigastric (discomfort, churning, nausea)

Generalised seizures — seizures that rapidly spread throughout bilateral networks.

- Motor onset is subdivided into the above plus:
  - » Myoclonic-tonic-clonic
  - » Myoclonic-atonic
- Absence seizures can be divided into:
  - » Typical — staring with brief loss of consciousness, accompanied by eyelid fluttering and automatisms like lip-smacking or chewing. Lasts <1 min, many times daily; triggered by hyperventilation.
  - » Atypical — slow onset, marked changes in tone
  - » Myoclonic
  - » Eyelid myoclonia — forced upward jerking of eyelids during an absence seizure

A 'drop attack' is a descriptive term but not a specific seizure type. Patients typically have sudden stiffening or jerking of the body, resulting in a forceful fall to the ground. This can be a spasm or a tonic or myoclonic seizure.

Aetiologies

- Structural
  - » Hippocampal sclerosis
  - » Brain tumours
  - » Malformations of cortical development

  - » Vascular malformations
  - » Glial scarring (including stroke and traumatic brain injury)
- Genetic
- Infectious
- Metabolic
  - » Inborn errors of metabolism
  - » Acquired, e.g. nutritional failure, organ failure, toxins
- Immune
- Neurodegenerative
- Unknown

Epilepsy Syndromes

A complex of signs and symptoms, investigation findings (EEG, magnetic resonance imaging [MRI]), treatment response and prognosis that define a unique epileptic condition.

1. Idiopathic Generalised Epilepsies (IGE)

- Consists of either one or a combination of: Absence, myoclonic, tonic-clonic and myotonic-tonic-clonic; these may have asymmetric features.
- Normal development but may have associated attention deficit hyperactivity disorder (ADHD), learning and mood disorders.
- EEG shows classical generalised spike-wave discharges accentuated in sleep.
- Usually anticonvulsant-responsive with 80% responding to appropriate anti-epileptic drugs (AED).

A. Childhood absence epilepsy (CAE)

- School-age children aged 4 to 10 years (peak 6–7 years), 2–8% of all cases of epilepsy (if older age onset, consider juvenile absence epilepsy).
- Multiple daily absence seizures: Brief (<1 minute) staring and unresponsiveness, behavioural arrest, sometimes with eyelid fluttering, oral or manual automatisms with immediate return to normal activity afterwards.
- Induced by hyperventilation (3 to 5 minutes).
- Treatment with ethosuximide or sodium valproate. Made worse by carbamazepine.
- 60% remits by early adolescence, others may evolve to other IGE syndromes.

B. Juvenile myoclonic epilepsy (JME)

- Commonest adolescent and adult onset IGE, typical age range 10 to 24 years (peak 12–18 years).
- Early morning sudden myoclonic jerks ('clumsiness'), generalised tonic-clonic seizures. 33% have absence seizure.
- Sleep deprivation worsens myoclonus.
- Interictal EEG — Generalised polyspike and spike-and-wave discharges at 4–6 Hz; photosensitivity is common.
- Valproate usually controls seizures but treatment may be lifelong.
- Carbamazepine and phenytoin aggravate myoclonic and absence seizures.

C. Juvenile absence epilepsy (JAE)

- Characterised by absence seizures with onset from 8 to 20 years of age (peak 9 to 13 years)
- May also have generalised tonic-clonic seizures (80%). Less commonly, adolescents may present with generalised tonic-clonic seizures before the onset of absences
- Interictal EEG — Generalised polyspike and spike-and-wave discharges at 4–6 Hz (clinical absences can be provoked by hyperventilation)
- Valproate usually controls seizures but treatment may be lifelong. Ethosuximide can help with absence seizures but does not protect against generalised tonic clonic seizures
- Carbamazepine and phenytoin can exacerbate seizures

D. Generalised tonic-clonic seizures alone (GTCA)

- Typical age onset: 10 to 25 years, with 80% having their first GTC in the second decade.
- Generalised tonic-clonic seizures, other seizure types are exclusionary.
- Seizures are infrequent, usually yearly or less.
- EEG: Generalised spike or polyspike waves >3–3.5 Hz, 50% only showing in sleep.
- Responsive to sodium valproate but treatment may be lifelong.

2. Self-limited Focal Epilepsies

- Accounts for up to 25% of paediatric epilepsies.
- Normal birth and development
- Behavioural and neuropsychological deficits may occur during the course of active epilepsy but usually improve after seizures remit
- No significant structural lesion on neuroimaging.
- Usually drug-responsive, remission occurs by adolescence.
- Seizures are usually focal motor or sensory, with or without impaired awareness; may sometimes evolve to bilateral tonic-clonic seizures.

A. Rolandic epilepsy/Benign epilepsy with centrotemporal spikes (BECTS)

- Estimated 15% of all childhood epilepsies; age of onset 5 to 10 years.
- Typically, infrequent seizures in sleep, sometimes awake/asleep, rarely only when awake.
- Simple partial seizures of the face, oropharynx and upper limb, at times with secondary generalisation.
- EEG: Centrotemporal spikes
- Treatment: e.g. sodium valproate indicated if frequent seizures or cognitive impairments.
- Excellent prognosis with remission by mid-teenage years.

B. Panayiotopoulos Syndrome/Early onset occipital epilepsy

- Accounts for 5% of all childhood epilepsies; age range 1 to 14 years with 70% between 3 and 6 years old.
- Infrequent focal autonomic seizures with or without impaired awareness. Vomiting is the commonest feature (often mistaken for gastroenteritis), often associated with pallor, flushing, malaise, nausea and abdominal pain. Can evolve to eye/head version, hemiclonic or bilateral tonic-clonic seizures.
- 70% occur in sleep, seizures are often prolonged, lasting >30 minutes.
- EEG: Multifocal spike or sharp-slow discharges over posterior regions
- Self-limited, with most seizures resolving within 3 years of onset

C. Childhood occipital epilepsy (Gastaut type)

- Onset of seizures between 15 months and 19 months of age, with peak onset between 8 and 9 years of age (slightly later than Panayiotopoulos Syndrome)
- Focal sensory visual seizures occur. These have rapid onset and are usually brief (typically lasting only seconds or <3 minutes, rarely do they last up to 20 minutes).
- Typically, visual phenomena are described as small multi-coloured circles in the peripheral vision
- Other occipital lobe seizure features include ictal blindness, visual hallucinations or orbital pain
- Seizures can spread outside the occipital lobe, resulting in hemiparaesthesia, or evolution into hemiclonic or generalised tonic clonic seizures
- Seizures are usually easily controlled, especially with carbamazepine
- EEG: Occipital spike or spike and wave is seen in the interictal EEG
- Remission occurs within 2–4 years in 50–60% of patients

3. **West Syndrome**
   - Epileptic encephalopathy of infancy (seizures are so severe that the brain function and development are affected)
   - Incidence: 1 in 4000–6000 live births
   - Peak frequency: 3 to 7 months of age, 93% before 2 years
   - Epileptic spasms (flexor, extensor, mixed) can be asymmetric or have focal features, e.g. tonic eye or head deviation. Cognition and developmental deterioration if untreated.
   - EEG: Hypsarrhythmia (disorganised generalised high amplitude sharp and slow waves) or modified hypsarrhythmia
   - Diagnostic work up: Awake and sleep EEG, brain magnetic resonance imaging/ spectroscopy, neurometabolic work up ± genetic testing
   - Prognosis: Guarded apart from idiopathic infantile spasm. 75–90% have developmental delay. Risk of developing Lennox–Gastaut syndrome.
   - Treatment:
     - » Oral prednisolone/Adrenocorticotropic hormone (ACTH)
     - » Vigabatrin
     - » Ketogenic diet
     - » Other medication, e.g. Topiramate, Pyridoxine

» Surgical treatment for underlying focal cortical dysplasias

4. Lennox–Gastaut syndrome

- Age of onset: 1 to 14 years
- Severe epileptic disorder with triad of:
  - » Multiple seizure types, typically tonic, atypical absence myoclonic and tonic-clonic seizures
  - » EEG: Diffuse, slow spike-and-wave 1–2.5 Hz complexes, slow background
  - » Diffuse and severe cognitive impairments, learning disability
- Status epilepticus common, especially non-convulsive forms
- Aetiology: Many causes, about 25% are cryptogenic
- Poor prognosis for seizure control and mental development
- Treatment:
  - » Medication: Sodium valproate, benzodiazepines, e.g. clobazam/nitrazepam, topiramate, but seizures are commonly refractory to medication
  - » Surgery: Corpus callosotomy for drop attacks, Vagus Nerve Stimulator

Approach

- Determine whether patient does or does not have seizures (seizures vs. non-seizures)
- Determine the seizure type or syndrome
- Determine aetiology where possible
- Assess co-morbidity
- Formulate a management plan

History

- Careful and detailed history is essential
- Clear description of semiology, pre- and post-ictal symptoms and duration, frequency of episodes
- Past medical history, including recent trauma and illness, associated symptoms, long-term medications
- Developmental history
- Social history
- Family history

Neurological and Physical Examination

Investigations

- Electroencephalography (EEG)
  - » Value: May help to localise seizure origin and assist in syndromic classification.
  - » Limitations: Cannot be used to make or exclude a diagnosis of epilepsy (epilepsy is a clinical diagnosis); easily affected by drugs, toxic or metabolic changes; does not elucidate cause.
    - ■ First EEG can be normal in 50% of persons with epilepsy.

    - ▪ A small percentage of normal children have epileptiform activity on EEG but never a seizure.
- Neuroimaging — computed tomography (CT) if emergency, MRI preferred
    - » Indicated in focal epilepsies, neurological deficits, young age, difficult-to-control seizures
    - » Not required in Rolandic epilepsy, childhood absence epilepsy
- Laboratory tests, lumbar puncture as indicated to elucidate genetic/metabolic/immune causes

Management

- Making a diagnosis of epilepsy is not necessarily the same as a decision to treat. Some seizures are minor and infrequent, and parents may choose to avoid the side effects of medication. Each treatment decision should be individualised between clinician and caregiver/patient.
- Aims: Stop or reduce seizures, maintain quality of life.
    - » Establish firm diagnosis of epilepsy before starting treatment.
    - » Consider seizure type, severity, recurrence risk, epilepsy syndrome, aetiology, co-morbidity and precipitants.
    - » Mainstay of treatment — anti-epileptic drugs (AEDs).
- Indications to treat:
    - » Recurrent frequent seizures (every few months or more), severity (tendency for status epilepticus, risk of injury), specific epilepsy syndromes.
    - » Presence of risk factors (e.g. epileptiform discharges on EEG).
    - » Accompanying neurological, neuropsychological or psychosocial problems.
- Initiate monotherapy using the appropriate medication, titrating up to a maintenance dose.
    - » Balance between drug efficacy and tolerability.
    - » Holistic approach — psychosocial management and epilepsy support are important.
    - » Refer for epilepsy counselling by pharmacy and specialty nurse; acute seizure advice ± standby rectal diazepam.
- Duration of therapy
    - » Syndrome diagnosis and treatment response are important considerations, with a minimum of 2 years in self-limiting epilepsy syndromes.
- Fifty per cent will respond to first anticonvulsant; ~20% to the second, the rest tend to be refractory and non-pharmacological treatments, such as epilepsy surgery, ketogenic diet or vagal nerve stimulation, etc., should be considered

Bibliography

1. Zupanc ML. (1996) Update of epilepsy in paediatric patients. *Mayo Clin Proc* **71**(9):899–916.
2. Commission on Classification and Terminology of the International League against Epilepsy. (1989) Proposal for revised classification of epilepsies and epileptic syndromes. *Epilepsia* **30**:389–399.

3. Scheffer I, Berkovic S, S Zuberi, *et al.* (2017) ILAE Classification of the epilepsies: Position paper of the ILAE commission for classification and terminology. *Epilepsia* **58**:512–521.
4. Pavone P, Polizzi, A, Marino SD, *et al.* (2020) West syndrome: A comprehensive review. *Neurol Sci* **41**:3547–3562.
5. Lamberink, *et al.* (2017) Individualised prediction model of seizure recurrence and long-term outcomes after withdrawal of antiepileptic drugs in seizure-free patients: A systemic review and individual participant data meta-analysis. *Lancet Neurol* **16**:523–531.
6. Balestrini S, Arzimanoglou A, Blumcke I, *et al.* (2021) The aetiologies of epilepsy. *Epileptic Disord* **23**(1):1–16.
7. Angurana SK, Suthar R. (2021) Efficacy and safety of levetiracetam vs phenytoin as second line antiseizure medication for pediatric convulsive status epilepticus: A systematic review and meta-analysis of randomised controlled trials. *J Trop Pediatr* **67**:1–14.

CHAPTER 92

Encephalopathy and Stroke

Lim Yi Xiu, Jocelyn; Terrence Thomas

Introduction

- Children with acute central nervous system (CNS) syndromes commonly present with acute encephalopathy. This may include a depression in consciousness (lethargy and drowsiness) or agitation and confusion.
  In infants and younger children, ask caregivers about a deviation from baseline activity.
- Look for focal manifestations: Seizures, motor weakness, sensory and autonomic deficits, speech abnormalities and visual disturbances.
- Systemic symptoms like fever, vomiting and decreased appetite may be present.
- Although stroke typically presents as a new onset neurological deficit (usually hemiplegia with/without aphasia) *without* encephalopathy, the general principles in assessment, stabilisation, time to neuroimaging and initial treatments are similar to a child with new onset encephalopathy.

Aetiologies

Table 19.6 Aetiologies of Acute Central Nervous Syndromes in Children

	Hyperacute *Minutes to Hours*	Acute *Hours to Days*	Subacute *Days to Weeks*	Chronic *Weeks to Months*
Neonate/ infants	Seizures Head trauma (consider non-accidental injury) Hypoxic-ischaemic injury Metabolic derangements (hypoglycaemia, hypo- or hypernatraemia)	Infection (bacterial, viral) Vascular (ischaemic stroke, cerebral venous thrombosis) Inborn errors of metabolism Hyperammonemia (e.g. urea cycle defects, aminoacidopathies)	Infection (TB, fungal, parasitic)	Neurometabolic disorders Genetic syndromes Epileptic encephalopathies Neoplasms (primary brain tumours, metastasis)

(Continued)

Table 19.6 (*Continued*)

	Hyperacute *Minutes to Hours*	**Acute** *Hours to Days*	**Subacute** *Days to Weeks*	**Chronic** *Weeks to Months*
Pre-schoolers/ Older children	Seizures Trauma Vascular (haemorrhagic or ischaemic stroke) Hypoglycaemia, DKA Drugs/toxins	Infection (bacterial, viral) Infection-triggered encephalopathy syndromes (MERS, ANE, AESD and HSES), FIRES, antibody-mediated encephalitis (usually NMDAR, MOG or GFAP), acute demyelinating encephalomyelitis (usually MOG, AQP4)	Infection (TB, fungal, parasitic) Infection-triggered encephalopathy syndromes (MERS, ANE, AESD and HSES), FIRES, antibody-mediated encephalitis (usually NMDAR, MOG or GFAP), acute demyelinating encephalomyelitis (usually MOG, AQP4) CNS Vasculitis (e.g. Takayasu, SLE)	Neurometabolic disorders Neoplasm (primary brain tumours, metastasis) Infections (TB, HIV)
Adolescents	Generalised seizures (post-ictal state) Head trauma Vascular (haemorrhagic or ischaemic stroke) Drugs/toxins ingestion DKA	Infection (bacterial, viral) Infection-triggered encephalopathy syndromes (MERS, ANE, AESD and HSES), FIRES, antibody-mediated encephalitis (usually NMDAR, MOG or GFAP), acute demyelinating encephalomyelitis (usually MOG, AQP4) Acute psychiatric disorders (schizophrenia, bipolar/mood disorder)	Infection (TB, fungal, parasitic) Infection-triggered encephalopathy syndromes (MERS, ANE, AESD and HSES), FIRES, antibody-mediated encephalitis (usually NMDAR, MOG or GFAP), acute demyelinating encephalomyelitis (usually MOG, AQP4) CNS Vasculitis (e.g. Takayasu, SLE)	Neoplasm (primary brain tumours, metastasis) Neurometabolic disorders Infections (TB, HIV)

TB: tuberculosis; DKA: diabetic ketoacidosis; MERS: Mild Encephalopathy with Reversible Splenial lesion; ANE: Acute Necrotising Encephalopathy; AESD: Acute Encephalopathy with biphasic Seizures and late reduced Diffusion; HSES: Haemorrhagic Shock and Encephalopathy Syndrome; FIRES: Febrile Infection-Related Epilepsy Syndrome; NMDAR: N-methyl-d-aspartate receptor; MOG: myelin oligodendrocyte glycoprotein; GFAP: Glial Fibrillary Acidic Protein; AQP4: anti aquaporin 4; CNS: central nervous system; SLE: systemic lupus erythematosus; HIV: human immunodeficiency virus

Clinical Examination

- Assess Airway, Breathing, Circulation with a set of vital signs: Heart rate, respiratory rate, blood pressure, oxygen saturation; do point-of-care test for electrolytes and blood glucose
- Determine Glasgow Coma Scale (GCS)
  - » Consider Children's Intensive Care Unit (CICU) admission if GCS <9 or rapidly deteriorating
  - » In those with GCS 14–15, perform a mini-mental state exam (see Tables 19.7 and 19.8)

Table 19.7 Glasgow Coma Scale and Modified Coma Scale for Infants

Glasgow Coma Scale		Modified Coma Scale for Infants	
Eye opening		**Eye opening**	
Spontaneous	4	Spontaneous	4
To speech	3	To speech	3
To pain	2	To pain	2
None	1	None	1
Verbal		**Verbal**	
Oriented	5	Coo/babbles	5
Confused	4	Irritable	4
Inappropriate words	3	Cries to pain	3
Non-specific sounds	2	Moans to pain	2
None	1	None	1
Motor		**Motor**	
Follows commands	6	Normal spontaneous movements	6
Localises pain	5	Withdraws to touch	5
Withdraws to pain	4	Withdraws to pain	4
Abnormal flexion	3	Abnormal flexion	3
Abnormal extension	2	Abnormal extension	2
None	1	None	1

Table 19.8 Mini-Mental State Examination

Orientation:
Date and place of birth
Country and place
Current time, day and date

Registration:
'I shall say 3 words for you to remember (e.g. watch, pen, book). Repeat them after I have said them.'

Mental Reversal:
Spelling 'WORLD' backwards; 5 serial 7s (serially subtract 7 from 100) or 5 serial 3s for younger children (serially subtract 3 from 20)

First Recall:
Recalling the 3 words the patient is asked to remember

Naming:
Objects; body parts

Three-stage Command:
E.g. 'Take this paper with your left hand, fold it in half, and hand it back to me'

Copying:
Copy a pair of intersecting pentagons

- Signs of meningism: Bulging fontanelle in an infant, nuchal rigidity or positive Kernig's sign in older children.
- Signs of raised intracranial pressure: Papilloedema, falling coma score, altered breathing patterns, abnormal pupil responses, Cushing's reflex with hypertension and bradycardia, decerebrate and decorticate posturing.
- Seizures may be subtle, e.g. tonic eye deviation, tonic posturing or minor clonic movements of the face or limbs.
- Observe for dyskinesia: Dystonia (oromotor or limb; ophisthotonus), chorea or motor stereotypies. Hyperkinetic (agitation) or negative (posturing) catatonic features may be present.

Investigations

Discuss investigations with neurologists. They should be tailored to each individual child based on history and examination findings.

Recommended Tests

- Full blood count, renal panel, liver function tests, electrolytes (calcium, magnesium, phosphate), erythrocyte sedimentation rate (ESR), C-reactive protein (CRP), plasma glucose, ammonia, thyroid function tests (TFT)
- Microbiological studies: Blood cultures, respiratory pathogen multiplex PCR, and mycoplasma throat swab/serology, cerebrospinal fluid (CSF) analysis (opening pressure, microscopy, culture, meningitis/encephalitis pathogen multiplex PCR)
- Immunological studies: Serum complements C3/C4, antinuclear antibody (ANA), double-stranded DNA (dsDNA), anti-thyroglobulin, anti-thyroperoxidase (TPO) antibodies (TFT can be normal) and anti-myelin oligodendrocyte glycoprotein (MOG) antibodies; paired CSF-plasma oligoclonal bands and anti-N-methyl-d-aspartate receptor (NMDAR) (± autoimmune encephalitis panel) antibodies; CSF blast cells.
- Genetic/metabolic investigations: Acylcarnitine profile, serum copper and caeruloplasmin; paired CSF and plasma lactate, amino acids; urine organic acids
- Electroencephalogram (EEG) may be considered if subclinical seizures are suspected

Neuroimaging

- Magnetic resonance imaging (MRI) brain with contrast is the preferred imaging modality. Add on MR Angiography or Venography if clinical suspicion of stroke as a cause of encephalopathy.
- Computed tomography (CT) brain helpful to exclude neurosurgical emergencies such as a space-occupying lesion or an intracranial bleed.

If MRI Brain demonstrates Arterial Ischaemic Stroke, add on the following investigations:

- Thrombophilia screen: Prothrombin Time (PT), Activated Partial Thromboplastin Time (APTT), International Normalised Ratio (INR), Protein C, Protein S, antithrombin III, Factor V Leiden, lupus anti-coagulant, anti-cardiolipin, serum homocysteine level. (Optional further tests: MTHFR [methylenetetrahydrofolate reductase], lipoprotein A, Prothrombin gene mutations)

- Evaluate for systemic vasculitides (consult Rheumatologist), e.g. Takayasu disease, anti-neutrophil cytoplasmic autoantibody (ANCA) vasculitides
- Cardiac assessment: Electrocardiogram (ECG) and 2D echocardiogram (with bubble study); carotid Doppler study.

Management

If child is ill, escalate care to High Dependency Unit or CICU

Supportive Care

1. Keep nil by mouth (NBM), minimise handling.
2. Maintain general homeostasis — normothermia, normal oxygen saturation and partial pressure of carbon dioxide (pCO2), glucose and electrolytes, heart rate and respiratory rate.
3. Maintain cerebral perfusion pressure (CPP) — adequate hydration with full maintenance intravenous (IV) fluids and normal blood pressure.
4. Elective intubation for cerebral protection if GCS <8 or rapidly dropping.
5. If agitated, consider IV lorazepam 0.05 to 0.1 mg/kg/dose Q8–12H (IV midazolam and/or morphine infusion if intubated).

Seizure Management

- As per Institution's Status Epilepticus protocol.
- Aim to stop all subclinical seizures.

Antimicrobials (see Hospital Antimicrobial guidelines)

- IV ceftriaxone 100 mg/kg Q24H
- IV acyclovir 10 mg/kg/dose Q8H
- IV ciprofloxacin 10 mg/kg Q8H (if suspected mycoplasma or rickettsial infection)

Immunotherapy (in immune encephalitis, demyelination or CNS vasculitis; consult Neurologist)

- IV methylprednisolone 30 mg/kg/day (max. 1 g) for 5 days ± oral (PO) prednisolone taper
- IV Immunoglobulins (IVIG) 2 g/kg over 2–5 days
- IV omeprazole 1 mg/kg Q12H or IV ranitidine 1 mg/kg Q8H or similar as gastric protection, if IV steroids are given.
- If active gastrointestinal bleed, may reduce IV methylprednisolone to 20 mg/kg/day (max. 1 g) or split into 10 mg/kg Q12H or Q8H doses

Tone Management (consult Neurologist)

- Either IV or PO clonidine, PO baclofen or benzhexol

Neurorehabilitation

- Physiotherapy, occupational therapy, speech and language therapy ± music therapy should be instituted as early as appropriate

Anticoagulation (If Arterial Ischaemic Stroke or Cerebral Sinovenous Thrombosis seen on MR imaging)

- Consult Haematologist, Neurologist ± Cardiologist (if cardiac disease present) for decision to anticoagulate.

General Principles (acute stroke period):

- Perform lumbar puncture for CSF studies prior to starting anticoagulation, if possible.
- Ensure no contraindications to anticoagulation.
- If carotid or proximal cerebral artery occlusion, cardiac aetiology or cerebral sinovenous thrombosis:
  - » Start with IV Standard (unfractionated heparin) or subcutaneous (SC) Enoxaparin [Follow current Institution Guidelines for anticoagulation]
  - » Aim for APTT 60–80 ms (standard heparin) or factor Xa 0.3–0.7 μ/ml (for both agents).
- If cerebral arterial malformations, e.g. Moya-moya syndrome, or small vessel focal cerebral arteriopathy: Start PO Aspirin 3–5 mg/kg/day.

Bibliography

1. Lim YXJ, Kwek SY, How CH, *et al.* (2020) A clinical approach to encephalopathy in children. *Sing Med J* **61**(12): 626–632.
2. Thompson C, Kneen R, Riordan A, *et al.* (2012) Encephalitis in children. *Arch Dis Child* **97**:150–161.
3. Mastrangelo M, Giordo L, Leuzzi V. (2022) Acute ischaemic stroke in childhood: A comprehensive review. *Eur J Pediatr* **181**:45–58.
4. Kossorotoff M, Chabrier S, Dinomais M. (2019) Arterial ischemic stroke in non-neonate children: Diagnostic and therapeutic specificities. *Neuropediatrics* **176**(1–2):20–29.

CHAPTER 93

Acute Flaccid Paralysis

Lim Yi Xiu, Jocelyn; Simon Ling

Introduction

Acute flaccid paralysis (AFP) is a clinical syndrome characterised by acute rapid onset of weakness and the lack of corticospinal tract signs. Flaccid suggests a picture of hypotonia and hyporeflexia, but the term indicates absence of spasticity, hyperreflexia and extensor plantar responses (i.e. the corticospinal tract signs) on examination. When referring to degree of weakness, 'paresis' generally indicates milder loss of motor strength and 'plegia' or 'paralysis' indicates severe loss of strength.

Aetiologies

AFP can be caused by a wide variety of conditions affecting the neuro-axis. Rather than detailing each of these, this chapter will give an overview of the clinical approach and reasoning. AFP in children can be a challenging neurologic emergency and some can progress rapidly to involve life-threatening bulbar or respiratory muscle weakness. Thus, an accurate diagnosis of the cause and timely appropriate investigation have implications for treatment and outcome. A logical approach focusing on the history, clinical examination and investigations helps to narrow the differential.

Approach

- First establish the presence of neurologic muscular weakness.
  - » Gait abnormality or inability to walk may be due to various causes, including joint pain, myalgia, incoordination or dyskinesia.
  - » Young pre-verbal children may present with non-specific symptoms such as irritability, poor feeding or refusal to walk.
  - » History, observation (bedside, in the ward) and neurological examination will determine weakness.

- **Detailed History**
  - » Onset and progression of weakness
    - ■ Hyperacute (within hours) — vascular (haemorrhagic or ischaemic)/traumatic/compressive
    - ■ Acute (hours to days) — infective/inflammatory

    - Subacute to chronic (days to weeks) — infective/inflammatory/infiltrative
  - Pattern/distribution of weakness
    - Symmetrical versus patchy
    - Proximal versus distal
    - Cervical versus thoracolumbar or lumbosacral spinal pattern
    - Cranial nerve involvement — ocular, facial, bulbar
  - Associated symptoms
    - Sensory deficits — sensory spinal level, paraesthesia/numbness (dermatomal versus distal)
    - Pain — muscle, joint, neuropathic
    - Autonomic features — urinary retention, constipation, temperature dysregulation, cardiac rhythm abnormalities, labile blood pressure
    - Central nervous system (CNS) symptoms — headache, encephalopathy, vomiting
    - Systemic features — fever, rash, oral ulcers
  - Recent exposures
    - Illnesses, trauma, drug/toxins
  - Existing systemic diseases and/or long-term medications

- **Clinical Examination**
  - Assess patient stability and vital signs — temperature, heart rate and rhythm, blood pressure, respiratory status.
  - Glasgow Coma Scale (GCS) status, cognition
  - Full neurological examination — motor, sensory, cranial nerves with the aim of localising the lesion.
    - Corticospinal tract signs are typically absent in the initial spinal shock stage, so acute spinal cord lesions can present as flaccid paralysis before upper motor neuron signs evolve.
  - Examine for palpable bladder, anal tone, abdominal reflexes.
  - Examine the back for step deformity, muscle tenderness.
  - Systemic features as guided by history.

- **Investigations as Determined by Clinical Features**
  - Magnetic Resonance Imaging (MRI) spine with contrast
  - Lumbar puncture
  - Cerebral spinal fluid analysis: Microscopy, culture, infective panel (e.g. Biofires)
  - Infective and autoimmune screen
  - Antibodies: Anti-AQP4 antibody (Ab) (Neuromyelitis optica), anti-myelin oligodendrocyte glycoprotein (MOG) Ab, Antiganglioside Ab (Guillain–Barré Syndrome [GBS] and its variants)
  - Consider nerve conduction studies if suspicious of neuromuscular junction disorders (e.g. botulism or myasthenia gravis) or radiculoneuropathies (e.g. GBS)

» AFP surveillance and reporting is required by the Ministry of Health (MOH) in Singapore to ensure continual eradication of polio
  - Stool samples for enterovirus × 2

Management

Treat a child with AFP as a neurological emergency.

Supportive

- Monitor vital signs, cardiac monitoring, if necessary.
- Respiratory and nutritional support if there is respiratory or bulbar weakness.
- Continued serial examination for disease progression.
- Urinary catheterisation and urology referral as indicated.
- Manage constipation if present.

Table 19.9 Differential Diagnoses in a Child with AFP

Site of Lesion	Disorder/Diagnosis
Spinal cord	• Compressive myelopathy (e.g. trauma, epidural abscess, haematoma, tumour) • Transverse myelitis or other inflammatory demyelinating disorder • Acute flaccid myelitis • Anterior spinal artery infarct (or other vascular ischaemia) • Fibrocartilaginous embolism
Anterior horn cell	• Viral myelitis affecting grey matter » Polio, enterovirus 71, enterovirus D68, West Nile, Japanese encephalitis
Nerve roots and peripheral nerves	• Guillain–Barré syndrome • Infections (Lyme, diphtheria) • Metabolic (porphyria) • Traumatic nerve injury
Neuromuscular junction	• Myasthenia gravis • Infant botulism • Toxicity/poisoning
Muscle	• Viral myositis • Inflammatory myopathy • Hypokalaemic periodic paralysis

Specific (depending on the cause):

- Timely neurosurgical referral and intervention if traumatic, vascular or compressive cause.
- Immunotherapy:
  » Guillain–Barré syndrome: Intravenous Immunoglobulin (IVIG) 2 g/kg over 2 days or plasma exchange (IVIG is first line because of the ease of administration; both are equally efficacious)

- » Transverse myelitis: IV high dose methylprednisolone 30 mg/kg/dose Q24H × 5 days followed by oral prednisolone taper
- Empirical antimicrobial coverage.
- Symptomatic medications, e.g. gabapentin for neuropathic pain, stool softeners for constipation, antibiotics for urinary tract infection prophylaxis.

Neurorehabilitation

- Physiotherapy, occupational therapy and speech language therapy
- Orthoses and aids as needed
- Bladder training

Prognosis

Eventual neurological recovery varies and depends on the cause and severity. Early immunotherapy generally confers a better prognosis for the conditions amenable to such treatment.

Bibliography

1. Marx A, Glass JD, Sutter RW. (2000) Differential diagnosis of acute flaccid paralysis and its role in poliomyelitis surveillance. *Epidemiol Rev* **22**(2):298–316.
2. Al-Ghamdi F, Ghosh PS. (2016) Clinical reasoning: A 2-year-old child with acute flaccid paralysis. *Neurology* **87**:e149–e154.
3. Murphy OC, Messacar K, Benson L, *et al.* (2021 Jan 23) Acute flaccid myelitis: Cause, diagnosis, and management. *Lancet* **397**(10271):334–346.
4. Leonhard SE, Mandarakas MR, Willison HJ, *et al.* (2019) Diagnosis and management of Guillain-Barre syndrome in ten steps. *Nat Rev Neurol* **15**:671–683.

CHAPTER 94

Cerebral Palsy

Ng Zhi Min; Yeo Tong Hong; Arjandas Mahadev; Choong Chew Thye

Introduction

- Cerebral Palsy (CP) describes a group of permanent, though not unchanging, disorders of movement, posture and motor function causing activity limitation that are attributed to non-progressive disturbances occurring in the developing foetal or infant brain. These are often accompanied by dysfunction in sensation, perception, cognition, communication and behaviour, epilepsy and secondary musculoskeletal problems.
- Cerebral palsy remains a clinical diagnosis. Evidence of motor dysfunction must be present; clinical findings and symptoms may evolve over time. Most patients exhibit symptoms as infants or toddlers.
- Incidence: Estimated 2–2.5 per 1000 live births, highest for babies before 1500 g and before the 28th week of gestation.

Causes and Risk Factors

Most cases are believed to be due to prenatal factors, with prematurity and low birth weight as significant risk factors. More than one aetiological factor is often identified.

Table 19.10 Causes and Risk Factors of Cerebral Palsy

Prenatal	Perinatal	Postnatal
• Infections • Vascular pathology • Placental insufficiency • Genetic factors • Maternal metabolic disturbances • Intrauterine exposure to toxins • Developmental brain lesions	• Prematurity • Infections • Foetal/neonatal stroke • Hypoxia-ischaemia	• Brain infections • Hypoxia-ischaemia • Toxic or metabolic encephalopathy, e.g. kernicterus, heavy metals • Traumatic brain injury- accidental or non-accidental • Seizures • Stroke

Classification

Different classification systems for CP serve different functions. Classification based on clinical findings is most widely used. It may be classified according to the extremities involved and/or characteristics of neurologic dysfunction.

1. **Spastic CP** (70%).
   At least two of:
      » Abnormal pattern of posture and/or movement
      » Increased tone (not necessarily constantly)
      » Pathological reflexes (hyperreflexia or abnormal Babinski response)
   - Quadriplegia: All four extremities equally involved
   - Diplegia: Legs more affected than arms
   - Hemiplegia: One-sided, arm more affected than leg
   - Monoplegia
2. **Dyskinetic CP** (10%)
      » Involvement of basal ganglia and extra-pyramidal tracts, characterised by an abnormal pattern of posture and/or movement.
      » Involuntary, uncontrolled, recurring, occasionally stereotyped movements of affected body parts.
   - Choreo-athetoid: Dominated by both chorea and athetosis
   - Dystonic: Dominated by involuntary movements and sustained abnormal posture
3. **Ataxic CP** (10%)
4. **Mixed CP** (10%)

In the evaluation of the severity of motor disorders in CP, the Gross Motor Function Classification System (GMFCS) is mostly widely used. This scale assesses a child's independence when performing basic motor function like walking or moving, with the aid of ancillary equipment (crutches, walking frames and wheelchairs).

Table 19.11 Gross Motor Function Classification System (GMFCS)

Level of Performance	Characteristics
I	Walks independently
II	Walks independently with mild limitations
III	Walks using ancillary equipment
IV	Moves on their own but with certain limitations; may use an electric wheelchair
V	Not able to move on their own; transported in a wheelchair by a carer

Associated Problems

- Intellectual disability
- Language and speech impairments
- Psychosocial behavioural problems
- Epilepsy
- Feeding and swallowing difficulties
- Hearing impairment
- Visual disorders, strabismus, refractive errors
- Scoliosis
- Pulmonary disease
- Poor growth and nutrition
- Orthopaedic problems, e.g. joint subluxations and dislocations and hip dysplasia
- Urinary disorders, e.g. voiding dysfunction

Approach

History

- Antenatal, perinatal, postnatal history
- Developmental history
- Exclude familial or neurodegenerative disorder masquerading as CP. Ask about regression of milestones, family history of similar affected siblings/relatives, consanguinity, episodic exacerbation of symptoms
- Social history, impact on family
- Others: Education, special aids
- Medications

Clinical and Neurological Examination

- Define the type of CP
- Assess mental and physical functional status
- Assess associated problems
- Growth, development and head circumference
- Dysmorphism
- Neurologic deficits, abnormalities of muscle tone, power and gait, brisk tendon reflexes, clonus, presence of involuntary movements, persistence of primitive reflexes, contractures

Laboratory Studies

- No specific tests to confirm the diagnosis of CP.

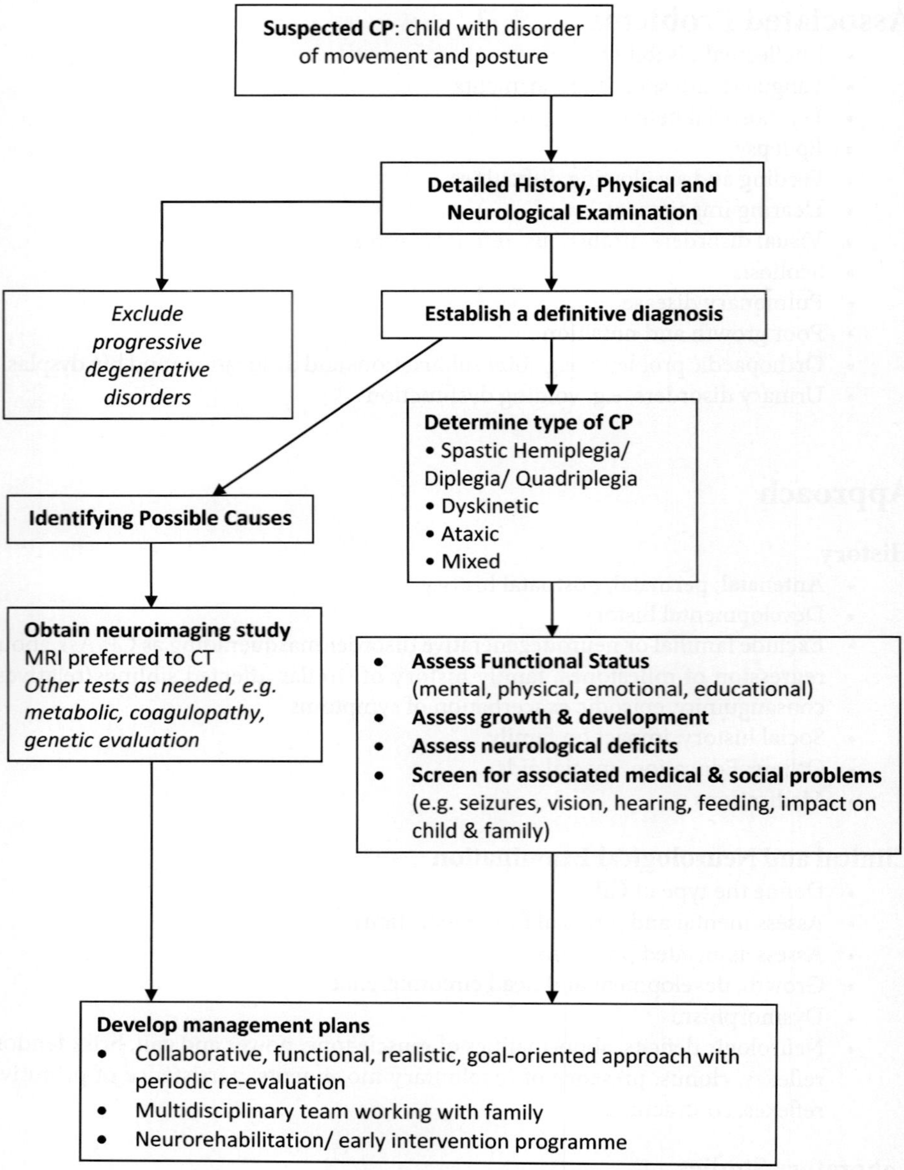

Figure 19.2 Evaluation and management of the child with Cerebral Palsy (CP).

- Neuroimaging should be performed to establish an aetiology and for prognostic purposes. Magnetic resonance imaging (MRI) is preferred to Computed Tomography (CT) scan.
- Children with atypical features in the history or neurologic examination should be thoroughly evaluated to exclude other conditions, including metabolic and

genetic disorders. Useful investigations include karyotype, metabolic testing, TORCH (Toxoplasmosis, Rubella, Cytomegalovirus, Herpes Simplex) screen in neonates.

- Children with hemiplegia or imaging evidence of cerebral infarction may have a prothrombotic coagulation disorder and may benefit from screening.

Management

Treatment goals are directed at reducing disability and maximising potential in all areas of development, including activities of daily living. Goals should be functional and realistic with periodic re-evaluation. Optimal management of the child with cerebral palsy requires a collaborative goal-oriented approach, in which a multidisciplinary team works with the family to address the child's medical, social, psychological, educational and therapeutic needs.

Treatment Modalities

- Rehabilitation therapy
  - » Physiotherapy
  - » Occupational therapy
  - » Speech therapy
  - » Behavioural therapy
- Mechanical devices to assist patients in sitting, walking or communicating, to prevent and correct deformities and control involuntary movements.
  - » Orthoses, serial casting, braces, special chairs
- Pharmacotherapy
  - » Anti-spasticity medications
    - i. Oral agents (baclofen, diazepam)
    - ii. Botulinum toxin A injections for focal spasticity
  - » Medications for seizures, involuntary movements
- Surgery
  - » Orthopaedic tendon lengthening, tendon transfer, bony fusion
  - » Neurosurgery, e.g. selective dorsal rhizotomy
  - » Gastrointestinal
- Special education may assist children with special needs
- Psychosocial therapy

Common Presentations to the Emergency Department/Reasons for Admission

- Respiratory problems, especially pneumonia
- Status epilepticus/uncontrolled seizures
- Unexplained irritability — consider acute infections, pain from fractures/subluxation, intestinal obstruction, brain trauma and possibility of non-accidental injury

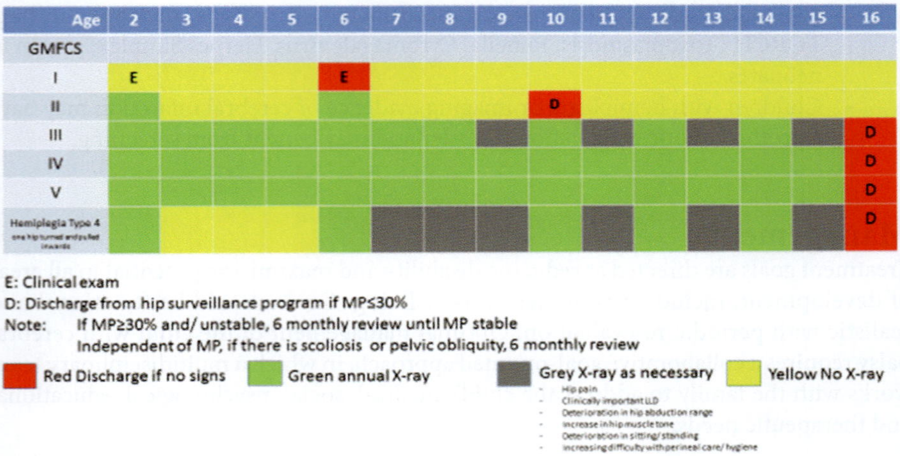

Figure 19.3 KKH hip surveillance schedule.

GMFCS — Gross Motor Function Classification System; MP — Hip Migration Percentage

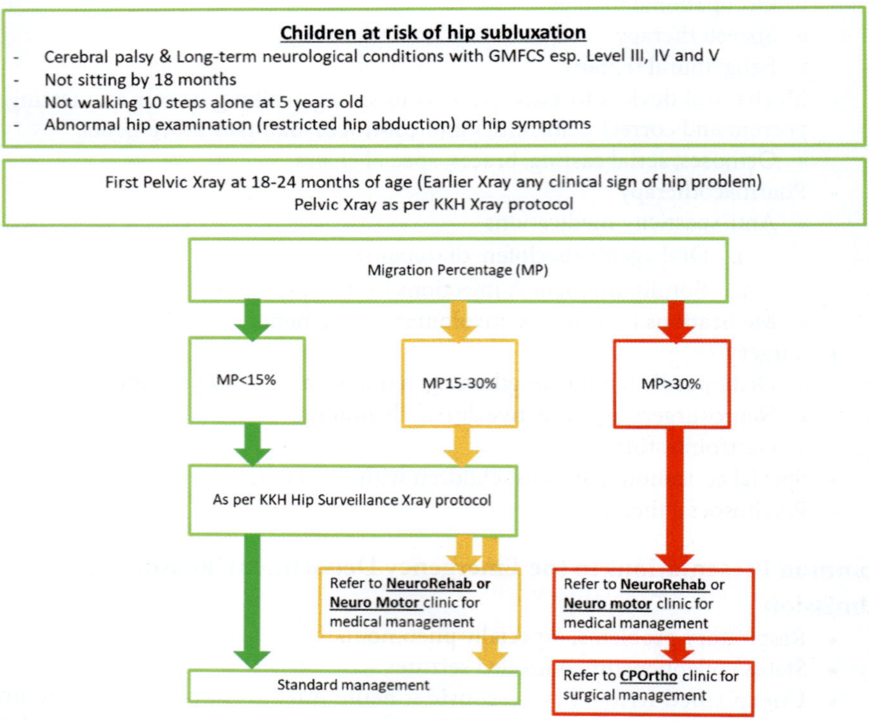

Figure 19.4 Management based on hip migration percentage (MP).

Migration Percentage (MP) is a radiographic measure of the amount of ossified femoral head that is not covered by the ossified acetabular roof.

KKH Hip Surveillance Programme

The KKH Hip Surveillance Programme aims to facilitate the timely identification of children with long-term neurological conditions (LTNC) who are at risk of hip displacement and dislocation. Refer to Figure 19.3 for the KKH Hip Surveillance Schedule.

Bibliography

1. Rosenbaum P, Paneth N, Leviton A, *et al.* (2007) A report: The definition and classification of cerebral palsy. *Dev Med Child Neurol* **109**:8–14.
2. Oskoui M, Coutinho F, Dykeman J, *et al.* (2013) An update on the prevalence of cerebral palsy: A systematic review and meta-analysis. *Dev Med Child Neurol* **55**(6):509–519.
3. ZM N, Jeremy BL, Yeo TH, *et al.* (2021 Feb) Causes, functional outcomes and healthcare utilisation of people with cerebral palsy in Singapore. *Ann Acad Med Sing* **50**(2):111–118.
4. Wimalasundera N, Stevenson VL. (2016) Cerebral palsy. *Pract Neurol* 16:184–194.
5. Delgado MR, Hirtz D, Quality Standards Subcommittee of the American Academy of Neurology and the Practice Committee of the Child Neurology Society, et al. (2010) Practice parameter: pharmacologic treatment of spasticity in children and adolescents with cerebral palsy (an evidence-based review): report of the Quality Standards Subcommittee of the American Academy of Neurology and the Practice Committee of the Child Neurology Society. *Neurology* 74:336.
6. Bjornson K, Hays R, Graubert C, *et al.* (2007) Botulinum toxin for spasticity in children with cerebral palsy: a comprehensive evaluation. *Pediatrics* 120:49.
7. Buckon CE, Thomas SS, Piatt JH. (2004) Selective dorsal rhizotomy versus orthopedic surgery: a multidimensional assessment of outcome efficacy. *Arch Phys Med Rehabil* 85:457–465.
8. Patel DR, Neelakantan M, Pandher K, Merrick J. (2020 Feb) Cerebral palsy in children: a clinical overview. Transl Pediatr 9(Suppl 1):S125–S135. PMID: 32206590; PMCID: PMC7082248.
9. Palisano R, Rosenbaum P, Bartlett D, Livingston M. (2007) Gross motor function classification system expanded and revised. In: Canchild Centre for Childhood Disability Research, Mcmaster University. Hamilton, ON: Institute for Applied Health Sciences McMaster University, p. b15.

CHAPTER 95

Movement Disorders

Yeo Tong Hong

Introduction

Movement disorders in childhood are frequently seen in a wide spectrum of neurological conditions, from benign, self-limiting transient phenomena to progressive disorders associated with significant disability. Clinical presentations may be acute, subacute or chronic.

They are often classified into two phenomenological groups:

(1) **Hyperkinesia/Dyskinesia** (including tics, myoclonus, dystonia, chorea, athetosis, tremors, and stereotypies).

(2) **Hypokinetic-rigid syndromes** (Parkinsonism)

The evaluation of movement disorders is usually clinical, either through history, examination and videos or patient's/caregivers' reports based on self-assessment.

Definitions

Tics are brief involuntary purposeless movements and/or sounds.

Myoclonus is a sudden, brief involuntary jerk of a muscle or a group of muscles.

Dystonia is characterised by sustained or intermittent muscle contractions causing abnormal, often repetitive, movements, postures or both. Typically patterned, twisting and may be tremulous, dystonia is often initiated or worsened by voluntary action and associated with overflow muscle activation.

Chorea is a rapid, abrupt, irregular, unpredictable, non-stereotyped, semi or non-purposeful movement.

Athetosis is a slow continuous stream of writhing movement, typically of the hands and feet.

Tremor is an involuntary, rhythmic, oscillatory movement of a body part.

Stereotypies are repetitive and purposeless movements.

History and Clinical Examination

- Normal or abnormal pattern of movements?
- Excessive or paucity of movements?

- Voluntary or involuntary?
- Paroxysmal? i.e. sudden onset and offset?
- Continual? i.e. repeated again and again?
- Continuous? i.e. without stopping?
- Changed over time? Wax and wean? Diurnal variation?
- Environmental stimuli? Emotional triggers?
- Abates with sleep?
- Suppressible?
- Premonition? Premonitory sensation or urge?
- Family history of similar or related conditions?
- Examination findings? Focal neurological deficit? Systemic involvement?
- Any parental/caregiver's video recordings?

Benign Movement Disorders of Childhood

A number of benign movement disorders of childhood are recognised, and they are transient in nature, and usually have a good long-term prognosis.

Neonatal Jitteriness

- High frequency and low amplitude tremor
- Location: Jaw and extremities
- Multiple factors, including metabolic disturbance, hypoxic-ischaemic encephalopathy (HIE), drug withdrawal
- Often mistaken for neonatal seizures
- Suppressed easily by gentle restraint
- No specific treatment; treat the underlying factors
- Usually resolves by 7 months

Benign Neonatal Sleep Myoclonus

- Self-limiting movement disorder
- Myoclonic jerks during non-rapid eye movement (NREM)/quiet sleep
- Stopped by arousal
- Usually resolves by 3 to 4 months

Benign Polymorphous Movement Disorders of Infancy (BPMDI) are part of a heterogeneous group of movement disorders, including shuddering attacks, benign myoclonus of early infancy, head nodding, benign infantile shaking body attacks, brief tonic contraction, benign non-epileptic infantile spasms and sleep-related infantile tremor.

Characteristic features:

- Onset: 4 to 7 months
- Paroxysmal, sometimes in clusters
- Brief
- Without impaired consciousness

- Several times on a daily basis
- Usually triggered by excitement, frustration or postural changes
- Normal developmental milestones and normal neurology
- Self-limiting

Transient Idiopathic Dystonia of Infancy

- Onset is usually before 5 months
- Hemidystonia — usually affecting single upper limb and trunk
- Persistent
- Abolished when infant moves purposefully
- Resolves without sequelae at 12 months

Motor Stereotypies/Stereotypic Movement Disorder

- DSM-5 Category: Neurodevelopmental Disorders
  - » Repetitive, seemingly driven, purposeless motor behaviour
  - » Early onset; > 4 weeks' duration
  - » Can interfere with normal activities or results in self-injury
  - » Not explained by another neurodevelopmental or psychiatric disorder
- Primary Motor Stereotypies
  - » Common amongst normal children
  - » Transient in nature; good prognosis
  - » Common behavioural stereotypies: Rocking, head banging, hair twisting, pencil tapping
  - » Complex stereotypies: Head nodding, hand shaking, opening/closing of hands, arm flapping, flexion/extension of wrists, mouth opening/facial grimaces
- Secondary Motor Stereotypies can be seen in children with autism, Rett syndrome, neurodegenerative disorders and metabolic disorders.

Table 19.12 Indications for Neurology Referral for Movement Disorders

Abnormal neurology/focal neurological deficit
History of epilepsy/epileptic seizures
Evidence of psychomotor regression
Diagnostic doubt as to the nature of the event
Clinical course no longer associated with existing diagnoses

Tic Disorders and Tourette Syndrome

- Tics are the most common movement disorder in childhood and can affect up to 20% of children.
- Tics are brief involuntary purposeless movements and/or sounds. Tics can either be 'simple' involving one muscle or 'complex' involving a group of muscles.
- Examples include:
  a. Simple motor tics — eye blinking, facial grimaces, head and neck jerks, and shoulder shrugs

   b. Complex motor tics — jumping, touching objects/clothes
   c. Simple vocal tics — grunting, coughing, sniffing and throat-clearing sounds
   d. Complex vocal tics — animal-like noises, swearing, etc.
- Some children experience premonitory feelings or sensations that are relieved by the execution of the tics.
- Tics are often transient and can be self-resolving within a few weeks or months. This is known as the Transient Tic Disorder.

Tourette Syndrome and Chronic Tic Disorder

- **Chronic Tic Disorder** is a condition in which a child experiences single or multiple occurrences of either motor or vocal tic for more than 1 year.
- **Tourette Syndrome** is a Chronic Tic Disorder, in which a child experiences both motor and vocal tics.
- Children with Tourette Syndrome can also have other conditions such as Anxiety, Obsessive Compulsive Disorder (OCD) and/or Attention Deficit Hyperactivity Disorder (ADHD).

Diagnosis

- Clinical history and careful observation.
- No role for laboratory tests or neuroimaging.
- Electroencephalography (EEG) is usually not indicated.
- Medications may induce tics, especially stimulants such as methylphenidate.
- *DSM-5* criteria for Tourette Syndrome are as follows:
  » A child or young person must have multiple motor and one or more vocal tics that happen regularly although not necessarily at the same time.
  » Tics occurring many times a day or intermittently for a period of more than 1 year.
  » Age of onset: <18 years old.
  » No other conditions that could cause tics.
- Some useful tools to measure outcomes include the Yale Global Tic Severity Score and ICF for sleep, pain and quality of life (QoL).

Management

- Majority of children with tics do not require medication.
- Psychological interventions, including anxiety/stress management, cognitive behaviour therapy, are helpful. Treatment for associated conditions, such as OCD and ADHD. These conditions may be more disruptive than the tics and require different treatments based on the symptoms.
- Medical options: Clonidine, Guanfacine, Aripiprazole, Risperidone

Dystonia and Status Dystonicus

Dystonia is characterised by sustained or intermittent muscle contractions causing abnormal, often repetitive, movements, postures or both. Typically patterned, twisting and may be tremulous. Dystonia is often initiated or worsened by voluntary action and associated with overflow muscle activation.

Status Dystonicus (SD) is defined as a movement disorder emergency characterised by severe episodes of generalised or focal dystonic with or without other hyperkinetic movements (e.g. chorea). Up to 60% of reported cases are children. SD is probably under recognised and can be fatal in up to 10% of cases.

It is important to recognise SD as the severe end of a continuum of deterioration through the application of **Dystonia Severity Action Plan (DSAP)** (Figure 19.5).

<table>
<tr><th>Grade</th><th>Description</th><th>Action</th><th>Dystonia Severity Action Plan (DSAP)</th></tr>
<tr><td>1</td><td>• Sits comfortably
• Normal sleep
• Stable on medication</td><td>• No assessment
• No change in individual Dystonia Action Plan</td><td></td></tr>
<tr><td>2</td><td>• Irritable and cannot settle
• Dystonic posturing interferes with sitting
• Can only tolerate lying</td><td>• Adjust medication as per individual Dystonia Action Plan
• Clinic review within 1-2 weeks</td><td rowspan="2">Brittle Dystonia Management Plan:
• As per existing individual Dystonia Action Plan
• Adjust individual Dystonia Action Plan to prevent deterioration through dystonia severity grades leading to status dystonicus
• Clinic review if required
• Suggestions:
o Benzhexol or L-dopa
o Gabapentin: esp. generalised dystonia
o Clondine: enteral/ IV /transdermal. Useful for sleep disturbance/ agitation
o Other: benzodiazepines (diazepam, clonazepam, nitrazepam), baclofen, tetrabenazine</td></tr>
<tr><td>3</td><td>• Sleep disturbed
• Unable to tolerate lying
• No signs of metabolic (e.g. pyrexia, dehydration) or respiratory compromise</td><td>• Clinic review within days
• Consider metabolic screen: CK, renal, liver and bone profile
• Escalate management
• +/- hospitalisation</td></tr>
<tr><td>4</td><td>• As per Grade 3
• Early multi-organ failure.
• Clinically as above with: Pyrexia, dehydration, abnormal electrolytes, myoglobinuria. CK>1000 IU/L</td><td colspan="2" rowspan="2">Status Dystonicus Management Plan:
1. Supportive Care
• Urgent admission: KKH HD or CICU
• Multisystem support as required
• Supportive care including IV hydration, anti-pyretics and analgesia
• Monitor Urea & Electrolytes, Renal, Bone and Liver profile, CK
• Identify and treat triggers (consider IV antibiotics)
2. Temporising measures
• Chloral hydrate to establish sleep
• Consider Enteral / IV clonidine (non-respiratory depressant)
• ± IVI midazolam
• ± General anaesthesia/ Paralytic agents
3. Dystonia-specific measures
• Consider oral medication trial: Benzhexol, L-dopa, Gabapentin, Baclofen, Benzodiazepines, Tetrabenazine
• Consider Neuromodulation (ITB, DBS) or Pallidotomy</td></tr>
<tr><td>5</td><td>• Severe generalised dystonia
• As per Grade 4 with full metabolic and renal decompensation and/ or cardiorespiratory compromise</td></tr>
</table>

CK - creatine kinase, HD – high dependency unit, CICU – Children's Intensive Care Unit, IV – intravenous, IVI – intravenous infusion, ITB - intrathecal baclofen, DBS – deep brain stimulation

Figure 19.5 Dystonia severity action plan (DSAP).

Patients at risk of SD are those with:

- Chronic dystonias (primary and secondary)
- Generalised quadriplegic cerebral palsy
- Neurodegenerative disorders (e.g. glutaric aciduria type 1 — GA1)
- Neurotransmitters disorders
- Post-acquired brain injury (e.g. traumatic brain injury, autoimmune encephalitis)
- Acute drug withdrawal (e.g. Baclofen or other anti-dystonic drugs)

Common triggers of SD: Pain, infection, surgery, drugs

Main features of SD:

- Hypertonia
- Abnormal dystonic posturing
- Preservation of consciousness
- Elevated creatine kinase (CK)
- Other complications — rhabdomyolysis, respiratory compromise

Initial management of SD

- Admission to HD/CICU
- **A**ddress precipitants
- **B**egin supportive care
- **C**alibrate sedation with a combination of oral chloral hydrate, oral or IV clonidine, and benzodiazepines (e.g. per rectal diazepam or IV midazolam); consider IVI clonidine/midazolam
- **D**ystonia specific therapy (under Neurologist's guidance)
  - » Clonazepam, Trihexyphenidyl, baclofen, L-dopa, Gabapentin, Tetrabenazine, Dantrolene
  - » Deep brain Stimulation/Intrathecal baclofen

Bibliography

1. Sanger TD, Chen D, Fehlings DL, *et al.* (2010) Definition and classification of hyperkinetic movements in childhood. *Mov Disord* **25**:1538–1549.
2. Fernadez-Alvarez E. (2018) Transient benign paroxysmal movement disorders in infancy. *Eur J Paediatr Neurol* **22**(2):230–237.
3. Lumsden DE, Lundy C, Fairhurst C, Lin JP. (2013) Dystonia severity action plan: A simple grading system for medical severity of status dystonicus and life threatening dystonia. *Dev Med Child Neurol* **55**:671–672.
4. Nakou V, Williamson K, Arichi T, *et al.* (2017) Safety and efficacy of high dose enteral, intravenous, and transdermal clonidine for acute management of severe intractable childhood dystonia and status dystonicus: An illustrative case-series. *Eur J Paediatr Neurol* **21**(6):823–832.

CHAPTER 96

Bell's Palsy

Lim Yi Xiu, Jocelyn; Terrence Thomas

Introduction

- Bell's palsy (BP) is an acute, peripheral facial nerve paralysis of unknown cause, making up about 50% of all paediatric facial nerve paralysis.
- Some proposed aetiologies include post-infectious inflammatory factors, vascular ischaemia and immunologic causes.
- Incidence in children aged 1 to 15 years is lower (6.1 per 100000 person-years) compared to adult (20 per 100000 person-years).
- The key to diagnosis lies in good clinical history and thorough clinical examination to exclude the other causes of facial nerve paralysis.

Table 19.13 Differential Diagnoses to Bell's Palsy in Children

Congenital	**Traumatic delivery:** Primiparity, birth weight >3.5 kg, forceps or caesarean section, prematurity **Syndromic:** Mobius syndrome, Goldenhar syndrome, Arnold-Chiari syndrome, syringobulbia **Genetic:** Hereditary myopathies: Congenital myaesthenic syndromes, myotonic dystrophy
Acquired	**Infectious:** Ramsay Hunt syndrome Ebstein–Barr virus, cytomegalovirus, adenovirus, rubella, mumps, HIV mycoplasma pneumonia, haemophilus influenza, tuberculosis, acute otitis media, chronic otitis media/cholesteatoma **Inflammatory:** Guillain–Barré Syndrome, Henoch–Scholein purpura, Kawasaki disease **Neoplastic:** Vestibular schwannomas, haemangiomas, rhabdomyosarcoma, temporal bone histiocytosis, leukaemia, parotid gland tumours **Traumatic:** Temporal bone fractures, iatrogenic

Note: It is most important to exclude other conditions that mimic presentation similar to BP. This can be achieved with thorough history-taking and competent clinical examination.

Clinical Presentation

- Acute onset of decreased forehead movement, incomplete eye closure, loss of nasolabial fold and asymmetric smile.
- Hyperacusis, decreased tearing and altered taste can also occur depending on site of facial nerve injury.
- Sparing of forehead muscles indicates a central upper motor neuron (UMN) lesion.
- In younger patients, observe facial movements and asymmetry while crying.
- Severity of paralysis can be assessed using the House–Brackmann (HB) facial nerve grading scale (according to the worst functioning branch) (see Table 19.14).
- Symptoms and signs suggesting an alternative aetiology:
  - » Gradual onset, progressive nature >3 weeks
  - » Ear discharge, tympanic membrane erythema, mastoid tenderness (acute otitis media)
  - » Vesicular rash and vestibulocochlear dysfunction (Ramsay Hunt syndrome)
  - » Other cranial neuropathies or neurological signs
  - » Other systemic features, e.g. hypertension, pallor, easy bruisability, lymphadenopathy, organomegaly, weight loss
- No investigations are necessary if there are no atypical features or red flags.
- Otherwise, investigations to consider include:
  - » Neuroimaging — CT or MRI brain
  - » ENT referral ± audiogram/tympanogram
  - » Autoimmune, malignancy or serological screen
  - » Lumbar puncture

Table 19.14 House–Brackmann (HB) Facial Nerve Grading Scale

Grade	Description
I	Normal
II	Mild dysfunction *Slight weakness, normal symmetry at rest*
III	Moderate dysfunction *Obvious but not disfiguring, synkinesis, symmetry at rest, complete eye closure with maximal effort, good forehead movement*
IV	Moderately severe dysfunction *Obvious and disfiguring asymmetry, significant synkinesis, incomplete eye closure, moderate forehead movement*
V	Severe dysfunction *Almost no movement*
VI	Total paralysis *No movement*

Management

- Treatment depends on underlying aetiology.
- Eye care to prevent corneal abrasions, exposure keratitis and vision loss: Eye patch and saline eye drops.
- While steroids and acyclovir have been shown to improve recovery in adults with BP, paediatric studies have remained inconclusive, with most studies showing no significant difference in recovery.
- Outpatient follow up in 4 to 6 weeks for resolution.
- If recurrent or persistent, refer to Neurology for further evaluation.

Prognosis

- Children with BP mostly recover well spontaneously and completely.
- Recovery in children is better (up to 90%) compared to adults (up to 70%), with most recovering within 3 months of onset.
- In general, a lower HB grade (II or less) and younger age at presentation (< 8 years old) confer a better prognosis with faster and more complete recovery.
- Persistent or recurrent lesions will need re-evaluation.

Bibliography

1. Lunan R, Nagarajan L. (2008) Bell's palsy: A guideline proposal following review of practice. *J Paediatr Child Health* **44**:219–220.
2. Gronseth GS, Paduga R. (2012) Evidence-based guideline update: Steroids and antivirals for bell palsy: Report of the guideline development subcommittee of the American Academy of Neurology. *Neurology* **79**(22):2209–2213.
3. Pitaro J, Waissbluth S, Daniel SJ. (2012) Do children with Bell's palsy benefit from steroid treatment? A systematic review. *Int J Pediatr Otorhinolaryngol* **76**:921–926.
4. Lee Y, Yoon HS, Yeo SG, Lee EH. (2020) Factors associated with fast recovery of bell palsy in children. *J Child Neurol* **35**(1):71–76.
5. Wang CS, Sakai M, Khurram A, Lee K. (2021) Facial nerve palsy in children: A case series and literature review. *Otolaryngol Case Rep* **20**:100297.

SECTION 20

ONCOLOGY

CHAPTER 97

Acute Leukaemia and Oncological Emergencies

Soh Shui Yen

Acute Leukaemia

Acute leukaemia is the most common malignancy in childhood. In general, there are two types of acute leukaemia in children — acute lymphoblastic leukaemia (ALL) and acute myeloid leukaemia (AML). Although urgent diagnosis and treatment are important, immediate supportive care is also necessary to monitor, prevent and treat complications such as acute tumour lysis syndrome, hyperleucocytosis or rarely disseminated intravascular coagulation (DIC).

Investigations for Patients Newly Diagnosed with Acute Leukaemia

Blood Tests

- Full blood count (FBC); peripheral blood film (PBF)
- Coagulation profile (PT and aPTT). Serum fibrinogen and D-dimer should be done in patients with suspected or possible DIC, e.g. in sepsis or acute promyelocytic leukaemia (APL).
- Biochemistries: Renal panel and electrolytes — including serum creatinine, potassium, calcium and phosphate; uric acid; lactate dehydrogenase (LDH); liver function test (LFT)
- Serum immunoglobulins — IgG, IgA, IgM
- Viral immunity status
  - » Mandatory: Hepatitis B surface antigen (HBsAg), Hepatitis B surface antibody (anti-HBs), Hepatitis B core total antibody (anti-HBc), Varicella–zoster virus (VZV) IgG
  - » Others: Hepatitis C total antibody (CMIA), Cytomegalovirus (CMV) IgG, Epstein–Barr virus (EBV), Viral Capsid Antigen (VCA) IgG, Herpes Simplex Virus (HSV) total antibody, Human Immunodeficiency Virus (HIV) screen, Measles IgG, Mumps IgG, Rubella IgG
- G6PD screen (if G6PD status unknown)
- Blood cultures (if febrile)
- Group and Cross Match

Imaging Studies

- Chest X-ray (CXR) — should be performed before the patient receives any sedation (to exclude mediastinal mass)
- Echocardiogram (prior to first dose of anthracyclines)

Bone Marrow Aspirate

- Bone marrow aspirate (BMA) examination or morphology
- BMA immunophenotyping (by flow cytometry)
- BMA cytogenetics
- Other investigations as required by the treatment protocol, e.g. flow cytometry analysis and/or molecular characterisation for subsequent monitoring of minimal residual disease (MRD); molecular genetic profiling. Trephine biopsy may be required if there is a dry tap.

Lumbar Puncture

The timing of the first lumbar puncture (LP) is specified by the treatment protocol and the patient's clinical condition. The first LP should be performed by an experienced practitioner to reduce the risk of traumatic or bloody tap. Ensure adequate platelet counts before LP: $>50 \times 10^9$/L; preferably $>100 \times 10^9$/L for the first LP. Do not perform LP on patients who have or are at risk of DIC. Adequate procedural sedation (or general anaesthesia) and analgesia are also important to help reduce the risk of traumatic LP. Send the cerebrospinal fluid (CSF) for the following investigations:

- CSF profile
- CSF cytospin for blasts

Following collection of CSF samples, intrathecal chemotherapy (e.g. methotrexate) is administered.

Immediate Supportive Management

A child suspected to have acute leukaemia should receive the following supportive management:

1. Monitoring and management of tumour lysis syndrome and hyperleucocytosis (see 'Oncological Emergencies')
2. Blood product support
   a. Platelet transfusion as guided by the clinical condition:
      - If the patient is asymptomatic: Keep platelets more than 10–20 $\times 10^9$/L.
      - If the patient is febrile or septic or having hyperleucocytosis: Keep platelets more than 20–30 $\times 10^9$/L.
      - If there is bleeding or DIC: Keep platelets more than 50 $\times 10^9$/L, or even higher ($>$50–100 $\times 10^9$/L) if there is severe bleeding or if the patient is undergoing invasive procedures.

b. Red cell (RBC) transfusion is generally indicated for patients who are symptomatic from moderate–severe anaemia (Hb <6–7 g/dL). In patients with high white blood cell (WBC) count, RBC transfusion may contribute to hyperviscosity. Therefore, RBC transfusion should be avoided, especially in asymptomatic patients, until the WBC is lower.

c. Coagulopathy (e.g. DIC) in patients with hyperleucocytosis or APL should be aggressively managed: Transfuse fresh frozen plasma (FFP) and cryoprecipitate to keep PT/aPTT within normal range and fibrinogen above 1.0–1.5 g/L. Maintain platelets above 30–50 × 10^9/L. Have a low threshold for urgent Computed Tomography (CT) Head in patients with neurologic symptoms worrisome for possible intracranial haemorrhage. In patients with suspected APL, all trans retinoic acid (ATRA) should be started as soon as possible.

3. Start broad spectrum intravenous (IV) antibiotics if patient is febrile or septic.

Oncological Emergencies

Tumour Lysis Syndrome

Tumour lysis syndrome (TLS) is a metabolic emergency that results from massive tumour cell destruction, leading to biochemical derangements that overwhelm the body's excretory mechanisms.

Laboratory TLS, as defined by Cairo-Bishop, is 2 or more of the following within 3 days before and 7 days after the commencement of chemotherapy:

- hyperuricaemia ≥476 μmol/L or 25% increase from baseline
- hyperkalaemia ≥6.0 mmol/L or 25% increase from baseline
- hyperphosphataemia ≥2.1 mmol/L or 25% increase from baseline
- hypocalcaemia ≤1.75 mmol/L or 25% decrease from baseline.

In clinical TLS, deposition of uric acid and phosphate in the kidney results in acute renal impairment. Severe electrolyte derangements such as hyperkalaemia and hypocalcaemia can lead to cardiac arrhythmias, tetany and seizures and can be life-threatening. Clinical TLS is therefore defined by the presence of laboratory TLS, together with one or more clinical complications: renal impairment (serum creatinine ≥1.5 times upper limit of normal), seizures, cardiac arrhythmias or sudden death.

Patients with acute leukaemia and high white cell count (>50 × 10^9/L) are at risk of developing TLS. Other malignancies with high risk of tumour lysis include high grade bulky lymphomas, e.g. Burkitt lymphoma/leukaemia. Patients with underlying renal impairment are at higher risk of developing TLS.

Hyperleucocytosis

Hyperleucocytosis is defined as a WBC count higher than 100×10^9/L. Hyperleucocytosis increases blood viscosity (hyperviscosity), especially in the microcirculation, and leads to leucostasis, which is the aggregation of blasts in the blood vessels. Leucostasis is more common in AML as myeloblasts are larger in size compared to lymphoblasts. Leucostasis symptoms most often involve the lungs and the central nervous system. Symptoms reflect tissue or organ congestion and ischemia, and can, therefore, include respiratory distress, desaturation, headache, confusion, drowsiness, seizure, visual disturbance, stroke, renal impairment, cardiac impairment, bowel ischemia, priapism, and so on. The risk of symptomatic leucostasis is higher in ALL with WBC $\geq 300 \times 10^9$/L and in AML with WBC $\geq 100 \times 10^9$/L (especially in M4/M5 subtypes).

Management of TLS and Hyperleucocytosis

- Hydrate with IV dextrose/saline at 3 L/m^2/day for at least 72 hours. Patients with very low WBC may be given less fluids.
- Do not add potassium or phosphate to IV fluids.
- Start oral (PO) allopurinol 100 mg/m^2/dose TDS and continue for up to 7 days and until peripheral blasts are reduced and serum uric acid level is normal.
- Reduce dose in renal impairment. Consider recombinant urate oxidase (rasburicase) in patients with high risk of tumour lysis or established TLS or renal impairment (see Box on the next page).
- Urine alkalinisation is no longer routinely recommended but may be considered if there is metabolic acidosis. Alkalinisation increases solubility of uric acid in the urine and prevents crystallisation in the renal tubules. However, over-alkalinisation causes crystallisation or precipitation of xanthine, hypoxanthine and phosphate, and also worsens hypocalcaemia. To alkalinise, add 15 ml 8.4% sodium bicarbonate ($NaHCO_3$) to each 500 ml of IV dextrose/saline and subsequently adjust the amount of added $NaHCO_3$ to keep the urine pH 6.5–7.5. Urine pH should be measured at each void when the patient is on alkalinisation. Do not alkalinise when patient is on rasburicase.
- Specific electrolyte abnormality (hyperkalaemia, hyperphosphataemia) should be treated accordingly. Hypocalcaemia is not treated unless it is symptomatic.
- If clinical TLS develops or fails to improve with the above measures, urgent renal dialysis will be necessary.
- Hyperleucocytosis should be managed by hydration to reduce hyperviscosity, as well as prompt initiation of chemotherapy for cytoreduction. Leucopheresis may be considered for patients with symptomatic leucostasis not responding to the above supportive care, if prompt chemotherapy cannot be initiated. Leucopheresis is not recommended in asymptomatic patients and is contraindicated in APL. Red cell transfusions may worsen hyperviscosity and should be avoided.
- Clinical and laboratory monitoring.

Use of Recombinant Urate Oxidase (Rasburicase) in Tumour Lysis Syndrome

- Indications:
  - » Patients with high risk of TLS:
  - » ALL or AML with WBC ≥100 × 10^9/L
  - » Burkitt lymphoma or lymphoblastic lymphoma
  - » Bulky high grade lymphoma — bulky disease as defined as elevated LDH ≥2× upper limit of normal, or large tumour mass, e.g. >10 cm in adults, or organ infiltration
  - » High grade haematologic malignancy with pre-existing renal dysfunction
  - » Patients with established TLS
- Contraindications: G6PD-deficiency, haemolytic anaemia, hypersensitivity
- Dose: IV 0.15–0.2 mg/kg/dose Q24H for 1–7 days, to be decided each day by a senior physician.
- For 96 hours after the last dose of rasburicase, blood samples for uric acid measurement should be sent to the laboratory immediately without delay, and preferably transported in cool condition (e.g. with cooling packs). Uric acid results may be falsely low post-rasburicase if there is a delay in measurement, and especially if the blood samples are at room temperature.
- Do not administer concurrent allopurinol when rasburicase is being used.

Monitoring

- Monitoring during hyperhydration: Strict intake/output monitoring with fluid tally every 4–6 hours during hyperhydration. Ensure urine output >100 ml/m^2/h (or >4 ml/kg/h for infants). IV furosemide 0.5 mg/kg/dose may be needed if there is concern about fluid overload (e.g. positive fluid balance exceeding 600 ml/m^2/day). Monitor weight while on hyperhydration.
- Daily blood tests during first week of induction: FBC, Renal Panel, Calcium, Phosphate, Uric Acid
- Close monitoring (every 4–6 hours, or less frequently if low risk of TLS) of serum potassium, phosphate and calcium until disease load has reduced and no evidence of tumour lysis.
- Patients with high risk of TLS may need more frequent monitoring of FBC, uric acid, renal panel and/or coagulation tests.

Febrile Neutropenia

Oncology and hematopoietic transplant patients are immunocompromised as a result of cancer treatment and immunosuppressive therapies. Febrile neutropenia is a medical emergency as the progression of infection in neutropenic patients can be very rapid, especially with gram-negative organisms. Prompt attention and administration of appropriate broad spectrum antibiotics (within 60 minutes of presentation) and good supportive treatment are critical for a favourable outcome.

- Fever is defined as a single temperature of ≥38.3°C or two or more episodes of ≥38°C (sustained over a 1-hour period).
- Significant or moderate neutropenia refers to ANC ≤500 cells/μl (0.5 × 10^9/L), or one that is expected to fall below 500 cells/μl (0.5 × 10^9/L) over the next 48 hours. This is the working definition for most febrile neutropenia guidelines. However, our institution guideline will use ANC of <1000 cells/μl (1 × 10^9/L) as the cut-off.
- Presence of indwelling vascular access devices and mucosal barrier injuries (e.g. from chemotherapy or radiation) are additional risk factors for infections in immunocompromised patients.

History and Clinical Examination

- Perform a thorough history-taking and physical examination to look for aetiology or focus of infection, paying special attention to the skin, mucosal surfaces (oral cavity, perineum), central line sites. DO NOT perform rectal examination in patients suspected to have neutropenia.
- Obtain the oncology and transplant history, as well as the information on recent and ongoing medications.
- Measure and monitor vital parameters (pulse rate, respiratory rate, blood pressure, oxygen saturation).
- Look for symptoms and signs that may suggest severe sepsis, such as altered mental state, lethargy, poor peripheral perfusion (capillary refill time >3 seconds), respiratory distress, decreased urine output.

Investigations

- FBC
- Group and cross match
- Routine biochemistries: Renal panel and electrolytes, LFT
- C-reactive protein
- Blood cultures — Aerobic and anaerobic
  - » One set from central lines — Port-a-cath; each lumen of central venous catheters (e.g. Hickman, PICC).
  - » One set percutaneously from peripheral veins — This is mandatory for febrile patients without central lines, but may be omitted in stable patients with central lines. If peripheral blood cultures are taken, they should be drawn simultaneously with 'Central' blood cultures, to enable evaluation of differential time to positivity (DTP).
  - » Each specimen should be clearly and correctly labelled (e.g. aerobic culture from small lumen).
- Urinalysis, urine culture and urine fungal smear in patients in whom a clean-catch midstream specimen is readily available. Urine collection must not delay initiation of antibiotics.

- Imaging (e.g. CXR) and other investigations (e.g. respiratory viruses, stool investigations, coagulation profile) as clinically indicated and must not delay initiation of antibiotics.

High-Risk Factors in Patients with Febrile Neutropenia

- Haematopoietic Stem Cell Transplant (HSCT) within 6 months and/or still on immunosuppressants
- ALL on induction or re-intensification phases
- AML
- High grade lymphomas, e.g. Burkitt
- High-risk neuroblastoma
- Relapsed/progressive malignancy on intensified treatment
- Down syndrome
- Recent overwhelming sepsis
- Clinically unwell — chills/rigours, hemodynamic instability, altered mental state, respiratory distress

Initial Management

- General supportive and resuscitative measures as required.
- Monitor parameters (heart and respiratory rate, blood pressure) at least 4 hourly. Look out for inappropriate tachycardia (impending shock) or tachypnoea (pneumonitis/chest infections).
- Review the patient's ongoing medications:
  - Stop any ongoing chemotherapy, e.g. PO 6-mercaptopurine or 6-thioguanine.
  - Prophylactic antimicrobials (e.g. co-trimoxazole for Pneumocystis prophylaxis, acyclovir for HSV prophylaxis), if present, should be continued.
  - If the patient is on granulocyte colony-stimulating factor (GCSF), this should be continued till neutrophil recovery.
  - Steroids should be continued. Abrupt discontinuation during sepsis may trigger an adrenal crisis.
- Prompt initiation of empirical broad-spectrum antibiotic within 60 minutes of presentation:
  - Piperacillin–tazobactam is a recommended first-line empirical monotherapy agent for febrile neutropenia as it has broad spectrum gram-negative (including antipseudomonal), gram-positive and anaerobic cover. It is also well tolerated and has a good toxicity profile.
  - If the patient is clinically unstable (e.g. haemodynamic instability — hypotension, excessive tachycardia), or when a resistant infection is suspected, antibiotic cover should be broadened to include a second gram-negative agent (e.g. aminoglycoside amikacin) and/or glycopeptide (vancomycin). Consider escalating piperacillin–tazobactam to meropenem.
- Blood product support may be necessary:

- » Maintain Hb >8 g/dL in patients with febrile neutropenia; if there is bleeding, maintain >9 g/dL.
- » Maintain platelets ≥20 × 10^9/L in patients with febrile neutropenia. If there is bleeding, maintain ≥50 × 10^9/L, or ≥100 × 10^9/L for life-threatening bleeds, including intracranial haemorrhage, massive gastrointestinal haemorrhage).

- Other supportive care
  - » Fever increases insensible fluid losses. Ensure that the child receives adequate IV/PO fluids.
  - » Correct electrolyte abnormalities.
  - » Do not administer rectal enemas or suppositories to neutropenic patients.

Ongoing Management

- If the patient is responding to initial empirical antibiotic(s): Discontinue the second gram-negative agent (e.g. amikacin) and glycopeptide (vancomycin) after 24–72 hours unless continued therapy is supported by relevant positive microbiology results.
- If the patient has persistent fever but is clinically stable: Consider repeat blood cultures and other evaluations as clinically indicated. It is not recommended to modify initial antibiotics based solely on persistent fever.
- If the patient has persistent fever and becomes clinically unstable: Repeat blood cultures. Repeat other evaluations as clinically indicated. Antibiotic cover should be broadened to include a second gram-negative agent (e.g. amikacin) and/or glycopeptide (vancomycin). Consider escalating piperacillin–tazobactam to meropenem.
- Empirical antifungal therapy:
  - » Patients at high risk of invasive fungal disease (IFD): AML, high-risk ALL, relapsed acute leukaemia, allogeneic HSCT, prolonged profound neutropenia (ANC ≤0.1 × 10^9/L for >7 days), high-dose corticosteroids (≥2 mg/kg/day or ≥20 mg/day of prednisolone or equivalent, for ≥2 weeks). All other patients are considered IFD low-risk.
  - » In IFD high-risk patients with prolonged (≥96 hours) febrile neutropenia not responding to broad-spectrum antibiotics:
    - ▪ CT Chest; abdominal ultrasound; other imaging only if there are localising signs or symptoms.
    - ▪ Initiate empirical antifungal therapy — ambisome or caspofungin.
- Adjust antimicrobial regimen based on clinical, radiological (if any) and/or microbiology results:
  - » If cultures are negative at 48 hours: Discontinue empirical antibiotics (i) if the patient is afebrile for ≥24 hours, and (ii) when there is evidence of marrow recovery (especially in patients with high-risk factors).
  - » If cultures are positive: Definitive antimicrobial therapy should be given for at least 7–14 days. Removal of central line and longer duration of systemic antimicrobial therapy may be necessary for complicated central line-associated blood stream infection (CLABSI).

Anterior Mediastinal Mass

The mediastinum is the central part of the thoracic cavity and can be the site of involvement of the several tumours such as:

- Anterior mediastinum: Lymphoma (Hodgkin or non-Hodgkin), malignant germ cell tumour, teratoma, thymoma, mediastinal extension of thyroid tumours.
- Posterior mediastinum: neuroblastic tumours (i.e. neuroblastoma, ganglioneuroblastoma, ganglioneuroma), neurofibroma.

Anterior mediastinal masses (AMM) can have aggressive behaviour and may cause life-threatening structural compression on the airways (trachea, carina, bronchus, bronchial branches), the heart and the great vessels (pulmonary vessels, superior vena cava).

History and Clinical Examination

- Onset and duration of symptoms.
- Close monitoring for airway/respiratory/haemodynamic instability.
- Neck/face/upper extremities: Engorged neck vessels, facial and neck swelling and congestion — Pemberton sign, upper limb swelling, lymphadenopathy, neck mass, syncope, cyanosis.
- Chest: Cough, dyspnoea, tachypnoea, orthopnoea, noisy breathing (stridor or wheeze), chest pain/discomfort. There may be signs of pleural and/or pericardial effusion.
- Systemic: Fever, night sweat, weight loss.
- Other: Hepatosplenomegaly, Horner syndrome (involvement of sympathetic ganglia), genetic syndrome (e.g. Klinefelter).

Initial Evaluation and Management

- General supportive and resuscitative measures as required. Maintain spontaneous respiration.
- Allow the child to assume the most comfortable position. Establish the 'position of comfort' or 'position of rescue'. Avoid procedures that will cause agitation or distress to the child.
- Immediate referral to multi-disciplinary team: Oncologist, surgeon, intensivist, anaesthetist.
- The minimum level of care and monitoring in the initial period is the High-Dependency Unit. The child should be in the Children's Intensive Care Unit if there is any clinical concern or radiologic evidence of significant airway obstruction or vascular compression.
- Avoid placement of IV cannula in the upper limbs, especially in patients with superior vena cava (SVC) obstruction.
- Initial investigations (to be with urgent multi-disciplinary discussion):
  - » FBC, PBF, renal panel and electrolytes, uric acid, LDH, alpha-fetoprotein (AFP), human chorionic gonadotropin (HCG)
  - » PT, aPTT, Group and Cross Match
  - » CXR postero-anterior and lateral

» CT neck/chest/abdomen
» Ultrasound doppler of neck vessels
» Echocardiogram
» Urine vanillylmandelic acid (VMA)/creatinine and homovanillic acid (HVA)/creatinine (for posterior mediastinal mass)

Table 20.1 Anterior Mediastinal Mass — High-Risk Features Which Have Been Shown to Be Associated with Complications

Clinical Findings	CT Findings	Echo Findings
• Any respiratory distress: Orthopnoea, dyspnoea, noisy breathing, cough • Upper body oedema • Syncope or cyanosis • Abnormal vital parameters: Desaturation, hypotension, inappropriate tachycardia	• Mediastinal mass ratio >45% • Tracheal compression >50% • Severe carinal or bronchial compression • Severe SVC or great vessel compression • Pericardial effusion	• Pericardial effusion • Pulmonary artery (PA) outflow obstruction • Impaired ventricular function

- Multi-disciplinary management is necessary to plan the best and safest way to perform the necessary diagnostic evaluations.
  » A tissue biopsy is required for histopathological diagnosis, unless the diagnosis can be made from elevated serum tumour markers (AFP and HCG) or from PBF and flow cytometry (lymphoblastic leukaemia/lymphoma).
  » General anaesthesia and heavy sedation are avoided, especially in patients with any high-risk features.
  » Local anaesthesia with the child in spontaneous respiration and in a position of comfort may suffice to allow less invasive diagnostic procedures on accessible sites to be performed safely — e.g. cervical lymph node biopsy, bone marrow aspiration/biopsy, pleural tap.
- Although sufficient diagnostic work-up is ideal prior to commencing definitive cancer treatment, patients with life-threatening airway and vascular compression may require urgent steroids or chemotherapy or radiotherapy. Tissue biopsy should still be obtained once it is safe enough to do so, otherwise these interventions may result in rapid tumour response and adversely affect accurate and timely diagnostic confirmation.
- Other oncologic evaluations and procedures as appropriate: Tumour lysis monitoring and management, central line placement, other diagnostic work-up (e.g. LP, PET scan).

Spinal Cord Compression

Spinal cord compression can be caused by tumours such as paravertebral neuroblastic tumours, bone or soft tissue sarcoma, myeloid sarcoma, lymphoma, germ cell tumours, primary or secondary intraspinal tumours. These can occur at initial presentation of the malignancy or at disease progression or recurrence. Spinal cord compression can also be caused by haematoma from traumatic lumbar punctures, especially in patients with thrombocytopenia or coagulopathy. The signs and symptoms may be insidious and non-specific initially, especially in young children. A high index of suspicion and prompt appropriate evaluation and management can improve short- and long-term neurological and spinal outcomes.

History and Clinical Examination

- Onset and duration of symptoms
- Oncologic history; recent spinal procedures
- Pain — back pain; radicular pain radiating to limbs
- Numbness or paraesthesia; sensory level may be present
- Weakness
- Bladder/bowel symptoms — retention of urine, constipation, loss of continence

Initial Evaluation

- Close monitoring of clinical signs/symptoms to look for rapid progression.
- Urgent magnetic resonance imaging (MRI) of whole spine.
- Urgent multi-disciplinary referral: Spine surgery, neurosurgery, oncology, neurology.
- Urgent laboratory investigations:
  - » FBC, renal panel and electrolytes, LFT, LDH, uric acid, AFP, HCG
  - » PT, aPTT, group and cross match
  - » Urine HVA/creatinine; urine VMA/creatinine
- Other imaging and laboratory investigations as necessary, for example, MRI brain, CT chest, BMA/trephine.

Initial Management

- Nil-by-mouth. Give adequate IV fluids but avoid hyperhydration, which may in some situations increase peri-tumoral swelling and worsen cord oedema.
- Consider dexamethasone if there is evidence of neurological deficit.
  - » Initial 1–2 mg/kg (max. 10 mg), followed by 0.25–0.5 mg/kg (max. 4 mg) Q6H.
  - » Haematologic malignancies may respond rapidly to steroids, and hence definitive diagnostic procedures should not be delayed once steroids have been administered.
- Discuss diagnostic and surgical procedures — biopsy for histological diagnosis, versus debulking and decompressive laminectomy; central line placement; other diagnostic procedures, e.g. bone marrow evaluation, biopsy of accessible site (if available and feasible).
- Further management of spinal cord compression include surgical debulking and decompressive laminectomy or emergency chemotherapy or emergency radiotherapy. The exact modality of choice will require urgent discussion on clinical and disease factors.
  - » Patients with severe presentation or rapid progression may require emergency surgical intervention.

» For patients with chemo-sensitive malignancies (such as lymphoma, neuroblastoma, Ewing sarcoma, rhabdomyosarcoma, myeloid sarcoma), chemotherapy is as effective as surgery in relieving cord compression. Biopsy of an accessible tumour, followed by urgent initiation of chemotherapy is generally the preferred strategy.

» For patients with disease progression or recurrence, prognosis and goals of care would have to be considered when planning further treatment intervention.

Bibliography

1. Jones GL, Will A, Jackson GH, *et al.* (2015) Guidelines for the management of tumour lysis syndrome in adults and children with haematological malignancies on behalf of the British Committee for Standards in Haematology. *Br J Haematol* **169**:661–671.
2. Sanz MA, Fenaux P, Tallman MS, *et al.* (2019) Management of acute promyelocytic leukemia: Updated recommendations from an expert panel of the European LeukemiaNet. *Blood* **133**:1630–1643.
3. Abla O, Angelini P, Di Giuseppe G, *et al.* (2016) Early complications of hyperleukocytosis and leukapheresis in childhood acute leukemias. *J Pediatr Hematol Oncol* **38**:111–117.
4. Lehrnbecher T, Robinson P, Fisher B, *et al.* (2017) Guideline for the management of fever and neutropenia in children with cancer and hematopoietic stem-cell transplantation recipients: 2017 update. *J Clin Oncol* **35**:2082–2094.
5. Freifeld AG, Bow EJ, Sepkowitz KA, *et al.* (2011) Executive summary: Clinical practice guideline for the use of antimicrobial agents in neutropenic patients with cancer: 2010 update by the infectious diseases society of America. *Clin Infect Dis* **52**:427–431.
6. McLeod M, Dobbie M. (2019) Anterior mediastinal masses in children. *BJA Ed* **19**:21–26.
7. Brenn BR, Hughes AK. (2019) The anesthetic management of anterior mediastinal masses in children: A review. *Int Anesthesiol Clin* **57**:E24–E41.
8. Pearson JK, Tan GM. (2015) Pediatric anterior mediastinal mass: A review article. *Semin Cardiothorac Vasc Anesth* **19**:248–254.
9. Sabnis A, Finlay JL, Mueller S. (2015) Neurologic emergencies BT — Supportive care in pediatric oncology: A practical evidence-based approach. In: Feusner JH, Hastings CA, Agrawal AK (eds.). *Supportive Care In Pediatric Oncology: A Practical Evidence-based Approach*. Springer Berlin Heidelberg, pp. 71–96.
10. Loblaw DA, Mitera G, Ford M, Laperriere NJ. (2012) A 2011 updated systematic review and clinical practice guideline for the management of malignant extradural spinal cord compression. *Int J Radiat Oncol Biol Phys* **84**:312–317.

CHAPTER 98

Infection Prophylaxis in Immunocompromised Patients

Mya Soe Nwe

Introduction

The following are **general measures** to reduce infections in immunocompromised oncology and haematopoietic stem cell transplant (HSCT) patients:

- All staff and visitors should wear a surgical facemask and practice hand hygiene. Sick staff/visitors should not enter the oncology/HSCT ward.
- Patients with active contagious diseases (e.g. respiratory illness, shingles, chickenpox) should be nursed in single isolation rooms away from the other immunocompromised patients.
- Patients are advised to follow food safety measures. In general, food should be well cleaned and eaten fresh. All meat and eggs should be thoroughly cooked. Dairy products, honey and juices should be pasteurised.
- Patients should practise frequent hand washing and regular baths to maintain personal hygiene and cleanliness, with special attention to oral cavity and perianal area.
- Plants, including fresh or dried flowers, are not allowed in the oncology/HSCT rooms because of the possible presence of fungal moulds and spores.
- Patients at risk of invasive mould infections (e.g. allogeneic HSCT recipients, patients with severe combined immunodeficiency) are nursed in single rooms with double doors, HEPA (high efficiency particulate air) filtration, positive air pressure and high rates of room air exchanges (>12 exchanges per hour).

Post Viral Exposure Prophylaxis

Chickenpox

- Varicella (chickenpox) is an extremely contagious infection due to the varicella-zoster virus (VZV), found only in humans.
- Transmission is by respiratory contact with airborne droplets, or direct contact or inhalation of aerosols from vesicular fluid of skin lesions of varicella, or by a transplacental route.

Table 20.2 Antimicrobial Guidelines for Paediatric Haematology/Oncology Patients

Patient Group	Antibacterial	Antifungal	Antiviral	*Pneumocystis jirovecii*
Acute myeloid leukaemia [newly diagnosed or relapsed]	Levofloxacin or ciprofloxacin (depending on age, see dosing table) during neutropenia	Posaconazole during neutropenia	Acyclovir if HSV seropositive, and during fludarabine containing courses	Co-trimoxazole
Acute lymphoblastic leukaemia (ALL)	No routine prophylaxis except in infant ALL	No routine prophylaxis for standard/ intermediate-risk protocol	No routine prophylaxis for standard/ intermediate-risk protocol	Co-trimoxazole Substitute co-trimoxazole with IV pentamidine during high-dose methotrexate courses to avoid drug-drug interaction.
		High-risk protocol/ relapsed ALL: Micafungin or liposomal amphotericin B during 4-drug induction and re-induction chemotherapy courses, until count recovery Posaconazole during fludarabine and clofarabine containing courses, until count recovery	High-risk protocol/ relapsed ALL: Acyclovir if HSV seropositive, and during fludarabine, clofarabine containing courses	
All other childhood cancers	No routine prophylaxis	No routine prophylaxis	No routine prophylaxis	Co-trimoxazole Most childhood cancers treatment protocols recommend for PJP prophylaxis, except for osteosarcoma.
Allogeneic haematopoietic stem cell transplant (HSCT)	No routine prophylaxis	Micafungin during conditioning chemotherapy, posaconazole when able to take orally	Acyclovir for 1 yr	Co-trimoxazole from engraftment
Autologous HSCT	No routine prophylaxis	Fluconazole during neutropenia	Acyclovir for 6 mth	Co-trimoxazole from engraftment

Table 20.3 Antimicrobial Prophylaxis Dosing Regime

	Drug	Spectrum	Dosing	Notes
Antibacterial prophylaxis	Ciprofloxacin	• Gram-negative including *Pseudomonas aeruginosa* • Levofloxacin has improved gram-positive coverage compared to ciprofloxacin • Do not cover anaerobes	>1 to <6 mth: PO 10 mg/kg BD	Prophylaxis may increase bacterial resistance, limit use to neutropenia period in selected group of patients.
	Levofloxacin		≥6 mth to 5 yr old: PO 10 mg/kg BD (max. 250 mg/dose) ≥5 yr old: PO 10 mg/kg OD (max. 750 mg/dose)	
Antifungal prophylaxis	Fluconazole	• Covers *Candida albicans*, *C. tropicalis*, *C. parapsilosis* • Variable activity against *C. glabrata* • Not active against *C. krusei* and moulds	PO/IV 6 mg/kg OD (max. 400 mg/dose)	Not for patients who require mould-active prophylaxis, e.g. alloHSCT, AML, high-risk ALL.
	Liposomal amphotericin B (Ambisome)	• Broad spectrum, including *Candida* and *Aspergillus* spp. (except *A. terreus*), *Mucorales*	IV 1 mg/kg thrice a week or IV 2.5 mg/kg twice a week	Monitor for renal toxicity (increased serum creatinine, urea, hypomagnesaemia, hypokalaemia)
	Micafungin	• Active against *Candida* and *Aspergillus* spp.	IV 2 mg/kg OD (max. 100 mg/dose)	Well tolerated.
	Posaconazole	• Active against *Candida* and *Aspergillus* spp., *Mucorales*	Suspension: - <13 yr old: PO 4 mg/kg TDS (max. 200 mg/dose) - ≥13 yr old: PO 200 mg TDS *Absorption of suspension is highly dependent on food and acidic pH, hence may not be suitable for patients with inadequate oral intake.* Delayed Release Tablet: - 5–7 mg/kg BD x 1/7 followed by	• Suspension and tablets are not interchangeable in doses. • Therapeutic Drug Monitoring: Check trough level 1 week after initiating, aim for levels of >0.7 mg/L for prophylaxis. • Strong CYP3A4 inhibitor — beware of potential drug-drug interactions with chemotherapy, e.g. vincristine, doxorubicin thiotepa.

			- 5–7 mg/kg OD (max. 300 mg/dose; round to nearest 50 mg, do not crush tablet) *Delayed release tablet has better absorption profile, but is only suitable for patients who can swallow tablets.*	
Antiviral prophylaxis	Acyclovir	• Covers for HSV and VZV	PO 40 mg/kg BD (max. 800 mg/dose) ≥40 kg: IV 250 mg/m² Q12H <40 kg: IV 250 mg/m² Q8H	Ensure adequate hydration, especially for IV therapy to prevent crystalluria and nephrotoxicity.
PJP[1] prophylaxis	Co-trimoxazole (sulfamethoxazole-trimethoprim)	• Active against PJP	PO 2.5 mg TMP/kg/dose BD (max. 80 mg TMP/dose), twice a week	• Drug of choice for PJP prophylaxis. • Avoid in patients with sulpha allergy or G6PD deficiency. • AVOID concurrent co-trimoxazole and high-dose methotrexate therapy — increase risks of methotrexate toxicities. Stop co-trimoxazole 1 week prior to high-dose methotrexate.
	Pentamidine	• Active against PJP	IV 4 mg/kg every 2–4 weekly	• Monitor for hypotension. Ensure patient lies supine during infusion to minimise risk of hypotension.

[1] *Pneumocystis Jirovecii* (previously *Pneumocystis* Carinii Pneumonia).
Pneumocystis jirovecii (PJP) can cause severe life-threatening pneumonitis in immunocompromised patients with severe lymphopenia and neutropenia. Prophylaxis is indicated for patients undergoing treatment for malignancy, patients undergoing HSCT, patients with severe combined immunodeficiency, patients undergoing intensive chemotherapy for certain brain and solid tumours, and patients receiving moderate–high doses of systemic corticosteroids for longer than 4 weeks. Prophylaxis should continue for at least 3–6 months after the end of chemotherapy or immunosuppression.

Post-exposure prophylaxis (PEP) includes VZIG (VZ immune globulin) or VZ vaccine, but not acyclovir currently (except in unusual circumstances; consult Infectious Disease specialist)

1) VZ vaccine: It is contraindicated if the patient is on active chemotherapy or high-dose steroids (should have their steroids discontinued for at least 1–3 months before receiving VZ vaccine) and for those with recent administration of blood, plasma or immune globulin, including IVIG (should have IVIG 11 months before receiving the VZ vaccine).
2) Varicella Immune globulin (VZIG): It is indicated if an immunocompromised patient is exposed to active chickenpox within 96 hours (up to 10 days) of exposure.

Dose (specific to Varitect® CP, intravenous (IV) preparation of VZIG):

- 25 IU/kg, or 1 ml/kg (compared with 125 IU for every 10 kg body weight for intramuscular (IM) preparation)
- There is no maximum dose for Varitect® CP
- Do NOT overdose, as this may lead to fluid overload and hyperviscosity

Administration:

- IV
- Infuse at 0.1 ml/kg/h for the first 10 minutes and monitor for side effects; if tolerated well, may increase to 0.2 ml/kg/h for the next 10 minutes, then 0.5 ml/kg/h for another 10 minutes and subsequently to 1 ml/kg/h till completion

Possible Side Effects:

- Local reactions — pain, redness, swelling (uncommon)
- Systemic reactions — fever, headache, malaise, chills, nausea, vomiting, arthralgia (uncommon)
- In cases of adverse reactions, reduce the rate or stop the infusion till symptoms disappear
- Severe reactions — angioneurotic oedema, anaphylaxis (rare); aseptic meningitis, reversible haemolysis (very rare)
- For acute anaphylaxis, give intramuscular adrenaline 0.01 ml/kg (1:1000), repeating every 15 minutes if necessary

The incubation period is 21 days (if VZIG is not given), or 28 days (if VZIG is given). During this period, it may be necessary to consider withholding intensive chemotherapy.

Treatment

If chickenpox should develop, IV acyclovir should be given for at least 7 days, until all lesions have crusted and with no appearance of new lesions for 48 hours. The dose of IV acyclovir is 500 mg/m^2/dose Q8H (or 10 mg/kg/dose Q8H for children younger than 1 year), given with adequate hydration.

Measles

- Measles is a highly contagious, acute infection caused by the measles virus (MV) and usually seen in children
- Transmission is by direct contact with respiratory secretions of infected persons or airborne droplets

Post-exposure prophylaxis (PEP) includes Human Immune Globulin (IG) or measles, mumps and rubella (MMR) vaccine

MMR vaccine is contraindicated in immunocompromised patients.

Immune globulin (IG): IV/IM

Contraindications/Precautions:

- Hypersensitivity to immune globulin or any component of the formulation
- GAMASTAN® must not be given intravenously, and must not be administered intramuscularly in cases of severe thrombocytopenia and in other disorders of haemostasis, and in IgA deficient patients with antibodies against IgA.

Dose:

- IV Immunoglobulin:
  - » Immunocompromised: 400 mg/kg as a slow infusion

<u>OR</u>

- IM Immunoglobulin (GAMASTAN® 2 ml vial)
  - » Usual dose: 0.25 ml/kg
  - » Immunocompromised: 0.5 ml/kg
  - » Maximum dose: 15 ml

Administration:

- IV (current preparation)
  - » Infuse at 0.5 ml/kg/hr for the first 15 minutes and monitor for side effects; if tolerated well, may increase to 1 ml/kg/hr for the next 15 minutes, then 2 ml/kg/hr for another 15 minutes and subsequently to 4 ml/kg/hr till completion
- IM (GAMASTAN® 2 ml)
  - » If anatomically feasible, the full dose should be administered at a single site
  - » Otherwise, the dose can be re-distributed to multiple sites to reduce local pain and discomfort

Possible Side Effects:

- Local reactions — pain, redness, swelling, itching, rash (IM: common)
- Systemic reactions — chills, headache, fever, vomiting, nausea, dizziness, low blood pressure, tachycardia, arthralgia, hyperhidrosis, pallor, paraesthesia, back pain
- In cases of adverse reactions, reduce the rate or stop the infusion till symptoms disappear
- Severe: Anaphylactic/anaphylactoid reactions, thromboembolic events, aseptic meningitis, acute renal failure, transfusion-related acute lung injury (rarely)

- For acute anaphylaxis, give IM adrenaline 0.01 ml/kg (1:1000), repeating every 15 minutes if necessary

The incubation period is 14 days, during which chemotherapy should be withheld if possible.

Splenectomy/Asplenia

Splenectomised patients or those with other causes of asplenia or impaired splenic function are at risk of developing severe sepsis from encapsulated bacteria such as *Streptococcus pneumoniae, Haemophilus influenzae* and *Neisseria meningitidis.*

Prevention of Post-Splenectomy Sepsis

The patient who has undergone splenectomy or who is functionally asplenic needs to be educated about the need for prompt medical attention after the onset of fever.

Immunisations

- Immunisation with pneumococcal, meningococcal and conjugate *H. influenzae* type b vaccines.
- If a patient will be undergoing elective splenectomy, the pneumococcal, meningococcal and *H. influenzae* vaccines should be administered at least 14 days prior to surgery. If it is not possible to administer these vaccines prior to splenectomy, they can be given after the 14th post-operative day.

Antibiotic Prophylaxis

Post-splenectomy, antibiotic prophylaxis is advised. Antibiotic prophylaxis also applies to patients with asplenia or functional asplenia (e.g. sickle cell disease, post-splenic irradiation or graft vs. host disease). Duration of antibiotic prophylaxis is still controversial, but should be until a minimum age of 5 years and at least 1–2 years post-splenectomy, or longer (until age 18 years, or even lifelong) for higher-risk patients.

Antibiotics Prophylaxis for Invasive Dental Procedure

Immunocompromised patients should receive standard antibiotic prophylaxis against infective endocarditis during invasive procedures such as gastrointestinal or genitourinary operations and invasive dental procedures (refer to Table 7.13 in Chapter 28: 'Infective Endocarditis').

Vaccination

Vaccination for Close Contacts of Immunocompromised Patients

- Household contacts should *not* receive oral polio vaccine (OPV). Individuals with recent OPV (within 4–6 weeks) should not come into close contact with immunocompromised patients.

Table 20.4 Recommendations for Additional Vaccine Requirements in Splenectomised/Asplenic Patients

Vaccine	Age at Start of Vaccine Course		
	<12 months	12–23 months	≥24 months (2 years)
MenACWY, meningococcal conjugate[d] Choice of MenACWY should depend on the age of the child at first vaccination, as the licensed minimum age of Menveo®, Menactra® and Nimenrix™ differs	**Menveo®**: 2-dose or 4-dose primary series, depending on age **Nimenrix™**:[2] 2-dose primary series **Booster dose:** Single dose 3 yr after primary vaccination, thereafter every 5 yr (<7 yr of age) Single dose every 5 yr (≥7 yr of age)	**Menveo®**: 2-dose primary series **Nimenrix™** 1-dose primary series **Booster dose:** Single dose 3 yr after primary vaccination, thereafter every 5 yr (<7 yr of age) Single dose every 5 yr (≥7 yr of age)	**Menveo®**, **Menactra®**[1]: 2-dose primary series **Nimenrix™** 1-dose primary series **Booster dose:** Single dose 3 yr after primary vaccination, thereafter every 5 yr (<7 yr of age) Single dose every 5 yr (≥7 yr of age)
PCV13, pneumococcal conjugate	Age appropriate vaccination as per current National Childhood Immunisation Programme. For incomplete/delayed vaccinations: • ≤6 mth of age: 2- or 3-dose primary series • 7–11 mth of age: 2-dose primary series • 12–23 mth of age: 1-dose primary series Booster dose (after 1 yr of age): Single dose		If not previously immunised: • 2–5 yr of age: 1-dose primary series + booster 8 wk apart • ≥6 yr of age: Single dose
Hib, *Haemophilus influenzae* type b	Age appropriate vaccination with combination of 5-in-1 and 6-in-1 vaccines. For children with incomplete/delayed vaccinations: • ≤6 mth of age: 3-dose primary series • 7–11 mth of age: 2-dose primary series • 12–23 mth of age: 1-dose primary series Booster dose (after 1 yr of age): Single dose		If not previously immunised: • 2 to <5 yr of age: 1-dose primary series + booster 8 wk apart • ≥5 yr of age: Single dose
PPSV23, pneumococcal polysaccharide[3]			If not previously immunised: 1-dose primary series + booster 5 yr later Final dose at ≥65 yr
Inactivated influenza	Annually from 6 mth of age • <9 yr of age: 2-dose primary series in the first season of receipt, then yearly single dose • ≥9 yr of age: 1-dose primary series, then yearly single dose		

[1] Menactra® should be administered at least 4 weeks after completion of the PCV series.

Do not administer Menactra® to those less than 2 years of age because of possible interference with the response to PCV13 vaccine.

[2] Whenever possible, Menactra®/Nimenrix™ and a tetanus toxoid (TT) containing vaccine (e.g. DTaP-HBV-IPV/Hib) should be co-administered or Menactra/Nimenrix™ should be administered at least 1 month before the TT-containing vaccine.

[3] When both PCV13 and PPSV23 are indicated, administer PCV13 first. PPSV23 should be administered at least 8 weeks after the last dose of PCV13.

Table 20.5 Antibiotic Prophylaxis for Asplenia

First Line Antibiotics	Alternatives
PO Penicillin V • <3 yr of age: 125 mg twice daily • ≥3 yr of age: 250 mg twice daily	PO Erythromycin (if penicillin allergy/G6PD deficient) • 4 mth to <3 yr of age: 125 mg twice daily • ≥3 to 8 yr of age: 250 mg twice daily • ≥8 yr of age: 500 mg twice daily
PO Amoxicillin • 10 mg/kg/dose twice daily (max. 500 mg/dose)	PO Bactrim (Trimethoprim [TMP]-sulfamethoxazole) • 4 mg/kg/dose (TMP component) twice daily (max.: 160 mg TMP/dose)

- Close contacts (including staff, family members and visitors) who are VZV-seronegative should receive the varicella vaccine, but should avoid contact with immunocompromised patients if they develop vaccine-associated skin lesions, until the skin lesions clear.
- If an infant in the household has received the rotavirus vaccine, the highly immunocompromised patient should avoid handling the infant's diapers for 4 weeks after the vaccination.

Bibliography

1. Children's Oncology Group. (2004) *Supportive Care of Children with Cancer: Current Therapy and Guidelines from the Children's Oncology Group, 3rd ed.* Johns Hopkins University Press.
2. Centers for Disease Control and Prevention; Infectious Disease Society of America; American Society of Blood and Marrow Transplantation. (2000) Guidelines for preventing opportunistic infections among hematopoietic stem cell transplant recipients — Recommendations of CDC, the Infectious Disease Society of America, and the American Society of Blood and Marrow Transplantation. *MMWR Recomm Rep* **49**(RR-10):1–125, CE1–7.
3. Tomblyn M, Chiller T, Einsele H, *et al.* (2009) Guidelines for preventing infectious complications among hematopoietic cell transplantation recipients: A global perspective. *Biol Blood Marrow Transplant* **15**:1143–1238.
4. Science M, Robinson PD, MacDonald T, *et al.* (2014) Guideline for primary antifungal prophylaxis for pediatric patients with cancer or hematopoietic stem cell transplant recipients. *Pediatr Blood Cancer* **61**:393–400.
5. Doring M, Muller C, Johann P-D, *et al.* (2012) Analysis of posaconazole as oral antifungal prophylaxis in pediatric patients under 12 years of age following allogeneic stem cell transplantation. *BMC Infect Dis* **12**:263.
6. Patel SR, Chisholm JC, Heath PT. (2008) Vaccinations in children treated with standard-dose cancer therapy or hematopoietic stem cell transplantation. *Pediatr Clin N Am* **55**:169–186.
7. Rubin LG, Levin MJ, Ljungman P, *et al.* (2014) 2013 IDSA clinical practice guideline for vaccination of the immunocompromised host. *Clin Infect Dis* **58**(3):e44–e100.
8. Kroger AT, Sumaya CV, Pickering LK, Atkinson WL. (2011) General recommendations on immunization: Recommendations of the advisory committee on immunization practices (ACIP). *MMWR* **60**(2):1–60.

CHAPTER 99

Lymphadenopathy

Prasad Ramanakrishnan Iyer; Chan Mei Yoke

Differential Diagnoses

- Infections
  - » Bacterial: *Staphylococcus aureus*, *Streptococcus pyogenes*, Bartonella (Cat Scratch Disease), Brucellosis, Tularaemia
  - » Viral: Epstein–Barr virus, Cytomegalovirus, Human immunodeficiency virus, Measles, Rubella
  - » Mycobacterial: *Mycobacterium tuberculosis*, *Mycobacterium avium-intracellulare*, *Mycobacterium scrotulareum*
  - » Protozoan: Toxoplasmosis, Malaria
  - » Fungal: Histoplasmosis, Coccidiomycosis, Cryptococcus, Aspergillosis
- Autoimmune conditions
  - » Juvenile chronic arthritis
  - » Systemic Lupus Erythematosus
- Immunodeficiency syndromes
  - » Chronic granulomatous disease
  - » Hyper-IgE syndrome (Job Syndrome)
  - » Leucocyte adhesion deficiency
- Malignant conditions
  - » Leukaemia/lymphoma
  - » Metastatic solid tumours, e.g. neuroblastoma
- Miscellaneous
  - » Kawasaki Disease
  - » Kikuchi Disease
  - » Sarcoidosis
  - » Histiocytosis
  - » Storage disease, e.g. Gaucher disease, Niemann-Pick Disease
  - » Medications, e.g. phenytoin

History

- Age of patient, duration of symptoms
- Travel history exposure to insects, animals, sick persons
- Recurrent infections, recurrent skin sepsis, immunisation status
- Constitutional symptoms, e.g. fever, loss of appetite, loss of weight

- Rash, arthralgia
- Drug history
- Travel history; exposure to insects, animals, sick persons

Clinical Examination

- Examine enlarged lymph node for: Size, warmth, tenderness, overlying skin erythema, fluctuancy, mobility
- Other lymph node involvement: Cervical, occipital, axillary, epitrochlear, inguinal, popliteal
- Presence of pallor, jaundice
- Joints for swelling, tenderness, limited range of movement
- Skin for vasculitis, petechiae, purpura
- Abdomen for hepatosplenomegaly, intra-abdominal masses
- Localised infection

Investigations and Management

See Table 20.6.

Features that may prompt lymph node biopsy in a child with lymphadenopathy:

- Lymph node size >2 cm or increasing in size
- Supraclavicular lymphadenopathy
- Abnormal chest X-ray
- Presence of systemic signs and symptoms: Fever, night sweats, weight loss, hepatosplenomegaly

If lymph node biopsy is to be done, consult oncologist and ID physician first.

The biopsy specimen is usually sent for the following:

- Histology (inform pathologist beforehand if lymphoma is suspected as a fresh specimen is often required)
- Gram stain, culture and sensitivity
- Acid Fast Bacillus (AFB) smear/AFB culture and sensitivity, AFB Polymerase Chain Reaction (PCR)
- Fungal smear/fungal culture

Table 20.6 Investigations and Management of Lymphadenopathy

Signs and Symptoms	Conditions Suspected	Investigations	Management
Isolated cervical lymphadenopathy, otherwise well	Viral lymphadenitis	None needed	Observe. Await resolution in up to 4–6 wk.
Fever, lethargic, upper respiratory tract infection, pharyngitis, otitis media	*S. aureus* infection *S. pyogenes* infection	Full blood count (FBC), Blood culture (C/S), Ultrasound scan if suppuration suspected	Augmentin. Incision and drainage if abscess formation.
Oral mucositis, dental abscess	Anaerobic oral flora	FBC, Blood C/S	Augmentin
School-going age group, fever, lethargy, white exudates on tonsils, hepatosplenomegaly, generalised lymphadenopathy	Infectious mononucleosis-like syndrome	FBC, Liver function test, EBV IgM, CMV IgM	Symptomatic treatment (Avoid Ampicillin)
Usually 1–5 yr old, usually multiple unilateral, firm lymph nodes. May undergo rapid suppuration or rupture and form cutaneous sinus tracts.	Non-tuberculous mycobacterium infection	Mantoux test (50% may be positive) Excision biopsy	Complete surgical excision. Antibiotics (Clarithromycin ± Rifampicin) for patients: • With established sinus tracts • At high risk for facial nerve damage if excision is done • With intra-parotid adenitis • With incomplete LN excision
Unilateral or bilateral firm, discrete, non-tender lymph nodes, often fixed to underlying tissues, may progress to become matted. May be associated with low-grade fever and systemic symptoms.	Tuberculous adenitis	Mantoux test Chest X-ray (normal in 70% of cases) FBC, Erythrocyte sedimentation rate (ESR), Lymph node biopsy	Two months of Rifampicin, Isoniazid and Pyrazinamide followed by 4 mth of Rifampicin and Isoniazid
Fever, vasculitic rash, arthralgia, arthritis, hepatosplenomegaly, generalised lymphadenopathy	Autoimmune condition	FBC, ESR C3, C4 ANA, anti-dsDNA	Steroid therapy
Fever, loss of appetite, loss of weight, petechiae, pallor, hepatosplenomegaly, supraclavicular lymph node enlargement	Malignant condition	FBC, Peripheral blood film, ESR LDH, uric acid Chest X-ray Excision biopsy	Treat underlying malignancy
Fever, rash, conjunctivitis, red lips, strawberry tongue, unilateral cervical lymph node enlargement, swollen or erythematous hands or feet, BCG scar erythema or induration	Kawasaki Disease	FBC, Blood C/S C-reactive protein, ESR 2D Echocardiogram	IV Immunoglobulin High-dose aspirin

CHAPTER 100

Paediatric Palliative Care

Chan Mei Yoke; Wynn Yi Yi

The World Health Organization (WHO) defines palliative care (PC) as 'active total care of patients whose disease is not responsive to curative treatment. Control of pain, of other symptoms and of psychological, social and spiritual problems is paramount. The goal of PC is the achievement of the best quality of life for patients and their families'. WHO also recommends that paediatric palliative care (PPC) for children begins when life-limiting illness is diagnosed and continues regardless of whether the child receives treatment directed at the disease. It involves giving support to the family and including them in decision-making regarding PC needs of the child.

Clinical skills in history-taking and examination are essential. Investigations are carried out only if the result will contribute to the patient's management. Care of palliative patients always involves assessment and re-assessment to ensure maximal relief of symptoms. Patients and their families are intimately involved in decision-making regarding treatment options and care.

Paediatric Patients Suitable for PPC

Children with these four categories of diseases may benefit from a referral to PPC:

- Diseases where cure is possible but can fail, e.g. cancer, organ failure — heart, liver or kidney or infections.
- Incurable diseases but child can live for an extended time, e.g. cystic fibrosis, Duchenne muscular dystrophy, human immunodeficiency virus/acquire immunodeficiency syndrome, cardiovascular anomalies, extreme prematurity.
- Progressive conditions from the diagnosis without curative options, for example, neuro-degenerative, progressive metabolic disorders, chromosomal abnormalities, advanced metastatic cancer on first presentation.
- Irreversible, non-progressive with severe disability, e.g. cerebral palsy, genetic disorders, congenital malformations, brain/spinal cord injury.

Many are non-malignant and some of the conditions, e.g. genetic disorders, which are extremely rare with diagnosis specific to childhood, may have affected more than one child in the family. Some have uncertain prognosis and the course may stretch for years, requiring lifelong palliative needs.

Earlier integration of PC has improved clinical outcomes and provided an extra layer of support to the child and family. Referral can be initiated in the following conditions:

- Upon diagnosis of life-threatening fetal condition (peri-natal PC).

- At the time of new life-threatening diagnosis with poor prognosis, e.g. diffuse intrinsic pontine glioma, Stage IV Neuroblastoma.
- New diagnosis with complex pain and/or symptom management issues.
- When disease becomes refractory to treatment.
- Disease progression with development of life-threatening complications (organ failure or prolonged intubation).
- Complex clinical course with complications requiring multiple admissions.

Adult versus PPC

The paediatric palliative model of care is integrated and seamless throughout initial diagnosis, active curative treatment and symptom relief, sharing care with community, home and inpatient PC and bereavement services. It is important to gradually move from curative treatment to PC without rigid boundaries.

The adult model of 6 months prognosis as referral criteria cannot apply in PPC. The focus of care may be more 'aggressive' as well, in that there may be more hospitalisations, and 'active' treatment may be ongoing. A parent should never have to choose between PC and hope for a cure.

PPC focuses on symptoms control, maintaining a good quality of life and supporting families when a child has a condition that is highly likely to end in premature death at any time prior to adulthood. PPC is not confined to end-of-life care but is incorporated throughout the disease trajectory as part of the continuum of care.

Providing PPC for children with life-limiting illness requires attention to the physical, developmental stage, psychosocial, ethical, spiritual and relational phenomena that are unique to children. Children undergo continual developmental changes and their age-dependent cognitive abilities will impact their medical, social, emotional needs and understanding of illness and death. They have changing information needs, recreational and educational needs and modes of coping with stress. Child life specialists, play therapists and behavioural specialists can facilitate through activities that assist with emotional distress and can provide important understanding into the fears and wishes of the child.

A child with a life-threatening disease may strain or challenge existing relationships within the family. Role reversal, overly enmeshed relationships, family dynamics and conflicts between family members are common and cause significantly impact on the child's quality of life. Assessment of family function and efforts to resolve conflict or dysfunction is thus essential.

Emphasis is placed on excellent communication skills with both patients and their families. This requires sensitivity to the child's developmental stage and to the language, culture and illness understanding of both the patient and family. PPC entails taking time to assess parents' awareness of their child's condition and explore their concerns, practical challenges, care preferences and facilitate discussion for future wishes and care. It is also important to clarify with regard to the preferred place of care as families may prefer the child to be at home rather than in a hospice.

'Parallel care planning' refers to the development of plans that allow for unpredictability in the course of the condition. There will be concurrent plans for potential survival and plans for deterioration and death. This allows clinical teams and parents an opportunity to review care plans according to the child's disease progression and needs, but also spare parents and family from the sense of abandonment and anxiety when the child's condition deteriorates and death becomes imminent.

Barriers to PPC

Children may be referred late or not at all to PPC due to barriers such as:

- Physician's prognostic paralysis regarding the child's illness.
- Stigma surrounding death and PC by both the physician and parents.
- Misunderstanding of purpose of PPC, e.g. abandonment or giving up and stopping all treatment.

PPC can help with the following categories of needs:

- Symptom management, e.g. pain, vomiting, breathlessness, excessive secretions.
- Psychosocial support, e.g. identify the child and family's fears, coping and communication styles.
- Spiritual support, e.g. review child's hopes, dreams, values, life meaning, role of prayer and ritual and beliefs regarding death.
- Discussion of Advance Care Plan with parents and child (if child is old enough).
- Preparation and support of the child and family for end-of-life care, including management of end-of-life symptoms and selection of preferred location of death.
- Facilitates and coordinates continuity of care across settings to ensure a smooth transition from hospital to home or hospice.
- Bereavement support for the family following the death of the child.

Conclusion

PPC aims to improve the quality of life for children of all ages with life-threatening illnesses and their families regardless of age (i.e. new born to young adults), stage of illness (i.e. curative treatment, chronic stage, recovery, terminal stage) and outcome (i.e. death or survival).

PPC adopts a holistic approach to provide the child and his/her family needs in all dimensions (physical, psychosocial, spiritual and practical) of care, which is consistent with the goals of the child and family. On-going regular assessment of their needs is essential and requires collaboration and coordination with all healthcare teams across different settings (hospital, home and hospice), with the aim to provide 'seamless' transitions for children with life-threatening conditions.

Bibliography

1. World Health Organization. (2018) Integrating palliative care and symptom relief into paediatrics: A WHO guide for health care planners, implementers and managers, World Health Organization, Geneva.
2. American Academy of Pediatrics. (2000) Committee on bioethics and committee on hospital care. Palliative care for children. *Pediatrics* **106**(2 Pt 1):351–357.

SECTION 21

PSYCHIATRY

CHAPTER 101

Agitated and Violent Patients

Radha Srikanth; Ong Say How

Introduction

Violent and agitated behaviour can be the manifestation of many psychiatric as well as medical conditions. It is often not essential and, in fact, not possible to establish and manage the cause of the agitation and aggression before managing the behaviour.

Risk Factors

- Patients with psychosis or bipolar affective disorder.
- Children with non-accidental injury (NAI) or have reason to fear for their own safety due to their own trauma.
- Patients with disruptive behaviour disorders like conduct disorder, attention deficit hyperactivity disorder (ADHD), impulsivity, etc.
- Patients who have misused substances/acute intoxication.
- Children with high levels of anxiety can also present with agitation and violent behaviour.

Approach to Managing Behavioural Disturbance in Children and Adolescents

- All aggressive and violent children and adolescent should have a comprehensive diagnostic evaluation.
- Physical restraint can be emotionally traumatic for children; hence, behavioural strategies or seclusion should be preferred.
- First-line management — De-escalation
- Second-line management — Seclusion and restraint
- Third-line management — Use of oral medications such as benzodiazepines and antihistamines. If there is a history of psychotic illness, intramuscular injection of haloperidol can be used.
- The lowest possible dose of medications should be used.
- A senior medical staff should be involved in decision-making for using medications.
- If the child or adolescent continues to be unmanageable, the child psychiatrist on-call must be consulted and if safety is a concern, admission to psychiatric inpatient unit should be considered.

Verbal De-Escalation When a Child is Restrained

- Talk to the child
- Use a calm space
- Listen to the child
- Acknowledge his feelings of anger
- Set time limits
- Motivate him — 'I want you to calm down', 'I want you to help me to calm you down'
- Use relaxation techniques — ask the child to take deep breaths and relax his muscles. Demonstrate this to the child.
- Distract the child by changing the focus to positive things.

Rapid Tranquillisation

- Defined as 'the use of psychotropic medication to control agitation, threatening or destructive psychotic behaviour'
- Aims
  - » Reduce the risk of physical harm to other patients, staff and the patient
  - » Reduce the distress to the patient caused by acute agitation
  - » Calm the patient and not sedate. (However, sometimes sedation is unavoidable.)
- Side effects
  - » Paradoxical reactions, including hyperactive/aggressive behaviour have been occasionally reported with benzodiazepine use. This may be more likely to occur in children/adolescents and patients with developmental delay or organic brain syndromes.
  - » The most serious acute complication of benzodiazepines remains respiratory depression.
  - » Children and adolescents are more likely to be antipsychotic-naïve and there is a greater risk of dystonic reaction and other acute side effects.
  - » The most commonly encountered problems (can happen even after a single dose) after administration of haloperidol are:
    - ▪ Acute dystonia,
    - ▪ Oculogyric crisis (type of acute dystonia, which includes blepharospasm, periorbital twitches and protracted staring episodes), and
    - ▪ Akathisia.
- The parameters to be monitored when medications are given to manage agitated and violent behaviour are:
  - » Blood pressure
  - » Heart rate
  - » Respiratory rate
  - » Temperature
  - » Oxygen saturation

Table 21.1 Medications (rapid tranquillisation)

Suggested Oral (PO) Medications	Suggested Intramuscular (IM)/Intravenous (IV) Injections
Children 6–12 yr old: • PO promethazine 0.5–1 mg/kg (max. 50 mg) stat • PO hydroxyzine 0.6 mg/kg (max. 25 mg) stat • PO lorazepam 0.05–0.1 mg/kg (max. 1 mg) stat. May repeat dose 30–60 min later. (Max. 2 mg/24 hr). **Above 12 yr old:** • PO promethazine 12.5–25 mg stat • PO hydroxyzine 12.5–25 mg stat • PO lorazepam 1–2 mg stat. May repeat dose 30–60 min later. (Max. 4 mg/24 hr.)	**Consult Child Psychiatrist before giving any IM or IV injections** **Children 6–12 yr old:** • IM or IV diphenhydramine 1 mg/kg/dose stat (max. 50 mg) • IM or IV lorazepam 0.05 mg/kg/dose (max. 1 mg). May repeat dose 30–60 min later. (Max. 2 mg/24 hr). **If psychotic/history of psychosis:** • IM haloperidol 0.025–0.075 mg/kg/dose (max. 3 mg). May repeat dose 30–60 min later, up to four times a day. (Max. 0.15 mg/kg/d.) **Above 12 yr old:** • IM or IV diphenhydramine 50 mg stat • IM or IV lorazepam 0.5–1 mg (max. 1–2 mg) stat. May repeat dose 30–60 min later. (Max. 4 mg/24 hr.) **If psychotic/history of psychosis:** • IM haloperidol 2.5–5 mg stat. May repeat dose 30–60 min later, up to 4 times a day. (Max. 0.15 mg/kg/d.)

Conclusion

- Always give the child an opportunity after the incident to address any concerns due to the whole incident.
- Remember to talk to parents to explain the management.
- A root cause analysis of how the violence started in the first place would produce valuable information.
- Concerns raised must be followed up and the child may need referral to specialists who can deal with the issues in detail.

Bibliography

1. Ellison JM, Blum NR, Barsky AJ. (1989) Frequent repeaters in a psychiatric emergency service. *Hosp Community Psychiatry* **40**:958–960. In: Pereira S, Gard D and Brandford D (eds.) *Rapid Tranquilisation of Acutely Disturbed Patient*, Royal College of Psychiatrists, CPD online, May 2009.
2. Pereira S, Gard D, Brandford D. (eds.) (2009) Rapid tranquilisation of acutely disturbed patient, Royal College of Psychiatrists, CPD online.

CHAPTER 102

Self-Harm and Suicidal Behaviours

Ong Say How

It is not uncommon for troubled adolescents to be referred for self-harm and suicidal behaviour. Deliberate self-harm (DSH) is also known as non-suicidal self-injury (NSSI). The motivations for carrying out self-harm are often multiple and certainly multi-factorial, with interpersonal conflicts and disputes being frequent precipitating factors. Individuals who have impulsive traits, poor frustration tolerance, anxiety, depression, conduct disorders and borderline personality traits are more predisposed to engaging in self-harm behaviour.

Self-harm is a set of maladaptive behaviour used to cope with intense and negative feelings, and could range from cutting, overdosing, peeling/scratching of skin, hitting and biting of self, etc. Individuals with self-harm behaviour are not suicidal in intent per se but the risk of suicide is elevated in this group of patients: 60 to 100 times higher than in the general population. As the frequency of self-harm increases, so do the risk of suicidal thoughts and plans. The recurrence of self-harm behaviour also increases with a past history of self-harm.

Self-harm typically happens when other means to self-soothe fail or the individual does not know how to do so. A common misconception is that self-harming adolescents are seeking attention. They are not.

Observe the following when attending to individuals who self-harm:

- Attend to the injury and assess whether surgical intervention or superficial first-aid is required. Be mindful to check for cuts in obscure locations on the body such as thighs. Self-cutting in the inner thighs could be a sign of prior or existing sexual abuse.
- Even if surgical intervention is not needed, decide whether admission is required, especially for individuals coming from complex family and social backgrounds, when there is concomitant high suicide risk or when the adolescent is visibly distressed over an ongoing stressor that will not go away any time soon. Admit the adolescent if you are uncertain, as it is better to err on the side of caution.
- If admission is not required, consider referring the patient to the Psychology Service outpatient clinics. Many individuals with self-harm behaviour benefit from cognitive behavioural therapy (CBT) and antidepressants (e.g. selective serotonin reuptake inhibitors).
- Stay calm as the attending doctor. Do not judge or criticise the behaviour of the adolescent. Let them know that even though you cannot help solve their problems, you or someone in the hospital/clinic could lend a listening ear.

- If there is a chance you are able to engage the adolescent in greater depth, use the HEADSS assessment to assess in greater details the presence of adverse psychosocial factors. This screen can be used to guide further management like referrals to other services.

Adolescents who self-harm do not stop the behaviour overnight. Many continue to do so for years before they either reduce the frequency of self-harm or stop completely. Improvements in self-harm is likely attributed to their developing maturity and self-esteem with time.

Fortunately, the suicide rate for youth in Singapore remains low at about 1.3 per 100000 (2011) compared to other countries. Reasons behind the low rate include availability of youth outreach, effective healthcare and emergency response systems, low poverty rate and high education attainment, firearms ban and strict anti-drug policies. However, there are still individuals who choose suicide to resolve their problems. Up to 70% of suicide completers had a mental disorder prior to suicide. About 30% of completed suicides have a past history of suicide attempts. Repeat suicide attempt rates are high: 16% at 1 year and 23% at over 4 years.

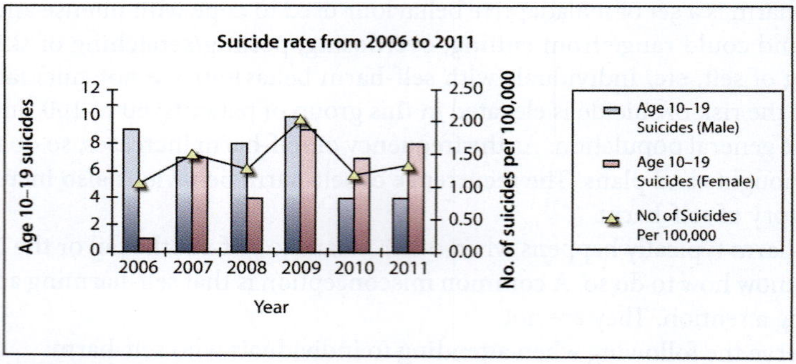

Source: IMH, 2012.

Figure 21.1 Suicide rate from 2006 to 2011.

Suicide Risk Assessment

The major risk factors for suicide amongst adolescents (adapted from Cash and Bridge [2009]) are as follows:

- Previous suicide attempt
- Psychopathology
  - » Especially major depressive disorder, bipolar disorder, conduct disorder and substance use disorders
  - » Psychiatric co-morbidity, especially the combination of mood, disruptive and substance use disorders

- » Dysfunctional personality traits (especially antisocial, borderline, histrionic and narcissistic traits)
  - » Feelings of hopelessness and worthlessness
  - » Impulsive aggression: The tendency to react to frustration or provocation with hostility or aggression
- Family factors
  - » A family history of depression or suicide
  - » Loss of a parent through death or divorce
  - » Family discord
- Physical and sexual abuse
- Lack of a support network, poor relationships with peers and feelings of social isolation
- Suicidal intention (in terms of motivation and planning such as writing suicide note, last acts, attempts to conceal suicide)
- Availability of lethal means and lethality of method used
- Lack of relief after being saved
- Having been exposed to suicide (e.g., suicide or suicide attempt in family members or friends; media reporting)
- Gender (males age 15–19 years) and ethnicity (Indians and Chinese)

It has been shown that psychiatrists are no better than general physicians in predicting suicide. Hence, possessing the necessary knowledge and skills in performing an adequate suicide risk assessment is extremely helpful in guiding your management of the suicidal patient.

Management of Inpatient Suicidal Patients

- Commence on a Monitoring/Observation Record Chart
- Hourly observation on:
  - » Whereabouts of patient
  - » What is patient doing
- Referral to Child Psychiatrist on duty
- Nurse in a bed visible to nurses and nearest to nurses' station
- Curtains open at all times
- Remove hand-rub from the foot of bed
- Accompany to toilet/bathroom by nurses/parents/caregivers
- Not allowed out of the ward unless accompanied by the parents/ caregivers
- Upon consulting the Child Psychiatrist on duty and if the decision is to transfer to tertiary psychiatry hospital (adolescent still at high risk for suicide but otherwise medically stable), ward team to initiate referral
- Remove suicide precaution if the adolescent is no longer at high suicide risk and upon instruction by the reviewing child psychiatrist

Table 21.2 Management of Suicidal Patients at Children's Emergency in Our Institution

Patient's Condition	Office Hours	After Office Hours
• Suicidal patients » Who are **cleared** of medical concerns, e.g. non-toxic overdoses, minor lacerations (not requiring T&S or post T&S), OR » Who have only psychiatric symptoms without medical issues.	• Call the Child Psychiatrist on-call and discuss a management plan. » Low suicide risk → child psychiatrist may recommend: ▪ An early follow-up appointment at the child psychiatry outpatient clinic. ▪ Parents must be willing to ensure close supervision, accept responsibility for safety and for bringing the child for follow up. ▪ Referral to MSW to follow up on case as well » High suicide risk→ child psychiatrist may recommend referral to an A&E in a tertiary psychiatry hospital (via ambulance). ▪ Inform A&E in the tertiary psychiatry hospital.	• Low suicide risk → referral to child psychiatry outpatient clinic can be done. Referral to MSW to follow-up on case as well. Parents must still ensure close supervision, accept responsibility for safety and for bringing the child for follow-up. • High suicide risk or risk assessment is uncertain → patient should be referred to an A&E in a tertiary psychiatry hospital for suicide assessment. The need for admission is dependent on the on-site assessment. » If highly suicidal, the patient should be sent in an ambulance (some parents may not be able to bring patient to the tertiary psychiatry hospital or are ambivalent about such as referral, both of which may cause unnecessary delay). ▪ Inform the tertiary psychiatry hospital about the transfer to the A&E for assessment. » If parents refuse to go, consult Child Psychiatrist on-call, who would then be able to advise on patient's management. ▪ The case manager should be informed by Children's Emergency the next working day so that he/she can follow up with clinic appointment booking and other necessary arrangements, if any.
• Suicidal patients » With medical/surgical concerns, e.g. toxic ingestions, surgical wounds requiring operative exploration/repair OR » Unable to rule out organic pathologies, i.e. requiring inpatient monitoring and management.	• Resuscitate and stabilise as necessary. • Admit with suicide precautions (see below) *Please highlight this in the admission notes and inform the admission and nursing staff to allow the necessary bed and staffing requirements to be prepared.*	

Bibliography

1. Chia BL. (1999) *Too Young to Die — An Asian Perspective on Youth Suicide.* Madurai: Times Book International.
2. Spirito A, Esposito-Smythers C. (2006) Attempted and completed suicide in adolescence. *Ann Rev Clin Psychol* **2**:237–266.
3. Owens D, Horrocks J, House A. (2002) Fatal and non-fatal repetition of self-harm. Systematic review. *Br J Psychiatry* **181**:193–199.
4. Cash SJ, Bridge JA. (2009) Epidemiology of youth suicide and suicidal behaviour. *Curr Opin Pediatry* **21**(45):613–619.

CHAPTER 103

Mental Health

Vicknesan Jeyan Marimuttu; Roselyne Shirley Pat Fong; Poon Ngar Yee; Hong Ling Feng; Paulette Reyes Po; Loh Hong Yan, Abigail

Anxiety Disorder

Introduction

Anxiety disorders are one of the most common psychiatric disorders in children and adolescents, but they often go undetected or untreated.

It is normal for children and adolescents to feel worried from time to time. However, it is considered a disorder when the individual's feelings of nervousness and anxiousness become excessive and persistent to the extent that they begin to interfere with their school, home or social life.

The prevalence of any anxiety disorder in youth ranges from 2 to 4%, with 6–12 months' estimates between 10% and 20%, and lifetime estimates being only slightly higher.

Presentation

The impact of anxiety symptoms in young children may be clinically significant, even if the full criteria are not met. These symptoms of anxiety can be in the form of thoughts, physical sensations or behaviours. Some examples include:

- Physical sensations
  - » Headache or giddiness
  - » Nausea or complaining of tummy aches
  - » Racing heart beat
  - » Chest tightness and feeling breathless
  - » Sweating more than usual
  - » Urgency and frequency of using toilet
- Behaviour associated with anxiety
  - » Being clingy
  - » Repeatedly asking parents and friends for reassurance
  - » Frequent crying
  - » Increase irritability or being out of control during outburst
  - » Going to great lengths to avoid what they perceive to be anxiety-provoking situations, e.g. school refusal due to bullying issues
  - » Insomnia or waking up with nightmares
  - » Poor appetite

- Anxious thoughts
  - » Finding it hard to concentrate on tasks
  - » Repeatedly worrying about the same problem

Treatment

The type of treatment offered will be dependent on the child's age and the cause of their anxiety.

- **Non-pharmacological treatment**

  Evidence-based psychological interventions can be effective treatments for anxiety disorder. They are recommended as the first-line treatment in preference to pharmacological treatment.
  - » Counselling: This can help the child understand what the cause of their anxiety is and allow them to work though the situation.
  - » Therapy: There are various type of therapy depending on the child's age and presentation. These include Behavioural Therapy, Cognitive Behavioural Therapy (CBT), Art Therapy, Sand Tray and Symbol Play Therapy. CBT is a talking therapy that is often used for older groups of children. This form of therapy can help the child to manage their anxiety by changing the way they think and behave.
- **Pharmacological treatment**

  Pharmacological interventions are usually not offered as first-line treatment for children and youth who suffer from anxiety disorders. Medications are reserved for situations where evidence-based therapy (e.g. CBT) alone is not adequate to reach the desired outcome or in situations where therapy is not a feasible option.
  - » The following factors must be taken into account:
    - ▪ The age of the patient
    - ▪ Risk: The likeliness of accidental overdose or deliberate self-harm using medications
    - ▪ Tolerability or side effects reported
    - ▪ Interaction with other medication used by the patient
    - ▪ Preference of the patient
    - ▪ Costs
  - » **Antidepressants** should be the only pharmacological intervention used for longer term management of anxiety disorders.
    - ▪ Selective Serotonin Reuptake Inhibitors (SSRIs) are the medication of choice for the treatment of anxiety disorders in children and adolescents. Studies support that SSRI such as fluoxetine and sertraline have proven efficacy in the management of anxiety disorders.
    - ▪ Serotonin-Norepinephrine Reuptake Inhibitors (SNRIs), e.g. venlafaxine and duloxetine have also been approved by the FDA for treatment of paediatric generalised anxiety disorder. This class of medication is generally less well tolerated compared to SSRIs. Nevertheless, this class of medication can be considered as a third-line

treatment for anxiety disorder when two consecutive trials with different SSRIs prove to be ineffective.
- Important note: Treatment with SSRIs and SNRIs appear to be associated with an increase in suicidal ideation and self-harm in a minority of people under the age of 30. It is therefore vital to monitor the risk of suicidal ideation and self-harm closely, especially in the first month after starting medication or after any increase in dosage.
- People starting on antidepressants should also be informed about the delayed onset of effect, the time course of the treatment and possible discontinuation/withdrawal symptoms.

» Other Medications
- Hydroxyzine is an antihistamine that has been used for patients presenting with milder anxiety symptoms.
- Propranolol is a beta-blocker drug used to slow the heart rate and reduce blood pressure. It can help with physical sensations of anxiety such as palpitation and tremors. However, it may not be suitable for patients who suffer from asthma or low blood pressure.
- Benzodiazepines (BDZ): This category of medication is not supported by controlled trials in children and may lead to paradoxical disinhibition in some. Nevertheless, it may be considered in certain clinical situations. Important note: BDZ are only recommended for short-term usage and to be used only when necessary, as prolonged use may result in dependency.

Practical Tips to Help Parents and their Child in Dealing with Anxiety

- Teach the child or parents to recognise signs of anxiety
- Encourage the child to manage their anxiety and to ask for help when needed
- Many children find routines reassuring; when possible, try to stick to a regular daily routine, which makes the child feel more in control and that life is being more predictable.
- Create a 'worry box' using an empty tissue box. Get the child to write or draw about their worries and put them into the box.
- Relaxation breathing technique — improper breathing technique may lead to an imbalance of oxygen and carbon dioxide level in the body, which can contribute to anxiety attacks. Simple relaxation techniques such as taking in a slow deep breath for a count of 3, holding it for another count of 3 and breathing out for the count of 3, and repeating the whole thing 3 times.
- Apps: Headspace, Clear Fear, Calm
- Progressive muscle relaxation exercise
  - » Step 1: Lie down or sit in a comfortable position
  - » Step 2: Gently close your eyes (can keep them open if the child prefers)
  - » Step 3: Take in a slow deep breath

» Step 4: With the rest of the body relaxed, clench the fists (tightening muscle) for a few seconds, and then relax (loosening the muscle). Repeat this for two times.
» Step 5: Repeat Step 4 with the other parts of the muscles in our body. From the top of the head to the tips of the toes.

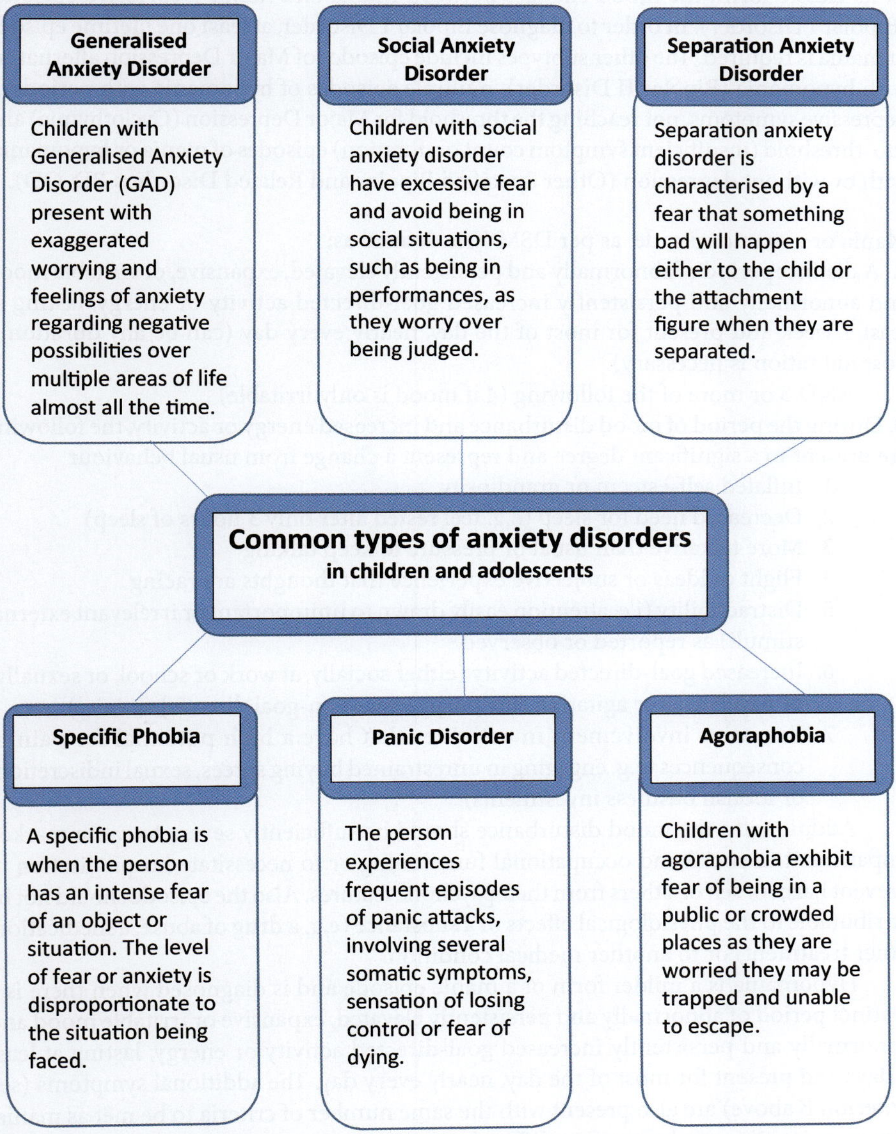

Figure 21.2 Common type of anxiety disorders in children and adolescents.

Bipolar Disorder

Introduction, Definition and Subtypes

Bipolar Disorder is a mood disorder that is characterised by cyclic changes in mood. In its classic form, the mood changes between Mania and Major Depressive episodes (Bipolar I Disorder). In order to diagnose Bipolar I Disorder, at least one lifetime episode of mania is required. The other subtypes include episodes of Major Depression alternating with hypomania (Bipolar II Disorder), multiple episodes of hypomania with periods of depressive symptoms, not reaching the threshold for Major Depression (Cyclothymia) and sub-threshold (insufficient symptom count or duration) episodes of mania or hypomania, with or without depression (Other Specified Bipolar and Related Disorders BD-OD).

Mania or a manic episode, as per DSM V, is defined as;
A. A distinct period of abnormally and persistently elevated, expansive, or irritable mood and abnormally and persistently increased goal-directed activity or energy, lasting at least 1 week and present for most of the day, nearly every day (can be any duration if hospitalisation is necessary).

AND 3 or more of the following (4 if mood is only irritable)

B. During the period of mood disturbance and increased energy or activity, the following are present to a significant degree and represent a change from usual behaviour

1. Inflated self-esteem or grandiosity
2. Decreased need for sleep (e.g. feel rested after only 3 hours of sleep)
3. More talkative than usual or pressure to keep talking
4. Flight of ideas or subjective experience that thoughts are racing
5. Distractibility (i.e. attention easily drawn to unimportant or irrelevant external stimuli) as reported or observed
6. Increased goal-directed activity (either socially, at work or school, or sexually) or psychomotor agitation (i.e. purposeless non-goal directed activity)
7. Excessive involvement in activities that have a high potential for painful consequences (e.g. engaging in unrestrained buying sprees, sexual indiscretions or foolish business investments)

Additionally, the mood disturbance should be sufficiently severe to cause marked impairment in social and occupational functioning or to necessitate hospitalisation to prevent harm of self or others from their psychotic features. Also the episode should not be attributable to the physiological effects of a substance (e.g. a drug of abuse, a medication, other treatment) or to another medical condition.

Hypomania is a milder form of a manic episode and is diagnosed when there is a distinct period of abnormally and persistently elevated, expansive or irritable mood and abnormally and persistently increased goal-directed activity or energy, lasting at least 4 days and present for most of the day, nearly every day. The additional symptoms (see criterion B above) are also present with the same number of criteria to be met as mania. However, importantly, hypomania differs from mania, in that the symptoms are not severe enough to cause marked impairment to social and occupational functioning. There also should not be a necessity for hospitalisation.

Epidemiology and Aetiology

A meta-analysis about the epidemiology of Bipolar Disorder in youth around the world reported that the overall rate was 1.8% (Van Meter *et al.*, 2011). If sub-threshold symptoms are included, prevalence rates are between 5.7 and 13.3%. Bipolar Disorder can have its onset in childhood, but its prevalence is much higher during adolescence. Similar to adults, studies in clinical populations suggest that the rates of bipolar spectrum disorders in youth are equally common in males and females.

Bipolar Disorder is highly heritable, with twin and family studies showing a concordance rate of 70% amongst identical twins. Multiple susceptibility genes are likely to be involved but have not have been fully elucidated. Stress and traumatic experiences can trigger an episode of Bipolar Disorder but episodes can also arise without any trigger.

Presentation

Children and adolescents with Bipolar Disorder can show a continuum of symptoms from sub-syndromal to full syndromal, with more frequent mood episodes as well mixed mood symptoms (when compared to adults). A sub-syndromal presentation can manifest with an insufficient symptom count (as per above criteria) or insufficient duration of symptoms. Hence, initial presentation in youth may not fulfil diagnosis for a Bipolar I or II disorder but may be classified as Other Specified Bipolar and Related Disorders (BD-OD) or a Bipolar Spectrum disorder. The most common presentation in youth is a sub-syndromal presentation. Retrospective studies in adults with Bipolar Disorder have reported that 10–20% had the onset before 10 years of age and up to 60% before the age of 20. As such, Bipolar Disorder often initially presents before adulthood with possible sub-threshold symptoms that can make diagnosis challenging. Untreated Bipolar Disorder in youth is associated with poor academic performance, impaired family and peer relationships, chronic mood symptoms, disruptive behaviour disorders, anxiety disorders, substance misuse disorders, hospitalisation, suicide attempts and completed suicides. Approximately 50% of youth with sub-syndromal presentation convert into Bipolar I Disorder or Bipolar II disorder later on in life (Axelson *et al.*, 2011).

Diagnosis and Treatment

Refer patients with suspected Bipolar Disorder to see a Child and Adolescent Psychiatrist.

Psychoeducation is important to help the young person and family understand the cause, varying symptoms, course of the illness, treatments and the consequences on different areas of life if untreated.

In terms of pharmacotherapy, the main aim is to stabilise the mood and prevent relapses. Second-generation atypical antipsychotics, sodium valproate, lamotrigine and lithium have been found to be efficacious. Antidepressants, like the SSRIs, should be used with caution in depressive episodes within a Bipolar Disorder as they may precipitate a manic episode.

In terms of psychosocial treatments, individual psychotherapy can be helpful to enhance insight into the disorder, sleep hygiene (poor sleep can trigger a relapse), problem-solving skills and self-care. Working with the family to enhance their understanding of the illness as well as any communication difficulties can also be beneficial. Liaison with schools can help adjust academic expectations, provide additional academic and pastoral support.

Conclusion

In conclusion, Bipolar Disorder in children and adolescents can present with sub-threshold symptoms with more frequent mood episodes compared to adults. Such presentations can be highly impactful, both in terms of the experience of the mood symptoms and how they affect daily function, academic performance, family and peer relationships.

Depression

Introduction

Depression is a mood disorder with core symptoms consisting of pervasive and persistent sadness, loss of interest and enjoyment. In children and adolescents, irritability may also be a core symptom. Other associated symptoms include decreased concentration, sleep disturbance, change of appetite or weight, excessive fatigue, excessive guilt, increased tiredness, psychomotor agitation or retardation, thoughts or acts of self-harm, suicidal thoughts or behaviours. Both ICD-10 and DSM-V require that symptoms be present for more than 2 weeks and have significant impact on functioning.

Depression can be categorised into severity depending on the symptoms and level of impairment in functioning. Subtypes include Major Depressive Disorder being the commonest, Dysthymia, which is a chronic milder depression lasting over a year, and psychotic depression, which is rare before mid-adolescence and is a more severe form of depression with psychotic symptoms. However, even milder forms of depression in adolescence are a risk factor for depression in adulthood.

In childhood, prevalence in various studies reported between 0.5 and 2.5% with an equal male to female ratio, whereas in adolescence, prevalence increases to between 2 and 8% with a female to male ratio of 2 to 1.

Aetiology

- Predisposing factors
  - » Genetic: Increased risk when there is a family history of depression or bipolar mood disorder
  - » Gender: Equal risk for males or females before puberty, subsequently, increased risk in females
  - » Temperament: Child's cognitive or behavioural style, e.g. tendency to blame self
- Precipitating Factors
  - » Environmental: Stressful life events, including parental ill health and/or family conflict, bullying, physical, emotional and/or sexual abuse
- Perpetuating Factors
  - » Ongoing stressors
  - » Delay in seeking help due to lack of understanding, stigma, etc.
  - » Comorbid disorders, e.g. anxiety or conduct disorder, substance abuse

Assessment

- Parental Interview
  - » Enquiry about presenting concerns, presence of symptoms of depression, premorbid functioning, assess any impairment of functioning (deterioration in academic results, social withdrawal, etc.), risk assessment (enquiry about deliberate self-harm, suicidal ideation or behaviour)
  - » Presence of physical symptoms to suggest underlying organic illness
  - » Any medication prescribed that may be impacting on mood
  - » Ask about behavioural changes or reported symptoms to suggest presence of mood swings, psychotic symptoms or other comorbid psychiatric disorder
  - » Family history, including psychiatric illness such as depression or bipolar disorder
  - » Family functioning, stressors
  - » History of abuse or neglect
  - » Somatic symptoms: Loss of appetite, sleep disturbance, decreased energy, headaches, chest or abdominal pain
- Separate interview with the child or adolescent
  - » Confirm information obtained from parental interview
  - » Elicit any relevant information that the child may not be comfortable discussing in front of parents, any history of abuse or neglect, alcohol or substance misuse
  - » Assess mental state, ask about self-harm and suicidal ideation, presence of psychotic symptoms
- Information from school
  - » Past and current functioning, academically and socially
- General physical examination
  - » Assess if reporting symptoms suggestive of a physical illness as well as to exclude a physical cause of depression
- Differential diagnosis
  - » Organic illness, Bipolar Mood Disorder, Psychosis, Eating Disorder
- Comorbidity
  - » Anxiety Disorder, Conduct Disorder, Psychosis, Obsessive-compulsive Disorder, Drug and alcohol abuse
- Investigations
  - » Baseline blood investigations: Full blood count (FBC), renal and liver profile, thyroid function test

Treatment

Biopsychosocial interventions include healthy diet and excercise.

Psychological: Mild depression may improve with psychoeducation and supportive counselling as well as addressing any environmental stressors, including those within the family or in school.

With at least moderate or more severe depression, presence of active suicidal intent or severe self-harm should give rise to consideration of whether inpatient psychiatric care is required for crisis intervention. If inpatient admission is not deemed necessary, referral for individual cognitive behavioural or interpersonal therapy is recommended. Medication may also be prescribed concomitantly specially in moderate to severe depression.

Pharmacological: Antidepressants should ideally be used alongside psychological therapy. SSRIs such as fluoxetine and escitalopram are usually prescribed after psychoeducation about the fact that medication takes two to four weeks to take effect. Side effects to look out for include nausea, headache, abdominal pain, insomnia, increased agitation and rarely worsening of suicidal ideation. The risk of suicidal ideation is far outweighed by the benefit conferred by treatment with antidepressants. Nevertheless, a careful discussion about safety and contingency planning is done with the teenager and carers prior to starting on antidepressant medication.

A review appointment will usually be offered within a month to monitor for side effects. If pharmacological treatment is effective, it is usually continued for at least 6 months to a year after symptoms have remitted and normal functioning is achieved. Subsequently, a joint decision is ideally made by the young person and parent in agreement with the psychiatrist about an appropriate time to gradually reduce and stop the medication.

Schizophrenia Spectrum and Other Psychotic Disorders

Introduction

Psychosis is a mental illness characterised by positive and negative symptoms that affects an individual's functioning. Psychosis in the younger population is associated with more severe symptomatology and poorer functioning. Early detection and treatment can help with overall prognosis. Treatment entails biological, psychological and social components.

Epidemiology

The worldwide prevalence of early-onset psychosis (defined as onset before 18 years old) has been estimated at 0.5% of the population across epidemiologic studies, and that of childhood-onset (defined as onset before 13 years old), psychosis is even lower, at about 1 in 10000.

Pathogenesis

Neurochemical abnormality hypothesis is characterised by imbalances of various neurotransmitters, most commonly that of dopamine and, hence, the use of antidopaminergic agents to treat psychosis. Other neurotransmitters, which are postulated to be involved include glutamate, serotonin and GABA. Genetic vulnerability, environmental factors, obstetric complications, trauma, social adversities and substance use are other factors that may contribute to the risk of acquiring a psychotic illness.

Symptoms

Diagnosis of schizophrenia is made based on the DSM-V classification and is characterised by at least two of the following symptoms, with at least one being (1), (2) or (3) present during a one-month period:

1. Delusions (which are defined as firmly held false belief that is in contrary to that of the wider community)
2. Hallucinations (which can happen in any of the five sensory modalities but more commonly auditory and visual)
3. Disorganised speech
4. Grossly disorganised or catatonic behaviour
5. Negative symptoms (which are defined as diminished emotional expressions)

There also needs to be disruption of functioning in various aspects such as work, education or self-care for at least a significant portion of a 6-month period and it is below what was previously achieved.

Differential Diagnoses

Other diagnoses to consider when a child presents with the above symptoms may include the following:

- Medical diseases that may present with psychotic symptomatology
  - » Seizure disorder
  - » Encephalitis
  - » Central nervous system tumour
  - » Chromosomal abnormalities (e.g. 22q11.2 deletion syndromes)
  - » Substance or medication induced
  - » Autoimmune disorder, e.g. systemic lupus erythematosus
  - » Metabolic disorder
- Delirium
  - » Characterised by waxing and waning symptoms associated with evidence of substance ingestion, metabolic derangement, etc.
- Non-psychotic children
  - » Pseudo-psychotic symptoms such as delusional thinking, hallucinations and looseness of association may occur in healthy non-psychotic children, especially before age 6. History, including decline in cognitive functioning, attention and presence of negative symptoms, would be more indicative of psychosis.
- Post-traumatic stress disorder
  - » Symptoms of hypervigilance and flashback may be misinterpreted as paranoia and hallucinations.
- Autism spectrum disorder (ASD)
  - » Impairment of social communication, which occurs in ASD may be misinterpreted as negative symptoms. Understanding the developmental history and baseline thought processes would be useful to distinguish between the two.
- Mood disorders
  - » Careful history looking at mood episodes would be useful.

Assessment

A thorough medical history and physical examination is important in the assessment of all patients presenting with psychotic symptoms.

- Systematic features to screen for:
  - Neurological: Headache, recent head injury, abnormal movements and/or coordination, hearing or visual impairment, fits or fainting, altered consciousness.
  - Respiratory: Dyspnoea
  - Cardiovascular: Chest pain, palpitations
  - Gastrointestinal: Nausea, vomiting
  - Genitourinary: Urinary symptoms, menstrual history for females
- A good mental state examination and history will help elicit pertinent features.
  - Psychotic symptoms
    - Hallucinations: Nature/description, modality, timing and frequency, intensity and impact of the experiences
    - Beliefs: Odd or bizarre beliefs, paranoid or persecutory content; determine intensity of beliefs (fleeting thoughts vs. overvalued ideas vs. delusional intensity)
    - Other phenomena: Control or passivity phenomenon (motor, volition, thought insertion/broadcast)
  - Mood screening, including anxiety symptoms
  - Other functional aspects
    - Sleep disruptions
    - Appetite changes
    - Daily self-care and activities (e.g. going to school)
    - Orientation
    - Attention and concentration
    - Screen for cognitive function and memory problems (this would be more suggestive of organic disease)
- Physical examination
  - A full physical examination is essential in the initial work-up.
  - This includes a neurological examination, particularly for:
    - Gait changes
    - Motor and sensory deficits
    - Coordination issues (e.g. hand–eye coordination)
- Investigations
  - Investigations will further aid in diagnosis and management of patients presenting with psychosis.
  - Blood tests
    - Routine — FBC, renal panel and electrolytes (including calcium), liver function test, thyroid function test, glucose.
    - Autoimmune panel, if psychotic symptoms are accompanied by neurological signs, antecedent systemic symptoms and/or other suspicions of autoimmunity

        - Consider if indicated — parathyroid hormone, tumour markers, 24-hr cortisol/catecholamines
    - » Urinary tests
        - Microscopy and culture, if screening for infection
        - Drug screen (if suspicious for substance use, particularly stimulants and cannabis)
    - » Radiological/Procedural
        - CT or MRI Brain
        - CXR, when there is suspicion of comorbid respiratory/cardiovascular issues
        - EEG if indicated (Temporal Lobe Epilepsy, in particular, has associations with psychosis)

Treatment

Initial treatment is largely determined by risk assessment. Risks include:

- The risk they currently pose to themselves — self harm, reputational, impact on family and peer relationships, school going, forensic/police involvement
- Risk of violence — the nature of risk and any association with current
- Degree of insight retained
- Whether transfer to a psychiatric ward is warranted to assess and manage the acute symptoms (with or without use of the Mental Health Care and Treatment Act [MHCT])
- Also consider the child's current social circumstances and the level of support available to them, including the need for rehabilitation or re-socialisation arrangements

If starting treatment inpatient

- First line includes use of second-generation antipsychotic (SGA), e.g. olanzapine, risperidone, quetiapine at an effective dose
- Use long-acting BDZ, e.g. diazepam to control anxiety/behavioural disturbance
- Other options: Low-potency first-generation antipsychotic (FGA), depot injections (rare)

Provide information and discuss the benefits vs. possible side effects of each drug, including:

- Metabolic (including weight gain and diabetes)
- Extra-pyramidal (including akathisia, dyskinesia and dystonia)
- Cardiovascular (including prolonged QT interval)
- Hormonal (including increasing prolactin levels)
- Other (including unpleasant subjective experiences)

Consideration to treat other symptoms such as mood or anxiety with antidepressants or anxiolytics.

Bibliography

1. Axelson DA, Birmaher B, Strober MA, *et al.* (2011) Course of subthreshold bipolar disorder in youth: Diagnostic progression from bipolar disorder not otherwise specified. *J Am Acad Child Adolesc Psychiatry* **50**(10):1001–1016.e3.
2. Van Meter AR, Moreira AL, Youngstrom EA. (2011) Meta-analysis of epidemiologic studies of pediatric bipolar disorder. *J Clin Psychiatry* **72**(9):1250–1256.
3. Maughan B, Collishaw S, Stringaris A. (2013) Depression in childhood and adolescence. *J Can Acad Child Adolesc Psychiatry* **22**(1):35–39.
4. Thapar A, Pine DS, Leckman JF, *et al.* (2015) *Rutter's Child and Adolescent Psychiatry Textbook, 6th ed.* Wiley-Blackwell.
5. Najjar S, Steiner J, Najjar A, *et al.* (2018) A clinical approach to new-onset psychosis associated with immune dysregulation: The concept of autoimmune psychosis. *J Neuroinflammation* **15**(1):40.
6. Semple D, Smyth R. (2019) *Oxford Handbook of Psychiatry, 4th ed.* Oxford: OUP Oxford.
7. Skehan B, Dvir Y. (2021) Schizophrenia in children and adolescents: Epidemiology, pathogenesis, clinical manifestations, course, assessment, and diagnosis. *UpToDate.* https://www.uptodate.com/contents/schizophrenia-in-children-adolescents-epidemiology-pathogenesis-clinical-manifestations-course-assess[]ment-and-diagnosis

SECTION 22

RESPIRATORY

CHAPTER 104

Chronic Cough

Biju Thomas

Introduction

Cough is one of the commonest symptoms with which children present for medical attention. Up to 10% of preschool and primary school children may have chronic cough without wheeze at some point in time.

Definition

Acute cough due to common infective causes usually resolve by 3–4 weeks. Occasionally, post infective cough may last longer (3–8 weeks) as in the case of pertussis or **post-viral cough**. Young children may get recurrent viral respiratory tract infections (up to 6–8 episodes per year) causing **recurrent cough,** and this may be confused with chronic cough, if the symptom-free intervals between episodes are short. Although **chronic cough** may be defined as a cough lasting longer than 4 weeks, a definition using a duration of more than 8 weeks may be more appropriate in identifying children with chronic cough that may require further investigations. Chronic cough may be classified into **specific cough** (in which there is an identifiable cause) and **non-specific cough** (persistent isolated dry cough in otherwise well children with no signs of respiratory disease and normal investigations).

Evaluation

The differential diagnoses for chronic cough in children is wide-ranging. The diagnosis depends on meticulous and accurate history-taking and targeted investigations based on specific pointers in the history. A **detailed history** addressing the following questions should be undertaken.

- How and when did the cough start?
- What is the nature (e.g. brassy, croupy, barking, paroxysmal, staccato, bizarre and honking) and quality (dry or wet) of the cough?
- Is the cough an isolated symptom? If not, what are the associated symptoms?
- Are there any obvious triggers (e.g. exercise, feeding) or diurnal variation?
- Is there a family history of respiratory symptoms, disorders or atopy (asthma, allergic rhinitis, eczema)?
- Is there any contact history with tuberculosis (TB) or other infectious diseases?

- Is the child on any long-term or regular medication, what treatment has the child had for the cough and what effect have they had on the cough frequency and severity?
- Is there exposure to tobacco smoke?
- Does the cough cease when asleep or when distracted?

Physical examination: Children with chronic cough should have a thorough physical examination that includes an assessment of growth (weight, height, body mass index), ENT and respiratory examination. A normal physical examination DOES NOT rule out significant pathology. Certain features in the history or examination raise suspicion of serious underlying respiratory disease, and these are listed in Table 22.1.

Table 22.2 lists the causes of chronic cough in children in relation to pointers in the history suggestive of specific aetiology and suggested investigations. A simplified algorithm for the assessment and management of the common causes of chronic cough is given in Figure 22.1.

Management of chronic-specific cough depends on the underlying aetiology. Detailed description of the assessment and management of various causes of chronic-specific cough is beyond the scope of this chapter.

Table 22.1 Features in History/Examination that Suggest Serious Underlying Respiratory Disease in Children with Chronic Cough

- Neonatal onset of cough
- Chronic wet (productive) cough
- Haemoptysis
- Cough started and persisting after a choking episode
- Cough that occurs during or immediately after feeding
- Feeding difficulties or known swallowing dysfunction
- History of contact with tuberculosis
- Underlying neuromuscular disease
- Underlying cardiac abnormalities
- Accompanying features suspicious of immune deficiency, e.g. persistent oral thrush, skin fungal infection, chronic diarrhoea, family history of primary immunodeficiency
- Recurrent pneumonia or other significant infections, e.g. ear, sinus, deep skin, organ or bloodstream
- Failure to thrive
- Digital clubbing
- Abnormal chest shape
- Abnormal respiratory examination findings

Table 22.2 Differential Diagnoses of Chronic-Specific Cough in Children

Diagnoses	Pointers in History	Physical Findings	Suggested Investigations
Asthma/wheezing disorders	Recurrent episodes of cough, wheezing and shortness of breath. Cough/symptoms may be exercise-induced. Response to bronchodilators. History of atopic diseases such as eczema or allergic rhinitis and family history of atopy.	Usually normal. Wheeze may be heard with exacerbations. Other features include chest hyperinflation and signs of eczema/allergic rhinitis.	Usually none Spirometry (children $\geq$ 5 yr old) may show bronchodilator reversibility Consider skin prick test for environmental allergens.
Allergic rhinitis/rhinosinusitis	Chronic nasal congestion, blockage, sneezing, nasal irritation. History of atopic diseases such as eczema or asthma and family history of atopy.	Allergic shiners, allergic salute, inflamed and hypertrophied nasal turbinates.	Usually none Consider skin prick test for environmental allergens.
Protracted bacterial bronchitis	Chronic 'wet' cough Otherwise well child History of preceding viral respiratory infection may be present.	'Ruttles' (coarse large airway noises on auscultation suggesting excessive airway secretions) — parents may describe this as they can 'feel the phlegm in the chest' when they put their hand on the child's chest.	CXR usually normal, may show perihilar infiltrates and/or peribronchial cuffing. Cough swab/sputum culture
Infections Pertussis Pertussis like - Parapertussis, Adenovirus, Mycoplasma, Chlamydia Tuberculosis	History suggestive of recent infection. Paroxysmal cough (± whoop) Staccato cough: Chlamydia in infants Tuberculosis: History of contact, may be associated with recurrent fever, loss of weight and/or night sweats	Usually non-specific. Children with TB may have failure to thrive, lymphadenopathy.	CXR If TB is suspected, consider Mantoux test, Quantiferon/T-spot TB test, gastric aspirate for AFB smear/TB culture, sputum culture (if the child can expectorate) for AFB smear/TB culture
Chronic suppurative lung disease a. Immune deficiencies b. Recurrent aspiration c. Bronchiectasis d. Retained inhaled foreign body	a. History of recurrent pneumonias, particularly if confirmed radiologically. b. History suggestive of gastroesophageal reflux disease, history of coughing on feeding (consider structural lesions	Variable, depending on the underlying problem. Clubbing, failure to thrive, abnormal chest shape and abnormal respiratory examination findings.	a. Immunology work up: FBC, IgG, IgA, IgM, IgE, antibodies to tetanus, Hib & pneumococci, lymphocyte subset analysis. b. pH/impedance study, if gastroesophageal reflux is suspected. Other investigations, such

e. Primary ciliary dyskinesia [PCD] — Rare f. Cystic fibrosis [CF] — Rare	such as tracheo-esophageal fistula, laryngeal cleft), swallowing dysfunction, neuromuscular disease c. Chronic 'wet' cough, haemoptysis d. History suggestive of foreign body inhalation e. Chronic rhinosinusitis, recurrent ear infections, neonatal onset of cough f. Failure to thrive, recurrent chest infections, features of malabsorption, nasal polyps, history of meconium ileus, rectal prolapse	Up to 40–50% of patients with PCD may have dextrocardia ± situs inversus.	as milk isotope scan, upper GI contrast study and videofluoroscopy, may be considered as appropriate. c. Imaging: CXR ± HRCT chest. HRCT is the imaging of choice in suspected bronchiectasis, as CXR can be normal. Flexible bronchoscopy and bronchoalveolar lavage (BAL) for identification of microorganisms d. If foreign body is suspected, a rigid ± flexible bronchoscopy is recommended. e. PCD: Nasal brushing for PCD studies, genetic test for PCD mutations f. CF: Sweat test, CF genetic test, faecal elastase
Structural airway lesions a. Tracheobronchomalacia ± infection b. Airway compression, e.g. lymph node, vascular ring c. Tracheo-esophageal fistula, laryngeal cleft	a. Barking or brassy cough, cough may be associated with wheeze, cough may be wet if there is associated infection. b. Cough associated with abnormal respiratory noises — wheeze/stridor c. History of coughing/choking on feeding		a. Bronchoscopy, BAL b. If external compression of airway is suspected, CT ± CT angiogram may be required. c. Special imaging studies — such as upper GI contrast study or videofluoroscopy may be required.
Others Tobacco smoke exposure Increased cough receptor sensitivity Psychogenic cough Habit cough/vocal tics Non-asthmatic eosinophilic bronchitis Interstitial lung disease (ILD) Bronchiolitis Obliterans (BO) Side effects of medications, e.g. ACE inhibitors Otogenic causes, e.g. Arnold's ear-cough reflex Cardiac failure Cytotoxic drugs/radiation	History relates to the underlying condition/cause. Psychogenic cough: Bizarre honking cough, increases with attention and decreases when distracted/asleep, child exhibits a paradoxical absence of psychological distress despite having the disruptive coughing. Symptoms often improves with suggestion therapy.	Physical examination findings vary according to the underlying condition/cause. Normal examination in psychogenic/habit cough.	Investigations are guided by the clinical suspicion (e.g. CT chest in suspected BO, CT chest ± lung biopsy in suspected ILD). Spirometry in children ≥6 yr.

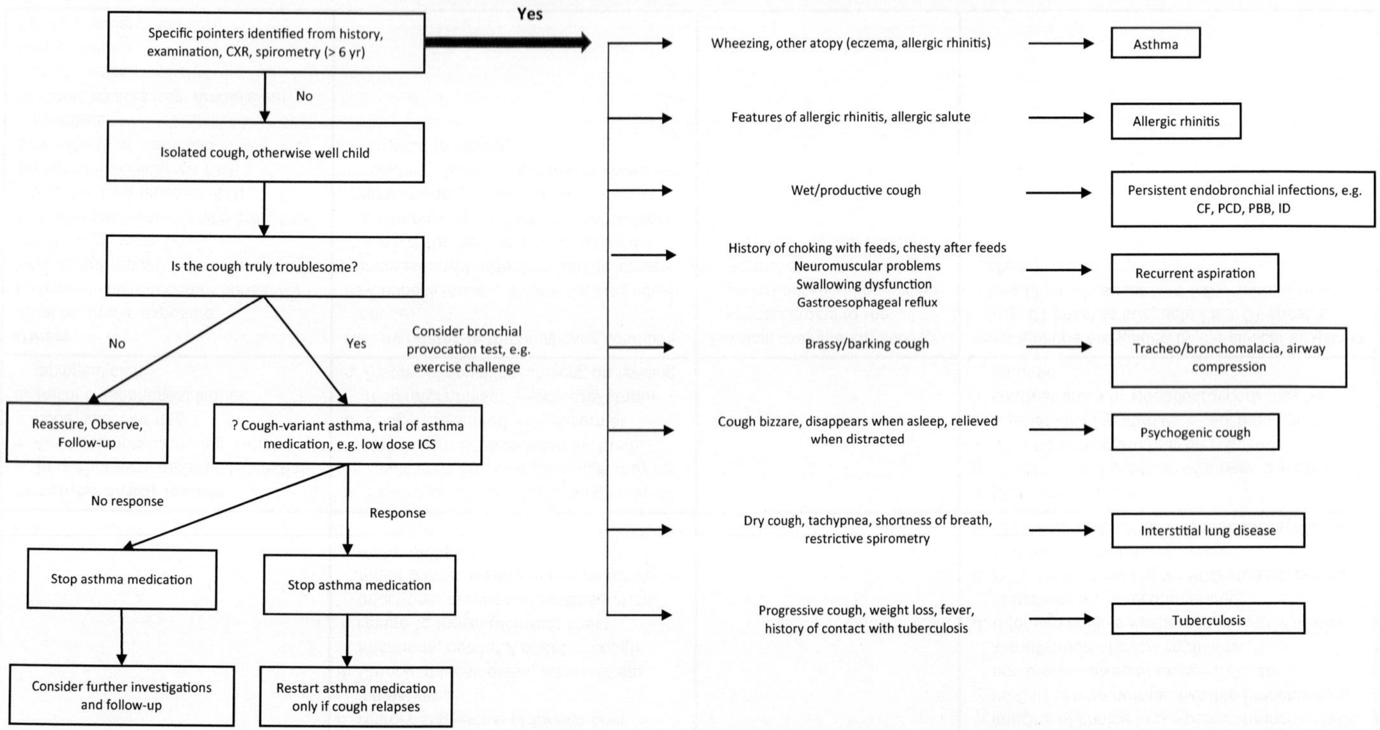

Figure 22.1 Simplified overview of assessment and management of the common causes of chronic cough (>8 weeks).

CF: cystic fibrosis; CXR: Chest X-ray; ICS: inhaled corticosteroids; PBB: protracted bacterial bronchitis; PCD: primary ciliary dyskinesia; ID: immunodeficiency.

Chronic Non-Specific Isolated Cough

This term denotes a chronic isolated dry cough that may be seen in a significant number of otherwise well children, with no signs/symptoms of underlying significant illness and normal investigations. The cause is usually not identifiable, though a small proportion of such children may have asthma. Some may have heightened cough receptor sensitivity (e.g. post-viral cough). If the cough is not troublesome, parental reassurance with a period of watchful observation with no diagnostic tests or treatment can be considered. These children need careful follow-up to ensure that their cough is resolved and no specific pointers have developed. Empirical anti-asthma, anti-allergic rhinitis or anti-gastroesophageal reflux therapies are unlikely of benefit and are generally not recommended. If a trial of empirical therapy is commenced, careful follow-up and assessment of response to therapy in a time-framed manner are warranted and the treatment should be stopped if the response is questionable.

Bibliography

1. Weinberger M, Fischer A. (2014) Differential diagnosis of chronic cough in children. *Allergy Asthma Proc* **35**(2):95–103.
2. Acosta R, Bahna SL. (2014) Chronic cough in children. *Pediatr Ann* **43**(8):e176–e183.
3. Gupta A, McKean M, Chang AB. (2007) Management of chronic non-specific cough in childhood: An evidence-based review. *Arch Dis Child Educ Pract Ed* **92**(2):33–39.
4. Chang AB, Glomb WB. (2006) Guidelines for evaluating chronic cough in pediatrics: ACCP evidence-based clinical practice guidelines. *Chest* **129**(1 Suppl):260S–283S.
5. Shields MD, Bush A, Everarad ML, *et al.* (2008) BTS guidelines: Recommendations for the assessment and management of cough in children. *Thorax* **63**(3):iii1–iii15.

CHAPTER 105

Asthma

Teoh Oon Hoe, Chay Oh Moh

Definition

- Heterogeneous disease characterised by chronic airway inflammation
- Characterised by a history of respiratory symptoms of wheeze, shortness of breath, chest tightness and cough that vary over time and in intensity, associated with variable expiratory airflow limitation

Diagnosis

- Often based on a thorough history and physical examination in young children
- Therapeutic response to bronchodilator and/or controller treatment or the presence of bronchodilator response on spirometry in older children may further help to establish the diagnosis
- Asthma should be considered in individuals with the following typical features, especially if there is positive family history of asthma or personal history of atopy:
  - » More than one symptom of wheeze, shortness of breath, cough or chest tightness
  - » Symptoms often worse at night or in the early morning
  - » Symptoms vary over time and in intensity
  - » Symptoms triggered by viral infections, exercise, allergens, weather changes, laughter, smoke or pollution
- For children below 5 years old, a probability-based approach to diagnosis is suggested by the Global Initiative for Asthma (GINA) guideline as episodic wheezing and cough are also common in young children without asthma, especially those below 2 years old. In children with the following symptom pattern, GINA suggests that most would have asthma:
  - » Personal history of atopy (allergic sensitisation, atopic dermatitis, food allergy) or family history of asthma
  - » More than three episodes of wheeze per year or severe episodes and/or night worsening
  - » Between episodes, child has cough, wheeze or heavy breathing during play or when laughing
  - » Symptoms (cough, wheeze, heavy breathing) for more than 10 days during upper respiratory tract infections

- For children who have atypical symptoms/signs or do not respond as expected to therapy, especially those below 1 year old, differential diagnoses need to be considered and excluded

Differential Diagnoses

- Recurrent viral wheeze
- Pulmonary tuberculosis
- Recurrent aspiration (e.g. gastroesophageal reflux, swallowing dysfunction)
- Chronic rhinitis/sinusitis
- Foreign body inhalation
- Chronic lung disease (e.g. bronchiectasis, interstitial lung disease, bronchopulmonary dysplasia)
- Airway structural abnormalities (e.g. tracheobronchomalacia, tracheobronchial stenosis)
- Airway compression/obstruction (e.g. mediastinal mass, vascular rings, bronchial tumours)
- Genetic disorders (e.g. cystic fibrosis, primary ciliary dyskinesia)
- Congenital or acquired immunodeficiency
- Cardiac conditions (e.g. heart failure, congenital heart disease)
- Vocal cord dysfunction, hyperventilation, dysfunctional breathing
- Pulmonary embolism, pulmonary arterial hypertension

History

- Personal history of atopy — allergic rhinitis, eczema, allergic conjunctivitis
- Family history of atopy — asthma, allergic rhinitis, eczema, allergic conjunctivitis
- Triggers (e.g. viral infections, house dust mites, animal dander, tobacco smoke, pollution, physical activity, stress)
- Exposure to environmental tobacco smoke, smoking history in adolescents
- Assessment of asthma control/severity
  - » Frequency and severity of exacerbations — use of written asthma action plan (WAAP), level of medical care attended
  - » Daytime and nocturnal asthma symptoms
  - » Physical activity-related asthma symptoms, activity limitation due to asthma
  - » Reliever medication use
  - » Questionnaire-based asthma control tests (e.g. Asthma Control Test, Asthma Control Questionnaire, Test for Respiratory and Asthma Control in Kids)
- Medications
  - » Understanding of asthma action plan, controller and reliever medications prescribed
  - » Adherence to controller medications
  - » Reasons for non-adherence (e.g. steroid phobia, child/parental over-estimation of asthma control, inconvenient medication regime)

    » Inhaler technique assessment
- Assess co-morbid conditions (e.g. allergic rhinitis, eczema, allergic conjunctivitis, obesity)
- 'Red flag' symptoms (e.g. chronic moist/productive cough, symptoms onset after choking episode, noisy inspiration, persistent tachypnea even at rest, syncopal episodes)

Clinical Examination

- Growth parameters — obesity, failure to thrive ('red flag' sign)
- Signs of co-morbid atopic conditions (e.g. dry eczematous skin, pale and edematous nasal turbinates, infraorbital shiners)
- Signs of chronicity — Harrison's sulci, barrel chest
- Air entry, wheeze and bronchodilator response, signs of respiratory distress
- Signs of complications of treatment — oral thrush, reduction in linear growth, Cushingoid features (long-term systemic or high-dose inhaled corticosteroids [ICS])
- 'Red flag' signs (e.g. clubbing, coarse crepitations, cardiac murmur, loud second heart sound, stridor, biphasic wheeze)

Investigations

- In children above 5 to 6 years old, peak expiratory flow assessment and spirometry can be helpful for diagnosis at presentation and an assessment of asthma control on follow-up.
- Other investigations are not mandatory for the asthma diagnosis but are important for the exclusion of differential diagnoses, especially in young children or in the presence of 'red flag' symptoms and signs.
    - » Chest X-ray — useful for exclusion of differential diagnoses (e.g. foreign body, pneumothorax, bronchiectasis, persistent lobar collapse, lymphadenopathy).
    - » Peak expiratory flow (PEF) assessment — performed with a peak flow meter. A PEF >80% of predicted PEF for height is considered to be within normal limits, but it is important to take into consideration the personal best and the trend of percentage-predicted PEF on serial measurements. Serial measurements may provide a better objective assessment of response to treatment.
    - » Spirometry — bronchodilator response with an increase of forced expiratory volume in 1 second (FEV1) of more than 12% suggests a diagnosis of asthma or partly controlled/uncontrolled asthma in a child with a clinical presentation consistent with asthma. FEV1 has greater sensitivity that PEF. Advise to avoid the use of bronchodilators before performing spirometry (6 hours before for short-acting beta-agonists [SABA], and 12 to 24 hours before for long-acting beta-agonists [LABA]).

» Bronchial provocation tests — mannitol/exercise challenge tests are not routine investigations. They may be useful in the clinical setting when spirometry is inconclusive for asthma or the evaluation of asthma as the cause of exercise-induced symptoms when spirometry is normal. Refer to a paediatric pulmonologist for bronchial provocation tests.
» Fractional concentration of exhaled nitric oxide (FeNO) — FeNO is elevated in eosinophilic asthma, but also in non-asthma conditions (e.g. allergic rhinitis). FeNO may help guide diagnosis and management of asthma in certain situations, but there is no established guideline available at this point to recommend routine use.
» Skin prick tests — assess for sensitisation to allergens, e.g. house dust mites, cat dander, dog dander, mould. May be useful for advising trigger avoidance/interventions. Advise to stop the use of antihistamines 7 days before a skin prick test.

Assessment of Asthma Severity, Control and Risk Factors

- The GINA asthma control assessment includes asthma symptom control assessment and an assessment of future risk of adverse outcomes — refer to the current GINA guideline for details and updates.
  » Asthma symptom control assessment is based on daytime and nocturnal asthma symptoms, reliever medication use, and activity limitation, and classified as 'well controlled', 'partly controlled' or 'uncontrolled'.
  » Important risk factors for poor asthma outcomes in children include low FEV1 (especially if <60% predicted), smoking or exposure to tobacco smoke, poor treatment adherence, history of severe exacerbation, Children's Intensive Care Unit (CICU) admission or intubation. Having one or more risk factors increases the risk of exacerbations even if symptoms are well controlled.
  » The GINA guideline advocates that asthma severity be assessed retrospectively from the level of treatment required to control symptoms and exacerbations.

Asthma Medications and Management

- All children diagnosed with asthma should be prescribed reliever medications, e.g. salbutamol metered dose inhalers (MDI) for use when having asthma symptoms/exacerbations.
- For safety reasons, the GINA and the Agency of Care Effectiveness (ACE) guidelines for asthma do not recommend treatment for asthma for adults, adolescents and children (6 years old and above) with SABA alone without an ICS controller medication.
  » ICS controller medication can be administered either as regular daily treatment or in mild asthma with as-needed SABA whenever needed for asthma symptoms.

- » In adults and adolescents with mild asthma, as-needed ICS-formoterol can be administered as reliever therapy when needed for asthma symptoms. In adults, adolescents and children 6 years old and above with moderate to severe asthma, ICS-formoterol is an option for both daily **m**aintenance **a**nd as-needed **r**eliever **t**herapy, referred to in short as MART.
- Children whose asthma symptom control is assessed as 'partly controlled' or 'uncontrolled' should be initiated on treatment with regular daily controller medications, e.g. ICS, leukotriene receptor antagonists (LTRA), or ICS/LABA combination therapy.
- In children 5 years old and below, regular controller therapy (e.g. ICS, LTRA) should be considered if the asthma symptoms are not controlled, if wheezing episodes are frequent (e.g. 3 or more episodes within 3 to 6 months) or if wheezing episodes are less frequent but more severe (e.g. 2 episodes requiring hospitalisation within a few months).
- The controller medications commonly used are ICS (fluticasone proprionate or budesonide), ICS/LABA combination therapy (salmeterol/fluticasone or formoterol/budesonide combination), and oral LTRA (montelukast). When considering montelukast, weigh the benefits against the risks before prescribing, and counsel patients/parents about the potential neuropsychiatric adverse effects on sleep and behaviour.
- The inhaled controller medications can be in form of MDIs or dry power inhalers (DPI), e.g. accuhaler or turbuhaler.
- The use of a spacer device with the MDI helps to deliver more medication to the lungs, decreases oropharyngeal deposition and addresses the challenge of coordinating MDI actuation and inhalation at the right time for children. Spacer devices are recommended for all children who are prescribed ICS in the form of MDIs.
  - » Children below 6 years old should always use their MDI together with spacers, while children above 6 years old have the additional option of DPIs to choose from if they are able to use the DPIs correctly.
  - » In children less than 3 to 4 years old, the spacer should be used with a face mask.
- Asthma education is an integral part of asthma management.
  - » The child and the caregiver must be educated on the disease, triggers and trigger avoidance and the use of the types of medication prescribed.
  - » The safety and importance of adherence to controller therapy needs to be emphasised, and the correct inhaler technique and maintenance of spacer devices need to be taught to the child and their caregiver.
- Individualised WAAP should be given and explained to each child and caregiver, to empower them to manage mild exacerbations at home and provide instructions on when they should seek medical attention.
- Smoking cessation advice and advice on setting up a smoke-free environment for the child should be given if the child/caregiver smokes or is exposed to environmental tobacco smoke.

Review of Controller Therapy

- Review response to treatment within 1–3 months after initiating controller therapy.
  - » Subsequent reviews can be every 3–6 months if there is good response.
  - » Younger children, children with uncontrolled asthma or children requiring high step controller therapy should be reviewed at closer intervals.
- If there is no or poor response, review controller adherence, inhaler device technique, ongoing trigger factor exposure, co-morbidity as contributory factors, before considering stepping up controller therapy.
- In general, if the asthma is partly controlled, consider stepping up controller therapy, and if the asthma is uncontrolled, controller therapy should be stepped up.
  - » The step of the controller therapy the child is at, the duration on the step of controller therapy, and the general trend of asthma control should be taken into consideration before stepping up controller therapy. For example, a 7-year-old child with a history of monthly hospitalisations for asthma started on and adherent with Step 4 controller therapy for 1 month may not need a further step up in controller therapy, even though his asthma may still be classified as 'uncontrolled' because of an attendance to the Children's Emergency (CE) for mild exacerbation 1 week before the clinic review.
- Review if the diagnosis of asthma is correct if treatment response is persistently poor or worsening or if there are 'red flag' signs or symptoms.
- If good asthma control is achieved and maintained for at least 3–6 months, controller therapy may be reduced stepwise to the lowest step required to maintain control.
  - » A child may lose asthma control when controller therapy is stepped down or ceased, so advice needs to be given to the child and caregivers to recognise symptoms of loss of asthma control and a follow-up review scheduled, so that controller therapy can be restarted or stepped up if there is worsening of asthma control.

High Risk Asthma

A small group of children may have asthma with high disease burden. They have frequent acute care attendances or admissions, and are at increased risk of asthma morbidity and mortality, and should be managed under the close supervision of paediatric pulmonologists. Following the 2008 Ministry of Health (MOH) Singapore's Management of Asthma Clinical Practice Guidelines, children at our institution with asthma who meet the following criteria are referred to a paediatric pulmonologist:

1. Poor asthma control
   a. Two or more exacerbations per month needing acute care
   b. Two or more hospitalisations for asthma within 3 months
   c. Requires reliever medication three times or more per week

   d. Severe exacerbation needing High Dependency Unit/CICU care
   e. Other risk factors (e.g. poor socioeconomic background, recalcitrant controller medication non-adherence)
2. Below 3 years and requires medium to high doses of ICS and not responding as expected
3. Requires high dose ICS
4. On prolonged low to moderate ICS for more than 6 months and remains symptomatic

Management of Acute Exacerbations

Refer to your institution's Asthma Clinical Pathway for management of acute exacerbations at the CE and in the ward. The general principles of management in the outpatient setting are as follows:

- Assess severity of the exacerbation — refer to Table 22.3 for a guide on assessing the severity of asthma exacerbation.
- Consider and exclude alternative diagnoses, associated complications, especially if 'red flag' history, symptoms or signs are present, e.g. foreign body aspiration, pneumonia, pneumothorax.
- Maintain oxygenation — maintain $SpO_2 \geq 95\%$ with oxygen supplementation
- Relieve bronchospasm with intensive bronchodilator therapy
  - » Salbutamol MDI 10 puffs (5 puffs if child <10 kg) with ipratropium bromide MDI 4 puffs (2 puffs if child <10 kg) every 20 minutes up to 3 cycles for mild to moderate exacerbation (As per our institution's CE Asthma Clinical Pathway)
  - » Nebulised continuous 0.5% salbutamol solution 1 ml (0.5 ml if child <10 kg) with 0.025% ipratropium bromide solution 1 ml (0.5 ml if child <10 kg) with at least 6 L/min oxygen if severe exacerbation with $SpO_2 < 90\%$ on oxygen supplementation (As per our institution's CE Asthma Clinical Pathway)
  - » If good response to treatment and meets the discharge criteria ($SpO_2 \geq 95\%$ in room air, mild end expiratory or no wheeze, mild or no retractions, not tachypnoeic on 4 hourly inhaled bronchodilator, adequate hydration and nutrition), discharge with salbutamol MDI 4 hourly (0.3 puffs/kg, minimum 2 puffs, maximum 8 puffs), to taper over a few days to as-needed basis. A WAAP should be provided.
  - » Arrange for admission, or refer/transfer to an Emergency Department if severe exacerbation on presentation, deterioration despite treatment, or does not respond well enough to meet discharge criteria.
  - » For severe exacerbation presenting at a hospital setting, may consider additional treatments — intravenous (IV) magnesium sulphate, IV salbutamol or IV aminophylline — refer to your institution's Asthma Clinical Pathway.
- Relieve underlying inflammation
  - » Oral prednisolone (1–2 mg/kg/day, maximum 40 mg/day) for moderate to severe exacerbations, for 3 to 5 days. Refer to your institution's Asthma Clinical Pathway for other indications for initiating oral corticosteroids.

Table 22.3 Assessment of Severity of Asthma Exacerbation

	Mild	Moderate	Severe or life-threatening
Breathless	On exertion	On talking	At rest
Speaks in	Sentences	Phrases	Words
Conscious level	Normal	May be agitated	Agitated/confused/drowsy
Accessory muscle use	Nil	+	++ Paradoxical thoracic-abdominal movement
Wheeze/rhonchi	Variable	Loud	Loud/silent
Pulse rate/min	<100	100–200	>200
Pulsus paradoxus	Nil	May be palpable, 10–25 mmHg	Palpable, >25 mmHg Nil if exhausted
Physical exhaustion	Nil	Nil	Yes (cyanosed)
SpO_2 in room air	≥95%	92–95%	<92%
PEF (predicted/personal best)	≥80%	60–80%	<60%
Respiratory rate	↑	↑↑	↑↑↑/↓(exhaustion)

- » IV hydrocortisone (4–5 mg/kg, maximum 100 mg/dose) for moderate to severe exacerbations and unable to retain oral corticosteroids.
- » Review controller therapy, step up until follow-up review if needed.
- Advise on symptoms and signs of recurrence and worsening of exacerbation, trigger avoidance.
- Review inhaler technique and provide WAAP.
- Arrange appropriate follow-up review.

Bibliography

1. Ministry of Health Singapore. (2008) Management of asthma, MOH Clinical Practice Guidelines 1/2008. https://www.moh.gov.sg/docs/librariesprovider4/guidelines/cpg_asthma.pdf
2. Global Initiative for Asthma. (2022) Global strategy for asthma management and prevention. www.ginasthma.org
3. Agency of Care Effectiveness. (nd) Asthma-optimising long-term management with inhaled corticosteroid, ACE Clinical Guidances. https://www.ace-hta.gov.sg/healthcare-professionals/ace-clinical-guidances-(acgs)/details/asthma-optimising-long-term-management-with-inhaled-corticosteroid

CHAPTER 106

Common Respiratory Conditions

Arun Pugalenthi, Teoh Oon Hoe

Croup (Acute Laryngotracheobronchitis)

- Croup is inflammation of the upper airway, larynx and trachea.
- Most commonly caused by the parainfluenza virus. Other viruses include the respiratory syncytial virus and adenovirus.
- Affects children 6 months to 5 years old, peak age between 6 months and 2 years old.
- Usually begins with symptoms of upper respiratory tract infection and fever, followed by a gradual onset of hoarseness, harsh 'barking' cough and stridor over 1 to 2 days.
- Croup symptoms usually worsen at night. The stridor usually worsens with crying or agitation. Symptoms resolve usually over a few days to a week.
- 'Red flag' symptoms and signs — sudden onset, toxic looking, drooling or dysphagia — consider alternative diagnosis, e.g. acute epiglottitis, retropharyngeal abscess, bacterial tracheitis, foreign body aspiration, angioedema.

Assessment

Assessment of severity is based on the Westley croup score:

Inspiratory stridor	Not present	0
	When agitated	1
	At rest	2
Intercostal recession	Mild	1
	Moderate	2
	Severe	3
Air entry	Normal	0
	Mildly decreased	1
	Severely decreased	2
Cyanosis	None	0
	With agitation	4
	At rest	5
Level of consciousness	Normal	0
	Altered	5

  - 2 or less suggests mild croup
  - 3–7 indicates moderate croup
  - 8 or higher indicates severe croup
- Regardless of the severity, all children with croup should be approached in a calm manner.
- Keep the child comfortable and avoid unnecessary distress.
- Avoid examination of the throat.
- Assess the degree of airway obstruction, not the loudness of stridor.
  - Beware of quietening stridor and increasing respiratory distress.
  - Assess work of breathing and effectiveness of respiration, look for recessions, tiring and falling of oxygen saturations.
- Biphasic stridor, dysphonia, drooling and dysphagia are all concerning.
- Clinical deterioration and altering consciousness is a sign of worsening severe upper airway obstruction.

Management

- Mild croup
  - Oral dexamethasone 0.15 mg/kg stat dose. Observe for 2 hours and re-assess Westley croup score. An additional dose of 0.45 mg/kg can be given, with consideration for discharge if Westley croup score <2 after another 2 hours.
- Moderate croup
  - Oral dexamethasone 0.6 mg/kg
  - Supplemental oxygen if SpO_2 <95%
  - Nebulised adrenaline (1:1000) 3ml:1ml normal saline if Westley croup score 4 or higher
- Severe croup
  - Nebulised adrenaline (1:1000) 3ml:1ml normal saline
  - Supplemental oxygen if SpO_2 <95%
  - Intramuscular/intravenous (IV) dexamethasone 0.6 mg/kg (max. 12 mg)
  - Consider intubation if altered sensorium or impending respiratory failure
  - Admit to Children's Intensive Care Unit (CICU)
- Admitted for mild to moderate croup
  - Minimal handling
  - Adequate hydration and nutrition — small frequent oral feeding, or IV hydration if required.
  - Supplemental oxygen if SpO_2 <95%
  - Monitor for worsening or recurrence of symptoms — if frequent repeated doses of nebulised adrenaline are needed, transfer the child to CICU.

Criteria for Discharge

Consider discharge if:

- Child not toxic, has adequate hydration and good oral intake.
- No stridor at rest, or minimal stridor only when agitated.

- Not in respiratory distress and SpO_2 ≥95%.
- Parents confident of care — advise caregivers to monitor closely and return if worsening of symptoms occurs.

Refer to your institution's Children Emergency (CE) Guidelines for further details for step-wise management.

Bronchiolitis

- Bronchiolitis is a viral lower respiratory tract infection.
- It is most commonly seen in infants between 3 and 6 months of age but can present in children up to 2 years.
- Most commonly caused by the respiratory syncytial virus. Other viruses include rhinovirus, parainfluenza virus, human metapneumovirus and adenovirus.
- Usually begins with symptoms of upper respiratory tract infection and fever, progressing to tachypnoea, wheezing and respiratory distress over a few days. Crepitations and/or wheezing are present on auscultation.
- Symptoms tend to worsen over the first 3–5 days of illness and peak between the 5th and 7th day of illness for most children. The symptom of cough resolves by 2–3 weeks in most children.
- Diagnosis is clinical

Risk Factors for Severe Bronchiolitis: Low Threshold for Admission and Close Monitoring

- Chronic lung disease
- Congenital heart disease
- Age <3 months
- Congenital airway abnormality, e.g. tracheal stenosis
- Immunodeficiency
- Neuromuscular disorder

Differential Diagnoses

- Pneumonia — fever late in the course of illness, localised signs
- Pertussis — consider in children presenting with apnoea, paroxysmal coughing spells or prolonged cough
- Viral induced wheeze — in children above 1 year, especially with recurrent episodes of wheeze
- Foreign body
- Congenital airway anomaly
- Cardiac anomaly

Investigations

- NOT routinely indicated in typical or mild disease
- Full blood count — only if there is concern of bacterial infection or sepsis

- Renal panel — only if there is concern with feeding, dehydration or commencing on IV fluids
- Blood culture — only if there are features of sepsis
- Viral testing — has little impact on outcome but may influence antibiotic prescription or guide isolation for infection control.
- Chest X-ray is not required for diagnosis, but indicated if
  - » Severe illness
  - » Diagnosis is uncertain
  - » Localised signs on auscultation
  - » Cardiac signs on examination

Management

Management of bronchiolitis is supportive and includes:

- Minimal handling
- Supplemental oxygen to keep SpO_2 ≥95%
- Adequate hydration and nutrition — small frequent oral feeding, nasogastric feeding or IV hydration, if required.
- Nasal suction is not routinely recommended — superficial nasal suction may be considered in those with moderate disease to ease work of breathing and improve feeding. Normal saline nasal drops can be considered.
- Do not routinely prescribe inhaled bronchodilators, nebulised adrenaline or hypertonic saline, antibiotics or oral steroids.
  - » A trial of nebulised adrenaline (1:1000) 3ml:1ml normal saline driven by 8 L/min oxygen may be given at CE for moderate disease, with view for discharge if there is good response.
  - » An inpatient trial of nebulised salbutamol (0.5 ml 0.5% salbutamol with 3.5 ml normal saline driven by 8 L/min oxygen) or salbutamol (100 mcg) Metered dose inhaler 2–4 puffs may be considered in children with history of atopy or in moderate /severe respiratory distress, to continue as needed 4–6 hourly ONLY if there is clinical response to intervention.
  - » Disease severity and response to intervention can be assessed with the aid of clinical scores for bronchiolitis, e.g. the modified Respiratory Index Score.
  - » Refer to your institution's Clinical Pathway for details.
- Chest physiotherapy is not routinely indicated.

The signs of deterioration that should be looked for are:

- Respiratory rate >60/min.
- Apnoea, bradypnoea or cyanotic episode despite supplemental oxygen.
- Persistent tachycardia.
- Drowsiness/lethargy.
- Increasing oxygen requirement to maintain oxygen saturations ≥95%.

Consider high flow nasal cannula (HFNC) on continuous positive airway pressure (CPAP) support if there is clinical deterioration or severe disease.

Consider discharge when SpO_2 ≥95% on room air when awake, the child is adequately hydrated and able to feed, with minimal or no retractions and end-expiratory or no wheeze. Caregivers should also be confident with the monitoring and care of the child before discharge.

Bibliography

1. Westley CR, Cotton EK, Brooks JG. (1978) Nebulized racemic epinephrine by IPPB for the treatment of croup: A double-blind study. *Am J Dis Child* **132**(5):484–487.
2. Gates A, Gates M, Vandermeer B, *et al.* (2018) Glucocorticoids for croup in children. *Cochrane Database Syst Rev* **8**(8):CD001955.
3. Ralston SL, Lieberthal AS, Meissner HC, *et al.* (2014) Clinical practice guideline: The diagnosis, management, and prevention of bronchiolitis. *Pediatrics* **134**(5):e1474–e1502.
4. Chong SL, Teoh OH, Nadkarni N, *et al.* (2017) The modified respiratory index score (RIS) guides resource allocation in acute bronchiolitis. *Pediatr Pulmonol* **52**(7):954–961.

CHAPTER 107

Pneumonia, Parapneumonic Effusion and Empyema

Biju Thomas, Teoh Oon Hoe

Pneumonia

- Lower respiratory tract infection involving the lung parenchyma.
- Affects all ages, higher incidence in children <5 years.
- Common causes of community-acquired pneumonia include viruses, *Mycoplasma pneumoniae* and *Streptococcus pneumoniae* (the most common bacterial cause). Table 22.4 summarises common infective aetiology and empiric antibiotic options for different age groups.
- Typically presents with fever, cough and tachypnoea ± signs of respiratory distress, but symptoms vary with age and infective aetiology. Young children may present with isolated fever, malaise, altered mental state, abdominal pain or vomiting.
- Adventitious sounds on auscultation may be subtle in young children with shallow breathing.
- 'Red flags' in history, symptoms and signs: Recurrent pneumonia (e.g. immunodeficiency, congenital airway/lung abnormality), pleuritic chest pain (empyema), night sweats and weight loss (pulmonary tuberculosis [TB]), clubbing, failure to thrive, chronic wet/productive cough (bronchiectasis) and significant background medical problems (malignancies, haemodynamically significant cardiac disease, neuromuscular disease, chronic lung disease, primary/secondary immune deficiency).
- For children who need inpatient management, commonly performed investigations include Chest X-ray (CXR), Full blood count, C-reactive protein and nasopharyngeal aspirate for respiratory viruses (multiplex PCR). Additional imaging (Ultrasound [US]/Computed Tomography [CT] of the chest) may be required in complicated pneumonia.
- Full blood count and C-reactive protein may help clinical decision-making regarding the need to commence antibiotics but are not specific in differentiating infective aetiologies. Blood culture is recommended before commencing intravenous (IV) antibiotics, though the yield is very low. Other investigations (Renal panel, Urine *S pneumoniae* antigen and Mycoplasma serology) may be required in selected cases.

- Consider repeat imaging and referral to respiratory medicine for children with persistent high fever or failure to improve/clinical deterioration despite having had 48 hours of treatment with appropriate antibiotics.
- Management:
  - » Indications for admission include significant tachypnoea, respiratory distress, $SpO_2 \leq 95\%$ in room air, tachycardia for age and temperature, poor perfusion and poor feeding.
  - » Maintain $SpO_2 \geq 95\%$ with supplemental oxygen.
  - » Supportive management: Maintain adequate hydration, control of fever.
  - » Monitoring: Temperature, Heart rate, Respiratory rate, SpO_2 and Blood pressure.
  - » Antimicrobial therapy is guided by the age, clinical presentation, presence of drug (penicillin) allergy, co-existing medical problems, prior antibiotic treatment, local antibiotic resistance patterns, as well as travel and contact history. Table 22.4 provides guidelines for the choice of empiric antibiotic therapy for children with normal immune function. Ideally, the first dose of antibiotic should be administered within 4 hours upon hospital arrival.
  - » Monitor serum sodium and watch for the syndrome of inappropriate secretion of anti-diuretic hormone if on IV fluids.
  - » Indications for referral to Respiratory Medicine/Infectious Disease Service: Persistent high fever or failure to improve/clinical deterioration despite having had 48 hours of treatment with appropriate antibiotics, complicated pneumonia (significant effusion OR effusion with US features of echogenic fluid ± loculations/empyema/necrotising pneumonia/pneumothorax/lung abscess), pre-existing significant lung disease and suspected TB/foreign body inhalation.
  - » There is no role for chest physiotherapy in previously healthy children presenting with pneumonia.
  - » Refer for chest physiotherapy if there is significant collapse and empyema post video-assisted thoracoscopic surgery (VATS).
  - » Convert to oral antibiotics when the child is afebrile for 24–48 hours.
  - » Follow-up CXR not necessary in previously well children with uncomplicated pneumonia. Indications for follow-up CXR (4–6 weeks later) include extensive atelectasis (e.g. ≥ one lobe), round pneumonia, complicated pneumonia (e.g. pleural effusion, empyema, extensive pneumonia, lung abscess), past history of recurrent CXR confirmed pneumonia and persistent symptoms/auscultatory signs on follow up.

Table 22.4 Empiric Antibiotics for Community Acquired Pneumonia (no drug allergy)

		1st Line	2nd Line if No Response ≥ 48–72 Hours	1st Line	2nd Line if No Response ≥ 48–72 Hours
Neonate	Grp B Streptococcus, *E.coli*, Listeria, Gram-negative bacilli	N/A	N/A	**IV Ampicillin +** **IV Gentamicin**	**IV Ampicillin +** **IV Cefotaxime**
1–3 mth	Viruses, *C.trachomatis*, *S.aureus*, *B.pertussis*, *S.pneumoniae*	**AFEBRILE**	**AFEBRILE**	**FEBRILE**	**FEBRILE**
		PO Clarithromycin*	**PO Amoxicillin**	**IV Ampicillin +** **IV Cloxacillin** **± PO Clarithromycin*** (if no response after 48 hr)	**IV Ceftriaxone +** **PO Clarithromycin*** **± IV Cloxacillin** (if suspect *S. aureus*)
3 mth–5 yr	Viruses, *S. pneumoniae*, *H. influenzae*, *M.catarrhalis*, *M. pneumoniae*	**MILD-MODERATE**	**MILD-MODERATE**	**SEVERE**	**SEVERE**
		If suspect S. pneumoniae, **PO Amoxicillin** **OR** If suspect Mycoplasma or H.influenzae, **PO Clarithromycin***	If no response to Amoxicillin, then reassess and switch/add on **Clarithromycin** If no response to Clarithromycin, then reassess and switch/add on **Amoxicillin**	**IV Ampicillin** If no response after 48–72 hr, **Add Clarithromycin*** If <1yr and suspect S. aureus), **Add IV Cloxacillin**	**IV Ceftriaxone +** **PO Clarithromycin*** If < 1 yr. and suspect S. aureus), **Add IV Cloxacillin**
≥ 5 yr	*M. pneumoniae* *S. pneumoniae*, *Chlamydophila pneumoniae*	**MILD-MODERATE**	**MILD-MODERATE**	**SEVERE**	**SEVERE**
		If suspect Mycoplasma, **PO Clarithromycin*** If suspect S.pneumoniae, **PO Amoxicillin**	If no response to Clarithromycin, then reassess and switch/add on **Amoxycillin** If no response to Amoxycillin, then reassess and switch/add on **Clarithromycin**	**IV Ampicillin** **+** **PO Clarithromycin***	**IV Ceftriaxone** **+** **PO Clarithromycin***

* If unable to tolerate Clarithromycin, consider PO Azithroymcin or IV Erythromycin.

Parapneumonic Effusion and Empyema

Definition

Parapneumonic effusion is defined as an abnormal collection of fluid in the pleural space in association with underlying pneumonia. Uncomplicated small parapneumonic effusions may be sterile exudates that often resolve with appropriate antibiotic treatment of the pneumonia. Occasionally, this could evolve into complicated parapneumonic effusions with fibrinopurulent changes and may require drainage in addition to appropriate antibiotic treatment. Empyema occurs when frank pus develops from a parapneumonic effusion, with organisation and formation of loculations and pleural peel. Empyema complicates about 1–2% of childhood pneumonia.

Aetiology

The most common organisms are *Streptococcus pneumonia, Mycoplasma pneumonia* and *Staphylococcus aureus*, depending on the age of the child. In neurologically impaired children and aspiration-related pneumonia, anaerobic bacteria may be the causative organism.

Diagnosis

Parapneumonic effusion is suspected when the CXR shows consolidation with pleural fluid accumulation in a febrile child with signs and symptoms of lower respiratory tract infection. Complicated parapneumonic effusion or empyema development should be suspected in children with persistent high fever or failure to improve/clinical deterioration despite having had 48 hours of treatment with appropriate antibiotics. Pleuritic chest pain and referred abdominal pain may be present. A referral to respiratory medicine is warranted for such children.

The choice of US thorax or CT chest for evaluation of the empyema should be discussed with the Respiratory Consultant and Paediatric Surgeon. In general, US thorax is preferred unless it is a complicated case or when surgery (VATS) is considered.

Differential Diagnoses of Pleural Effusion

- Transudative
  - » Heart failure
  - » Hypoalbuminemia, e.g. nephrotic syndrome, liver disease, protein losing enteropathy, malabsorption
- Exudative
  - » Pneumonia
  - » TB
  - » Connective tissue disease, e.g. systemic lupus erythematosus
  - » Malignant effusion
  - » Abdominal infection/inflammation, e.g. hepatic abscess, pancreatitis
- Chylothorax
- Other diagnoses, e.g. lung abscess, malignancy (pleuropulmonary blastoma)

Management

Refer to the Respiratory Medicine Service if a significant parapneumonic effusion (moderate/large effusion and/or echogenic fluid on imaging) or empyema is suspected. Management is often individualised, taking into consideration the clinical presentation, prior treatment, complexity of the effusion and patient factors. Figure 22.2 shows our institution's algorithm to guide management.

- Antibiotics: Empiric antimicrobial therapy is guided by the age, clinical presentation, presence of drug (penicillin) allergy, co-existing medical problems, prior antibiotic treatment, local antibiotic resistance patterns, as well as travel and contact history.
- High dose IV ampicillin is the first-line treatment if *S. pneumoniae* is suspected. Antibiotic choice should be reviewed once microbiological results are available or if there is poor response to the initial empiric treatment. Treatment should be IV until the child is afebrile for at least 24–48 hours and the chest drain (if

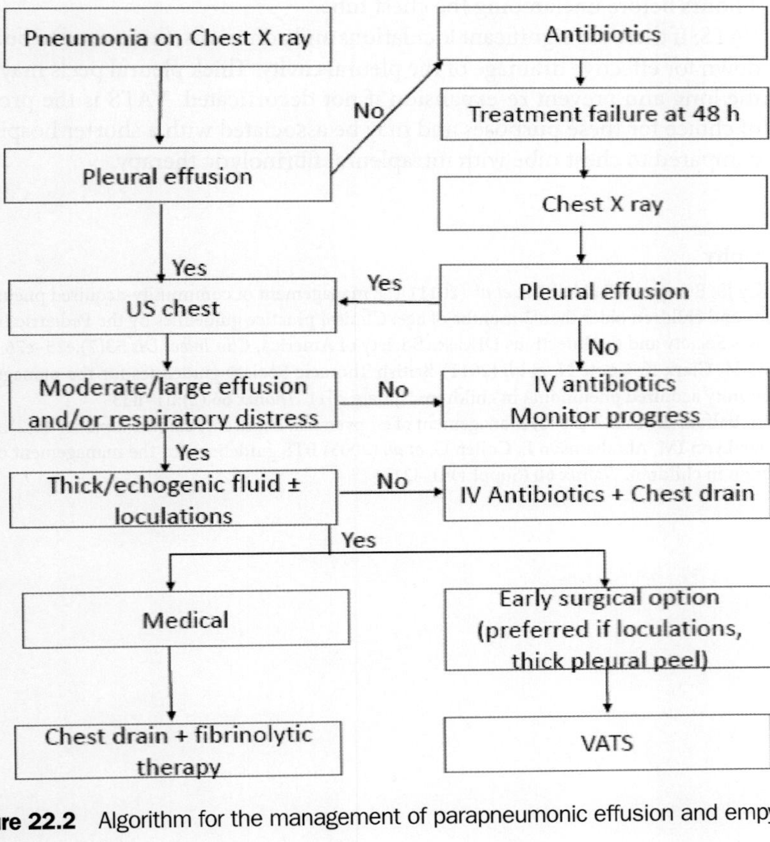

Figure 22.2 Algorithm for the management of parapneumonic effusion and empyema.

inserted) removed. In most cases, this would be for at least 7–14 days depending on severity of the disease and response to treatment and drainage. This is followed with oral antibiotics, and the total duration of antibiotic treatment should be at least 3–4 weeks.

- Chest tube drainage: Large parapneumonic effusions causing respiratory distress and complicated effusions require drainage in addition to antibiotics. As an alternative to a chest drain insertion by the medical team, ultrasound guided pigtail catheter placement by the interventional radiologist may be considered if the drainage is not urgent for relief of respiratory distress or if the size and location of the effusion is better accessed safely with ultrasound guidance.
- Intrapleural fibrinolytic therapy: If the pleural fluid is turbid or if there is evidence of early loculation on chest ultrasound, consider fibrinolytic therapy following chest tube insertion. Usually, intrapleural urokinase is given twice daily for 3 days. Each dose is 40000 U in 40 ml normal saline (10000 U in 10 ml normal saline if child <10 kg), to leave to dwell in the pleural cavity after instillation for 4 hours before unclamping the chest tube.
- VATS: If there are significant loculations and adhesions, these need to be broken down for effective drainage of the pleural cavity. Thick pleural peels may entrap the lung and prevent re-expansion if not decorticated. VATS is the procedure of choice for these purposes and may be associated with a shorter hospital stay compared to chest tube with intrapleural fibrinolytic therapy.

Bibliography

1. Bradley JS, Byington CL, Shah SS, *et al.* (2011) The management of community-acquired pneumonia in infants and children older than 3 months of age: Clinical practice guidelines by the Pediatric Infectious Diseases Society and the Infectious Diseases Society of America. *Clin Infect Dis* **53**(7):e25–e76.
2. Harris M, Clark K, Coote N, *et al.* (2011) British Thoracic Society guidelines for the management of community acquired pneumonia in children: Update 2011. *Thorax* **66** (2):ii1–ii23.
3. Jaffé A, Balfour-Lynn IM. (2005) Management of empyema in children. *Pediatr Pulmonol* **40**(2):148–156.
4. Balfour-Lynn IM, Abrahamson E, Cohen G, *et al.* (2005) BTS guidelines for the management of pleural infection in children. *Thorax* **60** (Suppl 1):i1–i21.

SECTION 23

RHEUMATOLOGY

CHAPTER 108

Joint Pain

Teh Kai Liang; Thaschawee Arkachaisri

History

- Location/Anatomic site of pain
- Duration of symptoms
- Number and pattern of joint involvement
- Functional impairment
- Time of the day with maximal discomfort: Morning, after activities or nocturnal
- Aggravating or relieving factors
- Associated signs or symptoms — for systemic diseases

Clinical Examination

- Arthritis: Signs of inflammation include swelling (effusion and/or synovial thickening), warmth, tenderness, erythema (usually absent without non-infectious chronic arthritis) and limitation in range of motion

Clinical Pearls

- Inflammatory causes: Infectious (septic) or non-infectious (reactive or idiopathic arthritis)/part of systemic diseases, malignancy associated arthritis, etc.
- Mechanical causes: Trauma, fracture, ligament or tendon tears, overuse, hypermobility, etc.
- Careful physical examination is important to identify areas of pathology. The site of pain may not correspond to the joints affected. For example, hip arthritis may be referred to as anterior thighs/knees.
- Presence of muscle atrophy usually indicates chronicity or denervation.
- Septic arthritis and trauma less likely to be polyarticular.
- Acute arthritis less than 6 weeks generally reflects aetiologies related to trauma or infection, while chronic arthritis reflects more inflammatory aetiology.
- The presence of systemic features like, fever, rashes, nail changes, oral ulcers, redness of eye and diarrhoea may suggest systemic illness.
- Arthritis with pain resulting in nocturnal night awakening should be evaluated further to rule out bone tumours or malignancy.

- Enthesitis-related arthritis is one of the most common forms of juvenile idiopathic arthritis locally. It is therefore important to ask about the presence of buttock pain, and if present, attention must be given to the examination of sacroiliac joints and entheses.
- Diagnosis of arthritis is clinical through careful physical examination. Patients with arthritis can have normal inflammatory markers and X-ray findings.

Nocturnal Pain

- Benign nocturnal pain of childhood or "growing pains"
  - » Pain never occurs during the day and only at night
  - » Affects 4–12 years old — male almost equal to female in distribution
  - » Usually lower limb and bilateral
  - » Relieved by massage and/or analgesics
  - » Normal joint examination and all investigations
- Bone tumours
  - » Benign tumours: osteoid osteoma, bone cyst, etc.
  - » Malignant bone tumours
    - ▪ Primary bone malignancy
    - ▪ Secondary bone tumours or metastasis — leukaemia, lymphoma, neuroblastoma

Table 23.1 Differentiation between Inflammatory and Mechanical Joint Pain

	Inflammatory Type	Mechanical Type
Onset	Usually insidious	Sudden
Morning stiffness	>30 min	None
Limitation of ROM	Gradual	Abrupt/Acute
Aggravation of pain	With rest	With use or movement
Joint swelling	Synovial hypertrophy, effusion, warmth	Effusion

Table 23.2 Transient Synovitis vs. Septic Arthritis

Number of Predictors*	Predicted Probability of Septic Arthritis (%)
0	<0.2
1	3.0
2	40.0
3	93.1
4	99.6

*4 predictors: 1. History of fever, 2. Non-weight bearing, 3. ESR >40 mm/hr, 4. Total WBC >12 K/ml. Adapted from Kocher MS, *et al*. (1999) *J Bone Joint Surg*.

Musculoskeletal Manifestations of Systemic Disease

- Infection: Infectious, reactive, rheumatic fever
- Malignancy: Leukaemia, lymphoma, neuroblastoma, bone/cartilaginous tumour
- Bone/connective tissue disorder: Osteochondrodysplasia, Marfan and Ehlers–Danlos syndromes
- Metabolic diseases: Mucopolysaccharidoses/mucolipidoses
- Haemophiliac arthropathy
- Endocrine: hypothyroidism, pancreatitis
- Immunodeficiency-associated arthritis
- Periodic Fever Syndromes/Autoinflammatory diseases

Bibliography

1. Kocher MS, Zurakowski D, Kasser JR. (1999) Differentiating between septic arthritis and transient synovitis of the hip in children: An evidence-based clinical prediction algorithm. *J Bone Joint Surg Am* **81**(12):1662–1670.
2. Nannery R, Heinz P. (2018) Approach to joint pain children. *Paediatr Child Health* **28**(2):43–49.

CHAPTER 109

Common Rheumatological Conditions

Teh Kai Liang; Thaschawee Arkachaisri

Juvenile Idiopathic Arthritis

- Idiopathic chronic arthritis that begins in childhood
- Different from adult rheumatoid arthritis (RA)
- Aetiology unknown. Genetic predisposition with environmental triggers leads to cytokine mediated inflammation (such as interleukin 1 [IL-1], interleukin 6 [IL-6] and TNF alpha). Possibly a complex genetic trait associated with human leukocyte antigen (HLA) genes and cytokine gene polymorphisms.
- In Singapore, the incidence is estimated to be 4–5/100000 children at risk, below the age of 16 years. Asian children lack the female predominance and uveitis described in the West.

Diagnosis

- Arthritis for ≥6 weeks (joint swelling, or two out of three of pain, warmth, restriction of movement)
- Onset before the age of 16
- Exclusion of secondary causes

International League of Associations for Rheumatology (ILAR) Classification

- Systemic juvenile idiopathic arthritis (JIA)
- Oligoarticular
  - » Extended oligoarticular JIA
  - » Persistent oligoarticular JIA
- Polyarticular
  - » Rheumatoid factor (RF)-positive JIA
  - » RF-negative JIA
- Psoriatic arthritis
- Enthesitis-related arthritis
- Undifferentiated JIA

Systemic JIA (13% of JIA patients locally)

- Arthritis with or preceded by daily spiking fever for 2 weeks (quotidian pattern documented for at least 3 days) and one or more of the following:
  - » Evanescent, erythematous rash
  - » Hepato/splenomegaly
  - » Generalised lymphadenopathy
  - » Serositis
- May be complicated by pericarditis and macrophage activation syndrome.
- Systemic features may precede the onset of arthritis.

Polyarticular Disease (15% of JIA patients locally)

- Arthritis affecting five or more joints during the first 6 months of disease
  - » RF-negative, typically younger age at onset.
  - » RF-positive, usually older girls/adolescents, mimics adult RA with early erosive disease.
- The presence of RF must be documented on at least two occasions at least 3 months apart.

Oligoarticular Disease (34% of JIA patients locally)

- Oligo-persistent disease: Classically younger girls with knee involvement, commonly antinuclear antibody (ANA) positive.
- Arthritis is usually easily treated with non-steroidal anti-inflammatory drugs (NSAIDs) or intra-articular steroid injection, but chronic uveitis is common and can lead to blindness if untreated.
- Oligo-extended disease, i.e. more than four joints after the first 6 months.

Enthesitis-Related Arthritis (35% of JIA patients locally)

- Arthritis and enthesitis, or arthritis or enthesitis with at least two of the following:
  - » Sacroiliac joint tenderness and/or inflammatory spinal pain
  - » Presence of HLA-B27
  - » Family history in one or more first-degree relative(s) of medically confirmed HLA-B27-associated disease
  - » Anterior uveitis that is usually associated with pain, redness or photophobia
  - » Onset of arthritis in a boy after 6 years of age

Juvenile Psoriatic Arthritis (35% of JIA patients locally)

- Arthritis and psoriasis or arthritis and at least two of the following:
  - » Dactylitis (sausage digit)
  - » Nail pitting or onycholysis
  - » Family history of psoriasis in a first-degree relative
  - » Arthritis may predate onset of psoriasis by many years

Complications

- Limb pain, swelling, deformity
- Loss of function, independence and ambulation

- Contracture, limb overgrowth, limb length discrepancy
- Osteoporosis, fracture, avascular necrosis
- Growth and pubertal delay (short stature, FTT)
- Uveitis, loss of vision, blindness
- Social and financial cost — loss of schooling, social development, poor self-image, hospitalisation

Clinical Evaluation

- History and physical examination aim to determine evidence of synovitis/arthritis/enthesitis, exclude secondary causes for limb symptoms (especially infection, malignancy, reactive arthritis) and assess subtype of arthritis, severity and complications
- History: Elicit inflammatory pain (especially morning stiffness)
- Physical Findings: Signs of chronicity, systemic features (including fever, rash, nail changes, organomegaly, lymphadenopathy, weight loss, tendonitis/enthesitis), measure limb length discrepancy
- No investigation is pathognomonic of JIA, but may be useful to rule out other differentials.
- Most patients with JIA do not have significantly raised inflammatory markers (except systemic JIA). If raised, will need to rule out other systemic illness
- Role of X-ray mainly to exclude other diseases (infection and malignancy), as bony changes in JIA are relatively late (including sclerosis, erosions, ankylosis)
- Ultrasound/MRI with contrast useful to assess hip, sacroiliac and temporomandibular joints
- Joint aspirate, if done, should be sent for cell count. Joint aspirate in JIA is neutrophil predominant, with negative gram stain and cultures.

Management Principles

- The goal is to suppress inflammation and prevent joint deformity and disability
- Physical — rest, pain relief, physiotherapy, occupational therapy
- Medical therapy
  - » Intra-articular joint injections
  - » NSAIDs
  - » Conventional disease-modifying antirheumatic drugs (DMARDs)
  - » Biological DMARDs (biologics against TNF, IL-1, IL-6)
  - » Targeted synthetic DMARDs (including JAK inhibitors)
- Eye review for uveitis and toxicity of medication
- Patient education, support (social, financial, emotional) — support club, social worker

Systemic Lupus Erythematosus

- Multi-systemic disease of immune dysregulation characterised by circulating antibodies to nuclear and other tissue antigens (99% positive ANA).

- Wide variety of clinical features, can evolve with time, affecting different organ systems; renal, neurological, cardiac disease and infection are major causes of mortality.
- Aetiology unknown, probably an interplay between genetic factors and environmental triggers.
- More common in females overall, possible due to hormonal differences. Equal sex distribution below the age of 5
- Sometimes familial.

Evaluation and Diagnosis

- Definite diagnosis of systemic lupus erythematosus (SLE) is made when four out of eleven of ACR classification criteria are present (at any time) and no alternative explanation exists.
- However, lupus should be considered when characteristic features occur in combination or evolve over time. Treatment should be started if clinical disease is significant, even if less than four criteria are met.
- High erythrocyte sedimentation rate (ESR) and normal C-reactive protein (CRP), low complement levels (especially C3) are suggestive of active SLE.

Other Features of SLE

- Constitutional — fever, malaise, loss of appetite, loss of weight
- Dermatological — alopecia, periungal erythema, vasculitis rash, livedo reticularis, Raynaud's Phenomenon, gangrene
- Liver, spleen, lymph node enlargement
- Musculoskeletal — arthritis, arthralgia, tenosynovitis, myopathy
- Cardiac — myocarditis, endocarditis, valvulitis, Libman–Sacks vegetations, cardiac failure, Ischaemic Heart Disease
- Respiratory — pneumonitis, pulmonary hypertension, pulmonary haemorrhage
- Gastrointestinal — colitis, peritonitis
- Thrombotic events, APS
- Neurological — central or peripheral manifestations
- Fundus — exudates, cytoid bodies, papilloedema, retinopathy

Renal Disease

- Nephritis is a major cause of morbidity and mortality in SLE.
- Can present clinically (as nephritic or nephrotic syndrome, mixed picture, hypertension, acute or chronic renal failure) or asymptomatic biochemical abnormality (haematuria, proteinuria, raised creatinine, abnormal creatinine clearance test)
- Renal biopsy — guide to management when considering immunosuppression such as cyclophosphamide or if there is doubt about the reversibility of renal damage to prognosticate
- Evaluation of lupus nephritis: Urinalysis for sediments and casts, measurement of glomerular function, serum creatinine and urea, measurement of proteinuria (using spot urine protein: creatinine ratio or 24-hour urine total protein)

Table 23.3 Criteria for the Classification of SLE (ACR 1997)

Criteria	Features/Explanations
Malar (butterfly) rash	Fixed erythema, sparing naso-labial folds
Discoid lupus	Red raised scaly patch, later may have atrophic scarring
Photosensitivity	
Oral or nasopharyngeal ulcerations	Painless usually
Non-erosive arthritis (two joints)	Tenderness, swelling, morning stiffness
Renal disorder	Persistent proteinuria >0.5 g/dL or 3+ cellular casts (red cell, Hb, granular, tubular, mixed)
Neurological disorder	Seizures or Psychosis (In the absence of offending drugs or metabolic derangements, e.g. uraemia, ketoacidosis, electrolyte imbalances)
Serositis	Pleuritis (pain, rub, effusion) Pericarditis (ECG, rub, effusion)
Haematological disorder	Haemolytic anaemia with reticulocytosis Leucopenia (<4000/mm^3) Lymphopenia (<1500/mm^3) Thrombocytopenia (<100000/mm^3) (in the absence of offending drugs)
Positive antinuclear antibody test	In the absence of drugs associated with 'drug-induced lupus'
Immunologic disorder	Antibodies to dsDNA Antibodies to Smith nuclear antigen Positive finding of antiphospholipid antibodies • IgG or IgM anticardiolipin antibodies • Lupus anticoagulant • False positive serologic test for syphilis for at least 6 mth (false positive VDRL) confirmed by Treponema Pallidum Immobilisation (TPI) or Fluorescent Treponemal Antibody (FTA) absorption test

- World Health Organization Classification of Lupus Nephritis (renal biopsy)
  - » Class I: Normal
  - » Class II: Minimal change (A)/mesangial glomerulitis (B)
  - » Class III: Focal and segmental proliferation
  - » Class IV: Diffuse proliferative glomerulonephritis (GN)
  - » Class V: Membranous GN
  - » Class VI: Glomerular sclerosis

Antiphospholipid Syndrome

- Antiphospholipid syndrome (APS) is present if one of the clinical manifestations and one of the laboratory tests on two or more occasions (at least 12 weeks

apart) are demonstrated — recurrent foetal loss or vascular thrombosis (arterial and venous) with lupus anticoagulant, anticardiolipin antibody or anti-beta 2 glycoprotein 1 antibody.
- Other features not included in the classification criteria include leg ulcer, livedo reticularis, haemolytic anaemia and thrombocytopenia.

Neurolupus

- Clinical features may be due to leucostasis, vasculitis, APS with thrombosis, infarct, haemorrhage
- May be overt (seizures, stroke) or subtle (mood change, behavioural change, deterioration in schoolwork)
- Central nervous system: Cerebrovascular disease (stroke/transient ischaemic attack), seizures, headache (excluding migraine and benign intracranial hypertension), demyelinating syndrome, movement disorder (chorea), acute confusional state, anxiety disorder, cognitive dysfunction, mood disorder, psychosis
- Peripheral nervous system: Acute inflammatory demyelinating polyradiculoneuropathy (Guillain–Barré Syndrome), autonomic disorder, mononeuropathy, single/multiplex, myasthaenia gravis, cranial neuropathy, plexopathy, polyneuropathy
- Investigations (Baseline)
  » Full blood count, reticulocyte count, ESR, CRP, urea, creatinine, ALT, AST, GGT, C3, C4, ANA, anti dsDNA, ENA profile, lupus anticoagulant, anticardiolipin antibody of immunoglobulin M (IgM)/IgG, TGAb, TRAb, TPOAb, anti-beta 2 glycoprotein 1 antibody of IgM/IgG
  » Urinalysis, spun urine for casts, urine protein/creatinine ratio

Management Principles

- Aim to bring disease under control and prevent progressive tissue damage
- Avoidance of triggering factors (sun or UV exposure, fatigue, intercurrent infection)
- Steroids remain the mainstay for the induction of remission and treatment of acute flares
- Maintenance medication thereafter to minimise steroid toxicity, choice of medication dependent on manifestations and systems involved
- Plasmapheresis for rapid removal of antibodies and immune complexes, together with steroids and cytotoxic drugs in life-threatening SLE

Differentiating between Lupus Flare and Infection

- Both can present with fever and ill health
- Infection can precipitate a flare out
- Infection important cause of mortality, so have a high index of suspicion
- Often, infection will have high CRP, but active lupus has normal CRP despite high ESR

- Look for evidence of active lupus: Rash, arthritis, serositis, low C3, high dsDNA titre
- If uncertain, may need to cover for both infection and active disease flare until investigations return

Juvenile Dermatomyositis

- Characterised by a diffuse microangiitis resulting in cutaneous manifestations and muscle weakness amongst other complications
- Not uncommon locally, under- and/or delayed diagnosis happens often
- Aetiology unknown. May be triggered by infection

Clinical Features

- Commonly presents with muscle tenderness and weakness, rash on face and extensor surface, constitutional symptoms
- Calcinosis, arthritis, muscle atrophy, alopecia common
- Gastrointestinal, respiratory and CNS disease potentially fatal
- Range of clinical features:
  - Constitutional: Fever, malaise, loss of appetite, loss of weight
  - Skin/mucosa: Heliotrope rash and periorbital oedema, malar rash, Gottron papules, erythroderma, erythematous rash, vasculitic rash, livedo, telangiectasia, periungal capillary changes, skin ulcers, oral ulcers, alopecia, panniculitis, calcinosis, subcutaneous fat atrophy (looks muscular), mechanic's hands (hyperkeratosis, fissures), palmar plantar hyperkeratosis
  - Muscle: Proximal muscle weakness, truncal weakness, speech (nasal), swallowing, breathing difficulty (shortness of breath, exertional dyspnoea)
  - Joints: Arthritis, arthralgia, contractures
  - Gastrointestinal tract: Gut vasculitis (potentially life-threatening), pancreatitis, hepatitis
  - Central nervous system: Vasculitis with seizures, stroke, chorea
  - Lung: Interstitial lung disease, pneumothorax, abnormal lung function
  - Cardiac: Pericarditis, myocarditis, arrhythmia
  - Infection: Prone to infections of skin (calcinotic lesions, S. aureus abscess), lung (suppurative, TB, Pneumocystis jirovecii pneumonia)
  - Other unusual presentations (fluid collections, e.g. seroma of back)

Diagnosis

- Bohan and Peter criteria — presence of all five makes diagnosis definite, four probable and three possible
  - Dermatologic features: Heliotrope rash, Gottron papules
  - Proximal and symmetrical muscle weakness
  - Elevated enzymes (CK, aldolase, AST, ALT, LDH)
  - Typical electromyogram findings
  - Muscle biopsy

- Invasive EMG and muscle biopsy are not done in children unless the diagnosis is uncertain. MRI helps to localise an ideal site for biopsy as muscle disease is patchy (vastus medialis of thigh is a good site). This modality has become a replacement for muscle biopsy in recent years.
- 'Dermatomyositis sine myositis' or Amyopathic juvenile dermatomyositis — characteristic skin disease (e.g. heliotrope rash, Gottron papules, vasculitis, calcinosis) without muscle disease could be a variant, or muscle disease may have subsided or may develop later
- Important to exclude other connective tissue disease (e.g. SLE, MCTD or overlap syndrome)

Evaluation at Diagnosis

- Baseline muscle enzymes, inflammatory markers
- Myositis specific and associated antibodies (myositis panel)
- Document rash, presence of Gottron papules and calcinosis, nailfold capillaritis, muscle power grading
- Objective evaluation of muscle weakness using Manual Muscle Testing (MMT) and Childhood Myositis Assessment Scale (CMAS)
- MRI of bilateral thighs
- Screen for major organ involvement — 2D echocardiogram, ECG, CXR, pulmonary function test/HRCT thorax, barium swallow and meal
- Eye examination/referral to ophthalmologist — baseline for steroid and hydroxychloroquine toxicity monitoring

Treatment

- Glucocorticoids
- Hydroxychloroquine for control of skin disease
- Immunosuppressants: Methotrexate, mycophenolate mofetil, azathioprine, cyclosporine, tacrolimus
- Intravenous immunoglobulin
- Biological and targeted therapies

Henoch-Schonlein Purpura

- Acute small vessel leucocytoclastic IgA1-mediated vasculitis
- The commonest small vessel vasculitis affecting children in Singapore
- History of preceding infection is implicated in the majority
- Self-limiting but can recur in up to a third of affected children

Clinical Presentation

- Cutaneous Purpura (Non-thrombocytopenic)
- Classically non-blanchable palpable purpura, predominantly affecting the dependent area, especially lower limbs and buttock
- Rash may vary from petechiae to ecchymosis, purpura and bullous type

- Rash may persist for weeks to months
- Bruise-like rash is due to deep-seated vasculitis. These ecchymoses are often associated with underlying subcutaneous oedema
- The presence of subcutaneous oedema may precede or be associated with gastrointestinal involvement.
- GI Involvement
  - » Secondary to bowel wall swelling
  - » May present with bloody stool, abdominal pain (colicky if intussusception presents), acute abdomen (if perforation occurs)
  - » GI symptoms may precede an onset of rash in a small number of children
- Arthritis/arthralgia
  - » Presence of arthritis may be confused with underlying subcutaneous oedema. Differentiation between arthritis and subcutaneous oedema is important in the management of patient
  - » May be migratory; involvement of knees and ankles are common
  - » Usually transient, does not result in deformity
- Renal Involvement
  - » Microscopic haematuria (common), proteinuria, renal impairment, end-stage renal failure
  - » May develop months after onset

Investigations

- Blood tests are often not needed unless clinical suspicion of thrombocytopenia/coagulation defect presents
- Elevated IgA level helps with diagnosis but a normal IgA level does not exclude diagnosis
- Urinalysis (to look for haematuria/proteinuria). Urine protein/creatinine ratio or 24 hours urine protein collection may be required.
- Abdominal ultrasound is sometimes required if history/clinical assessment is suggestive of intussusception (may also show thickened bowel wall, suggestive of enteritis/colitis)
- Skin biopsy is often not required (unless in atypical cases)

Treatment

- Supportive (adequate hydration, monitoring of GI and renal involvement)
- Use of steroids is still controversial. However, the use of steroid is well-accepted in patients who have abdominal pain. In some studies, steroid use has shown to reduce the duration and severity of abdominal pain, hospitalisation stay and the need for surgery.
- Early use of steroids does not prevent the progression of renal disease or change the course of illness.
- In the presence of subcutaneous oedema, steroids may be helpful in reducing the swelling and GI-associated complications.
- Serial urinalysis at routine clinic visit is required for 2 years from the disease onset, particularly important for the first 6 months.

- Immunosuppression therapy (cyclophosphamide or azathioprine) may be necessary in refractory or relapse cases or those with renal and/or major organ involvement.

Prognosis

- Self-limiting, good prognosis
- <1% develop end-stage renal failure
- Recurrence rate of 10–30%

Bibliography

1. Tanya M, Teh KL, Das L, *et al.* (2020) Juvenile idiopathic arthritis in Southeast Asia: The Singapore experience over two decades. *Clin Rheumatol* **39**(11):3455–3464.
2. Groot N, de Graeff N, Avcin T, *et al.* (2017) European evidence-based recommendations for diagnosis and treatment of childhood-onset systemic lupus erythematosus: The SHARE initiative. *Ann Rheum Dis* **76**(11):1788–1796.
3. McCann LJ, Livermore P, Wilkinson MGL, Wedderburn LR. (2022) Juvenile dermatomyositis. Where are we now? *Clin Exp Rheumatol* **40**(2):394–403.

CHAPTER 110

Drugs in Rheumatology

Teh Kai Liang; Thaschawee Arkachaisri

Introduction

A wide array of drugs is available for symptomatic, anti-inflammatory and immunomodulation of rheumatic disease to control pain, damage and progression:

- Nonsteroidal anti-inflammatory drugs (NSAIDs)
- Steroids
- Disease-modifying anti-rheumatic drugs
- Cytotoxics
- Biological agents
- Targeted therapies

Other modalities of treatment include:

- Plasmapheresis
- Intravenous Immunoglobulins
- Bone marrow/stem cell transplant

Clinical Pearls

- Patients on long-term steroids have suppression of hypothalamic-pituitary axis. Steroids should not be stopped abruptly, especially when the patient is sick. Stress dose may be depending on the clinical status.
- Other immunosuppressants should be stopped if:
  - » High fever more than 39°C
  - » Evidence of sepsis/bacterial infection
  - » Course of illness expected to be long for specific viruses (e.g. influenza, varicella)
  - » Unstable clinical status awaiting diagnostic tests to rule out infection
- If in doubt, contact on-call rheumatologist before stopping immunosuppressants

Nonsteroidal Anti-inflammatory Drugs (NSAIDs)

- First-line of treatment for arthritis (together with intra-synovial steroids)
- Inhibit the activity of COX enzymes
- Dose-dependent effects:
  - » Low dose: anti-platelet

  - Low-medium: anti-pyretic
  - Medium: analgesic
  - High: anti-inflammatory

Aspirin (Acetylsalicylic Acid)

- Dose:
  - Anti-inflammatory: 80–100 mg/kg/day (max. 3.6 g/day)
  - Anti-platelet: 3–5 mg/kg/day
- Adverse reactions:
  - Gastric irritation (50%)
  - Tinnitus and/or diminished hearing (15%)
  - Hepatotoxicity (50%, 15% cessation of therapy)
  - Reye's syndrome (rare)
  - Hypersensitivity (in asthma) (rare)
  - Salicylism

Cyclo-oxygenase-2 (COX-2) Selective Inhibitors

- Selectively inhibit COX-2 enzyme with minimal effect on COX-1 enzyme at recommended doses, thus safer (gastrointestinal) and comparably effective for acute and chronic pain relief
- Potentially useful in patients with:
  - Poor gastrointestinal tolerance of traditional NSAIDs
  - Low platelet patients
  - Sensitivity to traditional NSAIDs

Steroids

- Among the most potent anti-inflammatory drugs. Mainstay of treatment for many severe rheumatic diseases such as SLE, JDM, vasculitis and, rarely, arthritis.
- Dramatic effects but prolonged administration at high dose gives unacceptable toxicity, therefore limit the dose and duration of treatment.
- Use as induction therapy
- Irreversible adverse reactions in children include
  - Posterior subcapsular cataract
  - Osteonecrosis/AVN
  - Striae rubrae
- More susceptible to infection, e.g. tuberculosis (TB), herpes virus to avoid crowded places, seek treatment early if febrile, contact with chickenpox, measles. Signs of infection may be masked, so have a high level of suspicion
- Physical appearance changes: Cushingoid habitus, weight gain, rounded face, buffalo hump, acne, stretch marks, hirsutism
- Metabolic changes: Hyperglycaemia, hypercholesterolaemia, sodium and water retention, hypokalaemia, hypertension

- Neurological: Euphoria, depression, mood lability, psychosis, pseudotumour cerebri
- Musculoskeletal: Osteopenia, proximal myopathy, avascular necrosis

Disease Modifying Anti-Rheumatic Drugs (DMARDs)

- Onset of action slow over weeks or months

Methotrexate (MTX)

- Effective and generally well-tolerated in children
- Give with folic acid daily, avoid sulphur drugs and alcohol
- Side effects: Bone marrow suppression (megaloblastic anaemia, lymphopenia), hepatic (enzyme elevation), gastrointestinal, including nausea, oral ulcers

Sulphasalazine

- Before use: Ensure no allergy and/or G6PD deficiency
- Side-effects include rash, gastritis, liver dysfunction, renal dysfunction and bone marrow suppression

Hydroxychloroquine

- Anti-malarial drug with moderate anti-inflammatory properties
- G6PD deficiency — relative contraindication
- Side-effects: Macular degeneration, corneal deposit (therefore requires annual eye check), gastric irritation, skin rash (reversible, dark skin discoloration)

Immunosuppressives and Cytotoxics

Cyclophosphamide

- Alkylating agent with potent anti-inflammatory action, use limited by toxicity
- Side effects: Nausea and vomiting, myelo- and immunosuppression greatest in the second week post IV pulse (fall in total WBC), liver toxicity, haemorrhagic cystitis, long-term risk of secondary malignancies, gonadal damage with hormonal deficiency and sterility, SIADH

Mycophenolate Mofetil (MMF)

- Inhibits purine synthesis in T and B cells (selective non-competitive inhibitor)
- Side effects: Bone marrow suppression, gastrointestinal, weakness/numbness, tremors

Azathioprine

- Purine analogue
- Side-effects: Oral ulcers, gastrointestinal, bone marrow suppression, liver toxicity increased by enzyme deficiency (thiopurine methyltransferase [TPMT])

Cyclosporin A

- T-cell mediated immunosuppression (calcineurin inhibitor)
- Side effects: Alopecia, hirsutism, gingival hyperplasia, tremors, paraesthesia, hypertension, renal damage, nausea and vomiting
- Drug monitoring: Trough levels (150–250 mcg/ml, but do not correlate well clinically)

Intravenous Immunoglobulins

- First-line for Kawasaki disease, as adjunct therapy in other rheumatic diseases
- Dose:
  - » Replacement therapy: 400–500 mg/kg/dose
  - » Anti-inflammatory: 2 g/kg/dose
- Post IVIg haemolysis may occur, requiring a short course of oral prednisolone. To monitor FBC, retic and DCT.

Biologic Agents

Etanercept

- Tumour necrosis factor (TNF) receptor analogue — competitively binds TNF and inhibits natural receptors from binding
- Combination MTX and Etanercept increases efficacy with acceptable toxicity
- Side effects: Injection site reactions are not uncommon
- No increased rate of infection, but try to complete immunisation before starting etanercept; if in contact with chickenpox, give VZIG or PO/IV acyclovir

Infliximab

- Chimeric monoclonal antibody to TNF alpha
- Risk of anaphylaxis, reactivation of TB
- Contraindicated in TB, heart failure and during intercurrent infection

Adalimumab

- Humanised monoclonal antibody against TNF alpha
- Side effects similar to Etanercept

CHAPTER 111

Rheumatological Investigations

Teh Kai Liang; Thaschawee Arkachaisri

Erythrocyte Sedimentation Rate (ESR)

- Non-specific test that indicates the presence and intensity of inflammation
- Non-diagnostic but can be used to follow inflammatory activity
- Normal values
  - » Male: 1–10 mm/hr
  - » Female: 3–15 mm/hr

Table 23.4 Factors that Interfere with ESR Level

Increase	Decrease
Increase in fibrinogen, gamma or beta globulins	Abnormal RBC shape, i.e. sickle cell, spherocyte, microcytosis
Macrocytosis	Hypofibrinogenaemia
Hypercholesterolaemia	High WBC, polycythaemia
Drugs (dextran, methyldopa, penicillamine, throphylline, vitamin A)	Congestive heart failure
Technical factors	High dose adrenal steroids
Tilted tube	Cachexia
High room temperature	Drugs (aspirin, quinine, drugs causing high sugar level)
Female	Technical factors
Pregnancy	Low room temperature
Smoking	Delay test >2 hr
	Clotted blood sample
	Excess anticoagulation
	Bubbles in tube

Adapted from Wallach J. (2007) *Interpretation of Diagnostic Tests*, 8th ed.

C-Reactive Protein

- Appears within 24–48 hours with the peak at 72 hours. Half-life approximately 18 hours
- Increase indicates active inflammation except in SLE and related diseases unless infection is present
- Normal values: <10 mg/L

Rheumatoid Factor

- Antibodies against Fc portion of IgG
- Non-specific tests can be increased in certain infections and many other systemic autoimmune disorders
- Normal value: <10.3 U/ml

Antinuclear Antibodies

- Detected by immunofluorescence (IF) or ELISA
- Non-specific even for autoimmune disorders
- Could be positive in non-systemic autoimmune diseases, including infections, malignancy, old age, especially female, chronic active hepatitis
- Normal: <1:100 titre

Anti-dsDNA

- Present in 60–90% of childhood onset SLE (cSLE), ~90% of local cSLE
- Aids in SLE diagnosis and often fluctuates with lupus disease activity, especially lupus nephritis in some patients
- Crithidia assay detects antibodies that bind to double-stranded DNA located at Crithidia luciliae kinetoplast (a protozoan organism with a double-stranded circular DNA structure at one pole). This assay detects antibodies to double-stranded DNA almost exclusively.
- Should not be used alone in following cSLE patient's disease activity or predicting flare
- Normal: <25 U/ml (ELISA)

Antiphospholipid Antibodies (APA)

- Bind chiefly to negatively charged phospholipids like cardiolipin
- Three tests available that detect slightly different but overlapping populations of antibodies:
  - » Venereal Disease Research Laboratory test false positive — limited use
  - » Lupus anticoagulant — more sensitive functional coagulation assay
  - » Anticardiolipin antibodies
  - » Anti-beta 2 glycoprotein 1 antibodies
- Significant value: >40 GPL/MPL (IgG or IgM)

Antineutrophil Cytoplasmic Antibodies (ANCA)

- Binds to antigens in cytoplasm of neutrophils two patterns on alcohol-fixed IIF:
  - » Cytoplasmic ANCA (cANCA; cytoplasmic diffuse staining)
  - » Perinuclear ANCA (pANCA; peripheral staining around edge of nucleus)

- Anti-proteinase 3 (PR3) normal value: <10 U/ml
- Anti-myeloperoxidase (MPO) normal value: <20 RU/ml

Complements

- Complement cascade plays a central role in cell lysis, opsonisation of bacteria, clearance of immune complexes
- Elevated in inflammation as part of the acute-phase response
- Fall with immune complex consumption (especially active lupus nephritis, cytopenia, haemolysis)

Table 23.5 Complement C3, Serum Reference

Age	Gender	Reference Interval (g/L)
0–14 d	All	0.50–1.21
15 d–<1 yr	All	0.51–1.60
1–< 19 yr	All	0.83–1.52
19–80 yr	Male	0.82–1.85
19–80 yr	Female	0.83–1.93

Table 23.6 Complement C4, Serum Reference

Age	Gender	Reference Interval (g/L)
0–<1 yr	All	0.07–0.30
1–19 yr	All	0.13–0.37
19–80 yr	Male	0.15–0.53
19–80 yr	Female	0.15–0.57

SECTION 24

SLEEP MEDICINE

CHAPTER 112

Healthy Sleep in Children

Ting Chun Yi; Cheng Zai Ru

Introduction

Many people often mistake sleep as a period of inactivity that one passively enters at the end of a day's activities. Rather, there are many important physiological processes that actively take place during sleep. Sleep is essential for many vital functions such as growth hormone secretion, energy conservation, immune response modulation, cognition, physical performance, vigilance and mood regulation. Sleep is as crucial as the pillars of nutrition, exercise and social interactions are towards a healthy childhood.

Normal Sleep Development

Both sleep quantity and sleep quality are equally important. Good quality sleep in children can be defined by:

- The ability to fall asleep independently within 30 minutes of bedtime
- Maintaining sleep through the night
- Waking up refreshed

Newborns do not understand the concept of day or night and may wake every 1.5 to 3 hours. They may wake due to hunger, the need for a diaper change or to be carried.

A regular diurnal rhythm is usually established after 3 months, with gradual consolidation of sleep into the night and daytime sleep organised into naps. However, only 70% of 3-month-old babies regularly sleep throughout the night. This rises to about 90% by 9 months. Night awakenings in infants still happen often and many do not have the ability to sleep through the night. Daytime naps are usually dropped from around 3 to 5 years old.

Sleep quantity gradually decreases with age and can vary from person to person. Table 24.1 illustrates the general guidelines for total sleep requirements amongst children of varying ages.

Table 24.1 Sleep Requirements by Age (National Sleep Foundation)

Age Group	Recommended Sleep Durations (hours of sleep)
Newborn 0–3 mth	14–17
Infant 4–11 mth	12–15
Toddler 1–2 yr	11–14
Pre-schooler 3–5 yr	10–13
School age 6–13 yr	9–11
Teen 14–17 yr	8–10
Young adult 18–25 yr	7–9

Assessment of Sleep Problems

The BEARS questionnaire provides a practical guide in obtaining a comprehensive sleep history:

	Pre-school (2–5 years)	School-aged (6–12 years)	Adolescent (13–18 years)
Bedtime problems	P: Does your child have any problems going to bed? Falling asleep?	P: Does your child have any problems at bedtime? C: Do you have any problems going to bed?	C: Do you have any problems falling asleep at bedtime?
Excessive daytime sleepiness	P: Does your child seem overtired or sleepy a lot during the day? Does he/she still take naps?	P: Does your child have difficulty waking in the morning, seem sleepy during the day, or take naps? C: Do you feel tired a lot?	C: Do you feel sleepy a lot during the day? In school? While driving?
Awakenings during the night	P: Does your child wake up a lot at night?	P: Does your child seem to wake up a lot at night? Any sleepwalking or nightmares? C: Do you wake up a lot at night? Have trouble getting back to sleep?	C: Do you wake up a lot at night? Have trouble getting back to sleep?
Regularity and duration of sleep	P: Does your child have a regular bedtime and wake time? What are they?	P: What time does your child go to bed and get up on school days? Weekends? Do you think he/she is getting enough sleep?	C: What time do you usually go to bed on school nights? Weekends? How much sleep do you usually get?
Sleep-disordered breathing	P: Does your child snore a lot or have difficulty breathing at night?	P: Does your child have loud of nightly snoring or any breathing difficulties at night?	P: Does your teenager snore loudly or nightly?

C: Child; P: Parent

Other Corroborative History

- Sleep environment
  - » Sleep props, screen use, bedroom sharing arrangement
- Factors that disrupt sleep
  - » Acute: Recent illnesses, stressor, change in sleep schedule or naps
  - » Chronic medical conditions, e.g. eczema, asthma, allergic rhinitis
- Medical history
  - » Comorbid medical problems together with a child's distress will understandably present challenges for parents to implement behavioural strategies
- Developmental history
  - » Developmental delays should be accounted for, as sleep problems reflect the child's developmental age, not chronological age
- Family history
  - » Maternal depression, anxiety
  - » Family members with sleep disorders
- Social history
  - » Tolerance of family towards the child's behaviour at night, presence of consistence routines and/or caregivers
- Psychological history
  - » Child's temperament, e.g. daytime anxiety, insecure parent–child attachments

Clinical Examination

- Signs of chronic medical conditions affecting the child's sleep, e.g. asthma, eczema, allergic rhinitis
- Signs and presence of risk factors of obstructive sleep apnoea (OSA)

Investigations

- Diagnostic tests usually not indicated unless concerns of symptoms and signs of underlying OSA or medical disorders, e.g. reflux or restless legs syndrome

Common Paediatric Sleep Issues

Limit-Setting Issues

- Typically begin after age 2 years.
- Child able to independently climb out of their crib or bed
- Inadequate enforcement of bedtime limits by caregiver
  - » Requests are based on what the child has learned will elicit a parental response
  - » Bedtime refusal and stalling, resulting in a delay in sleep and inadequate sleep to meet the child's needs
  - » Delaying bedtime, e.g. watching more TV
  - » Prolonging bedtime routine, e.g. reading another bedtime story
  - » Curtain calls occurring after lights out, e.g. requests for another hug or drink of water

- » Bedtime refusal, e.g. refusal to get ready for bed, attempts to leave bedroom
- No limits
  - » Falling asleep while watching TV
  - » Giving the child the liberty to decide on screen use limits, allowing screen devices within easy reach of the child in the bedroom
- Inconsistent limits
  - » Intermittently allowing the child to choose where and when to fall asleep
  - » Limits change with the caregiver, e.g. conflicting styles amongst grandparents, domestic helper, parents

Sleep Onset Associations

- Inappropriate sleep onset associations that require parental intervention and cannot be re-established independently during the child's night awakening (e.g. rocking, nursing, swinging)
- During normal periodic night-time arousals, the child is unable to self soothe and return to sleep as these same conditions and associations are required for child to fall back to sleep

Management

- Developmentally appropriate and consistent sleep schedule
  - » Keep daytime naps till at least 3 to 5 years of age
- Consistent 20–30 minutes calming bedtime routine ending up in a darkened and cool bedroom free from screen devices
- Transitional objects
- Teaching the child to sleep independently and self-soothe
  - » Provides significant sleep benefits yet convey no long-term adverse effects on parent–child attachment or the child's emotions and behaviour
  - » Avoid responding to the infant's movements or sounds immediately during the night, allowing opportunity for the infant to self-soothe
  - » Methods:
    1. i. Extinction 'crying it out' — may be emotionally challenging for parents
    2. ii. Graduated extinction — similar to extinction, but with scheduled 'check-ins'
    3. iii. Fading of adult intervention
- Weaning off night-time feeds
- Reward charts (for pre-schoolers)
- When to refer:
  - » Child has symptoms of another underlying sleep disrupter (e.g. sleep-disordered breathing, restless legs)
  - » Clinically distressing and disruptive, not responding to initial first-line behavioural strategies

Parasomnias

Parasomnias are undesirable behaviours or events that disturb sleep and may occur during entry into sleep, within sleep or during arousals from sleep. Most parasomnias such as confusional arousals, sleepwalking and sleep terrors occur during NREM sleep, whereas nightmares occur during REM sleep. NREM-related parasomnias tend to occur in the first half of the sleep period, and children usually do not have recollection of the episode.

Risk Factors for Parasomnias

- Positive family history of parasomnias
- Associated conditions, e.g. migraine headaches, Tourette syndrome
- Factors that trigger disorders of arousal:
  - » Inadequate sleep
  - » Irregular sleep schedules
  - » Sleep disturbances, e.g. sleep-disordered breathing
  - » Caffeine

Types of Parasomnias

- **Confusional arousals**
  - » Onset 2 to 10 years of age, typically before age 5 years
  - » Child sits up in bed, cries and may appear agitated, distressed, disoriented or even inconsolable
  - » Episodes are brief, lasting for about 2 to 15 minutes
- **Sleepwalking**
  - » Onset 4 to 6 years of age, peak occurrence between ages 8 and 12
  - » Child may sit in bed, walk around the room or house or engage in other (sometimes bizarre) activities
  - » Child does not interact meaningfully with others, and speech is often unintelligible
  - » May persist till late adolescence or even adulthood
- **Sleep Terrors**
  - » Onset usually 4 to 12 years of age
  - » Sudden arousals from sleep that are accompanied by extreme fear, often involving crying, screaming and agitation
  - » Associated with autonomic manifestations such as facial flushing, hyperventilation, tachycardia, mydriasis and diaphoresis
  - » Child may resist comfort with escalation of symptoms (e.g. kicking, screaming) when caregiver intervenes
    - ▪ This may be distressing to watch but episodes present no harm to the child
  - » In most children, the episodes gradually improve spontaneously and decrease in frequency over the years and almost always resolve by late childhood
- **Nightmares**
  - » Onset 3 to 6 years of age, peak prevalence between ages 6 and 10

  - Vivid dreams that are associated with negative emotional responses such as fear, but these emotions are not as intense as sleep terrors
  - Child often fully awakes and has clear memory of the event (unlike NREM-related parasomnias)

Evaluation

- History
  - Usually benign
  - Ask for risk factors of seizures and other sleep problems
  - Find out about any recent acute sleep disruptors, e.g. illness, stressor, change in sleep schedule or naps
  - Development and child's behaviour are usually normal
  - Family history may be present
- Clinical examination: Generally normal
- Diagnostic tests: Polysomnography not routinely indicated unless concerned about an underlying sleep disorder. These arousal events are episodic and may not be captured in a single night study

Differential Diagnoses

- Nocturnal seizures: May involve stereotypic or tonic-clonic movements, happen multiple times per night, occur after the first third of the night and are usually associated with daytime sleepiness
- Nocturnal panic attacks: Child generally has similar episodes that occur in the daytime and the child has recollection of the episode the next day

Management

- Parental reassurance that parasomnias are generally benign and sleep-limiting and not indicative of an underlying psychopathology
- Pharmacotherapy is rarely indicated

Table 24.2 Main Clinical Characteristics of Parasomnias

	Confusional Arousal	Sleepwalking	Sleep Terrors	Nightmares
Peak time of occurrence	First third of sleep period	First third of sleep period	First third of sleep period	Last third of sleep period
Autonomic activity	No	Maybe	Increased	No
Arousal threshold	High	High	High	Low
Getting out of bed	Rare	Usual	Sometimes	No
Recall of event	No	No	No	Yes
Terminated by	Returning to sleep	Returning to bed and sleep	Returning to sleep	Usually awaken the sleeper

- For NREM-related parasomnias:
  - » Environmental safety:
    - ■ Safety measures — use of gates, locking the outside of doors and windows, removing sharp or dangerous objects
    - ■ Parent notification measures — attach bell to the bedroom door
  - » Healthy sleep habits:
    - ■ Ensure sufficient sleep (as inadequate sleep can trigger such episodes)
    - ■ Good sleep hygiene, avoid caffeine
  - » Parental response during an event:
    - ■ Avoid waking the child up as he/she is truly asleep, and attempts to awaken child usually increases agitation
    - ■ Guide the child back to bed
    - ■ Avoid trying to terminate the episodes
    - ■ Avoid next-day discussions — as child cannot recollect event and may cause undue anxiety, resulting in bedtime resistance
  - » Scheduled awakening
    - ■ May help to prevent partial arousal parasomnias, especially if the episodes occur nightly
    - ■ Parents wake their child 15 to 20 minutes before the expected time of occurrence, just to the point of arousal. This helps to modify the sleep state and thereby abort the episode
    - ■ Should be continued for 2 to 4 weeks but may be difficult for parents to implement practically
- For nightmares:
  - » Parental response: Offer comfort and reassurance
  - » Reduce likelihood of nightmares:
    - ■ Gently question child to identify any possible fearful experiences, and then try to minimise potential triggers
  - » Management of frequent nightmares
    - ■ Imagery rehearsal — develop an alternative ending to a frequently experienced dream and rehearsing that imagery during the day
    - ■ Systematic desensitisation — develop a hierarchy of fear-inducing activities from least to most frightening, and then pair these activities with a relaxing activity that counteracts the fear response
- When to refer:
  - » Night wakings resulting in injury to the child or exposure to potentially dangerous scenarios or nightmares that are extremely disruptive
  - » Very frequent episodes disrupting family members' sleep
  - » Has symptoms of another underlying sleep disorder, e.g. sleep-disordered breathing

Bibliography

1. National Sleep Foundation (nd) Recommended sleep durations. www.thensf.org
2. Mindell J, Owens J. (2009) *A Clinical Guide to Pediatric Sleep: Diagnosis and Management of Sleep Problems, 3rd ed.* Lippincott Williams & Wilkins.
3. Owens JA, Dalzell V. (2005) Use of the 'BEARS' sleep screening tool in a pediatric residents' continuity clinic: A pilot study. *Sleep Med* **6**(1):63–69.
4. Gradisar M, Jackson K, Spurrier N, *et al.* (2016) Behavioral interventions for infant sleep problems: A randomized controlled trial. *Pediatrics* **137**(6):e20151486.
5. Ophoff D, Slaats MA, Boudewyns A, *et al.* (2018) Sleep disorders during childhood: A practical review. *Eur J Pediatr* **177**(5):641–648.
6. Kotagal S. (2009) Parasomnias in childhood. *Sleep Med Rev* **13**(2):157–168.

CHAPTER 113

Obstructive Sleep Apnoea

Tan Yi Hua; Teoh Oon Hoe

Introduction

The incidence of obstructive sleep apnoea (OSA) is estimated to be 1.2–5.7% in children of all ages.

Paediatric obstructive sleep disordered breathing exists in a continuum:

- Primary snoring — snoring without associated apnoea, hypoventilation, hypoxaemia, hypercarbia, sleep disruption or daytime symptoms.
- Upper airway resistance syndrome — partial upper airway obstruction sufficient to cause sleep disruption and daytime symptoms with no observable obstructive events and gas exchange abnormalities.
- Obstructive hypoventilation — continuous partial upper airway obstruction during sleep with hypoxaemia and hypercarbia in the absence of cyclic discrete obstructive events.
- OSA — recurrent episodes of prolonged partial upper airway obstruction or intermittent complete or partial upper airway obstruction during sleep, usually associated with hypoxaemia, hypercarbia and sleep fragmentation.

Risk Factors and High Risk Groups

The most common risk factors in children are adenotonsillar hypertrophy, allergic rhinitis and obesity. Many other risk factors for OSA involve conditions that affect the neural control, size or collapsibility of the upper airway. Other important high risk groups are children with:

- Trisomy 21 (hypotonia, macroglossia, mid-face hypoplasia, obesity, hypothyroidism)
- Genetic disorders, e.g. achondroplasia, Prader–Willi syndrome, mucopolysaccharidoses
- Craniofacial abnormalities, e.g. Apert syndrome, Crouzon syndrome, Pierre–Robin sequence
- Upper airway abnormalities, e.g. laryngomalacia, glottic/subglottic stenosis, choanal stenosis, cleft palate
- Neuromuscular disorders, e.g. Duchenne muscular dystrophy, spinal muscular atrophy, myasthaenia gravis
- Spina bifida/Chiari malformation
- Prematurity

- Family history of OSA

Presentation

Habitual snoring (3 or more nights per week) is the key presentation in children with OSA. However, not all children with OSA present with a history of snoring, possibly due to limited awareness and observation by caregivers, or misinterpretation of snoring as other respiratory noises at night, e.g. wheezing, nasal congestion. Symptoms or signs suggestive of OSA in snoring children include:

- Observed cyanosis/apnoea, snorting, gasping during sleep
- Laboured/paradoxical breathing during sleep
- Unusual sleeping position, hyperextended neck
- Mouth breathing
- Restlessness and frequent awakening
- Diaphoresis
- Primary or secondary nocturnal enuresis or nocturia
- Difficulty getting up in the morning
- Unrefreshed after an overnight sleep
- Morning headaches
- Excessive daytime sleepiness
- Behavioural and learning problems, e.g. hyperactivity, inattention, aggressive behaviour, poor school performance
- Failure to thrive or obesity

Consequences of longstanding untreated significant OSA include:

- Neurobehavioural and cognitive impairment
- Growth failure
- Systemic hypertension, pulmonary hypertension, cor pulmonale
- Gastroesophageal reflux
- Insulin resistance and metabolic syndrome
- Obesity hypoventilation and death in severe cases

History

As children with OSA may have other co-existing sleep disorders, in addition to the risk factors and symptoms above, history should also include:

- Bedtime, wake time, sleep duration and regularity on weekdays and weekends
- Sleep hygiene, e.g. activity before sleep, sleep environment
- Bedtime problems, e.g. bedtime resistance, insomnia
- Parasomnias, e.g. sleepwalking, confusional arousals

If there is moderate to severe excessive daytime sleepiness (e.g. sleep attacks, falling asleep during exams, while talking to someone), consider narcolepsy and screen in the history for cataplexy (sudden loss of muscle tone triggered by strong emotions, e.g. laughter, surprise, anger), sleep paralysis and hypnagogic (sleep onset) hallucinations.

If there is restless sleep with reported leg movements, consider restless leg syndrome and periodic leg movement disorder and screen in the history for an urge to move the legs, accompanied by uncomfortable or unpleasant sensations in the legs. The urge and sensations often begin or worsen during periods of rest/inactivity (e.g. lying, sitting), are partially or totally relieved by movement (e.g. walking, stretching) and worse in the evening/night than during the day.

Clinical Examination

- Growth parameters, BMI — obesity, failure to thrive
- Blood pressure — hypertension
- Craniofacial features — mid-face hypoplasia, flat nasal bridge, facial asymmetry, retrognathia, micrognathia
- Nasal patency — signs of allergic rhinitis, deviated nasal septum, mouth breathing, hyponasal speech
- Oropharynx examination — tonsillar hypertrophy (using the Brodsky grading scale), oropharyngeal narrowing, large tongue, high-arched palate, Mallampati classification
- Noisy breathing — stridor, hoarse/weak voice
- Chest deformity — pectus excavatum
- Pulmonary hypertension — loud second heart sound

Investigations

If OSA is suspected, refer to the Sleep Clinic for review and scheduling of an overnight polysomnography (PSG), which is the gold standard for diagnosis of OSA.

While a PSG is generally preferred, there are real-world issues, including high costs, limited availability, longer wait time and tolerability of the many sensors placed on the body during PSG in very young children, especially those with special needs. Overnight oximetry is easier and less costly to perform, but has its limitations, e.g. low sensitivity, inability to differentiate between obstructive and central apnoea. The Sleep Clinic will discuss with parents about the investigation best suited to their child's situation.

Home unattended PSGs and other multichannel sleep apnoea tests are well established in the adult setting, but are not as well validated in paediatrics. These are emerging alternative investigations that may play an important role in time to come.

If narcolepsy is suspected, a multiple sleep latency test (MSLT) that is performed the next day after an overnight PSG can be considered.

Management

Management of each child depends on the cause(s) and severity of the OSA, extent of impairment from the OSA, and co-existing medical conditions (e.g. congenital heart disease, metabolic complications of obesity). Treatment options may involve one or a combination of the options below:

- **Tonsillectomy and adenoidectomy (T&A)** is the first-line treatment for children with adenotonsillar hypertrophy, with good response in most children. Outpatient surgery is not recommended in children with increased risk of post-operative respiratory complications, e.g. younger than 3 years, severe OSA, severe obesity, failure to thrive, co-existing cardiac/respiratory conditions, cor pulmonale, craniofacial abnormalities, neurological/neuromuscular disorders, Trisomy 21 and achondroplasia. These children require close post-operative monitoring. As they are also at higher risk of incomplete resolution of the OSA after T&A, a low threshold for repeat evaluation is recommended, especially if there are persistent or recurring symptoms. Nutritional counselling and physical activity advice should be provided to overweight children, as T&A may be associated with increased weight gain in children after surgery.
- **Continuous positive airway pressure (CPAP) therapy** is indicated for long-term use in children with significant OSA, where surgery has no role (e.g. OSA due to obesity without adenotonsillar hypertrophy), or children with significant residual OSA after T&A. Bi-level positive airway pressure may be used for better tolerance in severe OSA requiring high CPAP or children with certain neuromuscular disorders. Although CPAP therapy is effective, acceptance and adherence can be a limiting factor in children. CPAP education before initiation of CPAP, behavioural interventions and supportive interventions for side effects of CPAP use can help to improve adherence with CPAP therapy. Regular titration PSGs are necessary as pressure requirements can change in a growing child.
- **Medications** such as intranasal steroids and/or oral montelukast may be treatment options in children with mild OSA where parents do not wish to consider surgical options. Children on medications alone for treatment should be reviewed for response, and treatment options reconsidered if there is no improvement or worsening of the OSA. Medications that help with maintaining nasal passage patency, e.g. intranasal steroids and/or nasal saline are also important adjunctive therapy for OSA, particularly for children on CPAP therapy.
- **Weight loss** is an important part of management for overweight children with OSA. All overweight children should be given nutritional and physical activity counselling. Referral to a weight management clinic should be considered if a child has difficulty with weight management, metabolic complications of obesity or is morbidly obese.
- **Other surgical techniques** such as uvulopalatopharyngoplasty, epiglottoplasty, tongue base reduction, tracheostomy, mandibular advancement and other craniofacial surgery are treatment options considered only in a select group of children with complex OSA and not routinely performed.
- **Orthodontic procedures** such as rapid maxillary expansion may be considered in a select group of children with complex OSA related to maxillary constriction.

- **Myofunctional therapy** are specialised oral and oropharyngeal exercises strengthening dilator muscles of the upper airway that play a pivotal role in the patency of the airway during sleep. There is limited but positive evidence for its role as an adjunct treatment in mild to moderate OSA in children currently.

Most children with mild to moderate OSA due to adenotonsillar hypertrophy alone have good response to T&A with a complete resolution of symptoms. Repeat PSG after surgery to evaluate for residual OSA is indicated in children with partial resolution of symptoms, severe OSA and significant risk factors, e.g. Trisomy 21, morbid obesity. Children with high risk for OSA should have long-term follow up with the Sleep Clinic to monitor for recurrence, while children with low risk and resolution of symptoms after T&A can return to follow up with their primary care physicians.

Bibliography

1. Marcus CL, Brooks LJ, Draper KA, *et al.* (2012) Diagnosis and management of childhood obstructive sleep apnea syndrome. *Pediatrics* **130**(3):e714–e755.
2. Kaditis AG, Alonso Alvarez ML, Boudewyns A, *et al.* (2016) Obstructive sleep disordered breathing in 2- to 18-year-old children: Diagnosis and management. *Eur Respir J* **47**(1):69–94.
3. Ng DK, Huang YS, Teoh OH, *et al.* (2017) The Asian Paediatric Pulmonology Society (APPS) position statement on childhood obstructive sleep apnoea syndrome. *Paediatr Respirol Crit Care Med* **1**:26–38.
4. Tan YH, How CH, Chan YH, Teoh OH. (2020) Approach to the snoring child. *Sing Med J* **61**(4):170–175.

APPENDIX I

GROWTH CHARTS

PERCENTILES OF HEAD CIRCUMFERENCE-FOR-AGE GIRLS AGED 0 TO 24 MONTHS

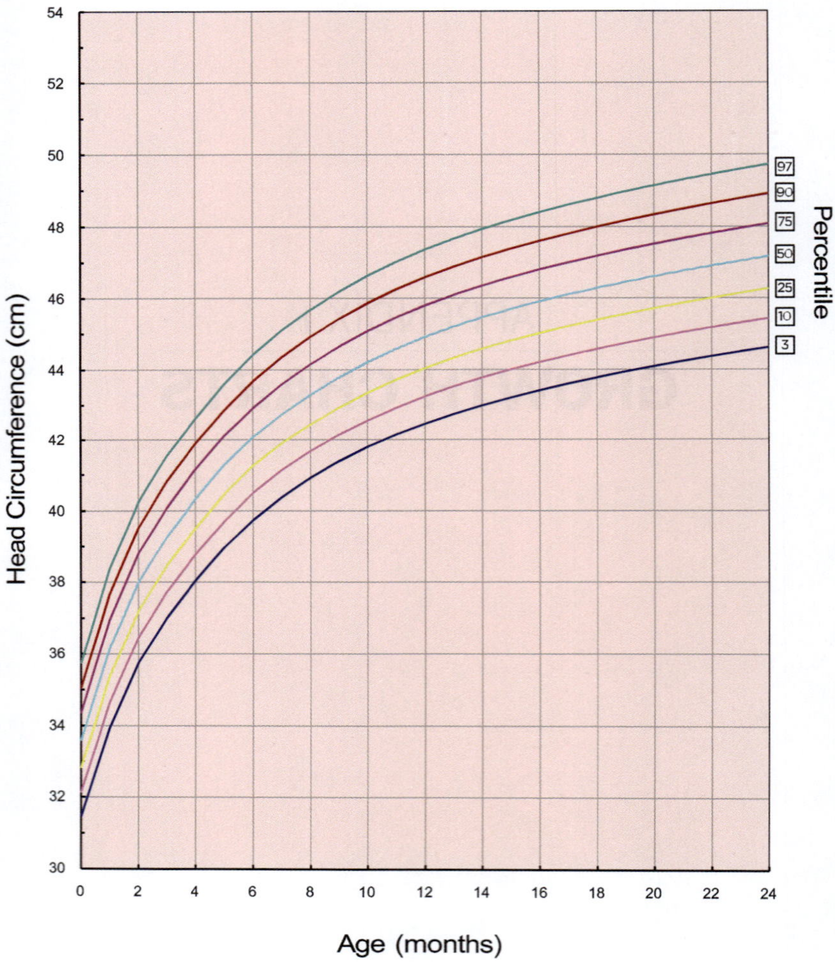

Anthropometric Study on Pre-School Children in Singapore, 2000
National Healthcare Group Polyclinics

PERCENTILES OF HEAD CIRCUMFERENCE-FOR-AGE BOYS AGED 0 TO 24 MONTHS

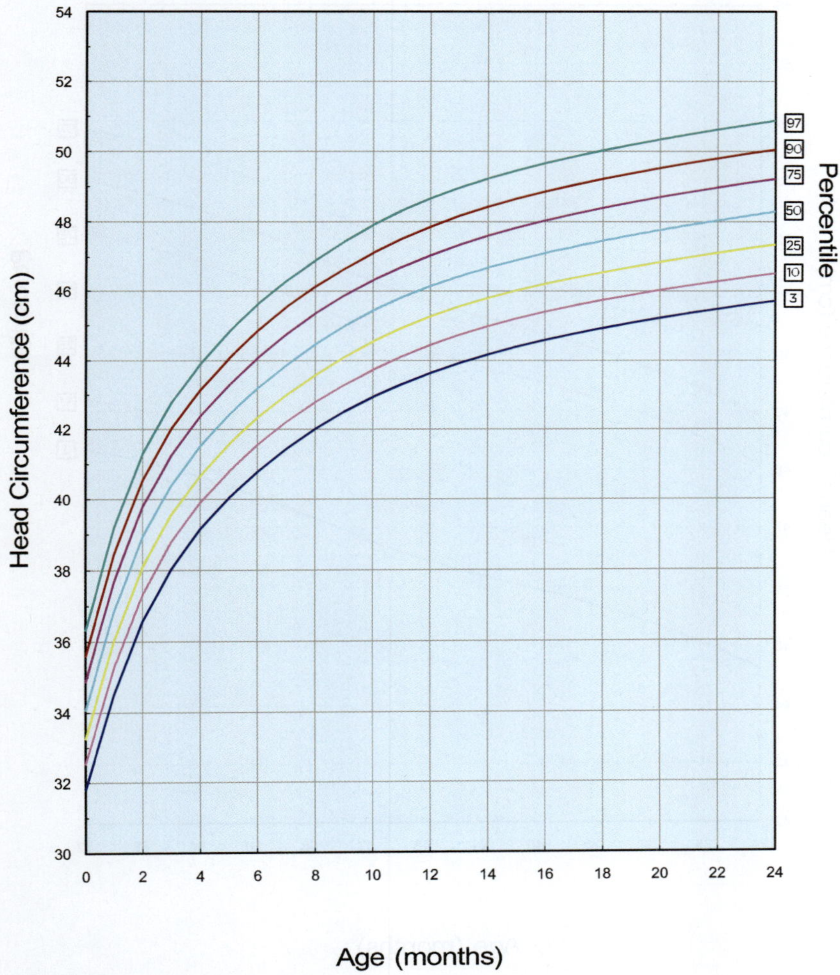

Anthropometric Study on Pre-School Children in Singapore, 2000
National Healthcare Group Polyclinics

PERCENTILES OF HEAD CIRCUMFERENCE-FOR-AGE GIRLS AGED 24 TO 72 MONTHS

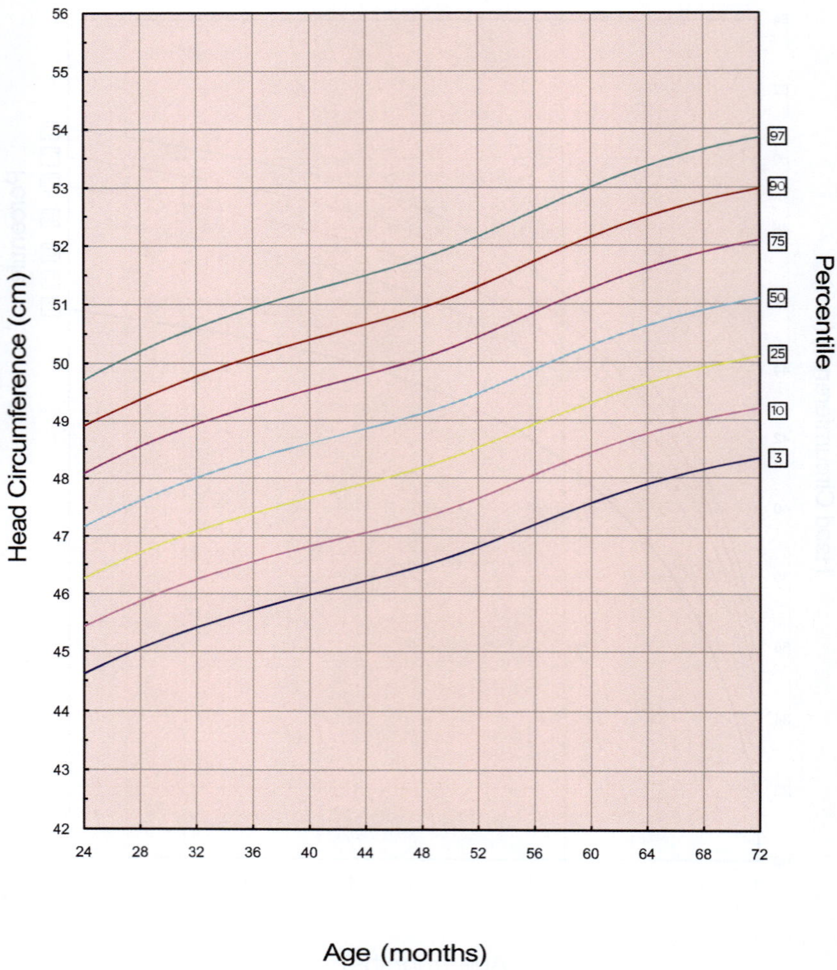

Anthropometric Study on Pre-School Children in Singapore, 2000
National Healthcare Group Polyclinics

PERCENTILES OF HEAD CIRCUMFERENCE-FOR-AGE BOYS AGED 24 TO 72 MONTHS

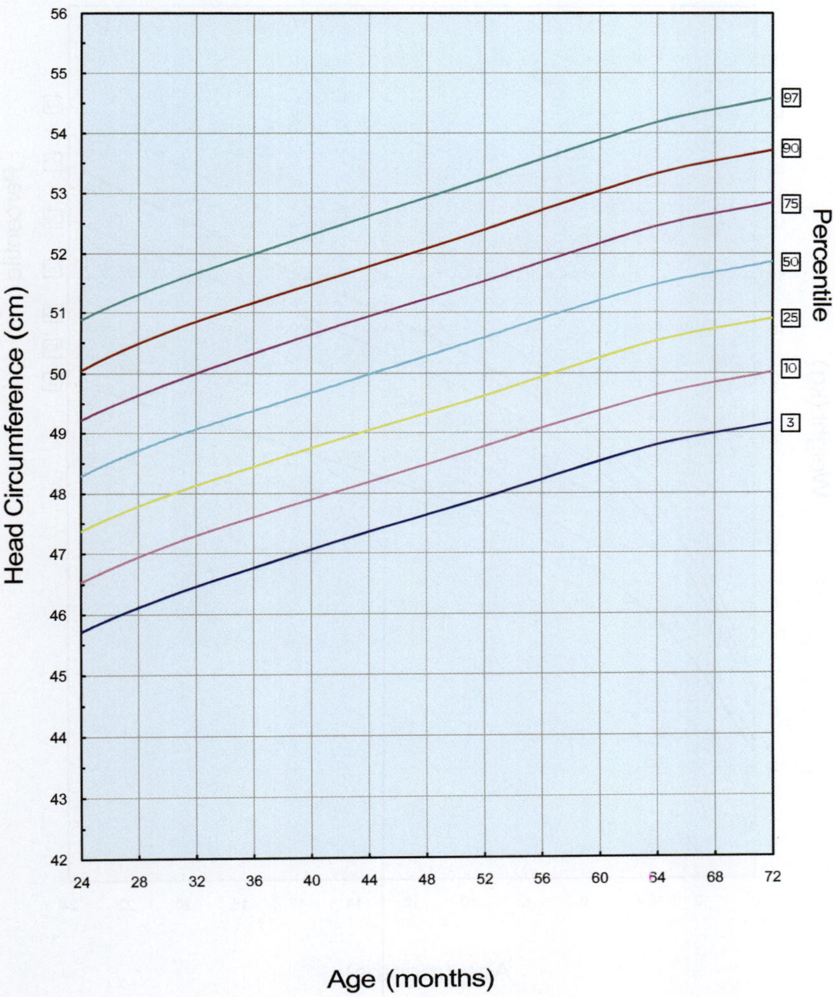

Anthropometric Study on Pre-School Children in Singapore, 2000
National Healthcare Group Polyclinics

PERCENTILES OF WEIGHT-FOR-AGE GIRLS AGED 0 TO 24 MONTHS

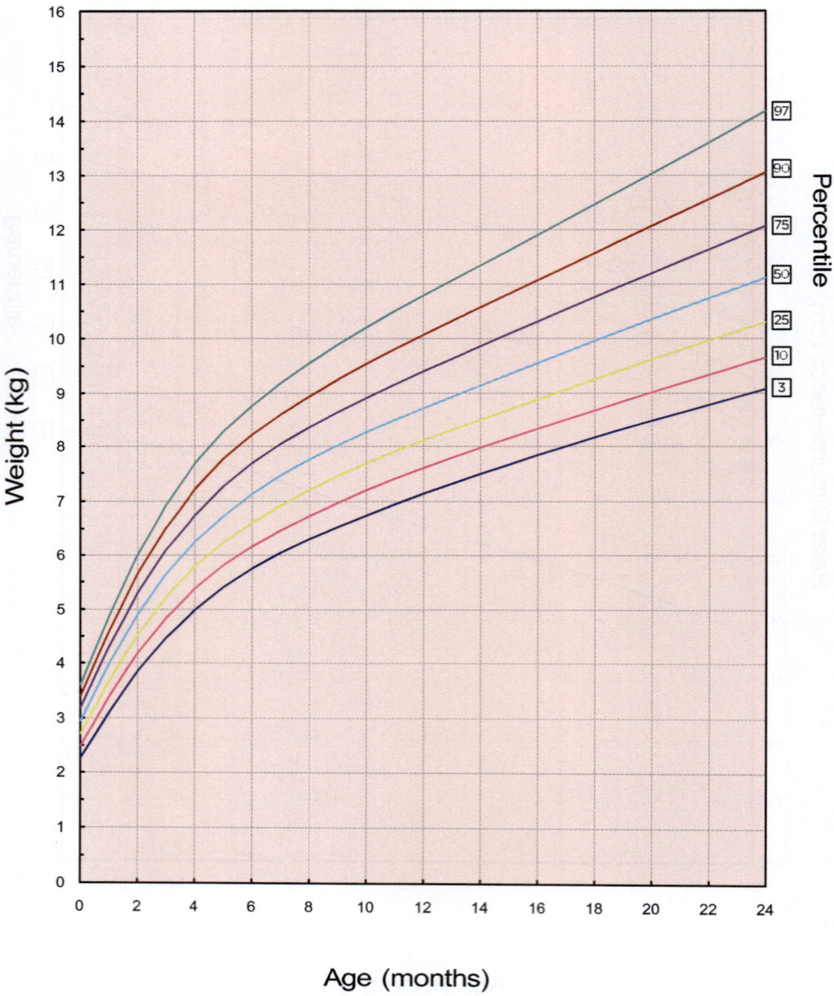

Anthropometric Study on Pre-School Children in Singapore, 2000
National Healthcare Group Polyclinics

PERCENTILES OF WEIGHT-FOR-AGE BOYS AGED 0 TO 24 MONTHS

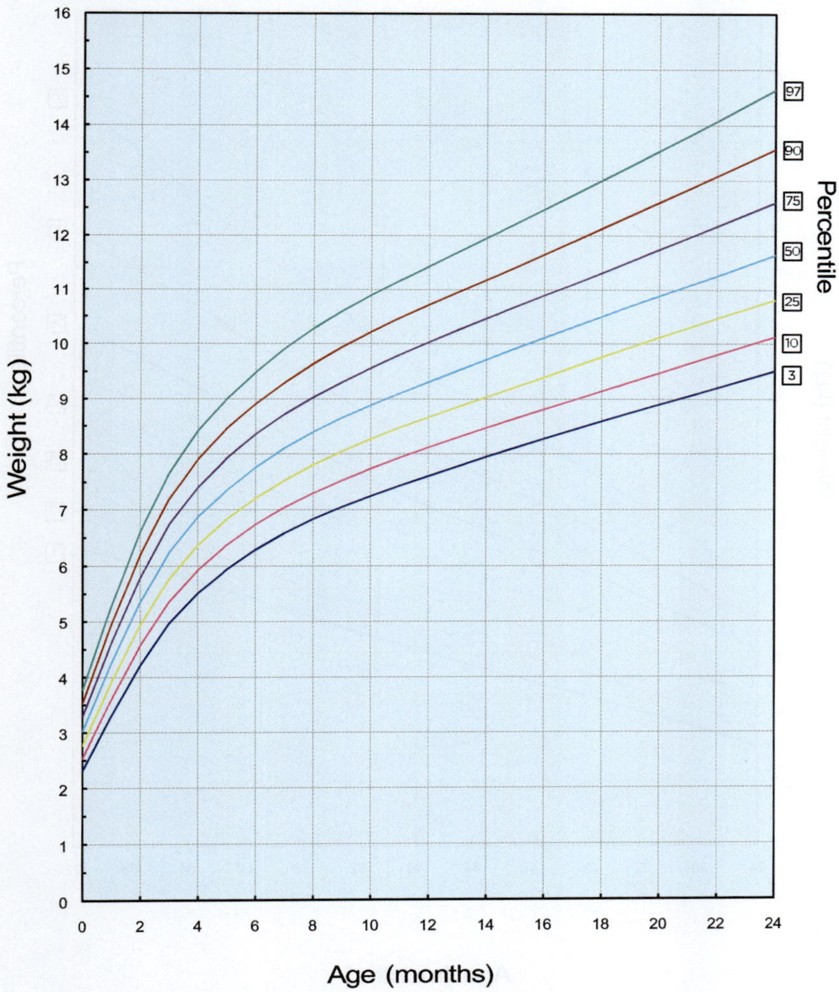

Anthropometric Study on Pre-School Children in Singapore, 2000
National Healthcare Group Polyclinics

PERCENTILES OF WEIGHT-FOR-AGE GIRLS AGED 24 TO 72 MONTHS

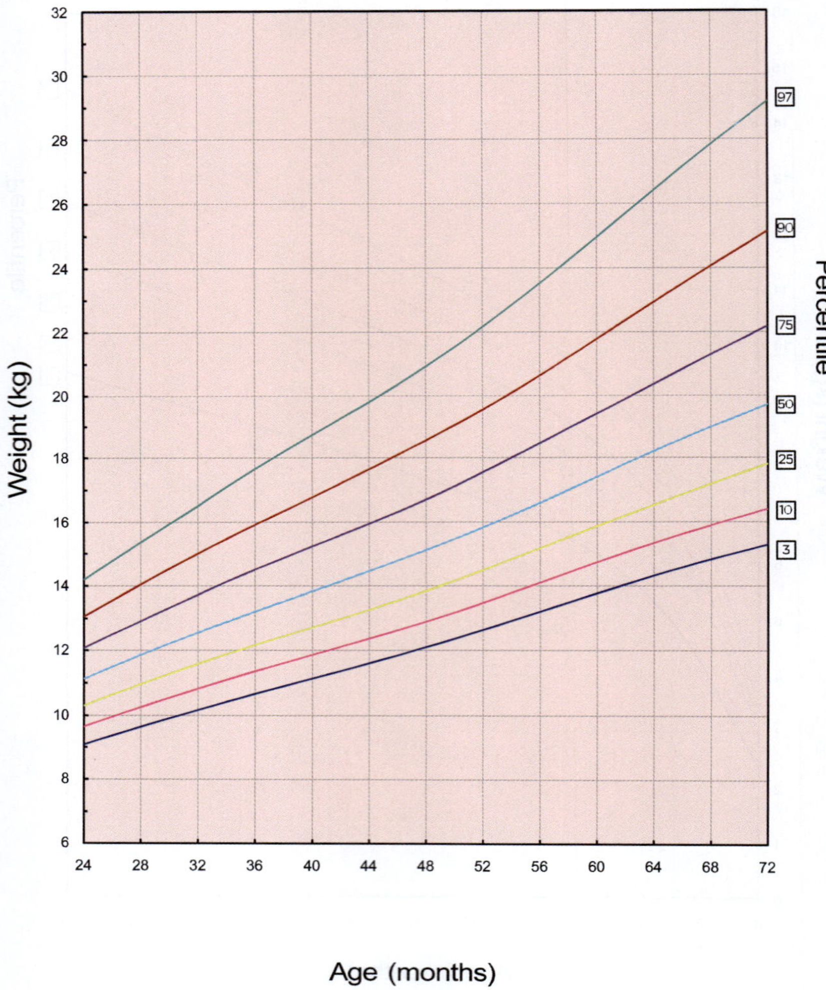

Anthropometric Study on Pre-School Children in Singapore, 2000
National Healthcare Group Polyclinics

PERCENTILES OF WEIGHT-FOR-AGE BOYS AGED 24 TO 72 MONTHS

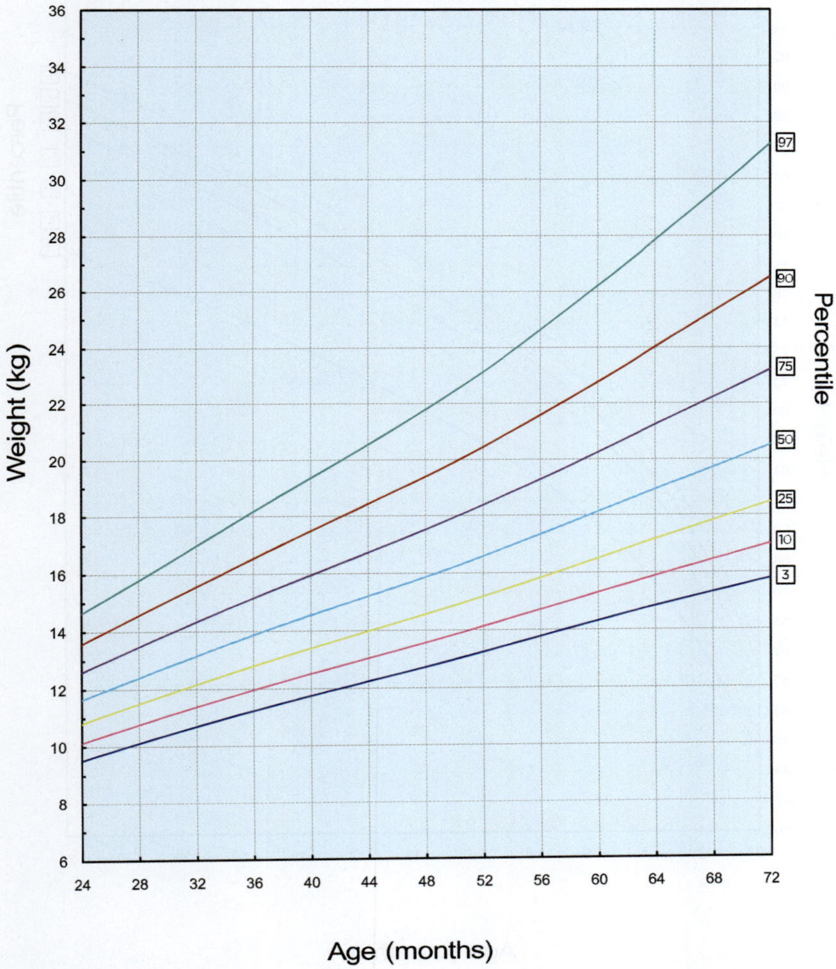

Anthropometric Study on Pre-School Children in Singapore, 2000
National Healthcare Group Polyclinics

PERCENTILES OF HEIGHT-FOR-AGE GIRLS AGED 0 TO 24 MONTHS

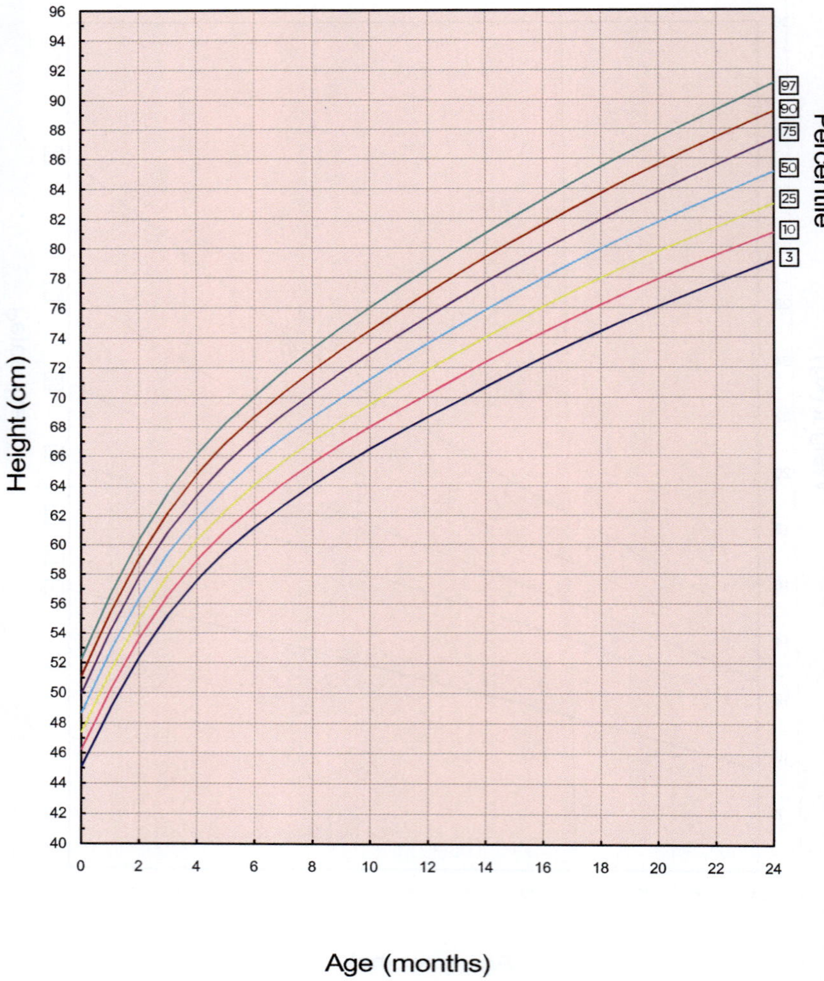

Anthropometric Study on Pre-School Children in Singapore, 2000
National Healthcare Group Polyclinics

PERCENTILES OF HEIGHT-FOR-AGE BOYS AGED 0 TO 24 MONTHS

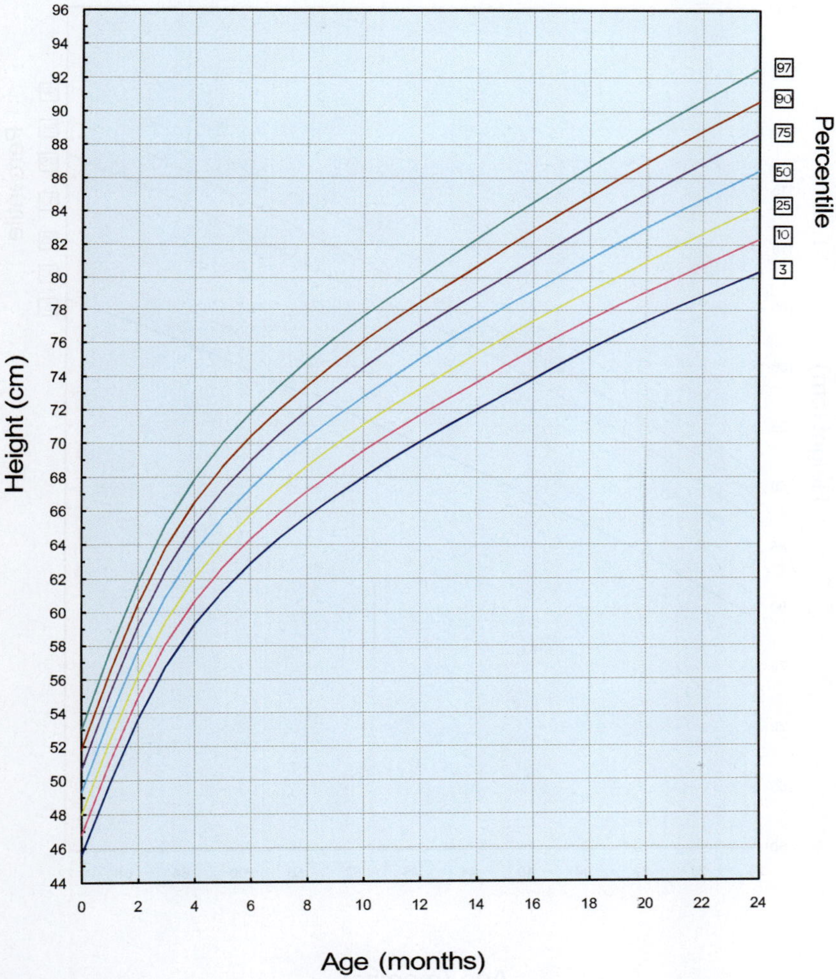

Anthropometric Study on Pre-School Children in Singapore, 2000
National Healthcare Group Polyclinics

PERCENTILES OF HEIGHT-FOR-AGE GIRLS AGED 24 TO 72 MONTHS

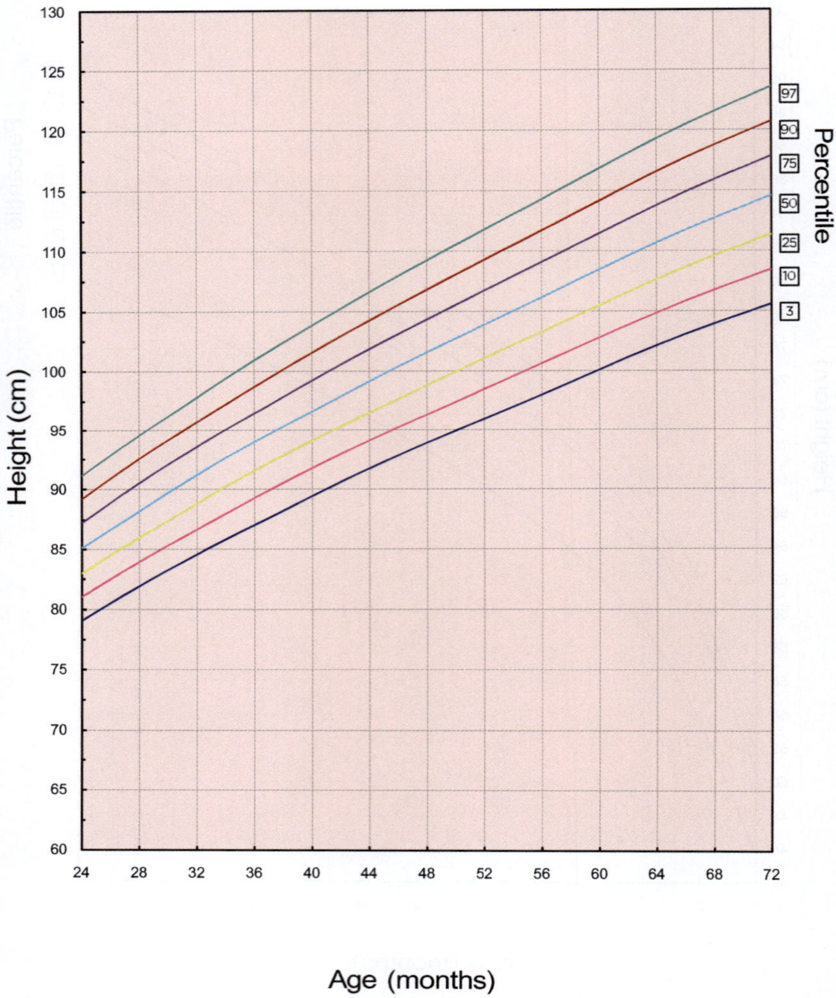

Anthropometric Study on Pre-School Children in Singapore, 2000
National Healthcare Group Polyclinics

PERCENTILES OF HEIGHT-FOR-AGE BOYS AGED 24 TO 72 MONTHS

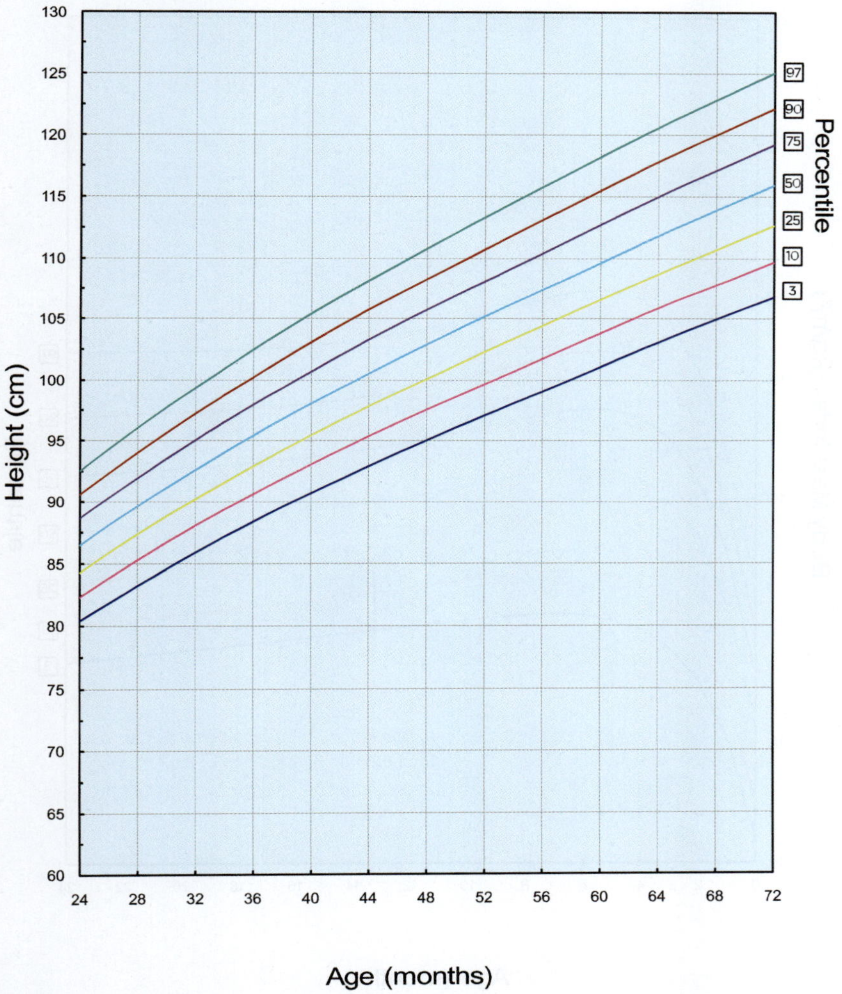

Anthropometric Study on Pre-School Children in Singapore, 2000
National Healthcare Group Polyclinics

PERCENTILES OF BODY MASS INDEX-FOR-AGE GIRLS AGED 0 TO 24 MONTHS

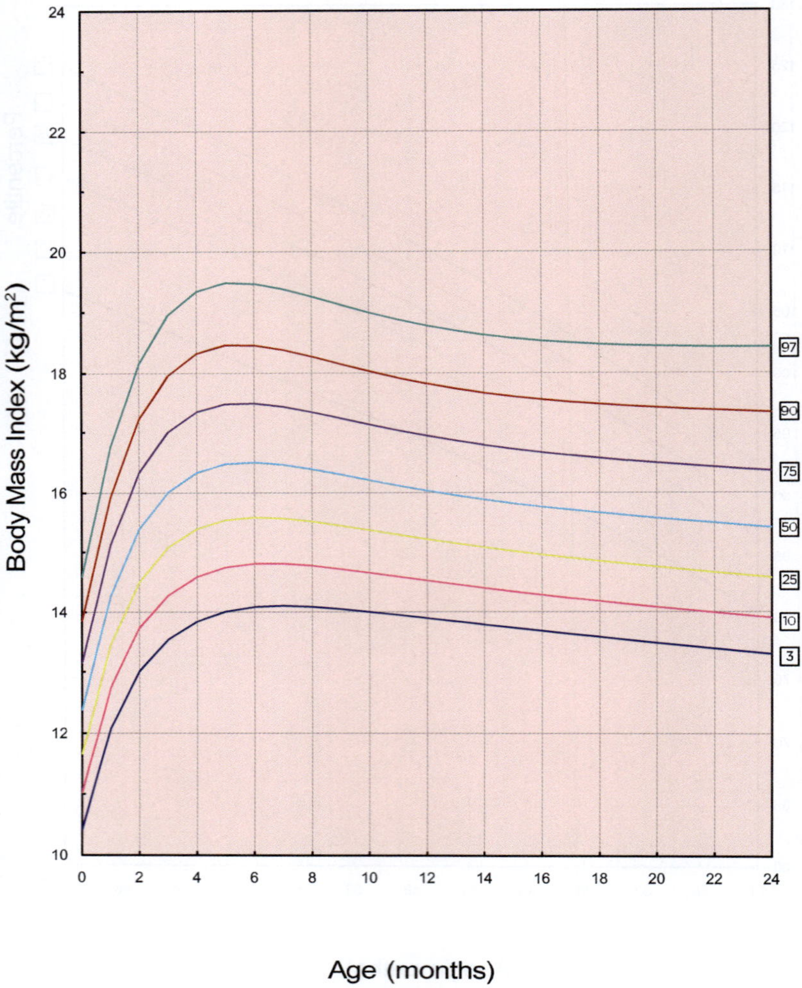

Anthropometric Study on Pre-School Children in Singapore, 2000
National Healthcare Group Polyclinics

PERCENTILES OF BODY MASS INDEX-FOR-AGE BOYS AGED 0 TO 24 MONTHS

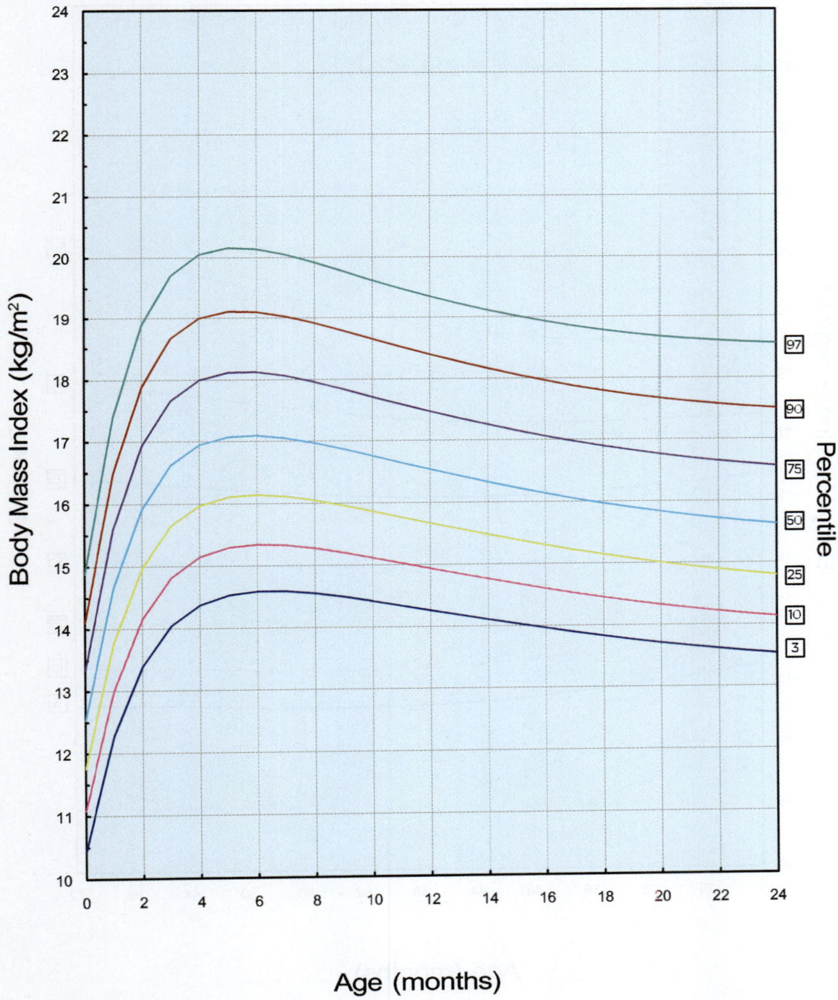

Anthropometric Study on Pre-School Children in Singapore, 2000
National Healthcare Group Polyclinics

PERCENTILES OF BODY MASS INDEX-FOR-AGE GIRLS AGED 24 TO 72

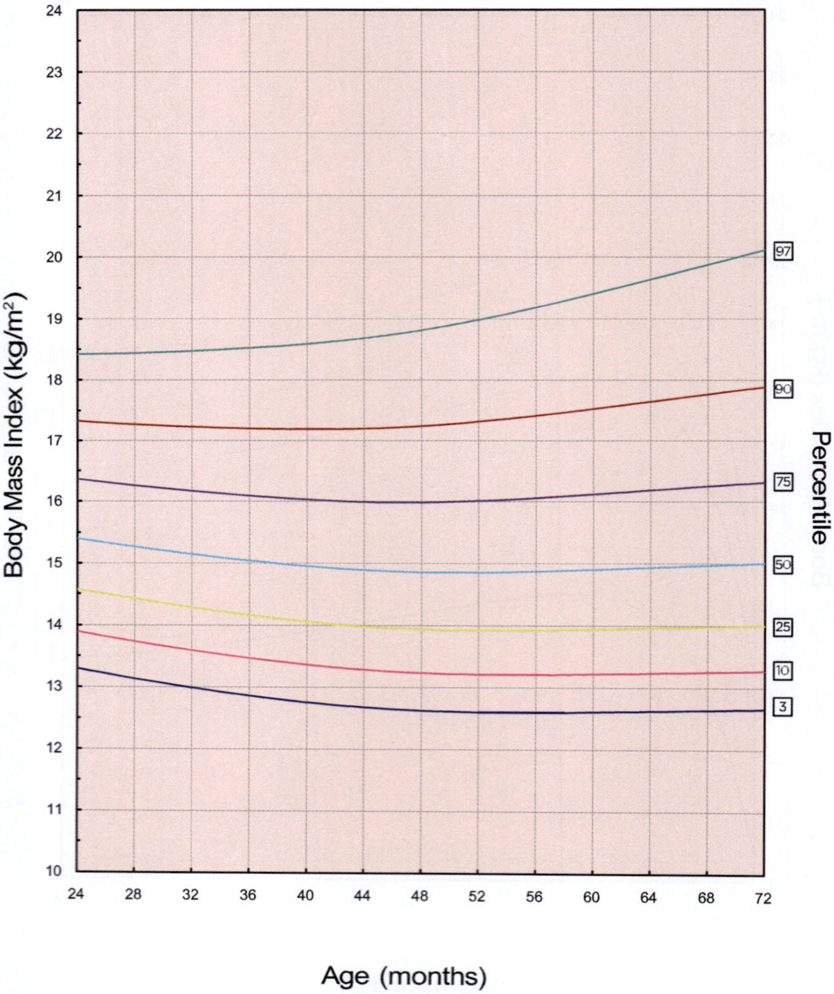

Anthropometric Study on Pre-School Children in Singapore, 2000
National Healthcare Group Polyclinics

PERCENTILES OF BODY MASS INDEX-FOR-AGE BOYS AGED 24 TO 72 MONTHS

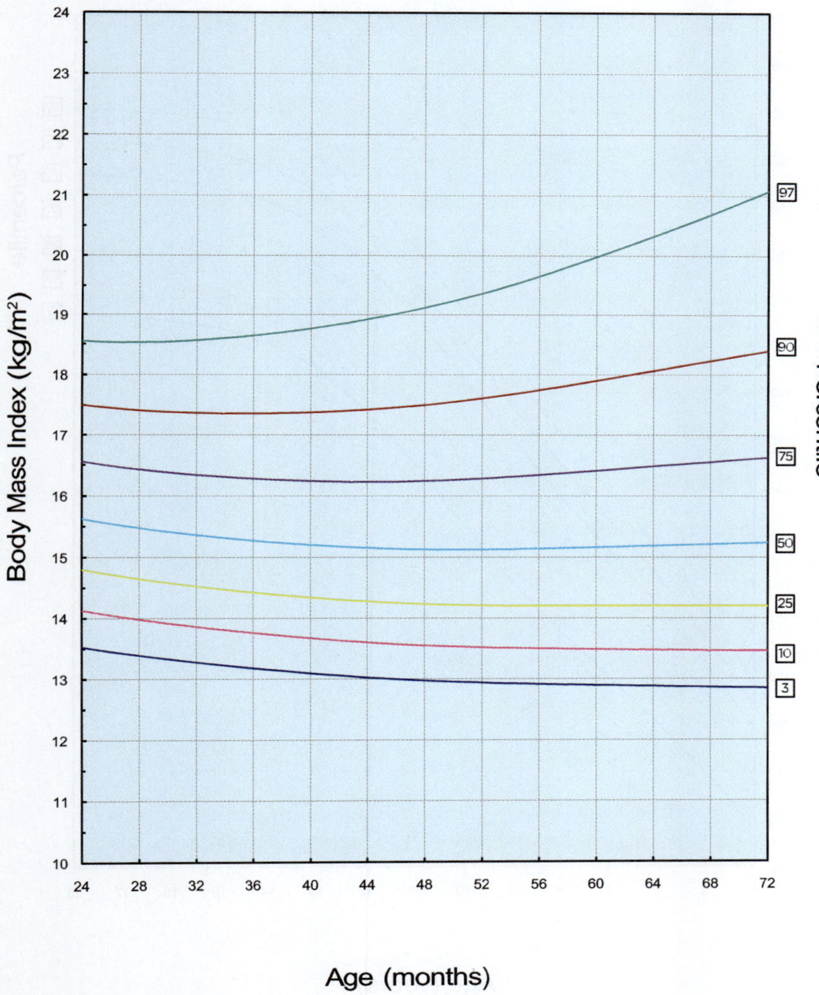

Anthropometric Study on Pre-School Children in Singapore, 2000
National Healthcare Group Polyclinics

PERCENTILES OF HEIGHT-FOR-AGE GIRLS AGED 4 TO 18 YEARS

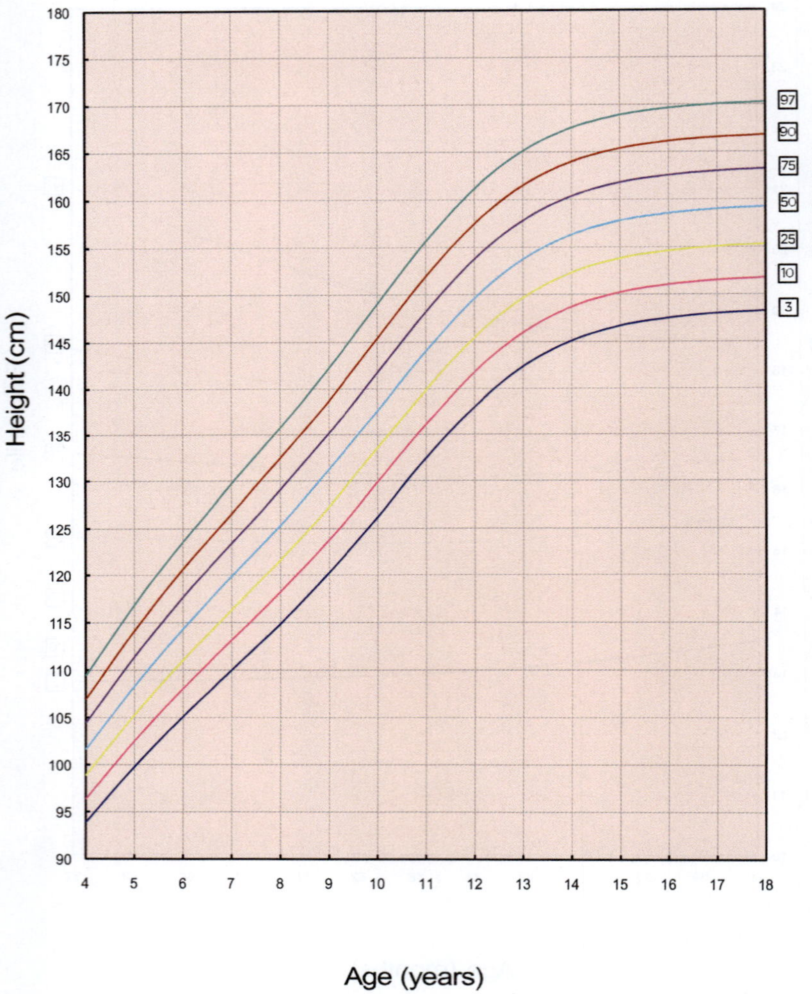

Anthropometric Study on School Children in Singapore, 2002
Health Promotion Board

PERCENTILES OF HEIGHT-FOR-AGE BOYS AGED 4 TO 18 YEARS

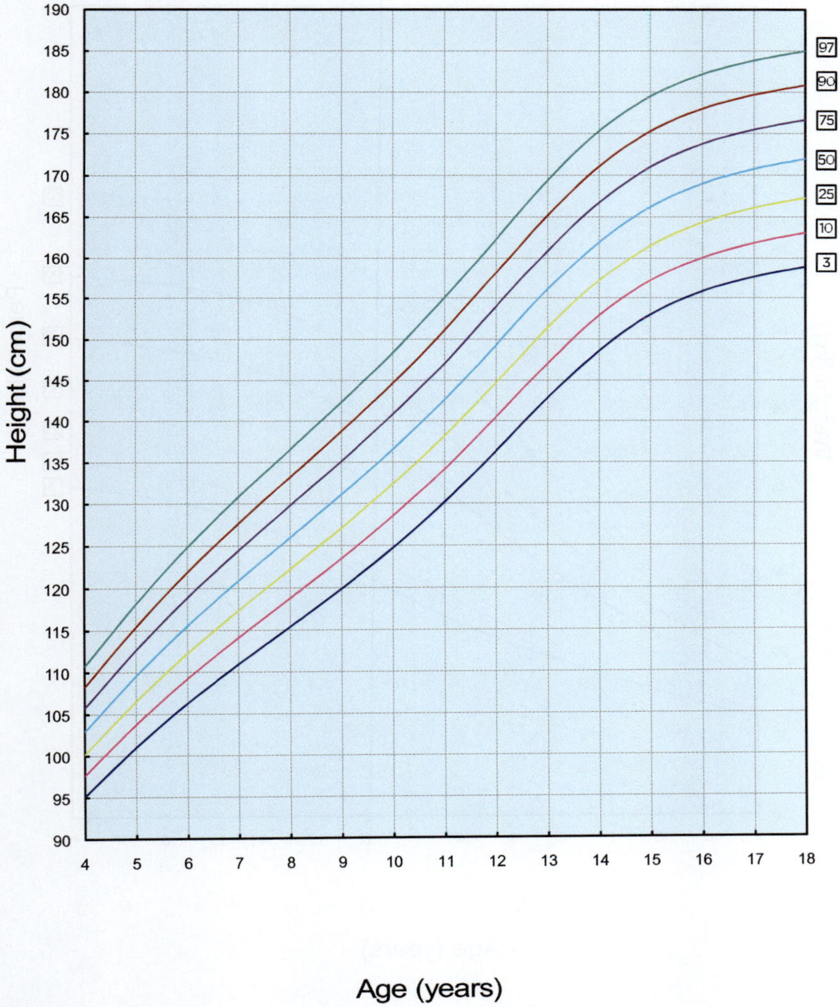

Anthropometric Study on School Children in Singapore, 2002
Health Promotion Board

PERCENTILES OF WEIGHT-FOR-AGE GIRLS AGED 4 TO 18 YEARS

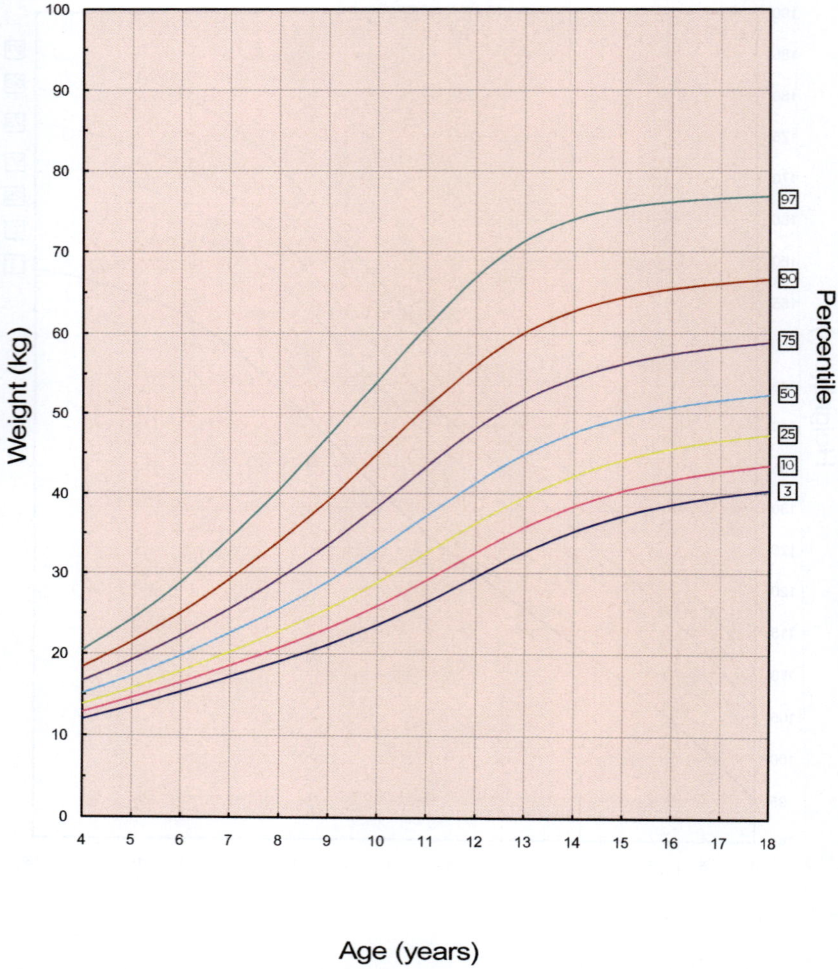

Anthropometric Study on School Children in Singapore, 2002
Health Promotion Board

PERCENTILES OF WEIGHT-FOR-AGE BOYS AGED 4 TO 18 YEARS

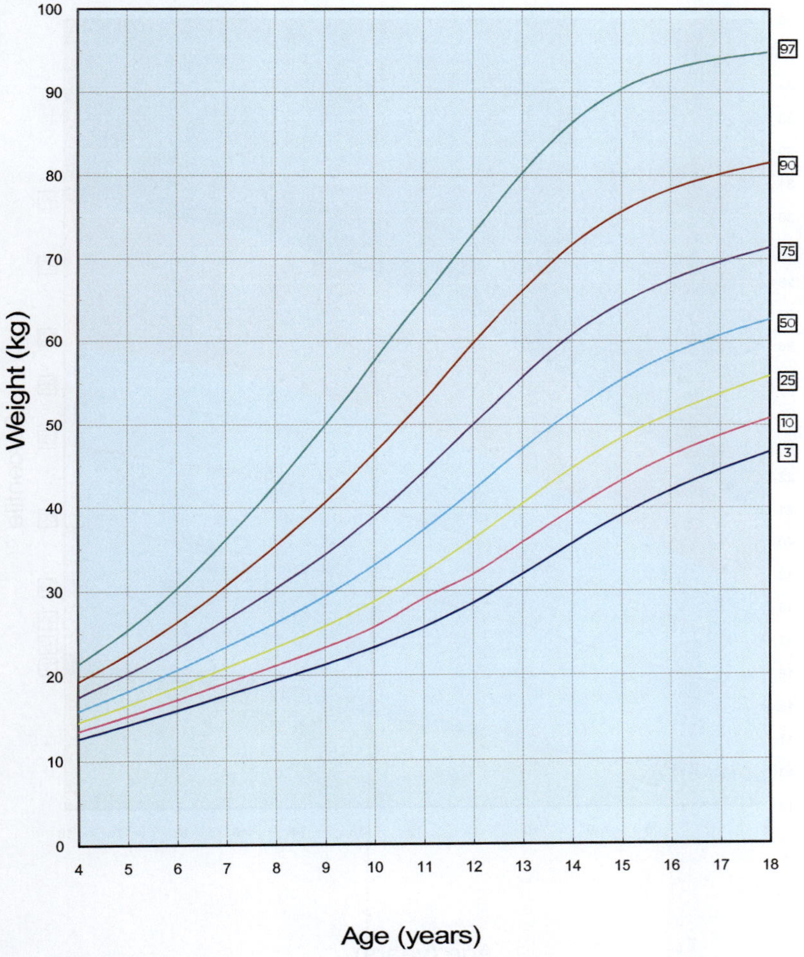

Anthropometric Study on School Children in Singapore, 2002
Health Promotion Board

PERCENTILES OF BODY MASS INDEX-FOR-AGE GIRLS AGED 6 TO 18 YEARS

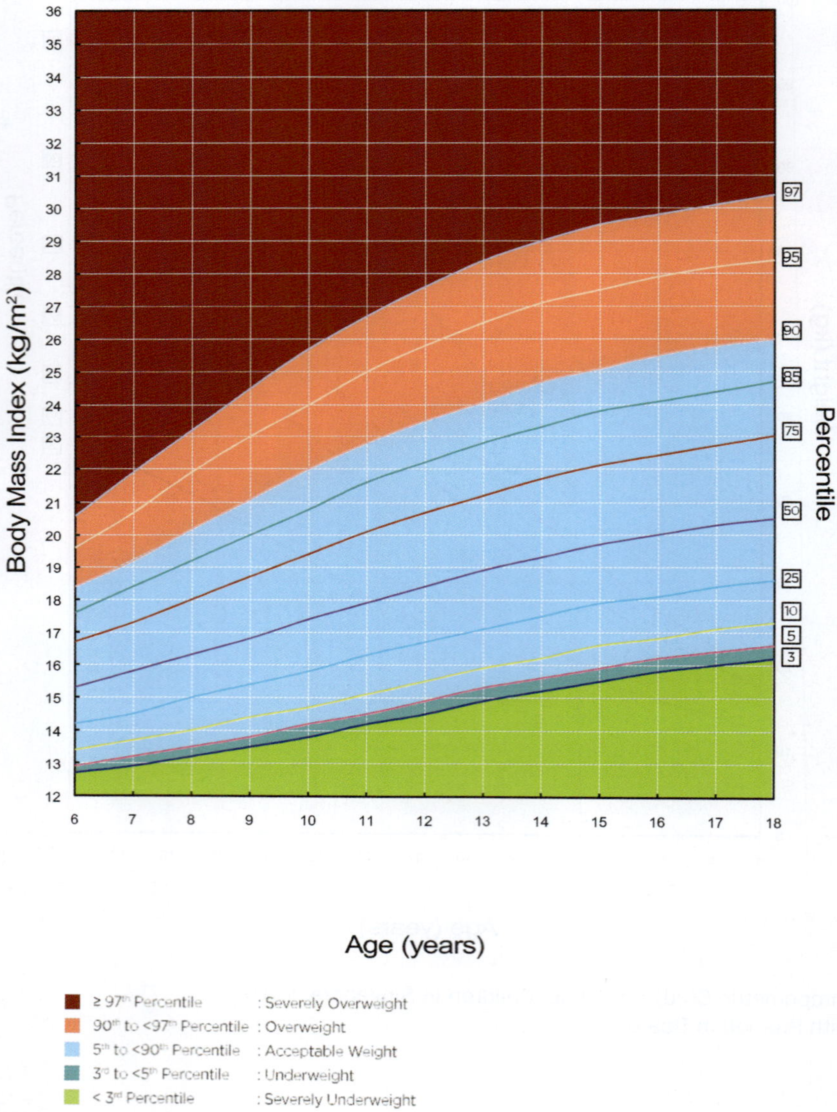

Anthropometric Study on School Children in Singapore, 2002
Health Promotion Board

PERCENTILES OF BODY MASS INDEX-FOR-AGE BOYS AGED 6 TO 18 YEARS

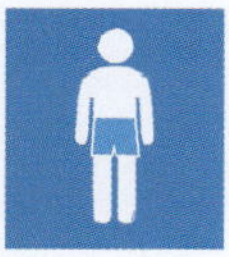

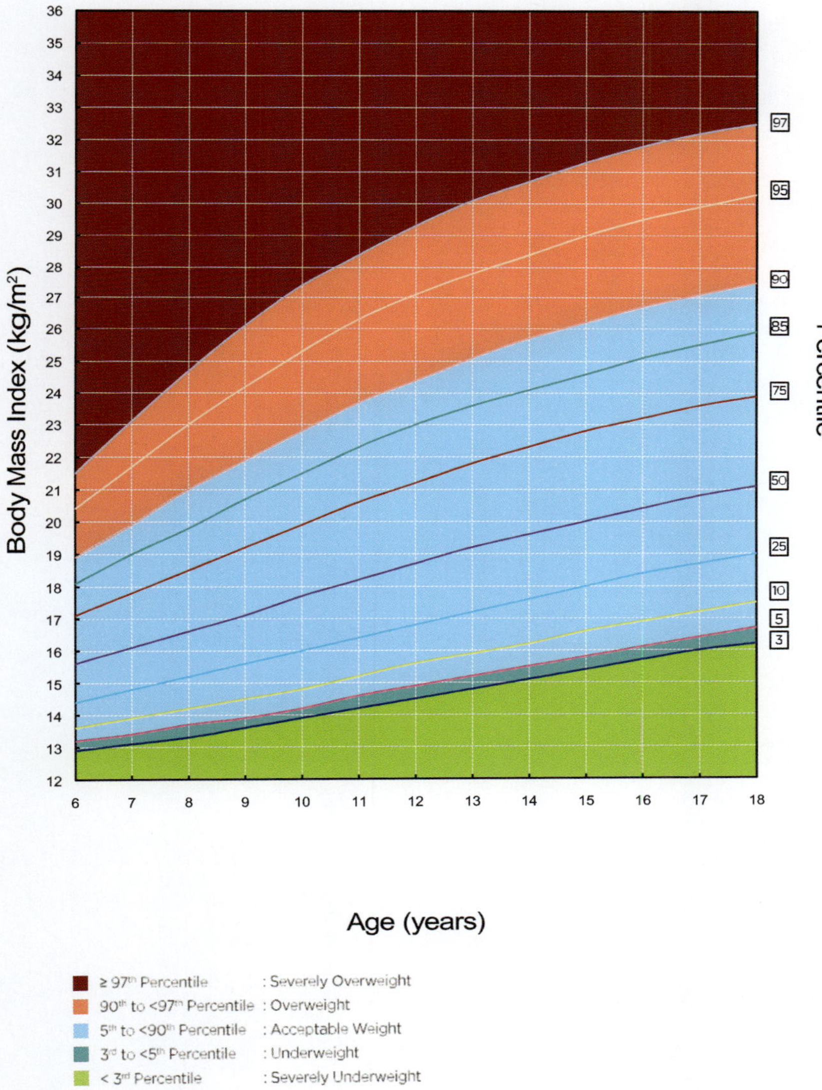

Anthropometric Study on School Children in Singapore, 2002
Health Promotion Board

APPENDIX II

DRUGS

Anti-infectives (Antibiotics, Antifungals, Antivirals, Antihelmintics, Antimalarials)

Ong Yue Ling, Rina; Seah Xue Fen, Valerie

Drug	Dosage	Remarks
	Antibiotics	
Amikacin	IV/IM 15–22.5 mg/kg/day Q8–24H Higher doses may be utilised for other indications (i.e. drug-resistant tuberculosis, infections caused by non-tuberculous mycobacteria, pulmonary infection in cystic fibrosis/bronchiectasis etc.).	Nephrotoxic and ototoxic. Therapeutic drug monitoring is recommended. Recommended therapeutic levels: - Target peak: 25–40 mcg/ml - Target trough: <10 mcg/ml (*ideal: 4–5 mcg/ml), *especially if existing nephrotoxic drugs or poor renal function
Amoxicillin	PO: Usual dose: 50 mg/kg/day Q8–12H Higher dose (for penicillin-resistant *Streptococcus pneumoniae* or severe infections): 80–90 mg/kg/day Q8–12H Max.: 4 g/day	Use higher oral doses for infections, which may be caused by intermediate susceptible/resistant *Streptococcus pneumoniae*, such as acute otitis media, pneumonia, sinusitis, etc.
Amoxicillin + Clavulanate (Brand Name: Augmentin)	PO: Usual dose: 50 mg (Amoxicillin)/kg/day Q8–12H Higher dose (for penicillin-resistant Streptococcus pneumoniae or severe infections): 80–90 mg (Amoxicillin)/kg/day Q8–12H Max.: 4 g (Amoxicillin)/day IV (Augmentin): 40 mg/kg/dose Q8H Max.: 1.2g/dose	Oral Amoxicillin-clavulanate (Augmentin) may be available in different preparations with different amoxicillin-to-clavulanate ratio. Dosing is usually based on the Amoxicillin component. Use higher oral doses for infections which may be caused by intermediate susceptible/resistant *Streptococcus pneumoniae*, such as acute otitis media, pneumonia, sinusitis etc.
Ampicillin	IV/IM: Mild to moderate infections: 100–200 mg/kg/day Q6H Severe infections (e.g. meningitis, endocarditis): 300–400 mg/kg/day Q4–6H Max.: 12 g/day	
Ampicillin + Sulbactam (Brand Name: Unasyn)	PO (as per Sultamicillin) <30 kg: 25–50 mg/kg/day Q12H ≥30 kg: 375–750 mg/dose Q12H IV/IM: Mild to moderate infections: 100–200 mg (Ampicillin)/kg/day Q6H	Oral Ampicillin-Sulbactam (Unasyn) is formulated as sultamicillin (the oxymethylpenicillinate sulfone ester of ampicillin). Dosing is based on the total Sultamicillin component.

(Continued)

Drug	Dosage	Remarks
Antibiotics		
	Severe infections: 300–400 mg (Ampicillin)/kg/day Q4–6H Max.: 12 g (Ampicillin)/day	IV Ampicillin-Sulbactam is a combination product formulated in a 2:1 ratio of Ampicillin and Sulbactam, dosing is usually based on the Ampicillin component.
Azithromycin	PO: For presumed atypical pneumonia: 10 mg/kg/day Q24H for 3 days, or Day 1 at 10 mg/kg/day Q24H then Day 2–5 at 5 mg/kg/day Q24H Max.: 500 mg/dose	Higher doses (up to 2 g/dose) may be indicated for other indications i.e. *Chlamydia trachomatis* or *Neisseria gonorrhoeae* infections.
Cefazolin	IV/IM: Mild–moderate infections: 25–50 mg/kg/day Q8H Severe infections: 100–150 mg/kg/day Q6–8H Max.: 12 g/day	
Cefepime	IV/IM: Mild/moderate infections: 100 mg/kg/day Q12H Severe infections: 150 mg/kg/day Q8H Max.: 2 g/dose; 6 g/day	
Cefotaxime	IV/IM: Mild-moderate infections: 50–180 mg/kg/day Q6–8H Severe infections: 200–300 mg/kg/day Q6–8H Max.: 12 g/day	
Ceftazidime	IV/IM: Mild-moderate infections: 90–150 mg/kg/day Q8H Severe infections: 200–300 mg/kg/day Q8H Max.: 12 g/day	
Ceftriaxone	IV/IM: Ophthalmia neonatorum: 50 mg/kg/dose single dose (max. 125 mg/dose) Mild-moderate infections: 50–75 mg/kg/day Q12–24H Severe infections (e.g. meningitis, penicillin-resistant pneumococcal pneumonia): 100 mg/kg/day Q12–24H Max.: 2 g/dose; 4 g/day	Avoid in hyperbilirubinemic neonates (especially if premature, or neonates <41 weeks postmenstrual age) and in neonates requiring calcium-containing solutions (e.g. parenteral nutrition).
Cefuroxime Axetil	PO: 20–30 mg/kg/day Q12H Max.: 500 mg/dose, 1 g/day	

(Continued)

(*Continued*)

Drug	Dosage	Remarks
Antibiotics		
Cephalexin	PO: Mild-moderate infections: 25–50 mg/kg/day Q6–8H Severe infections (e.g. osteomyelitis): 100–150 mg/kg/day Q6–8H Max.: 6 g/day	
Cefixime	PO: Usual dose: 8 mg/kg/day Q12–24H Max.: 400 mg/day	
Ciprofloxacin	PO: Usual dose: 20–30 mg/kg/day Q12H Severe infections: 40 mg/kg/day Q12H Max.: 750 mg/dose; 1500 mg/day IV: 20–30 mg/kg/day Q8–12H Max.: 400 mg/dose; 1200 mg/day	Contraindicated in G6PD deficiency. Fluoroquinolones: Not routinely first-line therapy in children. Possibility of increased musculoskeletal adverse effects but no strong evidence of sustained injury to developing bones or joints in children. May be considered only if no other alternatives available (e.g. multi-drug-resistant infection, oral step-down alternative). Weigh risks and benefits of use, proper counselling advised. Space at least 2 hours apart from iron and calcium containing supplements. May cause sun sensitivity. Avoid prolonged sun exposure, apply adequate sunscreen on exposed skin if outdoors.
Clarithromycin	PO: 15 mg/kg/day Q12H Max.: 500 mg/dose; 1000 mg/day	
Clindamycin	PO: 30–40 mg/kg/day Q6–8H Max.: 1800 mg/day IV/IM: Mild-moderate infections: 20 mg/kg/day Q6–8H Severe infections: 30–40 mg/kg/day Q6–8H Max.: 2700 mg/day	Oral Clindamycin should be taken with a full glass of water to avoid oesophageal irritation.
Cloxacillin	PO: 50–100 mg/kg/day Q6H Max.: 1 g/dose; 6 g/day IV/IM: Mild-moderate infections: 100 mg/kg/day Q6H Severe infections: 200–300 mg/kg/day Q4–6H Max.: 2 g/dose; 12 g/day	
Co-trimoxazole (Sulfamethoxazole-Trimethoprim)	PO/IV: Usual dose: 8–12 mg (TMP)/kg/day Q12H Severe infections (i.e. *Pneumocystis jirovecii*, meningitis): Up to 20 mg (TMP)/kg/day Q6–12H Prophylaxis (Urinary tract infection): 2 mg/kg/day Q24H Max.: 960 mg (TMP)/day	Dosing is usually based on the Trimethoprim (TMP) component. Contraindicated in G6PD deficiency. Avoid use in infants <2 months of age due to risks of hyperbilirubinemia and kernicterus.

(Continued)

Drug	Dosage	Remarks
Antibiotics		
Doxycycline	PO: 2.2 mg/kg/dose Q12H Acne: 50–100 mg Q12–24H Max.: 100 mg/dose; 200 mg/day	Risk of tooth staining and enamel hypoplasia (based on tetracycline). Not to be used in children <8 years old, unless no other alternatives available, and only for short durations (≤21 days) when appropriate. Weigh risks and benefits of use, proper counselling advised. Administer with plenty of fluid, and remain in an upright position following administration to reduce the risk of oesophageal irritation/oesophagitis. May cause sun sensitivity. Avoid prolonged sun exposure, apply adequate sunscreen on exposed skin if outdoors.
Erythromycin	PO (Erythromycin base): 30–50 mg/kg/day Q6–8H (Q12–24H for acne treatment) Anti-inflammatory: 25 mg/kg/day Q12H (max.: 500 mg/dose) Prokinetic dose: 3 mg/kg/dose Q6H Max.: 4 g/day IV (Lactobionate) 40–50 mg/kg/day Q6H (Lactobionate) Max.: 4 g/day	Use of erythromycin has been associated with infantile hyperpyloric sternosis (IHPS), monitor for non-bilious vomiting or irritability with feeding.
Ethambutol	PO: 15–25 mg/kg/day OM Max.: 2.5 g/day	May cause optic neuritis. Baseline vision tests are recommended.
Gentamicin	IV/IM: 5–7.5 mg/kg/day Q8–24H	Nephrotoxic and ototoxic. Therapeutic drug monitoring is recommended. Recommended therapeutic levels: - Target peak: 8–10 mcg/ml - Target trough: <2 mcg/ml (*ideal: <1 mcg/ml) *especially if existing nephrotoxic drugs or poor renal function
Isoniazid (INH)	PO: 10–20 mg/kg/day Q24H Max.: 300 mg/day	Monitor liver function tests while on Isoniazid. For patients at risk of isoniazid-induced neuropathy (e.g.: breastfed infants, diabetes, malnutrition), concomitant PO Pyridoxine is recommended.
Levofloxacin	PO/IV: <5 years old: 10 mg/kg/dose Q12H ≥5 years old: 10 mg/kg/dose Q24H Max.: 750 mg/day	Contraindicated in G6PD deficiency. Fluoroquinolones: Not routinely first-line therapy in children. Possibility of increased musculoskeletal adverse effects but no strong evidence of sustained injury to developing bones or joints in children. May be considered only if no other alternatives available (e.g. multi-drug-resistant infection, oral step-down

(Continued)

(*Continued*)

Drug	Dosage	Remarks
Antibiotics		
		alternative). Weigh risks and benefits of use, proper counselling advised. Space at least 2 hours apart from iron and calcium containing supplements. May cause sun sensitivity. Avoid prolonged sun exposure, apply adequate sunscreen on exposed skin if outdoors.
Linezolid	PO/IV: <12 years old: 10 mg/kg/dose Q8H ≥12years old: 10 mg/kg/dose Q12H Max.: 600 mg/dose	Risk of myelosuppression (may be duration-dependent, especially with >2 weeks of therapy).
Meropenem	IV: Usual dose [non-central nervous system (CNS) infection]: 20 mg/kg/dose Q8H Severe infection (i.e. CNS infection, septic shock): 40 mg/kg/dose Q8H Max.: 2 g/dose; 6 g/day	
Metronidazole	PO: 20–50 mg/kg/day Q8H Max.: 2250 mg/day IV: 22.5–40 mg/kg/day Q6–8H Max.: 4000 mg/day	May experience unusual, metallic taste or discolouration in the urine. Peripheral neuropathy may occur and may be prolonged even after drug discontinuation, due to the risk of cumulative neurotoxicity. It is associated with prolonged courses and/or at high doses.
Minocycline	PO/IV: 4 mg/kg/dose loading dose, then 2 mg/kg/dose Q12H Acne: 50–100 mg Q12–24H Max.: 200 mg/dose, 400 mg/day	Administer with plenty of fluid, and remain in an upright position following administration to reduce the risk of oesophageal irritation/ oesophagitis. May cause sun sensitivity. Avoid prolonged sun exposure, apply adequate sunscreen on exposed skin if outdoors. Not to be used in children <8 years old, unless no other alternatives available. Weigh risks and benefits of use, proper counselling advised.
Neomycin Sulphate	PO: 50–100 mg/kg/day Q8H Max.: 12 g/day	
Nitrofurantoin	PO: Lower-tract urinary tract infection: 5–7 mg/kg/day Q6H Max.: 400 mg/day Prophylaxis (Urinary tract infection): 1–2 mg/kg/day Q24H Max.: 100 mg/day	Contraindicated in G6PD deficiency. Not indicated for the treatment of pyelonephritis or perinephric abscess Not recommended for neonates (<1 month of age) due to the possibility of haemolytic anemia

(Continued)

Drug	Dosage	Remarks
Antibiotics		
Penicillin Benzathine	IM: Congenital syphilis: Single dose 50,000 units/kg/dose Max.: 2.4 million units/dose Rheumatic fever prophylaxis: ≤27 kg: 0.6 million units every 3–4 weeks >27 kg: 1.2 million units every 3–4 weeks	
Penicillin Crystalline G (Benzylpenicillin)	IV/IM: Usual dose: 100,000–300,000 units/kg/day Q4–6H Severe infection (i.e. GBS or non-GBS meningitis): Up to 500,000 units/kg/day Q4–6H Max.: 24 million units/day	
Penicillin V	PO: 25–75 mg/kg/day Q6–8H Prophylaxis in asplenia: <3 years old: 125 mg Q12H ≥3 years old: 250 mg Q12H Max.: 2000 mg/day	
Piperacillin/ Tazobactam	IV: 240–400mg (Piperacillin)/kg/day Q6–8H Max.: 16 g (Piperacillin)/day	Does not penetrate the blood brain barrier, not for meningitis/CNS infections.
Pyrazinamide	PO: 25–40 mg/kg/day Q24H Max.: 2000 mg/day	
Rifampicin	PO: Tuberculosis (active or latent): 10–20 mg/kg/day Q24H *Neisseria meningitidis* prophylaxis: 20 mg/kg/day Q12H x 2 days *H. influenzae* prophylaxis: 20 mg/kg/day Q12H x 4 days Max.: 600 mg/day	Urine, faeces, saliva, tears and sweat may be stained orange/red. Risk of hepatitis: Monitor liver function tests while on Rifampicin, especially if treatment is prolonged or given with other hepatotoxic drugs.
Trimethoprim	PO: Usual dose: 4–8 mg/kg/day Q12H Prophylaxis (Urinary tract infection): 2 mg/kg/day Q24H Max.: 200 mg/dose, 400 mg/day	Avoid use in infants <2 months old due to risks of hyperbilirubinemia and kernicterus.
Vancomycin	IV: 15 mg/kg/dose Q6–8H PO (*Clostridium difficile* infection): 10 mg/kg/day Q6H for 10–14 days Max.: 500 mg/dose, 2000 mg/day	Nephrotoxic and ototoxic. Therapeutic drug monitoring is recommended. Recommended therapeutic levels: - Target peak: 30–40 mcg/ml - Target trough: 10–20 mcg/ml - Target AUC/MIC: 400–600* *AUC/MIC is considered the optimal PK/PD efficacy target Each IV dose to be infused over a period of at least 60 minutes. Extend duration, with anti-histamines if Red Man Syndrome observed.

(Continued)

(*Continued*)

Drug	Dosage	Remarks
Antifungals		
Amphotericin B (Conventional)	IV Initial dose: 0.25–0.5 mg/kg/dose Q24H, then increase gradually daily until desired daily dose. Maintenance dose: 0.25–1.5 mg/kg/dose Q24H	Acute reactions (i.e. fever, chills, hypotension, nausea, vomiting, headache, tachypnoea) may occur 1–3 hours after starting the infusion, usually more common with the 1st few doses. Administer by slow IV infusion over at least 2–6 hours. Pre-medications may be required if mild adverse reactions experienced.
Amphotericin B (Liposomal)	IV: 3–5 mg/kg/day Q24H *Dose may be increased up to 10 mg/kg/day for severe infections.	Fever, chills, other acute infusion reactions are similar to conventional Amphotericin B, but less nephrotoxicity and hepatotoxicity.
Fluconazole	PO/IV: 6–12 mg/kg/dose Q24H Max.: 1600 mg/day	Risk of hepatitis: Monitor liver function tests while on Fluconazole, especially if treatment is prolonged or given with other hepatotoxic drugs.
Griseofulvin	PO: (Microsize): 10–25 mg/kg/day Q12–24H Max.: 1000 mg/day	Avoid prolonged sun exposure. Dose may differ for Ultrasize formulation — please consult specific product monograph/labelling for specific dosing.
Itraconazole	PO: 5–10 mg/kg/day Q12–24H (May be increased up to 15 mg/kg/day Q8H) Max.: 600 mg/day	Capsules and solution are not bioequivalent. Capsules are best if taken with food, while the solution should be taken on an empty stomach. Risk of hepatitis: Monitor liver function tests while on Itraconazole, especially if treatment is prolonged or given with other hepatotoxic drugs. Itraconazole trough serum concentrations may be monitored to ensure efficacy and reduce toxicity.
Nystatin	PO Neonate: 100000 units Q6H Infant: 200000–400000 units Q6H Child-Adolescent: 400000–600000 units Q6H	For oral thrush
Voriconazole	IV/PO: ≤14 years old AND <50 kg: 9 mg/kg/dose Q12H >14 years old OR ≥50 kg: Day 1: 6 mg/kg/dose Q12H x 2 doses, then Day 2 onwards: 4 mg/kg/dose Q12H	Monitor liver function tests, visual changes (especially >1 month of use) Therapeutic Drug Monitoring needed. Target trough levels for prophylaxis and treatment: 1–5 mg/L

(Continued)

Drug	Dosage	Remarks
Antifungals		
Micafungin	IV: 4 mg/kg/day Q24H (For severe/ CNS infections, dose may be increased to 6mg/kg/day (≥ 4 months) and up to 10-15 mg/kg/day (< 4 months)). Prophylaxis (Candida infection): 2 mg/kg/day Q24H	
Anidulafungin	IV: Loading dose 3 mg/kg/dose Q24H on Day 1, then 1.5 mg/kg/dose Q24H Max.: 200 mg/dose	
Pentamidine	IV: 4 mg/kg/dose Q2–4 weekly	For *Pneumocystis jirovecii* prophylaxis
Antivirals		
Acyclovir	PO: Varicella (uncomplicated): 20 mg/kg/dose Q6H for 5 days Herpes Simplex Virus (HSV) mucocutaneous, orolabial infection: 20 mg/kg/dose Q6H for 5–7 days HSV genital/labial (first episode): 20 mg/kg/dose Q8H for 7–10 days Eczema herpeticum: PO 20 mg/kg/dose Q8H Max.: 800 mg/dose, 4 g/day IV: Varicella (complicated), HSV encephalitis or HSV in immunosuppressed: 10 mg/kg/dose (or 500 mg/m^2/dose) Q8H HSV mucocutaneous, orolabial infection: 10 mg/kg/dose Q8H HSV genital/labial (first episode): 5–10 mg/kg/dose Q8H for 7–10 days Eczema herpeticum: IV 10 mg/kg/dose Q8H	IV: Crystalline nephropathy, rare occurrences of encephalopathy. May cause dizziness
Ganciclovir	IV: Induction dose: 5 mg/kg/dose Q12H Maintenance dose: 5 mg/kg/dose Q24H	Mainly for the treatment and prophylaxis of Cytomegalovirus infections. Monitor renal function, can cause bone marrow suppression.
Valganciclovir	PO: (BSA — Body Surface Area; CrCl — Creatinine Clearance) Induction Dose: (7 x BSA x CrCl) Q12H Maintenance Dose: (7 x BSA x CrCl) Q24H or Dose: 16 mg/kg/dose Q12H Max.: 900 mg/dose, 1800 mg/day	Mainly for the treatment and prophylaxis of Cytomegalovirus infections. Monitor renal function, can cause bone marrow suppression

(Continued)

(*Continued*)

Drug	Dosage	Remarks
Antivirals		
Ribavirin	Aerosolised: 6 g over 12–18 hours/day IV: 25 mg/kg/day Q8H on Day 1, then 15 mg/kg/day Q8H from Day 2–10. PO: 20–25 mg/kg/day Q8–12H	Limited experience in severe Respiratory Syncytial Virus (RSV) infection. Ribavirin (aerosolised) is FDA-licensed for use for treatment of severe RSV infection; whereas the use of oral and/or IV Ribavirin remains off-label. Bronchospasm has been reported with use of aerosolised Ribavirin. Haemolytic anemia has been reported, and usually occurs within 1–2 weeks of therapy. Dose adjustment or discontinuation may be required.
Oseltamivir	PO: Treatment: ≤8 months old: 3 mg/kg/dose Q12H >9 months old: 3.5 mg/kg/dose Q12H Prophylaxis: ≤8 months old: 3 mg/kg/dose Q24H >9 months old: 3.5 mg/kg/dose Q24H Max.: 75 mg/dose	For the treatment and prophylaxis (selected groups) of Influenza A and B virus. Rare occurences of neuropsychiatric events but causality has not been established.
Cidofovir	IV: 5 mg/kg/dose once weekly	Off-label use for the treatment of severe Adenovirus Infection, BK virus associated Haemorrhagic Cystitis or Ganciclovir- or Foscarnet-resistant Cytomegalovirus, Acyclovir-resistant Herpes Simplex Virus or Varicella Zoster infections. Monitor renal function. Ensure adequate hydration prior, during and after infusion. Concurrent PO Probenecid administration required (check G6PD status)
Antihelmintics		
Albendazole (Zentel)	PO: Pinworm, Roundworm, Whipworm: ≤2 years old: 200 mg ONCE, repeat in 2–3 weeks >2 years old: 400 mg ONCE, repeat in 2–3 weeks Hookworm: ≥8 months old: 200 mg Q24H for 3 days	
Mebendazole	PO: Pin-worm, thread-worm: ONCE, repeat in 2 weeks ≥6 months old AND ≤10 kg: 50 mg/dose ONCE ≥6 months old AND >10 kg: 100 mg/dose ONCE	

(*Continued*)

Drug	Dosage	Remarks
Antihelmintics		
	Round-worm, hook-worm and whip-worm ≥1 year old: 100 mg BD x 3 days OR 500 mg ONCE, then repeat in 3 weeks	
Antimalarials		
Artesunate	IV/IM: Treatment of severe malaria: 2.4 mg/kg/dose ONCE, and at 12 hours, then at 24 hours, 48 hours and 72 hours later (at least 24 hours apart, for 1–3 days), followed by appropriate oral therapy	Patients with P. vivax or P. ovale should received concomitant treatment with an antimalarial agent against Plasmodium liver hypnozoites, e.g. primaquine.
Chloroquine Phosphate	PO (Dose expressed as Chloroquine base; Chloroquine phosphate 16.7 mg = Chloroquine base 10 mg) Treatment: 10 mg/kg/dose (max. 600 mg/dose) followed by 5 mg/kg/dose (max. 300 mg/dose) at 6 hours, 24 hours and 48 hours later OR 10 mg/kg/dose Q24H on Day 1, followed by 10 mg/kg/dose Q24H on Day 2, and 5 mg/kg/dose Q24H on Day 3 (CDC 2021) Prophylaxis: 5 mg/kg/dose (max. 300 mg/dose) once weekly. Begin 1–2 weeks prior to exposure, and continue for at least 4 weeks after leaving endemic area.	Contraindicated in G6PD deficiency.
Mefloquine	PO (Dose expressed in terms of the salt, Mefloquine hydrochloride) Treatment: 15 mg/kg/dose (max. 750 mg/dose), followed by 10 mg/kg/dose (max. 500 mg) 6–12 hours later Prophylaxis: Weight-based dosing: 5 mg/kg/dose (max. 250 mg/dose) once weekly. Begin ≥2 weeks prior to exposure, and continue during travel and for at least 4 weeks after leaving endemic area. Fixed dosing: >9–19 kg: 62.5 mg, once a week >19–30 kg: 125 mg, once a week >30–45 kg: 187.5mg, once a week >45 kg/ adult: 250 mg, once aweek	
Primaquine Phosphate	PO (Dose expressed as Primaquine base; Primaquine phosphate 26.3 mg = Primaquine base 15 mg) Treatment (uncomplicated, or radical cure of P. vivax or P. ovale):	Contraindicated in G6PD deficiency. Use in combination with other appropriate antimalarial treatment, consult relevant guidelines to determine most appropriate agents.

(*Continued*)

(*Continued*)

Drug	Dosage	Remarks
Antimalarials		
	- Dose: 0.25–0.5 mg/kg/day Q24H for 14 days (CDC 2021) - Without G6PD deficiency: 0.5 mg/kg/dose (max. 30 mg) Q24H for 14 days - With G6PD deficiency: 0.75 mg/kg/dose once/week for 8 weeks (max. 45 mg/dose) Prophylaxis (short-duration travel <6 months, to areas with primarily P. vivax): 0 5 mg/kg/dose (max. 30 mg) Q24H. Begin 1–2 days prior to travel and continue while in the area with malaria risk, and for 7 days after departure. Terminal prophylaxis: 0.5 mg/kg/dose (max. 30 mg) Q24H fr 14 days after departure from endemic area.	
Malarone	PO: Treatment (uncomplicated P. falciparum or P. vivax): Given Q24H for 3 doses. 5–8 kg: 125 mg (atovaquone)/50 mg (proguanil) 9–10 kg: 187.5 mg/75 mg 11–20 kg: 250 mg/100 mg 21–30 kg: 500 mg/200 mg 31–40 kg: 750 mg/300 mg >40 kg: 1000 mg/400 mg Prophylaxis: Given 1–2 days prior to entering endemic area, continue throughout stay and for 7 days after leaving area. 5–8 kg: 31.25 mg(atovaquone)/12.5 mg (proguanil) 9–10 kg: 46.88 mg/18.75 mg 11–20 kg: 62.5 mg/25 mg 21–30 kg: 125 mg/50 mg 31–40 kg: 187.5 mg/75 mg >40 kg: 250 mg/100 mg	Start 1–2 days before entering endemic area and continue until 7 days after leaving.
Quinine Sulphate	PO (Dose expressed as Quinine sulfate salt; Quinine sulfate 324 mg = Quinine base 269 mg) Treatment (P. falciparum, P. vivax): 30 mg/kg/day Q8H for 3–10 days (max. 650 mg/dose)	

Gastrointestinal System (Antacids, Antireflux Agents & Antiulcerants, Anti-spasmodics, Laxatives, Drugs for Inflammatory Bowel Disease)

Nurashyura Binte Ishak; Mai Xiangrui

Drug	Dosage	Remarks
Antacids, Antireflux agents and Antiulcerants		
Antacid with Simethicone Tablet (Magnesium trisilicate 250 mg, Aluminium hydroxide 250 mg, Simethicone 30 mg)	>12 years old: PO 1–2 tab TDS.	Separate apart from other medications by 2 hours (may reduce absorption of other medications). Consider Eviline Forte for <12 years old.
Domperidone	PO: 0.2–0.4 mg/kg/dose Q8H (max. 10 mg/dose) Rectal: 0.75 mg/kg/dose Q12H (max. 30 mg/dose)	Use lowest effective dose for the shortest possible duration. Contraindicated in patients with cardiac disease. Suspension is to be used only if post-menstrual age ≥41 weeks AND post-natal age ≥ 28 days.
Magnesium hydroxide 400 mg, Aluminium hydroxide 400 mg, Simethicone 40 mg Suspension (Eviline Forte Suspension)	PO: 2–5 years old: 2.5 ml Q8H 5–12 years old: 2.5–5 ml Q6–8H ≥ 12 years old: 5–10 ml Q6–8H (max. 40 ml/day)	Separate apart from other medications by 2 hours (may reduce absorption of other medications).
Famotidine	PO: 1–3 month old: 0.5–1 mg/kg Q24H ≥3 month old: 0.5–1 mg/kg Q12–24H (max.: 40 mg/dose, 80 mg/day)	
Magnesium Carbonate (as Magnesium Carbonate 3% w/v Sodium bicarbonate 5% w/v)	PO: 1–2 years old: 2.5 ml/dose Q8H 2–5 years old: 5 ml/dose Q8H 5–10 years old: 7.5 ml/dose Q8H >10 years old: 10 ml/dose Q8H	Separate apart from other medications by 2 hours (may reduce absorption of other medications).
Omeprazole	PO: 0.4–1 mg/kg/dose Q12–24H (max. 40 mg/dose) IV: 1 mg/kg/dose Q8-Q12H (max. 40 mg/dose)	Take 30 minutes before meal for best effects.

(*Continued*)

(*Continued*)

Drug	Dosage	Remarks
Antacids, Antireflux agents and Antiulcerants		
Lansoprazole	For ≥ 1 year old only PO: ≤30 kg: 15 mg OM (max. 30 mg/day) >30 kg: 30 mg OM (max. 60 mg/day)	Take 30 minutes before meal for best effects.
Rabeprazole	For ≥12 years old only PO: 20–40 mg OD-BD	May be taken with or without food.
Simethicone Drops 100 mg/ml	PO: <2 years old: 0.2 ml Q2–6H (max. 12 doses/day) 2–11 years old: 0.4 ml Q2–6H (max. 12 doses/day) ≥12 years old: Consider using antacid tablet or Eviline Forte	Take before each feed for best effect.
Sucralfate (1 g Tablet)	PO: 1 month to 2 years old: 250 mg QDS 2–12 years old: 500 mg QDS >12 years old: 1 g QDS Alternative dosing: 40–80 mg/kg/day QDS (max. 1 g QDS)	Separate apart from other medications by 2 hours (except antacids, which may be taken 30 mins before or after).
Dioctahedral Smectite 3 g Sachet (Smecta)	≥2 years old: PO 1 sachet Q8–24H (max. 1 sachet TDS)	Separate apart from other medications by 2 hours (may reduce absorption of other medications).
Anti-Spasmodics		
Hyoscine butylbromide (Buscopan)	PO: 6–11 years old: 10 mg TDS ≥12 years old: 10–20 mg TDS-QDS 0.5 mg/kg/dose Q6–8H (max. 20–40 mg per dose)	Take ½–1 hour before food.
Trimebutine maleate (Suspension 72 mg/15 ml, Tablet 100 mg)	PO: <6 months old: 2.5 ml/dose Q8–12H 6 months to 1 year old: 5 ml/dose Q12H 1–5 years old: 5 ml/dose Q8–12H >5 years old: 10 ml/dose Q8–12H >12 years old: 15–30 ml/dose OR 100–200 mg tab/dose Q8–12H	Take ½–1 hour before food.
Laxatives		
Bisacodyl	PO Enteric Coated (EC) tablet: 3–12 years old: 0.3 mg/kg OD (max. 10 mg OD) ≥12 years old: 10–20 mg OD (max. 30 mg OD) PR Suppository: <12 months old: 2.5 mg OD 1–10 years old: 5 mg OD ≥10 years old: 5–10 mg OD (max. 10 mg OD)	Takes about 10–12 hours for tablet and 20–60 minutes for suppository to take effect.

(Continued)

Drug	Dosage	Remarks
Laxatives		
Fleet	Oral fleet: 5–9 years old: 7.5 ml once 10–11 years old: 15 ml once >11 years old: 15–45 ml once (max. 45 ml) PR Fleet Enema: 2 – <12 years old: 66.6 ml (Paeds enema) ≥12 years old: 133 ml (Adult enema)	Oral fleet may be mixed with Coca-Cola or syrup to mask taste.
Glycerin Infant suppository (2 g)	PR: <1 month old: 0.5 g (¼ supp) as needed 1 month–1 year old: 1 g (½ supp) as needed 1–12 years old: 2 g (1 supp) as needed >12 years old: 4 g (2 supp) as needed	Lubricate with some water before inserting into anus. Insert high into the rectum and retain it for at least 15 minutes.
Lactulose syrup	PO: 0.5 ml/kg/dose Q8–12H Alternative dosing Infant: 2.5–10 ml/day Older children: 40–90 ml/day	Drink plenty of water while on lactulose.
Macrogol/Polyethylene Glycol 4000 (Forlax®) 10 g Sachet	PO: Maintenance 1 – <12 months old: ½ sachet/day 12 months to <4 years old: ½–1 sachet/day 4 – <12 years old: 1–2 sachets/day ≥12 years old: 1–3 sachets/day Alternative dosing: 0.2–0.8 g/kg/day, round to nearest sachet	Every half sachet should be mixed in 50–60 ml of water, beverages, fruit juices or milk (but not soda), and consumed within 30 minutes as it will turn into gel-like consistency. Space at least 2 hours apart from other medications.
Sennosides	Sennosides 7.5 mg tablet PO: 2-<6 years old: 3.75–7.5 mg ON (max. 7.5 mg BD) 6–12 years old: 7.5–15 mg ON (max. 15 mg BD) ≥12 years old: 15–30 mg ON (max. 30 mg BD) Ex-lax 15 mg tablet PO: 2-<6 years old: 7.5–15 mg ON (max. 15 mg BD) 6–12 years old: 15 mg ON (max. 15 mg BD) ≥12 years old: 15–30 mg ON (max. 30 mg BD)	Ex-Lax 1 small square = 15 mg of sennosides
Inflammatory Bowel Disease		
Sulfasalazine	PO: 40–70 mg/kg/day (max. 1 g QDS)	Round to nearest 250 mg for ease of administration. To maintain induction dose as maintenance for several months.

(Continued)

(*Continued*)

Drug	Dosage	Remarks
Inflammatory Bowel Disease		
Mesalazine	PO: 60–80 mg/kg/day (max. 4.8 g/day) PR: (Enema, Foam or Suppository) 25 mg/kg/day (max. 1–4 g/day), round to nearest half suppository or foam actuation* *Higher PR doses up to 4 g have been used but it appears no more effective than 1 g/day	Enema, Foam or Suppository: Give last dose just before bedtime.
	Alternatively, PR Suppository (≥12 years) *Acute attack - Proctitis and rectosigmoid disease 500–1000 mg BD to TDS for 4–6 weeks. - Rectosigmoid and descending colon disease: 2 g/dose OD for 4–6 weeks, increase to BD if required. *Maintenance PR: 250–500 mg 2–3 times/day PR Enema/Foam (≥12 years) *Acute attack - Rectosigmoid disease: 1 g OD for 4–6 weeks - Rectosigmoid and descending colon disease: 2 g/dose OD to BD for 4–6 weeks *Maintenance - Rectosigmoid and/or descending colon disease: PR 1g daily	
Hydrocortisone Rectal Foam	PR: 1 applicator OD to BD	Limited data available for use in children.
Azathioprine	PO: 2–2.5 mg/kg/day	
6-Mercaptopurine	PO: 1–1.5 mg/kg/day	
Methotrexate	Subcutaneous: Start with 15 mg/m^2 (max. 25 mg), and may reduce dose 10 mg/m^2 (max. 15 mg) once well-controlled	Recommended to administer folic acid 24–72 hours after methotrexate as it may reduce side effects.
Infliximab	≥6 years old: IV Infusion 5–10 mg/kg at week 0, 2, 6 then Q8 weekly	Monitor Infliximab antibody and drug levels to direct therapy.

(*Continued*)

Drug	Dosage	Remarks
Inflammatory Bowel Disease		
Adalimumab	Moderate to severe Crohn's Disease: ≥6 years old 17–<40 kg: Subcutaneous 80 mg on Day 1, then 40 mg on Day 15, then 20 mg every 2 weeks from Day 29 ≥40 kg: Subcutaneous 160 mg on Day 1 (or split over Day 1 and 2), then 80 mg on Day 15, then 40 mg every 2 weeks from Day 29 Moderate to severe Ulcerative Colitis: ≥5 years old 20–<40 kg: Subcutaneous 80 mg on Day 1, then 40 mg on Day 8 and Day 15, then 40 mg every 2 weeks (or 20 mg every week) from Day 29 ≥40 kg: Subcutaneous 160 mg on Day 1 (or split over Day 1 and 2), then 80 mg on Day 8 and Day 15, then 80 mg every 2 weeks (or 40 mg every week) from Day 29	Monitor Adalimumab antibody and drug levels to direct therapy.

Cardiovascular System (Anti-arrhythmics, Anti-hypertensives, Diuretics, Other Cardiovascular Agents, Anticoagulants and Antiplatelets)

Poh Bao Hui; Wang Lay Nee

Drug	Dosage	Remarks
Anti-Arrhythmics		
Adenosine	SVT: IV, Intraosseous: 0.1 mg/kg/dose (max. 6 mg/dose). If not effective within 1–2 minutes, increase to 0.2 mg/kg/dose (max. 12 mg/dose)	For rapid bolus IV administration, administer over 1–2 seconds at peripheral IV site closest to patient's heart. Follow each bolus with 5–10 ml of normal saline flush.
Amiodarone	Tachyarrhythmias: IV 25 mcg/kg/min for 4 hours, then 5–15 mcg/kg/min	Close haemodynamic and ECG monitoring required during and after administration.
Atropine Sulphate	Bradycardia: IV, Intraosseous: 0.02 mg/kg/dose (min 0.1 mg/dose; max. 0.5 mg/dose), may repeat once in 5 minutes Endotracheal: 0.04–0.06 mg/kg/dose; may repeat once if needed	IV: Administer undiluted by rapid IV injection; slow injection may result in paradoxical bradycardia. Endotracheal: Administer undiluted followed by 5 ml (at least ≥ 1 ml for neonates) of normal saline after endotracheal administration.
Digoxin	Based on lean body weight and normal renal function for age. Decrease maintenance dose in patients with decreased renal function. Heart failure (Maintenance dose): <u>Preterm neonates</u> PO: 5 to 7.5 mcg/kg/day Q12H IV: 4 to 6 mcg/kg/day Q12H <u>Full-term neonates:</u> PO: 8 to 10 mcg/kg/day Q12H IV: 5 to 8 mcg/kg/day Q12H <u>1 to 24 months:</u> PO: 10 to 15 mcg/kg/day Q12H IV: 9 to 15 mcg/kg/day Q12H <u>2 to 5 years:</u> PO: 8 to 10 mcg/kg/day Q12H IV: 6 to 9 mcg/kg/day Q12H	Therapeutic drug monitoring: Digoxin serum concentrations are monitored because digoxin possesses a narrow therapeutic serum concentration range. Digoxin serum concentrations should be drawn at least 6–8 hours after the previous dose, regardless of route of administration (optimally 12–24 hours after a dose). For initiation of therapy with loading dose given: draw level within 12–24 hours after the initial loading dose administration. For initiation of therapy without loading dose given: draw level after 3–5 days of therapy.

(Continued)

Drug	Dosage	Remarks
Anti-Arrhythmics		
	<u>5 to 10 years:</u> PO: 5 to 10 mcg/kg/day Q12H IV: 4 to 8 mcg/kg/day Q12H <u>>10 years:</u> PO: 2.5 to 5 mcg/kg/day Q24H IV: 2 to 3 mcg/kg/day Q24H Tachyarrhythmias (e.g. supraventricular tachycardia): <u>Term neonates:</u> Oral: Initial digitalising dose: 20 to 40 mcg/kg/day Q8H for 2 to 3 doses followed by maintenance dose: 8 to 10 mcg/kg/day Q12H <u>Infants, Children, and Adolescents:</u> Initial (digitalising dose): IV: 10 to 12 mcg/kg/dose Q8H for 3 doses Oral: 13 to 17 mcg/kg/dose Q8H for 3 doses Maintenance: Oral: 8 to 10 mcg/kg/day divided once or twice daily (use twice daily dosing in infants and young children)	For maintenance therapy: - Draw trough concentrations just prior to the next dose or at a minimum of 6–8 hours after last dose. - Draw trough level within 5–7 days after any dosage changes. Reference range: Heart failure: 0.5–0.9 ng/ml Toxic: >2 ng/ml; Use serum concentration in conjunction with clinical symptoms and ECG to confirm diagnosis of digoxin toxicity. Use with caution in patients with renal impairment, monitor digoxin serum concentrations closely as time to steady state will be longer. When switching from intravenous to oral route, may need to increase dose by 20–25% to maintain the same serum digoxin concentration.
Flecainide	Arrhythmias: Initial: PO 1–3 mg/kg/day Q8H Usual maintenance range: PO 3–6 mg/kg/day Max.: PO 8 mg/kg/day	Refer to institution-specific guideline for monitoring parameters and dose titration. Reduce dose by 25–50% for patients with renal impairment GFR <35 ml/min/1.73m^2. Flecainide serum level and CYP2D6 gene testing should be performed when warranted. Use with caution as drug-drug interactions exist with QT-prolonging agents and other anti-arrhythmics such as amiodarone and digoxin (dose reduction may be necessary). Separate administration of flecainide from milk feeds and dairy products as they may reduce absorption of flecainide.
Lignocaine	Ventricular arrhythmias, pulseless ventricular tachycardia (VT), ventricular fibrillation (VF): IV, Intraosseous: Loading dose 1 mg/kg/dose followed by continuous infusion 15–50 mcg/kg/min (max. 20 mcg/kg/min for patients with shock, hepatic disease, cardiac arrest, or congestive heart failure) Endotracheal: Loading dose 2–3 mg/kg/dose	IV, Intraosseous: May administer second bolus if delay between initial bolus and start of infusion is >15 minutes. Endotracheal: Flush with 5 ml normal saline and follow with 5 assisted ventilations.

(Continued)

(Continued)

Drug	Dosage	Remarks
Anti-Arrhythmics		
Procainamide	IV, Intraosseous: 15 mg/kg over 30–60 minutes (max. total loading dose: 500 mg) IV Maintenance: 20–80 mcg/kg/min (max. daily dose: 2000 mg/24 hours) PO: 15–50 mg/kg/day Q3–6H (max.: 4000 mg/day)	Close haemodynamic and ECG monitoring required during and after administration. Stop infusion if hypotension occurs or QRS complex widen by >50% of baseline. Administer via a slow infusion to avoid toxicity from heart block, myocardial depression and QT interval prolongation. Routine use in combination with QT interval prolonging drugs is not recommended. Contraindicated in patients with complete heart block, second-degree AV block or various types of hemiblock (without a functional artificial pacemaker).
Propranolol	IV: 0.01–0.15 mg/kg/dose slow IV over 10 minutes (max. dose: 1 mg/dose for infants, 3 mg/dose for children and adolescents) PO: 0.5–4 mg/kg/day Q6–8H (max. daily dose: 16 mg/kg/day or 60 mg/day)	For IV, may repeat Q6–8H as needed. Monitor ECG and BP closely.
Sotalol	PO: Start at 2 mg/kg/day Q8H and increase dose by 1–2 mg/kg/day with 3 days interval between dosage increments Max.: 10 mg/kg/day; 320 mg/day	Monitor clinical response, heart rate and ECG (QTc interval, PR interval) with every dose increment.
Verapamil	SVT: IV, Intraosseous: 0.1–0.3 mg/kg/dose (max. 5 mg/dose); may repeat dose in 15–30 minutes if response inadequate, max. dose for second dose: 10 mg/dose PO: 2–8 mg/kg/day TDS (max. 480 mg/day)	Adverse effects: severe apnea, cardiac arrest, hypotension and myocardial depression
Anti-Hypertensives		
Amlodipine	PO 0.05–0.6 mg/kg/dose once daily (max. 10 mg/day)	
Atenolol	PO: 0.5–1 mg/kg Q12–24H (max. 2 mg/kg/day; 100 mg/day)	Use with caution in compensated heart failure.
Captopril	Heart failure/hypertension: PO: Infants: 0.3–3.5 mg/kg/day Q6–12H Children: 0.9–3.9 mg/kg/day Q8–12H Max.: 6 mg/kg/day; 150 mg/day	Use with caution in renal failure and hyperkalaemia.

(*Continued*)

Drug	Dosage	Remarks
Anti-Hypertensives		
Enalapril	Heart failure/hypertension: PO 0.1–0.5 mg/kg/day Q12H (max. 1 mg/kg/day; 40 mg/day).	Use with caution in renal failure and hyperkalaemia.
Glyceryl Trinitrate (Nitroglycerin)	IV continuous infusion: 0.5–10 mcg/kg/min	Use non-PVC administration sets as adsorption can occur.
Hydralazine	Hypertension: IV: 0.1–0.6 mg/kg/dose Q4–6H Max.: 20 mg/dose; PO: 0.25 mg/kg/dose Q6-8H Max.: 7.5 mg/kg/day; 25 mg/dose; 200 mg/day	Use is contraindicated in patients with coronary heart disease and mitral valve rheumatic heart disease. Avoid use in treatment of hypertension in patients with heart failure (with reduced ejection fraction) of ischemic origin if not used with a concomitant nitrate. May be associated with lupus-like syndrome in some patients.
Labetolol	PO: 1–2 mg/kg/dose Q6–8H Max.: 10–12 mg/kg/day; 2400 mg/day IV continuous infusion: 0.25–3 mg/kg/h	Use with caution in heart failure.
Nifedipine	PO: 0.25–0.5 mg/kg/dose Q6–8H Max.: 10 mg/dose; 3 mg/kg/day; 120 mg/day	
Nitroprusside Sodium	IV continuous infusion: 0.5–4 mcg/kg/min (max. 10 mcg/kg/min)	Monitor thiocyanate levels if requiring prolonged infusion (>3 days) or dose ≥4 mcg/kg/min or if patient has renal dysfunction. Avoid use in patients with hepatic failure as cyanide or thiocyanate metabolites may accumulate. If use is necessary, monitor cyanide blood levels closely. Monitor for cyanide toxicity via acid-base status and venous oxygen concentration.
Diuretics		
Frusemide	IV/PO: 0.5–2 mg/kg/dose Q6–24H Max.: IV: 6 mg/kg/dose; 200 mg/dose PO: 12 mg/kg/day; 600 mg/day IV continuous infusion: 0.1–2 mg/kg/h	Potentiates ototoxicity and nephrotoxicity of aminoglycosides when used concurrently. Monitor electrolytes closely as electrolytes disturbances such as hypokalaemia, hypomagnesemia, hypocalcemia may occur.
Hydrochlorothiazide	PO: 1–2 mg/kg/day Q12–24H (max. 200 mg/day)	Monitor electrolytes closely as electrolytes disturbances such as hypokalaemia, hypomagnesemia, hypercalcemia and hyponatraemia may occur.
Spironolactone	PO: 1–6 mg/kg/day Q12–24H (max. 400 mg/day)	Monitor electrolytes closely as electrolytes disturbances such as hyperkalaemia, hypomagnesemia, hypocalcemia and hyponatraemia may occur.

(*Continued*)

(Continued)

Drug	Dosage	Remarks
Other Cardiovascular Agents		
Adrenaline	Asystole/pulseless arrest/bradycardia: IV, Intraosseous: 0.01 mg/kg Max.: 1 mg/dose Endotracheal: 0.1 mg/kg Max.: 2.5 mg/dose May repeat every 3–5 minutes until return of spontaneous circulation if necessary Hypotension/shock: Continuous IV infusion: 0.1–1 mcg/kg/min.	Doses <0.3 mcg/kg/min generally produce beta-adrenergic effects while higher doses (>0.3 mcg/kg/min) generally produce alpha-adrenergic vasoconstriction. Caution between different strengths available: 1:1000 = 1 mg/ml (MUST be further diluted) 1:10000= 0.1 mg/ml (can be administered undiluted) Administration via central line is preferred. Vesicant: risk of extravasation (antidote: phentolamine)
Dobutamine	Continuous IV or intraosseous infusion: 0.5–20 mcg/kg/min	Contraindicated in hypertrophic cardiomyopathy with outflow tract obstruction.
Dopamine	Low dose: 1–5 mcg/kg/min (increase renal blood flow and urine output) Intermediate dose: 5–15 mcg/kg/min (increase renal blood flow, heart rate, cardiac contractility, cardiac output and BP) High dose >15 mcg/kg/min (alpha-adrenergic effects begin to predominate, vasocontriction, increased BP)	Haemodynamic effects of dopamine are dose-dependent. Administration via central line is preferred. Vesicant: Risk of extravasation (antidote: phentolamine)
Isoprenaline (Isoproterenol)	Severe bradycardia/AV nodal block: Continuous IV infusion: 0.05–2 mcg/kg/min	Dose-dependent vasodilation may be present due to unopposed beta2-agonism Contraindicated for use in angina, pre-existing ventricular arrhythmias, tachyarrhythmias, cardiac glycoside intoxication
Milrinone	Haemodynamic support/low cardiac output syndrome: Continuous IV infusion: 0.25–0.75 mcg/kg/min	
Noradrenaline	Hypotension/shock: Continuous IV infusion: 0.05–2 mcg/kg/min	Administration via central line is preferred. Vesicant: Risk of extravasation (antidote: Phentolamine)
Vasopressin	Hypotension/shock: Continuous IV infusion: 0.02–0.06 units/kg/h	Administration via central line is preferred. Vesicant: Risk of extravasation (antidote: Phentolamine)

(*Continued*)

Drug	Dosage	Remarks
Anticoagulants and Antiplatelets		
Aspirin	Antiplatelet effects: PO 1–5 mg/kg/dose Q24H Anti-inflammatory: PO 80–100 mg/kg/day Q6–8H	
Clopidogrel	PO 0.2–1 mg/kg/dose once daily	
Enoxaparin	Patients <2 months old*: Treatment: Subcutaneous 1.7 mg/kg/dose BD Prophylaxis: Subcutaneous 0.75 mg/kg/dose BD Patients ≥2 months old*: Treatment: Subcutaneous 1 mg/kg/dose BD Prophylaxis: Subcutaneous 0.5 mg/kg/dose BD *Based on chronological age	Refer to institution-specific guidelines for monitoring parameters and titrate dose of enoxaparin according to anti-factor Xa. For children who require doses that are less than a full syringe, institutions may practice dose rounding for ease of administration. Refer to institution-specific guidelines. Antidote: Protamine
Warfarin	For prophylaxis and treatment of thromboembolism (baseline INR 1–1.3): Initial dose on Day 1: PO 0.1 – 0.2 mg/kg/day once daily Max.: PO 5 mg/dose Use initial dose of PO 0.1 mg/kg for patients with multiple co-morbid conditions, liver dysfunction, thyroid dysfunction, hypoalbuminemia, higher risk of bleeding and poor nutritional status. Doses for Day 2–4 are dependant on patient's daily INR and the target INR.	Refer to institution-specific guidelines for monitoring parameters and for dose recommendation from Day 2 onwards. Titrate dose of warfarin according to target INR. Antidote: Vitamin K

Respiratory System (Anti-asthma Medications, Cold Medications, Nasal Preparations)

Tan Wei Wei; Cedric Poh Wei Ming

Drug	Dosage	Remarks
Anti-Asthma Medications		
Aminophylline	Loading dose: IV 5 mg/kg/dose over 30 minutes followed by Maintenance: Continuous infusion: IV 15–20 mg/kg over 24 hours OR 0.5–0.7 mg/kg/h, up to 1 mg/kg/h	For use in acute severe asthma exacerbation. Omit loading dose for patient on theophylline therapy. Therapeutic levels: 5–15 mcg/ml.
Budesonide 500 mcg/2 ml Respule 200 mcg/puff Turbuhaler	Dosing depends on asthma severity/control. Respule: ≤6 years old: 250–500 mcg daily >6 years old: 250–1000 mcg daily Turbuhaler: >6 years old: 200–1000 mcg daily	For children with asthma requiring long term controller therapy, inhaled corticosteroids (ICS) delivery via metered dose inhalers (MDI) and dry powder inhalers (DPI) are preferred. GINA 2020 (Budesonide DPI) <u>Children 6 to 11 years:</u> Low dose: ≤200 mcg/day Medium dose: 200–400 mcg/day High dose: >400 mcg/day <u>Children ≥ 12 years and Adults</u>: Low dose: ≤400 mcg/day Medium dose: >400–800 mcg/day High dose: >800 mcg/day
Budesonide/Formoterol Symbicort™ 80/2.25 mcg RAPIhaler (80 mcg budesonide/2.25 mcg formoterol) Symbicort™ 160/4.5 mcg Turbuhaler (160 mcg budesonide/4.5 mcg formoterol)	Dosing depends on the asthma severity/control. Usual Maintenance dose <u>RAPIhaler:</u> 2–4 puffs BD <u>Turbuhaler:</u> 1–2 puffs BD Quick relief of asthma symptoms for patient on Symbicort™ Maintenance And Reliever Therapy (SMART) regimen <u>RAPIhaler:</u> 2 puffs as needed in response to symptoms. If symptoms persist after a few minutes, another 2 puffs can be taken. Not >12 puffs on any single occasion.	Both Symbicort™ Turbuhaler and RAPIhaler are NOT licensed in children <6 years old, Symbicort™ RAPIhaler and Turbuhaler are ONLY approved for use as reliever as per SMART regimen for patients >12 years old unless under specialist care. RAPIhaler: Do NOT exceed max. of 12–16 puffs per day (inclusive of maintenance dose) during asthma exacerbation. Patient using >16 puffs daily should be advised to seek medical attention.

(Continued)

Drug	Dosage	Remarks
Anti-Asthma Medications		
	Turbuhaler: 1 puff as needed in response to symptoms. If symptoms persist after a few minutes, another 1 puff can be taken. Not >6 puffs on any single occasion.	Turbuhaler: Do NOT exceed max. of 6–8 puffs per day (inclusive of maintenance dose) during asthma exacerbation. Patient using >8 puffs daily should be advised to seek medical attention.
Fluticasone 50 mcg/puff EVOhaler 125 mcg/puff EVOhaler	Dosing depends on the asthma severity/control. Usual Maintenance dose: 50–200 mcg/day	GINA 2020 (Fluticasone MDI) Children ≤5 years: Low dose: 50 mcg/day Children 6 to 11 years: Low dose: ≤100 mcg/day Medium dose: 100–200 mcg/day High dose: >200 mcg/day Children ≥12 years and Adults: Low dose: ≤250 mcg/day Medium dose: >250–500 mcg/day High dose: >500 mcg/day
Salmeterol/Fluticasone Seretide™ ACCUhaler 50/100 mcg (50 mcg salmeterol/100 mcg fluticasone) Seretide™ EVOhaler 25/50 (25 mcg salmeterol/50 mcg fluticasone) Seretide™ EVOhaler 25/125 (25 mcg salmeterol/ 125 mcg fluticasone)	Dosing depends on the asthma severity/control. Usual Maintenance dose based on Fluticasone component: 100–250 mcg/day.	Seretide™ is NOT to be used during acute asthma attack. Seretide™ is NOT licensed in children <4 years old. Do NOT exceed max. of 100 mcg salmeterol/day.
Hydrocortisone	IV 4 mg/kg/dose Q6H (Max.: 100 mg/dose or 400 mg/day)	
Ipratropium Bromide: 20 mcg/puff MDI 500 mcg/ 2 ml nebulising solution	Ipratropium MDI: <10 kg: 2 puffs/dose up to Q20min for 3 doses ≥10 kg: 4–8 puffs/dose up to Q20min for 3 doses (8 puffs/ dose for moderate-severe exacerbation in children 6 years or older) Ipratropium nebulising solution: <10 kg: 0.5 ml/dose Q20min for 3 doses ≥10 kg: 1–2 ml/dose Q20min for 3 doses (2 ml/dose for moderate-severe exacerbation in children 6 years or older)	Administration via MDI with spacer is preferred over nebulisation. Administer with salbutamol for acute asthma exacerbation.
Ketotifen 1 mg/5 ml	6 months – 3 years old: PO 0.5 mg BD >3 years old: PO 1 mg BD	

(Continued)

(Continued)

Drug	Dosage	Remarks
Anti-Asthma Medications		
Magnesium Sulfate	Loading dose: IV 50 mg/kg over 30 minutes (max. 2 g/dose) Maintenance dose: Start at IV 20 mg/kg/h (range 20–40 mg/kg/h)	(Max. dose 40 g/day, max. infusion rate 40 mg/kg/h) Check Mg level routinely. Target serum Mg= 1.5–2.5 mmol/L
Montelukast 4 mg granules 5 mg and 10 mg tablet	PO: 6 months – 5 years old: 4 mg once daily 6–14 years old: 5 mg once daily ≥15 years old: 10 mg once daily	Counsel on rare but known neuropsychiatric adverse effects before prescription. For use of prevention of exercise-induced bronchoconstriction, administer dose at least 2 hours prior to exercise.
Prednisolone	PO 1–2 mg/kg/day Max.: 60 mg/day	For use in acute asthma exacerbation GINA 2020 (Prednisolone max. dose) Children 0–2 years: 20 mg/day Children 3–5 years: 30 mg/day Children 6–11 years: 40 mg/day Children ≥12 years and Adults: 40–50 mg/day A course of 3–5 days is usually sufficient unless otherwise advised by specialist.
Salbutamol 100 mcg/puff MDI 0.5% nebulising solution 5 mg / 5 ml injection	Salbutamol MDI: 0.2–0.3 puffs/kg/dose (min 2 puffs/dose, max. 10 puffs/dose for inpatient use, max. 6–8 puffs/dose in the written asthma action plan). Not more frequent than 4–6 hourly in written asthma action plan. Salbutamol 0.5% nebulising solution: 0.03 ml/kg/dose (max. 2 ml/dose) every 15 minutes to 6 hourly interval depending on severity of exacerbation and response Salbutamol injection: Loading dose: IV 5 mcg/kg diluted to 10 ml normal saline over 10 minutes Maintenance dose: IV 1–5 mcg/kg/min (max. rate 10 mcg/kg/min)	Administration via MDI with spacer is preferred over nebulisation for mild to moderate exacerbations. Close monitoring and review in a healthcare facility required if more frequent than 4 hourly. For acute exacerbations may administer up to 15 min interval with close review in healthcare facility, depending on severity of exacerbation and response.
Cold Medications		
Acetylcysteine 100 mg/sachet 600 mg effervescent tablet	PO 100 mg/sachet: 2–6 years old: 100 mg BD-TDS >6 years old: 100 mg–200 mg BD-TDS PO 600 mg effervescent tablet: >6 years old: 600 mg OD	Mucolytics are contraindicated in children <2 years old because of risk of aggravation of respiratory symptoms. Use with caution.

(*Continued*)

Drug	Dosage	Remarks
Cold Medications		
Bromhexine HCl	PO: 2 to <6 years old: 2 mg TDS or 4 mg BD (max. 8 mg/day) 6 to <12 years old: 4–8 mg TDS (max. 24 mg/day) ≥12 years old: 8 mg TDS (max. 24 mg/day)	Mucolytics are contraindicated in children <2 years old because of the risk of aggravation of respiratory symptoms. Use with caution.
Carbocisteine & promethazine (Rhinathiol® promethazine) 100 mg carbocisteine and 2.5 mg promethazine/5 ml syrup	PO: 2–5 years old: 2.5–5 ml QDS 6–12 years old: 7.5–12.5 ml TDS ≥12 years old: 12.5–15 ml TDS	Mucolytics are contraindicated in children <2 years old because of the risk of aggravation of respiratory symptoms. Use with caution.
Cetirizine	PO: 6 to <12 months old: 2.5 mg/dose OD (max. 2.5 mg/day) 1–2 years old: 2.5 mg/dose OD-BD (max. 5 mg/day) 2 to <6 years old: 2.5 mg BD or 5 mg OD (max. 5 mg/day) ≥6 years old: 5–10 mg OD (max. 10 mg/day)	
Chlorpheniramine Maleate	PO: 6 months to <2 years old: 0.1 mg/kg/dose BD ≥2 years old: 0.1 mg/kg/dose BD or TDS Max.: 4 mg/dose, 0.35 mg/kg/day	
Desloratadine	PO: 6–11 months old: 1 mg daily 1–5 years old: 1.25 mg daily 6–11 years old: 2.5 mg daily ≥12 years old: 5 mg daily	
Diphenhydramine 14 mg/5 ml syrup	PO: 2 to <6 years old: 2.5 ml/dose TDS Max.: 10 ml/day (28 mg/day) 6 to <12 years old: 5 ml/dose TDS Max.: 40 ml/day (112 mg/day) ≥12 years old: 10 ml/dose TDS Max.: 60 ml/day (168 mg/day)	Contraindicated in children <2 years old because of respiratory depression.
Fexofenadine	PO: Allergic rhinitis: 2–11 years old: 30 mg BD ≥12 years old: 60–90 mg BD (suspension) or 120–180 mg OD (tablet)	Can be used from 6 months old for treatment of chronic spontaneous urticaria.
Promethazine	PO: ≥2 years old: 0.2 mg/kg/dose TDS >12 years old: 10 mg TDS	Contraindicated in children <2 years old because of respiratory depression.

(*Continued*)

(*Continued*)

Drug	Dosage	Remarks
Nasal Preparations		
Sodium Chloride 0.9% Nose Drop /Spray	1 drop/spray in each nostril up to 4 times a day	Refer to product-specific labelling as some products contain other minerals and components.
Oxymetazoline Nasal Drop / Spray 0.01% 0.025% 0.05%	< 1 year old: 0.01% 1–6 years old: 0.025% >6 years old: 0.05%: Usual dosing: 1 drop into each nostril BD to TDS	Risk of rebound congestion increases when oxymetazoline is used continuously for more than 5 days. Stop for 2–3 days before using again if needed.
Betamethasone eye/nose drops	<2 years old: 1 drop in each nostril BD to TDS	Limit use to not more than 1 to 2 weeks. Prolonged treatment course increases risk of systemic side effects in view of relatively high bioavailability compared to other intranasal corticosteroids. Consider sodium chloride and/or sodium cromoglycate nasal drops as an option, or off-label use of mometasone or fluticasone furoate nasal sprays. After 2 years of age, switch to other safe and age-appropriate intranasal corticosteroid preparation.
Fluticasone Furoate Nasal Spray (27.5 mcg/spray)	2 to <12 years old Usual Starting Dose: 1 spray to each nostril ON ≥12 years old Usual Starting Dose: 1–2 sprays in each nostril ON The dose should be titrated to the lowest dose at which effective control of symptoms is maintained.	
Mometasone Furoate Nasal Spray (50 mcg/ spray)	2 to <12 years old Usual Starting Dose: 1 spray in each nostril ON ≥12 years old Usual Starting Dose: 1–2 sprays in each nostril ON The dose should be titrated to the lowest dose at which effective control of symptoms is maintained.	
DYMISTA® Nasal Spray (Azelastine 125 mcg and 50 mcg fluticasone propionate)	Adults, adolescents and children ≥ 6 year old: 1 spray in each nostril twice daily (morning and evening). Not licensed for use in children below 6 years old	

Central Nervous System (Anti-convulsants, Muscle Relaxants, Neuromuscular Drugs, Anti-pyretics and Analgesics, Drugs for Attention-deficit hyperactivity disorder)

Zhang Yifan; Eng Jing Jia; Lim Guo Yong

Drug	Dosage	Remarks
Anti-Convulsants		
Acetazolamide	PO 4–16 mg/kg/day divided TDS-QDS Max.: 30 mg/kg/day or 1 g/day, whichever lower	
Carbamazepine	PO: <6 years old: PO 5–20 mg/kg/day divided BD-TDS 6–12 years old: PO 200 mg/day Uptitrate weekly Max.: 35 mg/kg/day or 2.4 g/day (in adults)	Do HLA-B*1502 allele test for all Asian patients before starting therapy. Monitor for Steven Johnson Syndrome for up to 3 months. Therapeutic levels: 4–12 mcg/ml CYP3A4 Inducer, may increase clearance of other drugs. Monitor for haematologic and hepatic toxicity.
Clobazam	PO: <2 years old: 0.1–1 mg/kg/day 2–18 years old: 5 mg/day divided OD-TDS Max.: 60 mg/day or 0.4 mg/kg/dose BD-TDS	Do not stop abruptly, wean gradually by 5–10 mg weekly if required.
Clonazepam	PO: <10 years old or <30 kg: 0.01–0.03 mg/kg/day divided OD-QDS (max. 0.2 mg/kg/day) ≥10 years old or >30 kg: 1.5 mg/day divided OD-QDS (max. 20 mg/day)	Do not stop abruptly, wean dose gradually by ~25% weekly if required.
Diazepam	IV 0.15–0.2 mg/kg/dose (max. 10 mg), may repeat similar dose in 5 minutes if needed PR: 1 month–5 years old: 0.5 mg/kg 6–11 years old: 0.3 mg/kg ≥12 years old: 0.2 mg/kg Max.: 10–20 mg/dose; dose may be repeated in 4–12 hours if needed; do not use >5x/mth or more than once every 5 days.	IV Diazepam used in status epilepticus. Infuse at 1–2 mg/min. PR Diazepam used for seizures >5 minutes or cluster seizures. PR dose to be rounded to the nearest 2.5 mg increment (half enema).

(*Continued*)

(*Continued*)

Drug	Dosage	Remarks
Anti-Convulsants		
Ethosuximide	PO: <6 years old: 10 mg/kg/day 3–6 years old: 250 mg/day divided BD >6 years old: 250 mg BD Uptitrate every 4 days Max.: 40 mg/kg/day or 1.5 g/day (paeds) or 2 g/day (adults)	
Lamotrigine	With concurrent enzyme-inducing AEDs: Week 1 and 2: 0.6 mg/kg/day Week 3 and 4: 1.2 mg/kg/day Uptitrate by no more than 1.2 mg/kg/day every week after week 4, max. 400 mg/day (1–12 years old) or 700 mg/day (>12 years old) With concurrent Sodium Valproate: Week 1 and 2: 0.15 mg/kg/day Week 3 and 4: 0.3 mg/kg/day Uptitrate by no more than 0.3 mg/kg/day every week after week 4, max. 200 mg/day Without concurrent Sodium Valproate or any enzyme-inducing AEDs: Week 1 and 2: 0.3 mg/kg/day Week 3 and 4: 0.6 mg/kg/day Uptitrate by no more than 0.6 mg/kg/day every week after week 4, max. 400 mg/day	Higher initial dose, and/or rapid titration increases risk of skin hypersensitivity reactions.
Levetiracetam	IV: Load at 20–60 mg/kg/dose; then maintain at 30–60 mg/kg/day divided BD PO: 1–6 months old: 14 mg/kg/day divided BD 6 months to <16 years old: 20 mg/kg/day divided BD ≥16 years old: 500 mg BD Uptitrate every 2 weeks Max.: 60 mg/kg/day or 3 g/day	Additional benefit of PO/IV doses >3 g/day and 60 mg/kg/day has not been established.
Levocarnitine	PO 50 mg/kg/day Max.: 400 mg/kg/day or 3 g/day, whichever lower	For carnitine deficiency secondary to chronic valproate treatment.
Lorazepam	IV 0.1 mg/kg (max. 4 mg), may repeat similar dose in 5 minutes if needed	Used in status epilepticus. Infuse at 1–2 mg/min.
Midazolam	Intranasal (to divide dose between nares): 1–5 months old: 0.2 mg/kg (max. 10 mg) ≥6 months old: 0.2 mg/kg (max. 10 mg), may repeat once to a total max. of 0.4 mg/kg Buccal: ≥3 months old: 0.2–0.5 mg/kg (max. 10 mg)	Injection vial to be used for intranasal and buccal route. Used for seizures >5 minutes or cluster seizures.
Nitrazepam	PO 0.3–1 mg/kg/day divided TDS Uptitrate as tolerated to max. tolerable/effective dose	Do not stop abruptly, wean dose gradually if required.

(*Continued*)

Drug	Dosage	Remarks
Anti-Convulsants		
Oxcarbazepine	PO 8–10 mg/kg/day divided BD Uptitrate weekly Max.: 60 mg/kg/day or 2.4 g/day	Convert from carbamazepine to oxcarbazepine using 1:1–1.5
Phenobarbitone	IV: Load 20 mg/kg (max. 1000 mg/day) over 20 minutes, may repeat additional dose of 5–10 mg/kg after 10 minutes. Maintain at PO 3–6 mg/kg/day divided OD-BD Uptitrate as tolerated to max. tolerable/effective dose	IV Phenobarbitone used in status epilepticus for patients <1 year old or at risk of arrhythmias. Dilute with normal saline, infuse at max. 1 mg/kg/min or 60 mg/min. CYP3A4 Inducer, may increase clearance of other drugs. Therapeutic levels: 10–40 mcg/ml
Phenytoin	IV: Load 20 mg/kg over 20 minutes (max. 1.5 g), may repeat additional dose of 5–10 mg/kg after 10 minutes. Begin PO maintenance 12 hours later. PO: Load 15–20 mg/kg in 3 divided doses Q2–4H. Maintain at 5 mg/kg/day divided BD or TDS, uptitrate to response (max. 300 mg/day)	IV Phenytoin used in status epilepticus. Administer neat, infuse at max. 1 mg/kg/min or 50 mg/min, and monitor ECG and BP. Risk of extravasation as phenytoin is a vesicant. Phenytoin exhibit saturable metabolism, caution at high doses, in neonates, or patients with renal or hepatic impairment. CYP3A4 Inducer, may increase clearance of other drugs. Therapeutic levels: 10–20 mcg/ml
Piracetam	PO 30–160 mg/kg/day divided BD-QDS Uptitrate every 3–4 days Max.: 160 mg/kg/dose or 24 g/day	
Sodium Valproate	PO 10–15 mg/kg/day divided BD-TDS (immediate-release) or OD-BD (modified-release) Uptitrate weekly Max.: 60 mg/kg/day Total daily IV dose should be equivalent to the total daily PO dose and divided every 6 hours.	Monitor for hepatotoxicity (especially in children <2 years old) and thrombocytopenia. Therapeutic level: 40–100 mcg/ml
Topiramate	PO 1–3 mg/kg/day divided BD Uptitrate weekly Max.: 9 mg/kg/day or 400 mg/day (adults)	Risk of hyperthermia and renal stones, so ensure adequate fluid intake.
Vigabatrin	PO 50 mg/kg/day divided OD-BD Uptitrate at 25–50 mg/kg/day every 3 days Max.: 150 mg/kg/day	Consider limiting the treatment duration to 1 year in view of visual side effects.
Zonisamide	PO 1–2 mg/kg/day divided BD (2–4 mg/kg/day if for infantile spasms) Uptitrate every 2 weeks Max.: 12 mg/kg/day or 600 mg/day	Risk of hyperthermia and renal stones, so ensure adequate fluid intake.
Muscle Relaxants		
Edrophonium	Diagnosis of Myasthenia Gravis: <1 years old: IV 0.1 mg/kg, OR IM/SQ 0.15 mg/kg, may repeat at 0.15 mg/kg (max. total dose: 0.6 mg)	To standby atropine for the development of bradycardia, arrhythmia or hypotension: 0.02 mg/kg/dose (max. 0.5 mg/dose)

(*Continued*)

(Continued)

Drug	Dosage	Remarks
Muscle Relaxants		
	≥1 years old (≤34 kg): IV 1 mg, may be repeated every 30–45 seconds if no response (max. total dose: 5 mg) ≥1 years old (>34 kg): IV 2 mg, may be repeated every 30–45 seconds if no response (max. total dose: 10 mg) Reversal of nondepolarising neuromuscular blocking agents: IV 0.5–1 mg/kg/dose	
Neostigmine	Relaxant reversal (to use together with anticholinergic agent): IV 0.03–0.07 mg/kg/dose (max.: 0.07 mg/kg/dose or 5 mg/dose whichever lower)	Dose selection is dependent on half-life of the neuromuscular blocking agents or the first twitch response to the train-of-four (TOF) stimulus.
Pyridostigmine	PO 1–5 mg/kg/day in 3–6 divided doses (max. 7 mg/kg/day, or 1500 mg/day)	Short half-life of 1–2 hours.
Neuromuscular Drugs		
Baclofen	PO 0.6 mg/kg/day divided OD-TDS, uptitrate every 3 days Max. dose for Infants ≥4 months old and Children <2 years old: 40 mg/day; Children 2–7 years: 60 mg/day; >8 years old: 80–200 mg/day	Intrathecal balcofen may be considered for refractory dystonia or spasticity. Avoid abrupt withdrawal in therapy.
Benzhexol (Trihexyphenidyl)	PO 0.1–0.2 mg/kg/day divided OD-QDS, uptitrate weekly Max.: 2.6 mg/kg/day or 20 mg/day, whichever lower	
Clonidine	PO 1–2 mcg/kg/dose (frequency is patient dependent), uptitrate as tolerated to max. tolerable/effective dose	Patients on stable or higher doses may be converted to transdermal patch for more consistent release profile and convenience. Avoid abrupt withdrawal in therapy.
Gabapentin	PO 5–10 mg/kg/day divided TDS, uptitrate weekly Max.: 70 mg/kg/day or 3600 mg/day, whichever lower	Caution in renal impairment.
Madopar® (Levodopa 200 mg, Benserazide 50 mg)	PO 2 mg/kg/day (levodopa component) divided OD-QDS, uptitrate every 2–3 days Max.: 12 mg/kg/day or 800 mg/day (levodopa component), whichever lower	Response is most substantial in dopa-responsive dystonia.
Anti-Pyretics/Analgesics		
Acetysalicylic Acid (Aspirin)	PO: Anti-inflammatory (Kawasaki Disease): 80–100 mg/kg/day Q6–8H Antiplatelet: 3–5 mg/kg Q24H Analgesic: 10–15 mg/kg/dose Q4–6H (max. 4 g/day or 90 mg/kg/day whichever lower)	If an NSAID is also prescribed, administer NSAID 30 minutes to 2 hours after aspirin, or at least 8 hours before aspirin (exception: celecoxib, etoricoxib)
Celecoxib	≥2 years old: PO 2–4 mg/kg/day Q12–24H (max. 400 mg/day)	

(Continued)

Drug	Dosage	Remarks
Anti-Pyretics/Analgesics		
Diclofenac Sodium	PO/PR 0.3–1 mg/kg/dose Q8–12H (max. 50 mg/dose, 150 mg/day)	For Juvenile Idiopathic Arthritis (JIA), may go up to 200 mg/day
Etoricoxib	≥16 years old and/or ≥40 kg: 30–120 mg OD	
Ibuprofen	≥6 months old: PO 5–10 mg/kg/dose Q6–8H (max. for oral: 400 mg/dose, and 40 mg/kg/day or 1.2 g/day) ≥6 months old: IV 10 mg/kg/dose Q4–6H (max. for IV: 400 mg/dose, and 40 mg/kg/day or 2.4 g/day)	For JIA, may go up to 800 mg/dose, and 2.4 g/day
Indomethacin	≥2 years old: PO 0.5–1 mg/kg/dose BD-QDS (max. 4 mg/kg/day or 200 mg/day)	
Naproxen Sodium	≥2 years old: PO 5–10 mg/kg/dose Q8–12H (max. 550 mg/dose, and 15 mg/kg/day or 1.1 g/day)	
Paracetamol	IV/PO 10–15 mg/kg/dose Q4–6H (max. 1 g/dose, and 4 g/day or 75 mg/kg/day) PR 10–20 mg/kg/dose Q4–6H (max. 4 g/day or 90 mg/kg/day)	
Attention-deficit Hyperactivity Disorder (ADHD)		
Atomoxetine	≥6 years old: PO 0.5 mg/kg/day, uptitrate every 3 days to target dose of 1.2 mg/kg/day divided OD-BD Max.: 1.4 mg/kg/day or 100 mg/day	Do not open capsule as atomoxetine is an ocular irritant.
Methylphenidate	Immediate-release formulation: ≥6 years old: PO 5–10 mg/day (divided OD-BD), uptitrate weekly Max.: 60 mg/day (child); 80 mg/day (adult)	Modified and extended release formulations available (Ritalin® LA, Medikinet® MR, Concerta® ER). Caution in patients with seizures, tics/Tourette syndrome, or cardiovascular disorders.

Endocrine System

Tan Xin Yi; Christine Choo

Drug	Dosage	Remarks
Endocrine		
ACTH	IV: 0–1 month old: IV 15 mcg/kg (max. 125 mcg) 1–24 months old: IV 125 mcg ≥2 years old: IV 250 mcg	Short Synacthen test
Carbimazole	PO: 0–11 years old: Initial 0.75 mg/kg/day in single or divided doses until euthyroid, then gradually reduce to maintenance dose of 30–60% of initial dose. ≥12 years old: Initial 30 mg once daily in single or divided doses until euthyroid, then gradually reduce to maintenance dose of 30–60% of initial dose.	Monitor for bone marrow suppression.
Desmopressin Acetate (DDAVP)	Diabetes insipidus: PO: 1 month–2 years old: Initial 10 mcg 2–3 times a day. Usual dose range is 30–150 mcg daily. 2–11 years old: Initial 50 mcg 2–3 times a day. Usual dose range is 100–800 mcg daily. ≥12 years old: Initial 100 mcg 2–3 times a day. Usual dose range is 0.2–1.2 mg daily. Intranasal: 1 month–2 years old: Initial 2.5–5 mcg 1–2 times a day 2–11 years old: Initial 5–20 mcg 1–2 times a day ≥12 years old: Initial 10–20 mcg 1–2 times a day Nocturnal enuresis: PO 200 mcg ON (up to 400 mcg ON)	Monitor for hyponatraemia and fluid retention.
Fludrocortisone	PO 0.05–0.2 mg daily in 1–2 divided doses.	
Glucagon	Hypoglycaemia: IM/IV/Subcutaneous: Weight <25 kg: 0.5 mg Weight ≥25 kg: 1 mg IV continuous: 10–20 mcg/kg/h Hyperinsulinaemia: IM/IV: 0–1 month old: 0.2 mg/kg (max. 1 mg) 1 month–1 year old: 1 mg IV continuous:1–20 mcg/kg/h	For hypoglycaemic coma.

(*Continued*)

Drug	Dosage	Remarks
Endocrine		
Hydrocortisone Sodium Succinate	Adrenal crisis: IM/IV 100 mg/m^2, followed by 100 mg/m^2/day in 4 divided doses until the clinical condition stabilises. Peri-operative: Induction of anaesthaesia — IV hydrocortisone 50 mg/m^2, followed by 50–100 mg/m^2/day in 4 divided doses until the major stress period is resolved. Physiological replacement dose: Primary adrenal insufficiency: PO 9–15 mg/m^2/day in 3 divided doses. Secondary adrenal insufficiency: PO 8–10 mg/m^2/day in 3 divided doses.	Follow sick day plan provided by endocrinologists. Double to triple of physiological dose, or crisis dose, may be required depending on stress level.
Levothyroxine	To consult endocrinologist regarding dosing.	Dosing is variable and titrated according to thyroid function tests (TFT).
Pamidronate	To consult endocrinologist regarding dosing for osteogenesis imperfecta.	Monitor for osteonecrosis of the jaw.
Propylthiouracil	PO 5–10 mg/kg/day in 3 divded doses (max. 300 mg/day)	High risk for hepatotoxity in children. To be used in consultation with a specialist in children who are allergic to carbimazole.
Vasopressin	Diabetes insipidus: IM/Subcutaneous: 2.5–10 units Q6–12H IV continuous: 0.0005 units/kg/hr (max. 0.01 units/kg/h)	For diabetes insipidus.
Alfacalcidiol (One-Alpha/1-Hydroxy Vit D3)	PO/IV 0.025–0.05 mcg/kg once daily (max. 1 mcg/day)	
Calcitriol (Rocaltrol/1,25-Dihydroxy Vit D3)	PO: 1 month–11 years old: Initial 0.015 mcg/kg once daily, increased every 2–4 weeks (max. 0.25 mcg/day) ≥12 years old: Initial 0.25 mcg once daily, increased every 2–4 weeks. Usual dose 0.5–1 mcg/day	

Dermatology (Oral antihistamines, Drugs for Acne, Scabies and Head Lice, Infantile Haemangioma, Atopic Dermatitis, Complicated Vascular Anomalities, Severe Cutaneous Adverse Reactions, Vitiligo)

Chen Mee Kuan; Nicholas Teo

Drug	Dosage	Remarks
Oral Antihistamines		
Cetirizine	*Refer drug information under Respiratory System*	
Fexofenadine	PO: Chronic idiopathic urticaria: 6 months-< 2 years old: 15 mg BD 2–11 years old: 30 mg BD ≥12 years old: 60–90 mg BD (suspension) or 120–180 mg OD (tablet)	
Hydroxyzine	PO: 6 months – <6 years: 0.5–1 mg/kg/dose ON (max. 2 mg/kg/day or 50 mg/day, and 25 mg/dose) ≥ 6 years: 0.5–1 mg/kg/dose ON (max. 2 mg/kg/day or 100 mg/day, and 25 mg/dose)	
Acne		
Isotretinoin	≥12 years old: PO 0.2–1 mg/kg/DAY OD-BD (max. 2 mg/kg/day; 20 mg/day)	Max. cumulative dose of 120 mg/kg
Scabies and head lice		
Ivermectin	PO: Scabies due to *Sarcoptes scabie:* Adults & children ≥15 kg: 200 mcg/kg/dose To repeat dose in 7 to 14 days Head lice: Adults & children ≥15 kg: 400 mcg/kg/dose To repeat dose in 7 days	Limited literature available on the safety of ivermectin in children <5 years old and <15 kg.

(Continued)

Drug	Dosage	Remarks
Scabies and head lice		
Malathion 0.5% lotion	Scabies: ≥6 months old: Apply once for 24 hours and repeat application 7 days after initial treatment. Head lice: ≥2 years old: Apply once to hair and scalp for 8–12 hours before washing off with shampoo. May repeat application 7 days after initial treatment if live lice are observed.	
Permethrin 5% lotion	Scabies: ≥2 months old: Apply once for 8–14 hours before washing off with water and may repeat 7 days after initial treatment. Head lice: ≥2 months old: Apply once for 10 minutes and may repeat 7 days after initial treatment if live lice or nits are observed.	
Infantile Haemangioma		
Propranolol	PO 2–3 mg/kg/day, divided in 2–3 doses	Usually started at 1 mg/kg/day, then increased weekly in increments of 0.5–1 mg/kg/day
Timolol	Topical 1 drop BD (max.: 1 drop/kg/dose; 4–6 drops/day)	Ophthalmic XE 0.5% formulation is preferred for better retention and efficacy
Atopic dermatitis		
Azathioprine	PO 1–3 mg/kg/day OD (max. 3 mg/kg/day)	
Cyclosporine	PO 2–3 mg/kg/day, divided in 2 doses (max.: 5 mg/kg/day)	
Dupilumab	Subcutaneous: 6 months – <6 years (no loading dose): 5-<15 kg: 200 mg every 4 weekly 15-<30 kg: 300 mg every 4 weekly 6 to <18 years old: 15 to <30 kg: 600 mg once, then 300 mg every 4 weekly 30 to <60 kg: 400 mg once, then 200 mg every 2 weekly ≥60 kg: 600 mg once, then 300 mg every 2 weekly ≥18 years: 600 mg once, then 300 mg every 2 weekly	
Methotrexate	PO 0.2–0.4 mg/kg/week, divided in 1–2 days a week (max. 25 mg/dose/week)	
Prednisolone	PO 0.5–1 mg/kg/day OD (max. 60 mg/day)	May increase up to 2 mg/kg/day if required

(Continued)

(*Continued*)

Drug	Dosage	Remarks
Complicated vascular anomalies		
Sirolimus	PO 0.8 mg/m^2/dose BD	Titrate to maintain trough level at 10–15 ng/ml
Severe Cutaneous Adverse Reactions		
Cyclosporine	SJS/TEN: PO/IV 1–3 mg/kg/day, in 2 divided doses	To aim for lower dose if renal function is compromised
Hydrocortisone	DRESS: IV 4–5 mg/kg/dose Q6H (max. 100 mg/dose)	
Intravenous Immunoglobulin (IVIG)	SJS/TEN: IV 1 g/kg/day x 3 days	
Vitiligo		
Dexamethasone	PO: ≤11 years old: 2–2.5 mg/day, 2 days a week >11 years old: 5–10 mg/day, 2 days a week	
Prednisolone	PO 0.3 mg/kg/day OD (max. 60 mg/day)	

Vitamins & Minerals

Lim Kae Shin; Jamie Stephanie

Drug	Dosage	Remarks
Vitamin A	Vitamin A products may be expressed as retinol activity equivalents [RAE]; 1 unit of retinol (IU) = 0.3 mcg RAE PO: Vitamin A deficiency: 5000 – 10,000 units daily Higher doses may be used initially for treatment of severe deficiency, but monitor closely for acute toxicity. Measles: <6 months old: 50,000 units daily for 2 days 6–11 months old: 100,000 units daily for 2 days ≥12 months – 5 years old: 200,000 units daily for 2 days Xerophthalmia: Administer as a single dose, repeat the next day and again after at least 2 weeks for a total of 3 doses <6 months old: 50,000 units 6–12 months old: 100,000 units Children and Adolescents: 200,000 units	For very young children, the capsules may be cut open and contents squeezed into the mouth.
Vitamin B_{12} (Cyanocobalamin / Hydroxocobalamin)	Vitamin B_{12} deficiency: IM 250–1000 mcg daily or on alternate days for 1–2 weeks, then weekly until blood count normal, then every 1–3 months	Hydroxocobalamin is the preferred form of Vitamin B_{12} compared to cyanocobalamin as it is retained in the body longer and can be given at longer intervals of up to 3 months.
Vitamin B_6 (Pyridoxine)	Treatment of isoniazid-induced neuropathy: Neonates: 5–10 mg daily 1 month – 11 years old: 10–20 mg BD-TDS 12–17 years old: 30–50 mg BD-TDS Prevention of isoniazid-induced neuropathy, penicillamine-induced neuropathy in Wilson's disease: PO 1–2 mg/kg once daily (max. 50 mg/day) Pyridoxine-dependent seizures: IV 50–100 mg daily, if responsive, followed by oral maintenance dose up to 30 mg/kg/day	Deficiency of the B vitamins, other than Vitamin B_{12} is not common and is usually treated by multivitamin preparations or Vitamin B combination preparations.
Vitamin H (Biotin)	Biotin deficiency: PO 5–20 mg/day	

(*Continued*)

(Continued)

Drug	Dosage	Remarks
Folic acid	Folic acid deficiency: PO: Neonates: 25–50 mcg/day (up to 100 mcg) <4 years old: 100–300 mcg/day ≥4 years old: 500 mcg – 1 mg/day Folate-deficient megaloblastic anaemia: PO 500 mcg/kg (max. 5 mg) once daily	Most causes of folate deficiency are self-limiting, hence folic acid is not usually indicated for long-term use. In folate-deficient megaloblastic anaemia, daily supplementation up to 4 months will replenish body store.
Vitamin K_1 (Phytomenadione)	Vitamin K deficiency bleeding: Prophylaxis in neonates: ≤1.5 kg: IM/IV 0.5 mg >1.5 kg: IM 1 mg Alternative route (when IM route refused): PO 2 mg at birth and 2 mg at 1 week of life. For exclusively breastfed infants, 3rd dose of 2 mg at 4 weeks of age. Treatment in neonates: IM/IV: 1 mg/dose Correction may take 12 to 24 hours, other treatments may be necessary (e.g. fresh frozen plasma, platelets) Reversal of vitamin K antagonists (e.g. warfarin): When continued anticoagulation required or no significant bleeding: IV: 0.03 mg/kg/dose (max. 1 mg/dose) for 1 dose, dose may be repeated as necessary When continued anticoagulation NOT required or if significant bleeding: IV: 0.3 mg/kg/dose (max. 10 mg/dose) for 1 dose	IM therapy is preferred (vs. oral) as incomplete oral therapy may leave the infant at risk of Vitamin K deficient bleeding. IV route may be used in preterm neonates with very low birth-weight if IM is not possible; however, it may not provide the prolonged protection of the IM route (subsequent oral doses may be required). Vitamin K is fat soluble. Phytomenadione (Vitamin K) injection can be given orally.
Vitamin E (Alpha-tocopherol)	1 IU of the natural form (*d*-alpha-tocopherol) = 0.67 mg of alpha-tocopherol Vitamin E deficiency (due to malabsorption e.g. in cystic fibrosis, cholestasis): Children: PO 1 unit/kg/day (0.67 mg/kg/day), up to 25 units/kg/day (17 mg/kg/day)	Water-soluble Vitamin E formulations is more easily absorbed (vs. Vitamin E in oil preparations), and hence more beneficial in preventing deficiency. IM therapy should be considered in children with severe liver disease when response to oral therapy is inadequate.
Vitamin D_3 (Cholecalciferol)	Prevention of Vitamin D deficiency: PO 400–800 units/day Treatment of Vitamin D deficiency : PO 2000 units/day for 6–8 weeks to achieve adequate serum level 25(OH)D >20 ng/ml followed by maintenance dose of 400–1000 units/day	Vitamin D requires hydroxylation, by the kidney and liver to its active form. In those with severe liver or renal impairment, the hydroxylated derivatives alfacalcidol or calcitriol should be prescribed.

(*Continued*)

Drug	Dosage	Remarks
Magnesium (Mg)	1 mmol elemental Mg = 24 mg elemental Mg Mild hypomagnesemia: PO 10–20 mg/kg/dose elemental Mg up to 4 times daily Hypomagnesemia: *Dose expressed as magnesium sulfate* IV/IM 25–50 mg/kg/dose Q6H for 2–3 doses	Magnesium salts are not well absorbed in the gastrointestinal tract and may cause diarrhoea. Symptomatic hypomagnesemia should be treated either intravenously or intramuscularly.
Zinc	Zinc deficiency: PO 0.5–1 mg/kg/day of elemental zinc Acrodermatitis enteropathica: PO 0.5–1 mg/kg/dose BD of elemental zinc	Zinc deficiency can occur as a result of inadequate diet or malabsorption; excessive loss of zinc can occur in certain conditions such as burns or trauma.
Iron	Iron deficiency: PO: Prophylaxis: 2 mg/kg/day of elemental iron Treatment: 3–6 mg/kg/day of elemental iron in divided doses. Treatment should continue for another 3–4 months after a normal level has been reached to replenish iron stores. (usual adult dose 100–200 mg/day)	Iron may cause gastrointestinal disturbances and colour the stool black.

APPENDIX III

USEFUL FORMULAE

Useful Formulae

Emergency Intubation

Rapid Sequence Induction (RSI) drugs:

- Pre-medication: Atropine (consider)
- Sedation/analgesia: **Ketamine**/midazolam/morphine
- Neuromuscular blockade: **Suxamethonium**

Medications Suitable for Endotracheal Administration

Naloxone
Atropine
Ventolin (salbutamol) Neb
Epinephrine (adrenaline 1:1000)
Lignocaine

Formulae for Endotracheal Tube

Uncuffed ETT size (internal diameter) = [(age in years ÷ 4) + 4]
Cuffed ETT size (internal diameter) = [(age in years ÷ 4) + 3.5]
ETT length (oral) = [(age in years ÷ 2) + 12] cm
OR ETT internal diameter × 3
ETT length (nasal) = [(age in years ÷ 2) + 15] cm

Estimated Size/Length of ETT

Age	Weight (kg)	Size	Oral (cm)	Nasal
Neo	3	3.5	8.5	10
3m	5	3.5	10	12
1y	9	4.0	11	14
2y	12	4.5	12	15
4y	16	5.0	14	17
8y	24	6.0	16	20
12y	38	7.0	18	22

ETT size for neonates:

<1 kg	2.5 mm
1–2 kg	3 mm
>2 kg	3.5 mm

Normal Ranges

Maintenance Fluid Requirements

Fluids for neonates:

For INFANTS and OLDER:

1st 10 kg	4 ml/kg/h
Next 10 kg	2 ml/kg/h
Every kg >20 kg	1 ml/kg/h

Normal Urine Output

Neonates	>0.5 ml/kg/h
Infants and above	>1 ml/kg/h

Fluid Resuscitation

Bolus volume:	10–20 ml/kg
Fluid type:	0.9% saline, 5% albumin, blood, FFP
Total body blood volume:	80 ml/kg

Expected Systolic Blood Pressure

<1month of age:	SBP >60 mmHg
1month to 1 year:	SBP >70 mmHg

1 to 10 years:
SBP > 70 + (age in years × 2) mmHg

Burns

Burn Depth:
Superficial — dry, red, no blisters
Partial thickness — wet or dry, blisters
Full thickness — insensate (black/white eschar)
Beyond full thickness — extend to deep tissues
Estimate % BSA of burn: 1 child's palm = 1% BSA

Parkland Formula

Volume replacement (2nd/3rd degree burns):
In first 24 hours, total volume = 3–4 ml/kg per % BSA burn
Give half over first 8 hours after burn, half over the next 16 hours.

Rhythm Disturbances

Bradycardia

Stable
Close monitoring
Optimise oxygenation
Consider causes

Unstable — signs of shock present
CPR (chest compressions + BVM)
Adrenaline or Isoprenaline
Atropine (if vagal aetiology)
Consider pacing

Tachycardia

Stable
Narrow complex (SVT)
Adenosine
Amiodarone if refractory
Wide complex (VT)
Amiodarone
Consider lignocaine

Unstable — signs of shock present
Narrow complex (SVT)
Synchronised cardioversion
First dose 0.5–1 J/KG; second dose 2 J/kg
Wide complex (VT)
As per SHOCKABLE RHYTHMS

Pulseless Arrest — All Rhythms

Commence chest compressions and BVM with 100% O_2
Secure airway; obtain vascular access

Non-Shockable Rhythms

Asystole / Pulseless Electrical Activity
Adrenaline every 3–5 min
Consider Hs and Ts:
Hypoxaemia, Hypovolaemia, Hydrogen ions (acidosis), Hyper/hypokalaemia, Hypoglycaemia, Hypothermia
Thromboembolism, Tension pneumothorax, Trauma, Tamponade (cardiac), Toxins